Psychiatric Mental Health Nursing

Success

NCLEX®-Style Q&A Review

FIFTH EDITION

Cathy Melfi Curtis, MSN, RN-BC Retired

Psychiatric Mental Health Nurse
Sullivan's Island, South Carolina

Audra Baker Fegley, MSN, PMHNP-BC

Psychiatric Mental Health Nurse Practitioner
Knoxville, Tennessee

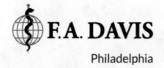

F.A. DAVIS

Philadelphia

F. A. Davis Company
1915 Arch Street
Philadelphia, PA 19103
www.fadavis.com

Printed in the United States of America

Last digit indicates print number: 10 9 8 7 6 5 4 3 2 1

Sponsoring Editor: Haleahy Craven
Content Project Manager: Veronica Neff
Design and Illustrations Manager: Carolyn O'Brien

As new scientific information becomes available through basic and clinical research, recommended treatments and drug therapies undergo changes. The author(s) and publisher have done everything possible to make this book accurate, up to date, and in accord with accepted standards at the time of publication. The author(s), editors, and publisher are not responsible for errors or omissions or for consequences from application of the book, and make no warranty, expressed or implied, in regard to the contents of the book. Any practice described in this book should be applied by the reader in accordance with professional standards of care used in regard to the unique circumstances that may apply in each situation. The reader is advised always to check product information (package inserts) for changes and new information regarding dose and contraindications before administering any drug. Caution is especially urged when using new or infrequently ordered drugs.

Library of Congress Cataloging-in-Publication Data

Names: Curtis, Cathy Melfi, author. | Fegley, Audra Baker, author.
Title: Psychiatric mental health nursing success : NCLEX-style Q&A review /
  Cathy Melfi Curtis, Audra Baker Fegley.
Description: Fifth edition. | Philadelphia : F.A. Davis, [2025] | Includes
  bibliographical references and index.
Identifiers: LCCN 2024013425 (print) | LCCN 2024013426 (ebook) |
  ISBN 9781719649742 (paperback) | ISBN 9781719653459 (epub) |
  ISBN 9781719653466 (PDF)
Subjects: MESH: Psychiatric Nursing | Test Taking Skills | Examination
  Questions
Classification: LCC RC440 (print) | LCC RC440 (ebook) | NLM WY 18.2 |
  DDC 616.89/0231076--dc23/eng/20240416
LC record available at https://lccn.loc.gov/2024013425
LC ebook record available at https://lccn.loc.gov/2024013426

The authors dedicate this book to nursing students whose eagerness to learn motivates us to teach mental health nursing concepts in a way that is clear and readily understood. Through the use of application and analysis test questions, we hope to enhance the students' critical-thinking skills and thereby promote excellence in their nursing practice.

—CATHY MELFI CURTIS, AUDRA BAKER FEGLEY

I would like to dedicate this book to the memory of my sister, Sally. She was also a nursing instructor and would have appreciated the time and effort that went into this book. Also, I would like to thank my children, Scott, Emily, and Katie, who were supportive and patient during the project development. I'm now available to babysit the grandchildren.

—CATHY MELFI CURTIS

This book is dedicated to my family and friends. To my mom, these last few years have been hard, but you have been there every step of the way. My son Dorian and daughter Nora June, I don't know what I would do without you all, you make my heart full. To my friend, Ashley, thanks for taking the trip or two to Charleston with me and sharing in the experience. Love you all.

—AUDRA BAKER FEGLEY

Contents

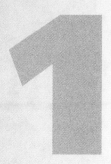

Critical Thinking and Clinical Judgment Related to Test Taking

INTRODUCTION

Nurses rely on critical thinking and clinical judgment to guide their actions in practice. This book is designed to help nurses practice the critical thinking and clinical judgment needed to be successful in psychiatric and mental health nursing. The practice questions in the upcoming chapters include an answers and rationales section. The rationales address the distractors in addition to the correct answers to further reinforce content. Tips for decision making in the testing environment are also included. This content also serves as a springboard for classroom discussion to demonstrate the steps in clinical decision making. Before attempting any of the question in this book, however, one must understand the difference between critical thinking and clinical judgment and become familiar with the NCSBN's Clinical Judgment Medical Model (CJMM).

Critical Thinking

Critical thinking is a cognitive strategy by which you reflect on and analyze your thoughts, actions, and decisions (Venes, 2021). Critical thinking often is integrated into traditional linear processes. Linear processes usually follow a straight line, from a beginning to a product at the end. Some linear-like processes, such as the nursing process, are considered cyclical because they repeat themselves. Some formal reasoning processes include the following:

- **Problem-solving**—involves identifying a problem, exploring alternative interventions, implementing selected interventions, and arriving at the end product, which is a solution to the problem.
- **Decision making**—involves carefully reviewing significant information, using methodical reasoning, and arriving at the end product, which is a decision.
- **Diagnostic reasoning**—involves collecting information, correlating the collected information to standards, identifying the significance of the collected information, and arriving at the end product, which is a conclusion or nursing diagnosis.
- **The scientific method**—involves identifying a problem to be investigated, collecting data, formulating a hypothesis, testing the hypothesis through experimentation, evaluating the hypothesis, and arriving at the end product, which is acceptance or rejection of the hypothesis.

- **The nursing process**—involves collecting information (assessment); determining significance of information and making a nursing diagnosis (analysis/diagnosis); identifying goals, expected outcomes, and planning interventions (planning); implementing nursing interventions (implementation/intervention); and assessing the client's response to interventions and comparing the actual to expected outcomes (evaluation), ultimately arriving at an end product, which is meeting a person's health-care and wellness needs.

Each of these methods of employing and processing information incorporates critical thinking. They all are influenced by intellectual standards, such as being focused, methodical, deliberate, logical, relevant, accurate, precise, clear, comprehensive, creative, and reflective. It is helpful to incorporate critical thinking into whatever framework or structure works for you.

Clinical Judgment

Nursing is an applied science that connects information in decision making. When a nurse enters a client's room, the client rarely asks the nurse to define a term or to recite a fact. Rather, the client presents the nurse with a set of data that the nurse must interpret, connect, and respond to. This process involves using clinical judgment.

Clinical judgment requires the nurse to look for meaning that may not be obvious or is implied rather than explicitly stated and to apply fragmented pieces of information into a unified whole that may be unique to each client. It's the process by which nurses make decisions, derived from nursing knowledge (including evidence, theories, ways/patterns of knowing), combined with other disciplinary knowledge, critical thinking, and clinical reasoning (American Association of Colleges of Nursing, n.d.).

NATIONAL COUNCIL OF STATE BOARDS OF NURSING CLINICAL JUDGMENT MEASUREMENT MODEL

To better measure students' abilities to use clinical judgment in their decision making, the National Council of State Boards of Nursing (NCSBN) has introduced next-generation questions to enhance the National Council Licensure Examination (NCLEX®); the enhanced examination is called the Next Generation NCLEX® (NGN). The NCSBN's CJMM involves:

1. **Recognizing cues.** What's abnormal? What puts the client at risk?
2. **Analyzing cues.** What could be happening? Or what might happen? Begin a list of hypotheses.
3. **Prioritizing hypotheses.** What is most likely? Or which hypothesis carries the highest risk to the client?
4. **Generating solutions.** What can I do?
5. **Taking action.** Where shall I start?
6. **Evaluating outcomes.** Did it help?

The intent of this model is to measure a graduate nurse's clinical judgment ability in various contexts so that novice nurses are better prepared for the clinical setting (NCSBN, 2019). At first, this model may seem intimidating, but the following strategies can help you build confidence in your abilities. In addition, Chapter 17 is devoted entirely to NGN-style case studies for practice.

MAXIMIZE YOUR CRITICAL THINKING AND CLINICAL JUDGMENT ABILITIES

Be Positive

Assuming responsibility for the care one delivers to a client and desiring a commendable grade on a nursing examination raise anxiety because a lot is at stake: to keep the client safe, to achieve a passing grade, to ultimately become a nurse, and to support one's self-esteem.

The most important skill that you can learn to help you achieve all of these goals is to be an accomplished critical thinker. We use critical thinking skills every day when we explore, "What will I have for breakfast?" "How can I get to school from my home?" and "Where is the best place to get gas for my car?" Once you recognize that you are *thinking critically* already, it is more manageable to think about thinking critically and then apply that thinking to clinical judgment. If you feel threatened by the idea of critical thinking, then you must do something positive to confront the threat. You need to be disciplined and work at increasing your sense of control, which contributes to confidence.

OVERCOME BARRIERS TO A POSITIVE MENTAL ATTITUDE

Supporting a positive mental attitude requires developing discipline and confidence. **Discipline** is defined as self-command or self-direction. The disciplined person will work in a planned manner, explore all options in an organized and logical way, check for accuracy, and seek excellence. When you work in a planned and systematic manner with conscious effort, you are more organized and therefore more disciplined. Disciplined people generally have more control over the variables associated with an intellectual task. Effective critical thinkers are disciplined, and discipline helps to develop confidence.

Confidence is defined as poise, self-reliance, or self-assurance. Confidence increases as one matures in the role of the student nurse. Understanding your strengths and limitations is the first step to increasing confidence. When you know your strengths, you can draw on them, and when you know your limitations, you know when it is time to contact the instructor or look for another resource to help you in your critical thinking. Either way, you are in control. For example, ask the instructor for help when critically analyzing a case study, share with the instructor any concerns you have about a clinical assignment, and seek out the instructor in the clinical area when you feel the need for support. Failing to use your instructor is burying your head in the sand. Learning needs must be addressed, not avoided. Although your instructor is responsible for your clinical practice and for stimulating your intellectual growth as a nursing student, you are the consumer of your nursing education. As the consumer, you must be an active participant in your own learning by ensuring that you get the assistance and experiences you need to build your abilities and confidence. When you increase your theoretical and experiential knowledge base, you will increase your sense of control, which ultimately increases your confidence. This applies not only to beginning nursing students but at every level of practice, especially because of the explosion in information and technology. When you are disciplined, you are more in control; when you are more in control, you are more confident; and when you are more confident, you have a more positive mental attitude.

Be Reflective

Reflection is the process of thinking back or recalling a situation or event to explore its meaning. Reflection helps you identify and understand the relationships between information, concepts, and principles, and to apply them in future clinical or testing situations. Reflection can be conducted internally as quiet, thoughtful consideration; in a one-to-one discussion with an instructor or another student; or in a group.

As a beginning nursing student, you are just starting to develop an experiential background from the perspective of a health-care practitioner. However, you have a wealth of experiences, personal and educational, that influence your development as a licensed nurse. Your personal experiences include activities using verbal and written communication, such as delegating tasks to family members or coworkers, setting priorities for daily activities, using mathematics when shopping or balancing a checkbook, and so on. A nursing program of study incorporates courses from a variety of other disciplines, such as anatomy and physiology, chemistry, physics, psychology, sociology, reading, writing, mathematics, and informatics. Every single experience is a potential valuable resource for future learning. Recognize the value that you bring to your nursing education and incorporate it into your reflective processes.

Engaging in reflection is a highly individualized mental process. One form of reflection is writing a journal. A **learning journal** (or a clinical diary) is a chronicle that includes cognitive learning, feelings, and attitudes. In addition, it requires you to actively develop skills related to assessing, exploring the meaning of critical incidents, documenting, developing insights into thoughts and actions that compose clinical practice, and evaluating. Journal writing is a rich resource that provides a written record of where you have been, where you are, and where you are going. It helps you to incorporate experiences into the development of your professional being. After an examination, explore your feelings and attitudes regarding the experience. Be honest with yourself. Did you prepare adequately for the test? Did you find the content harder or easier than content on another test? Were you anxious before, during, or after the test, and if so, was your anxiety level low, medium, or high? What would a low score or high score on the test mean to you? When you were confronted with a question that you perceived as difficult, how did you feel, and how did you cope with the feeling? You do not necessarily have to ask yourself all of these questions. You should ask yourself questions that have meaning for you.

Another form of reflection is making mental pictures. **Mental pictures** are visual images that can be recalled in the future. For example, when caring for a client who has Parkinson's disease, compare the client's signs and symptoms with the classic clinical manifestations associated with the disease. Then make a visual in your mind. Visualize the pill-rolling tremors, masklike face, drooling, muscle rigidity, and so on, so that, in the future, you can recall that picture rather than having to remember a memorized list of symptoms.

RETROSPECTIVE REFLECTION

Retrospective (after the event) reflection involves seeking an understanding of relationships between previously learned information and the application of this information in client care situations or testing experiences. This type of reflection helps you to judge your personal performance against standards of practice. A self-assessment requires the willingness to be open to identifying one's successful and unsuccessful interventions, strengths and weaknesses, and knowledge and lack of knowledge. The purpose of retrospective reflection is not to be judgmental or to second-guess decisions but rather to learn from situations. The worth of the reflection depends on the abilities that result from it. When similar situations arise in subsequent clinical practice, previous actions that were reinforced or modified can be accessed to have a current successful outcome.

A clinical post conference is an example of retrospective reflection. Students often meet in a group (formally or informally) after a clinical experience to review the day's events. During the discussion, students have an opportunity to explore feelings and attitudes, consider interventions and alternative interventions, assess decision-making and problem-solving skills, identify how they and other students think through a situation, and so on. You can also review your own thinking when reviewing a client experience by speaking aloud what you were thinking. For example:

> When I went into the room to take my postoperative client's vital signs, I realized that the client had an IV in the right arm. I knew that if I took a blood pressure in the arm with an IV it could interfere with the IV, so I knew I had to take the blood pressure in the left arm. When I looked at my client, he looked very pale and sweaty. I got a little nervous, but I continued to get the other vital signs. I put the thermometer in the client's mouth and started to take his pulse. It was very fast, and I knew that this was abnormal, so I paid special attention to its rhythm and volume. It was very thready, but it was regular. The temperature and respirations were within the high side of the expected range.

A beginning nursing student in this situation may immediately respond by saying, "I don't know what is going on here, so I better take this information to my instructor." A more advanced student might say, "What could be happening? Maybe the client is bleeding or has an infection. I think I should inform my instructor, but I'll inspect the incision first."

When you review an experience like this example, you can identify your thinking skills. Taking the blood pressure reading in the left arm and assessing the rate, rhythm, and volume of the pulse were habits because you did not have to figure out a new method when responding to the situation. Remembering the expected range for the various vital signs used the thinking skill of total recall because you memorized and internalized these values. Determining further assessments after obtaining the vital signs required inquiry. You collected and analyzed information and did not take the vital sign results at face value. You recognized abnormalities and gaps in information, collected additional data, considered alternative conclusions, and identified alternative interventions.

Another example of retrospective reflection is reviewing an examination. When reviewing each question, determine why you got a question wrong. For example, several statements you might make are:

- I did not understand what the question was asking because of the English or medical vocabulary used in the question.
- I did not know or understand the content being tested.
- I knew the content being tested, but I did not apply it correctly in the question.

When a limited English or medical vocabulary prevents you from answering a question correctly, you must spend time expanding this foundation. A list of English words that appear repeatedly in nursing examinations is included in a glossary at the end of this textbook. In addition, nursing/medical keyword lists have been included in each content area in this textbook. You can use these word lists to review key terminology used in nursing-related topics. To expand your vocabulary, keep English and medical dictionaries at your side when studying and look up new words, write flash cards for words you need to learn, and explore unfamiliar words with which you are confronted on tests.

LEARNING FROM MISTAKES

When you answered a question incorrectly because you did not understand the content, make a list so that you can design a study session devoted to reviewing this information. This study session should begin with a brief review of what you do know about the topic (5 minutes or less). The majority of your efforts should be devoted to studying what you identified as what you need to know. You should do this after reviewing every test. The test is over, so your anxiety level is reduced, and the way nursing-related content may be presented in a test question is fresh in your mind. Study sessions that are goal-directed tend to be more focused and productive.

Knowing the content being tested but applying the information incorrectly can be a frustrating experience. However, do not become discouraged. It is motivating to recognize that you actually know the content. Your next task is to explore how to tap into your knowledge successfully. Sometimes restating or summarizing what the question is asking places it into your own perspective, which helps to clarify the content in relation to the test question. Also, you can view the question in relation to specific past experiences or review the information in two different textbooks to obtain different perspectives on the same content. Another strategy to reinforce your learning is to use the left page of your notebook for taking class notes and leave the facing page blank. After an examination, use the blank page to make comments to yourself about how the content was addressed in test questions or add information from your textbook to clarify class notes. How to review thinking strategies in relation to cognitive levels of nursing questions is explored later in this chapter.

Examine your test-taking behaviors. For example, if you consistently changed your initial answers on a test, it is wise to explore what factors influenced you to change your answers. In addition, determine how many questions were converted to either right or wrong answers. The information you collect from this assessment should influence your future behaviors. If you consistently changed correct answers to incorrect answers, you need to examine the factors that caused you to change your answers. If you changed incorrect answers to correct answers, you should identify what mental processes you used to arrive at your second choice so that you can use them the first time you look at a question.

Reflection is an essential component of all learning. How can you know where you are going without knowing where you have been? Therefore, to enhance your critical thinking abilities, you must look at your past actions to better understand the next actions to take.

OVERCOME BARRIERS TO EFFECTIVE REFLECTION

Reflecting on your knowledge, strengths, and successes is easy, but reflecting on your lack of knowledge, weaknesses, and mistakes takes courage and humility. **Courage** is the attitude of confronting anything recognized as dangerous or difficult without avoiding or withdrawing from the situation. Courage is necessary because when people look at their shortcomings, they tend to be judgmental and can be their own worst critics. A nonjudgmental assessment of your own work is learned through practice and self-awareness. Working to stay positive promotes open-minded thinking, supports the reception of new information, and builds on self-confidence.

Humility is having a modest opinion of one's own abilities and knowledge. Humility is necessary because it is important to admit your limitations. Only when you identify what you do and do not know can you make a plan to acquire the knowledge necessary to be successful on nursing examinations and practice safe nursing care. Arrogance or a know-it-all attitude can interfere with maximizing your potential. For example, when instructors review examinations with students, the students who benefit the most are the ones who are willing to listen to their peers or instructor as to why the correct answer is correct. The students who benefit the least are the ones who consistently and vehemently defend their wrong answers. A healthy amount of inquiry, thoughtful questioning, and not accepting statements at their face value are important critical thinking competencies; however, a self-righteous or obstructionist attitude more often than not impedes rather than promotes learning.

Be Inquisitive

To **inquire** means to question or investigate. The favorite words of inquisitive people are *what, where, when,* and, most important, *how, why, if . . . then,* and *it depends.* When studying, ask yourself questions with these words to delve further into a topic under consideration.

HOW

You raise the head of the bed when a client is short of breath. You recognize that this intervention will facilitate respirations. Ask yourself, "*How* does this intervention facilitate respirations?" The answer could be, "Raising the head of the bed allows the abdominal organs to drop by gravity, which reduces pressure against the diaphragm, which in turn permits maximal thoracic expansion."

WHAT

You insert an indwelling urinary catheter and are confronted with the decision as to where to place the drainage bag. Ask yourself *what* questions: "*What* will happen if I place the drainage bag on the bed frame?" The answer could be, "Urine will flow into the drainage bag by gravity." "*What* will happen if I place the drainage bag on an IV pole?" The answer could be, "Urine will remain in the bladder because the IV pole is above the level of the bladder and fluid does not flow uphill; if there is urine in the bag, it will flow back into the bladder."

WHY

When palpating a pulse, you should use gentle compression. Ask yourself, "*Why* should I use gentle compression?" The answer could be, "Gentle compression allows you to feel the pulsation of the artery and prevents excessive pressure on the artery that will cut off circulation and thus obliterate the pulse."

Textbooks tend to say that in emergencies nurses should always assess the airway first. Ask, "*Why* should I assess the airway first?" There may be a variety of answers. "In an emergency, follow the ABCs (Airway, Breathing, Circulation) of assessment, which always begin with the airway. Maslow's hierarchy of needs identifies that physiological needs should be met first. Because an airway is essential for the passage of life-sustaining gases in and out of the lungs, this is the priority." Although all these responses answer the question *why,* only the last sentence really provides an in-depth answer. If your response to the original why question still raises another why question, you need to delve deeper. "*Why* do the ABCs of assessment begin with the airway?" "*Why* should physiological needs be met first?"

IF . . . THEN

When you are talking with a client about an emotionally charged topic, the client begins to cry. You are confronted with a variety of potential responses. Use the method of *if . . . then* statements. *If . . . then* thinking links an action to a consequence. For example, "*If* I remain silent, *then* the client may refocus on what was said. *If* I say, 'You seem very sad,' *then* the client may discuss the feelings being felt at the time. *If* I respond with an open-ended statement, *then* the client may pursue the topic in relation to individualized concerns." After you explore a variety of courses of action with the *if . . . then* method, you should be in a better position to choose the most appropriate intervention for the situation.

IT DEPENDS

You will recognize that you have arrived at a more advanced level of critical thinking when determining that your next course of action is based on the concept of *it depends*. For example, a client suddenly becomes extremely short of breath, and you decide to administer oxygen during this emergency. When considering the amount and route of delivery of the oxygen, you recognize that *it depends*. You need to collect more data. You need to ask more questions, such as, "Is the client already receiving oxygen? Does the client have a chronic obstructive pulmonary disease? Is the client a mouth breather? What other signs and symptoms are identified?" The answers to these questions will influence your choice of interventions.

When exploring the *how, what, where, when, why, if . . . then,* and *it depends* methods of inquiry, you are more likely to arrive at appropriate inferences, assumptions, and conclusions that will ensure effective nursing care.

These same techniques of inquiry can be used when practicing test taking. Reviewing textbooks that offer question responses with rationales is an excellent way to explore the reasons for correct and incorrect answers. When answering a question, consider why you think your choice is the correct answer and why you think each of the other options is an incorrect answer. This practice encourages you to focus on the reasons why you responded in a certain way in a particular situation. It prevents you from making quick judgments before exploring the rationales for your actions. After you have done this, compare your rationales with the rationales for the correct and incorrect answers in the textbook. Are your rationales focused, methodical, deliberate, logical, relevant, accurate, precise, clear, comprehensive, creative, and reflective? This method of studying not only reviews nursing content but also fosters critical thinking and applies critical thinking to test taking.

During or after the review of an examination, these techniques of inquiry also can be employed, particularly with those questions you got wrong. Although you can conduct this review independently, it is more valuable to review test questions in a group. Your peers and the instructor are valuable resources that you should use to facilitate your learning. Different perspectives, experiential backgrounds, and levels of expertise can enhance your inquiry. Be inquisitive and habitually curious.

OVERCOME BARRIERS TO BEING INQUISITIVE

Effective inquiry requires more than just a simplistic, cursory review of a topic. Therefore, critical thinkers must have curiosity, perseverance, and motivation. **Curiosity** is the desire to learn or know and is a requirement to delve deeper into a topic. If you are uninterested in or apathetic about a topic, you are not facing the challenge of new knowledge. Sometimes you may have to build your confidence to take on the study of a particular topic. Students frequently say they are overwhelmed by topics such as fluids and electrolytes, blood gases, or chest tubes. As a result, they develop a minimal understanding of these topics and are willing to learn by trial and error in the clinical area or surrender several questions on an examination. Pursuit of knowledge and understanding should be your norm. This approach supports competence. The attitude of lifelong learning amplifies your perseverance.

Perseverance means willingness to continue in some effort or course of action despite difficulty or opposition. Critical thinkers continue their learning until they have the information that satisfies their curiosity. To perform a comprehensive inquiry when studying requires time. Make a schedule for studying at the beginning of the week and adhere to it. This prevents procrastination later in the week, when you may prefer to rationalize doing something else and postpone studying. Studying for 1 hour a day is more effective than studying for 7 hours in 1 day. Breaks between study periods allow for the processing of information and provide time to rest and regain focus and concentration. The greatest barriers to perseverance are your own anxiety, discomfort, and negative thoughts.

While deadlines can feel intimidating, you can use a due date to your advantage. When working under a time limit, you may not have enough time to process and understand information. The length of time to study for a test depends on the amount and type of content to be tested and how much previous studying has been done. If you study for 2 hours every day for 2 weeks during a unit of instruction, a 1-hour review may be adequate for an examination addressing this content. If you are preparing for a comprehensive examination for a course at the end of the semester, you may decide to study for 3 hours a night for 1 to 2 weeks. If you are studying for an NCLEX® examination, you may decide to study for 2 hours a day for 3 months. Only you can determine how much time you need to study or prepare for a test. Perseverance can be enhanced by the use of motivation strategies.

Motivation strategies inspire, prompt, encourage, or instigate you to act. For example, divide the information to be learned into segments and set multiple short-term goals for studying. After you reach a goal, cross it off the list. This is also the time to use incentives. Reward yourself after an hour of studying. Think about how proud you will be when you earn an excellent grade on the examination. Visualize yourself walking down the aisle at graduation or working as a nurse during your career. Incentives can be more tangible (e.g., eating a snack, reading a book for 10 minutes, playing with your children, or doing anything that strikes your fancy). You need to identify the best pattern of studying that satisfies your needs; use motivation techniques to increase your enthusiasm; and then draw on your perseverance and determination to explore in depth the *how, what, where, when, whys, if . . . then,* and *it depends* of nursing practice.

Be Creative

Creative people are imaginative, inventive, innovative, resourceful, original, and visionary. To find solutions beyond common, predictable, and standardized procedures or practices, you must be creative. Creativity is what allows you to be yourself and individualize the nursing care you provide to each client. No two situations or two people are exactly alike. With the explosion of information and technology, the importance of thinking creatively will increase in the future because the old ways of doing things will be inadequate.

OVERCOME BARRIERS TO CREATIVITY

To be creative, you must be open-minded, have independence of thought, and be a risk taker. Being **open-minded** requires you to consider a wide range of ideas, concepts, and opinions before framing an opinion or making judgments. You need to identify your opinions, beliefs, biases, stereotypes, and prejudices. Everyone has both conscious and unconscious biases to some extent. However, they must be continually assessed, recognized, and compartmentalized. Unless these attitudes are placed in perspective, they will interfere with critical thinking and equitable patient care. In every situation, you need to remain open to all perspectives, not just your own.

When you think that yours is the only right opinion, you are engaging in egocentric thinking. *Egocentric thinking* is based on the belief that the world exists or can be known only in relation to the individual's mind. This rigid thinking reflects a lack of humility and obstructs the inflow of information, imaginative thinking, and the outflow of innovative ideas. An example of open-mindedness is one in which you have changed your mind after having had a discussion with someone else. The new information convinced you to reconsider your original thoughts and opinions.

Independence of thought means the ability to consider all the possibilities and then arrive at an autonomous conclusion. To do this, you need to feel comfortable with ambiguity. *Ambiguous* means having two or more meanings or being open to interpretation, so that something is therefore uncertain, unclear, indefinite, and vague. For example, a nursing student may be taught to establish a sterile field for a sterile dressing change by using the inside of the package of the sterile gloves. When following a sterile dressing change procedure in a clinical skills book, the directions may state to use a separate sterile cloth for the sterile field. When practicing this procedure with another student, the other student may open several 4×4 gauze packages and leave them open as the sterile fields. As a beginning nursing student, this is difficult to understand because of a limited relevant knowledge base and experiential background. Frequently, thinking is concrete and follows rules and procedures, is black and white, or is correct or incorrect. It takes knowledge and experience to recognize that you have many options and may still follow the principles of sterile technique.

To travel a different path requires taking risks. *Risk* means the chance of injury, damage, or loss. However, **risk taking** in relation to nursing refers to considering all the options, eliminating potential danger to a client, and acting in a reasoned, logical, and safe manner when implementing unique interventions. Being creative requires intellectual stamina and a willingness to go where no one has been before. Risk takers tend to be leaders, not followers.

LEARNING FROM ERRORS

The greatest personal risk of creativity is the blow to the confidence when confronted with failure. However, you must recognize that throughout your nursing career, you will be faced with outcomes that are successful as well as those that are unsuccessful. How you manage your feelings with regard to each, particularly those that are unsuccessful, will influence your willingness to take future creative risks. While successful outcomes build confidence, unsuccessful outcomes, when appropriately examined, should not be defeating or prevent future creativity. The whole purpose of evaluation in the nursing process is to compare and contrast client outcomes with expected outcomes. If expected outcomes are not attained, the entire process must be re-examined and then reperformed. You must recognize that:

- Unsuccessful outcomes do occur.
- Unsuccessful outcomes may not be a reflection of your competence.
- The successful outcomes far outnumber the unsuccessful outcomes.

CRITICAL THINKING AND CLINICAL JUDGMENT APPLIED TO TEST TAKING

Educational Domains

Nursing as a discipline includes three domains of learning—affective, psychomotor, and cognitive. The **affective domain** is concerned with emotional responses through attitudes, values, and the development of appreciations. An example of nursing care in the affective domain is the nurse quietly accepting a client's statement that there is no God without the nurse imposing personal beliefs on the client. The **psychomotor domain** is concerned with physical movement, coordination, and motor skills related to procedures or physical interventions. An example of nursing care in the psychomotor domain is the nurse administering an intramuscular injection to a client. The **cognitive domain** is concerned with recall, recognition of knowledge, comprehension, and the development and application of intellectual skills and abilities. An example of nursing care in the cognitive domain is the nurse clustering collected information and determining its significance. When discussing the application of critical thinking to test taking, the focus is on the cognitive domain.

Cognitive Levels of Nursing Questions

Questions on nursing examinations reflect a variety of thinking processes that nurses use when caring for clients. These thinking processes are part of the cognitive domain, and they progress from the simple to the complex, from the concrete to the abstract, and from the tangible to the intangible. There are four types of thinking processes represented by nursing questions:

- **Remembering-Level Questions**—the emphasis is on recalling information.
- **Understanding-Level Questions**—the emphasis is on understanding the meaning and intent of remembered information.
- **Applying-Level Questions**—the emphasis is on using previously acquired knowledge to solve problems and utilizing the information in new situations.
- **Analyzing-Level Questions**—the emphasis is on identifying reasons, causes, or motives to reach a conclusion or on attributing, organizing, or differentiating data/knowledge.

CRITICAL THINKING, CLINICAL JUDGMENT, AND THE NEXT GENERATION NCLEX®

Traditional NCLEX® test questions are primarily multiple-choice or alternate-format questions to test for critical thinking skills: audio, charts/exhibits, hot spot, multiple response, ordered response, and fill-in-the-blank. Most questions on the NCLEX® will still be presented in this traditional format. However, NGN question types are either standalone or unfolding cases. The unfolding cases guide the test taker through the six steps of the CJMM (NCSBN, 2019). Of course, not every test you encounter in your nursing studies will be the NCLEX®, but knowing the various question types can help frame your decision making on any test.

A multiple-choice question is called an **item.** Each item has two parts. The **stem** is the part that contains the information that identifies the topic and its parameters and then asks a question or forms the beginning portion of a sentence that is completed by the correct option. The second part consists of one or more possible responses, which are called **options.** One of the options is the correct answer, and the others are wrong answers (also called **distractors**).

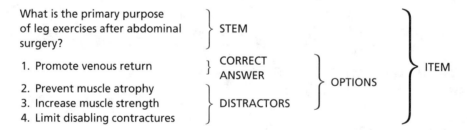

Traditional NCLEX® Questions

MULTIPLE-CHOICE QUESTIONS

In multiple-choice questions, a stem is provided (presenting a situation), and the test taker must choose among four possible responses. The test taker may be asked to choose the best response, the first action that should be taken, and so on. There are many ways that multiple-choice questions may be presented, including using charts, graphs, or pictures as options. Only one choice is the best response.

FILL-IN-THE BLANK QUESTIONS

Fill-in-the blank questions are usually reserved for drug calculations. The test taker may be asked to calculate a medication dosage, an IV drip rate, a minimum urinary output, or other factors. The question will include the units that the test taker should indicate in the answer.

MULTIPLE-RESPONSE QUESTIONS

The instruction to *select all that apply* follows a multiple-choice question stem that has more than one correct answer. This question requires the student to identify all the correct responses to the question. Questions will include up to five responses, and the test taker must select all of the provided responses that are correct. There may be two, three, four, or even five correct responses.

HOT SPOT ITEMS

Hot spots require the test taker to identify the correct response to a question referencing a picture, graphic, or other image. For example, a test taker may be asked to place an X on a particular location. It is important to be as precise as possible because there is only one best answer.

AUDIO

Some questions may require interpretation. For example, the test taker may be asked to interpret the sound on an audio file, recognize progression based on laboratory results, or perform calculations based on information given.

ORDERED RESPONSE

Ordered response is a drag-and-drop-style question in which all the options offered are correct and the test taker must put them in order. For example, the appropriate order may be setting priorities or steps in a process.

NGN Questions Formats

For NGN item types, the test taker must reference, analyze, and interpret the client data provided to answer the item stem. Item formats include variations on drag-and-drop, drop-down, multiple-choice, and multiple-response questions as well as highlighting and "bowtie" questions. NGN item types may be standalone or in the context of an unfolding case study that addresses the six steps of the CJMM. In the unfolding case studies, test takers are provided with the related electronic medical record, which may include the client's health history, nurses' notes, vital signs, and laboratory values. When nurses' notes have been updated, the test taker will be informed and asked to refer to the latest information.

MATRIX/GRID MULTIPLE CHOICE AND MULTIPLE RESPONSE

In matrix-style questions, the test taker is provided client data on which to base their decisions for the most appropriate response for each row. The test taker may be asked to consider such information as a list of potential orders and indicate whether they are anticipated, nonessential, or contraindicated for the client in the case study. If this item type is used in the context of evaluating outcomes, the test taker will be asked to indicate whether the client's condition has improved, has not changed, or has deteriorated.

EXTENDED DRAG-AND-DROP

Using patient data provided, the test taker uses their computer mouse to drag items from one box to the other. There are two styles of drag and drop questions: *Drag-and-drop cloze* requires the test taker to select the best word choice to complete a sentence. *Drag-and-drop rationale* requires the test taker to drag one condition and one client finding to complete the sentence.

ENHANCED HOT SPOT (HIGHLIGHTING)

Test takers are provided with patient data and asked to highlight content to determine the course of treatment. This may include such things as client risk, client conditions requiring follow-up, or client conditions that require advance preparation before receiving the client. When the test taker clicks on the selected section, it will show up yellow, as though highlighted manually with a felt-tipped pen.

DROP-DOWN QUESTIONS

Three styles of drop-down questions will appear on the NCLEX®. All provide patient data in the form of history and physical, laboratory results, flow sheet, orders, and/or nursing notes. All require the test taker to choose the most likely options to complete the statements.

BOWTIE

Bowtie questions are considered standalone rather than part of an unfolding case. Bowtie questions are built upon all six stages of CJMM. Responses fall into three categories: actions to take, potential conditions, and parameters to monitor. In this brief case study format, a case is provided, followed by three questions. The test taker is asked to select the highest priority and drag it to the center box, then select the best two *actions to take* and the two most important *parameters to monitor* (see Fig. 1.1).

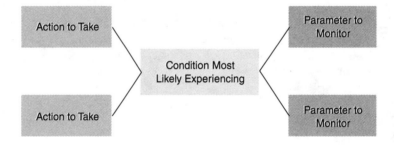

Option choices		
Action to Take	Potential Conditions	Parameters to Monitor
Option 1	Option 1	Option 1
Option 2	Option 2	Option 2
Option 3	Option 3	Option 3
Option 4	Option 4	Option 4
Option 5		Option 5

Figure 1–1. Sample bowtie item.

CRITICAL THINKING STRATEGY: THE RACE MODEL

Achieving success on nursing examinations is a bit like participating in a race; however, your success is based not only on speed but also on strategy and tactics. Although speed must be considered when taking a timed test to factor in the amount of time spent on each question as part of the test strategy, the emphasis should be on using critical thinking strategies to answer multiple-choice questions. The RACE model is a critical thinking strategy to use when answering nursing multiple-choice questions. As you apply the RACE model to every test question, this thinking process will become second nature. This methodical approach will improve your ability to critically analyze a test question and your chances of selecting the correct answer (Doherty, 2022).

The RACE model has four steps to answering a test question:

R—Recognize what information is in the stem.
* Recognize the keywords in the stem.
* Recognize who the client is in the stem.

A—Ask what the question is examining.
* Ask specifically what the question requires you to do.

C—Critically analyze the options in relation to the question asked in the stem.
* Critically scrutinize each option in relation to the information in the stem.
* Critically identify a rationale for each option.
* Critically compare and contrast the options in relation to the information in the stem and their relationships to one another.

E—Eliminate as many options as possible.
* Eliminate one option at a time.

The following discussion explores this critical thinking strategy in relation to the thinking processes represented in multiple-choice nursing questions. Thoughtfully read the cognitive requirements under each type of question (e.g., remembering, understanding, applying, and analyzing). It is important to understand this content to apply the critical thinking strategies inherent in each cognitive-level question. In addition, four sets of sample test questions are presented to demonstrate the increasing complexity of thinking reflected in the various cognitive levels, focusing on specific nursing content.

Remembering-Level Questions: Remember Information!

Knowledge is information that is filed or stored in the memory. It represents the elements essential to the core of a discipline. In nursing, this information consists of elements such as terminology and specific facts, including steps of procedures, phenomena, expected laboratory values, classifications, and the expected ranges of vital signs. This type of information requires no alteration from one use or application to another because it is concrete. The information is remembered or recognized in the form in which it was originally learned. This information is the foundation of critical thinking. You must have adequate, accurate, relevant, and important information on which to base your more theoretical, abstract thinking in the future.

Beginning nursing students find remembering-level questions the easiest because they require the recall or reiteration of information. Information may be memorized, which is done by repeatedly reviewing information or through repeated experiences with the information. Repetition is necessary because information is forgotten quickly unless reinforced. When answering remembering-level questions, you either know the information or you don't. The challenge of answering remembering-level questions is defining what the question is asking and tapping your knowledge.

USE A CRITICAL THINKING STRATEGY TO ANSWER
REMEMBERING-LEVEL QUESTIONS

1. What is the description of the interviewing technique of paraphrasing?
   1. Asking the client to repeat what was just said.
   2. Condensing a discussion into an organized review.
   3. Restating what the client has said using similar words.
   4. Asking goal-directed questions concentrating on key concerns.

Table 1–1. Critical Thinking Strategy for Remembering-Level Questions

Recognize keywords.	What is the **description** of the interviewing technique of **paraphrasing**?
Recognize who the client is.	There is no client in this question.
Ask what the question is asking.	What is the description of paraphrasing?
Critically analyze options in relation to the question.	To answer this question, you must know the definition or characteristics of paraphrasing. It is information that you must recall from your memory. You do not have to know other interviewing skills or their descriptions and characteristics to answer this question. **Rationales:** 1. Asking a client to repeat what was just asked is known as *clarifying*, not paraphrasing. 2. Reviewing a discussion is known as *summarizing*, not paraphrasing. 3. **Paraphrasing or restating is an interviewing skill in which the nurse listens for a client's basic message and then repeats the content of the message in similar words. This validates information from the client without changing the meaning of the statement and provides an opportunity for the client to hear what was said.** 4. Asking goal-directed questions that concentrate on key concerns is known as *focusing*, not paraphrasing.
Eliminate incorrect options.	Options 1, 2, and 4 are not examples of paraphrasing and can be eliminated.

Understanding-Level Questions: Understand Information!

Understanding is the ability to construct meaning from learning in order to explain, compare, interpret, summarize or classify. To be safe practitioners, nurses must understand information such as reasons for nursing interventions, physiology and pathophysiology, consequences of actions, and responses to medications. To reach an understanding of information in nursing, you must be able to translate information into your own words. Once information is rearranged in your own mind, you must interpret the essential components for their intent, corollaries, significance, implications, consequences, and conclusions in accordance with the conditions described in the original communication. The information is employed within its own context without being used in a different or new situation.

Beginning nursing students generally consider understanding-level questions slightly more difficult than remembering-level questions but less complicated than applying- and analyzing-level questions. Students often try to deal with understanding-level information by memorizing the content. For example, when studying local signs and symptoms of an infection, students may memorize the following list: heat, erythema, pain, edema, and exudate. Although memorization is a useful tool, it is far better to understand why these adaptations occur. Erythema and heat occur because of increased circulation to the area. Edema occurs because of increased permeability of the capillaries. Pain occurs because the accumulating fluid in the tissue presses on nerve endings. Exudate occurs because of the accumulation of fluid, cells, and other substances at the site of infection. The mind is a wonderful machine, but unless you have a photographic memory, lists of information without understanding often become overwhelming and confusing. The challenge of answering understanding-level questions is to comprehend the information at a level where you can restate it in your own words. See *TEST SUCCESS: Test-Taking Techniques for Beginning Nursing Students* for specific study techniques related to understanding-level questions.

USE A CRITICAL THINKING STRATEGY TO ANSWER UNDERSTANDING-LEVEL QUESTIONS

1. How does the interviewing technique of paraphrasing promote communication?
   1. Requires clients to defend their points of view.
   2. Limits clients from continuing a rambling conversation.
   3. Allows clients to take their conversations in any desired direction.
   4. Offers clients an opportunity to develop a clearer idea of what they said.

Table 1–2. Critical Thinking Strategy for Understanding-Level Questions

Recognize keywords.	How does the interviewing technique of **paraphrasing promote communication?**
Recognize who the client is.	There is no client.
Ask what the question is asking.	How does paraphrasing promote communication?
Critically analyze options in relation to the question.	The word in the stem that indicates that this is a comprehension level question is **promote**. What is the consequence of paraphrasing? You need to scrutinize each option to identify whether the description in the option correctly explains how paraphrasing works to promote communication. **Rationales:** 1. This describes the results of challenging statements that usually are barriers to communication. 2. This describes one purpose of the interviewing skill of focusing, which is the use of questions or statements to center on one concern mentioned within a wordy, confusing conversation. 3. This is the purpose of open-ended questions or statements. 4. **Paraphrasing involves actively listening for client concerns that are then restated by the nurse in similar words. This intervention conveys that the nurse has heard and understood the message and gives the client an opportunity to review what was said.**
Eliminate incorrect options.	Options 1, 2, and 3 do not accurately describe how paraphrasing works to promote communication and can be eliminated.

Applying-Level Questions: Use Information!

Applying is the ability to use known and understood information in new situations. It requires more than just understanding information because you must demonstrate, solve, change, modify, or manipulate information in ways beyond its originally learned form or context. With application questions, you are confronted with a new situation that requires you to implement information taken out of a familiar context to arrive at abstractions, generalizations, or consequences that can be used in the new situation to answer the question. Applying-level questions require you to make rational, logical judgments.

Beginning nursing students frequently find applying-level questions challenging because they require a restructuring of understood information into abstractions, commonalities, and generalizations, which are then applied to new situations (Nugent & Vitale, 2023). Although parts of your day are routine, every day you are exposed to new, challenging experiences where you apply your knowledge. Similarly, with applying-level questions, you will be confronted by situations that you learned about in a book, experienced personally, or relived through other students' experiences. Throughout your entire nursing career, you will encounter topics you have never heard about or experienced before. The challenge of answering applying-level questions is going beyond remembering to demonstrate knowledge of regulations and information in a creative way. See *TEST SUCCESS: Test-Taking Techniques for Beginning Nursing Students* for specific study techniques related to applying-level questions.

USE A CRITICAL THINKING STRATEGY TO ANSWER APPLYING-LEVEL QUESTIONS

1. A client scheduled for major surgery, who is perspiring and nervously picking at the bed linen, says, "I don't know if I can go through with this surgery." The nurse responds, "You'd rather not have surgery now?" Which interviewing technique was used by the nurse?
   1. Focusing.
   2. Reflection.
   3. Paraphrasing.
   4. Clarification.

Table 1–3. Critical Thinking for Applying-Level Questions

Recognize keywords.	A patient scheduled for major surgery, who is perspiring and nervously picking at the bed linen, says, **"I don't know if I can go through with this surgery."** The nurse responds, **"You'd rather not have surgery now?" Which interviewing technique was used by the nurse?**
Recognize who the client is.	The patient is the client.
Ask what the question is asking.	What interviewing technique is being used by the nurse when the nurse says in response to the client, "You'd rather not have surgery now?"
Critically analyze options in relation to the question.	The word in the stem that indicates that this is an application question is **used**. To identify which technique was used by the nurse, you have to understand the elements of a paraphrasing statement, and you need to be able to recognize a paraphrasing statement when it is used. Although it is helpful to understand the elements of the other interviewing techniques because it will help you eliminate incorrect options, it is not necessary to understand this information to answer the question. **Rationales:** 1. The example in the stem is not using focusing because the client's statement was short and contained one message that was reiterated by the nurse. Focusing is used to explore one concern among many statements made by the client. 2. The example in the stem is not using reflection because the nurse's statement is concerned with the content, not the underlying feeling, of the client's statement. An example of reflection used by the nurse is, "You seem anxious about having major surgery." 3. **The nurse used paraphrasing because the client's and nurse's statements contain the same message but are expressed with different words.** 4. The example in the stem is not using clarification. When clarification is used, the nurse is asking the client to further explain what is meant by the client's statement. An example of clarification used by the nurse is, "I am not quite sure that I know what you mean when you say you would rather not have surgery now."
Eliminate incorrect options.	Options 1, 2, and 4 can be eliminated because these techniques are different from the technique portrayed in the nurse's response in the stem.

Analyzing-Level Questions: Scrutinize Information!

Analysis is the separation of an entity into its constituent parts and examination of their essential features in relation to each other. Analyzing-level questions assume that you know, understand, and can apply information. They ask you to engage in higher-level critical thinking strategies. To answer analyzing-level questions, you first must examine each element of information as a separate entity. Second, you need to investigate and distinguish the differences among the various elements of information. In other words, you must compare and contrast information. Third, you must analyze the structure and organization of the compared and contrasted information to arrive at a conclusion or answer. Analyzing-level questions often ask you to set priorities and, in the stem, use words such as *first, initially, best, priority*, and *most important*.

Beginning nursing students find analyzing-level questions the most difficult to answer. Analysis questions demand scrutiny of individual elements of information as well as require identification of differences among elements of information. Sometimes students cannot identify the structural or organizational relationship of elements of information. The challenge of answering analysis-level questions is performing a complete scrutiny of all the various elements of information and their interrelationships without overanalyzing or reading into the question.

USE A CRITICAL THINKING STRATEGY TO ANSWER ANALYZING-LEVEL QUESTIONS

1. The mother of a terminally ill child says, "I never thought that I would have such a sick child." What is the best initial response by the nurse?
   1. "How do you feel right now?"
   2. "What do you mean by sick child?"
   3. "Life is not fair to do this to a child."
   4. "It's hard to believe that your child is so sick."

Table 1–4. Critical Thinking Strategy for Analyzing-Level Questions

Recognize keywords.	The mother of a terminally ill child says, "I never thought that I would have such a sick child." What is the **best initial response** by the nurse?
Recognize who the client is.	The mother is the client.
Ask what the question is asking.	Which is an example of the best interviewing skill to use when initially responding to a statement made by the mother of a sick child?
Critically analyze options in relation to the question.	Analysis questions often ask you to set priorities as indicated by the words **best initial response** in the stem of this question. To answer this question, you need to identify which interviewing techniques are portrayed in the statements in each option, understand how and why each interviewing skill works, compare and contrast the pros and cons of each technique if used in this situation, and identify which technique is the most supportive, appropriate, and best initial response by the nurse. **Rationales:** 1. Direct questions cut off communication and should be avoided. 2. This response focuses on the seriousness of the child's illness, which is not the issue raised in the mother's statement. 3. This statement reflects the beliefs and values of the nurse, which should be avoided. 4. **This is a declarative statement that paraphrases the mother's beliefs and feelings. It communicates to the mother that the nurse is attentively listening and invites the mother to expand on her thoughts if she feels ready.**
Eliminate incorrect options.	Options 1, 2, and 3 can be eliminated because they do not focus on the content of the mother's statement.

HOW TO APPROACH EXAMINATION QUESTIONS

There are several techniques a test taker should use when answering examination questions.

1. **Pretend the examination is a clinical experience.** First and foremost, test takers must approach critical thinking questions as if they were in a clinical setting and the situation were developing on the spot. The student taking an examination and a nurse working on a clinical unit both need the same critical thinking ability.
2. **Read the stem carefully before reading the responses.** There are several different types of questions on the NCLEX-RN® examination. Before answering any questions, the test taker must be sure to identify what the question is asking—that is, what is in the stem?
3. **Read nothing into the stem.** The response reflects only the information given in the stem. For example, if the stem does not say the client is anxious, the test taker must not select an answer that includes anxiety.
4. **Consider possible responses before answering.** After forming a clear understanding of the stem, but before reading the possible responses, the test taker should consider possible correct answers to the question. Test-question writers include only plausible answer options. A test writer's goal is to determine whether the test taker knows and understands the material. The test taker, therefore, must have an idea of what the correct answer might be before beginning to read the possible responses.
5. **Consider each possible response as a standalone true-or-false question.**
6. **When prioritizing answers, select either the client condition that threatens survival or the answer(s) that relate to ABC—airway, breathing, and circulation.**
7. **Read the responses.** Only after clearly understanding what is being asked and after developing an idea of what the correct answer might be, the test taker reads the options (distractors). The one response that is closest in content to the test taker's guess should be the answer that is chosen. The test taker should not second-guess themselves, as the first idea is almost always the correct response. Only if the test taker knows that they misread the question should the answer be changed.
8. **Read the rationales for each question.** In this book, rationales are given for each answer option. The learner should take full advantage of this feature. Read why the correct answer is correct. The rationale may be based on content, on interpretation of information, or on a number of other reasons. Understanding why the answer to one question is correct and others are not correct is likely to transfer over to other questions with similar rationales. Next, read why the wrong answers are wrong. The rationales may be based on a number of different factors, including the mistake of reading the question and/or answer options too quickly.
9. **Finally, read all test-taking tips in this book and others.** Some of the tips relate directly to test-taking skills, whereas others include invaluable information in general.

SUMMARY

In the end, the person who knows the material and applies it consistently will do the best on the test. There is no substitute for studying and making sense of the information for oneself. If the test taker uses this text as recommended, they should be well prepared to be successful when taking an examination in any or all of the content areas presented. As a result of strong study practices, the test taker should be fully prepared to function as a beginning registered professional nurse in the many areas of psychiatric mental health nursing.

REFERENCES

American Association of Colleges of Nursing. (n.d.). *Clinical judgement.* https://www.aacnnursing.org/essentials/tool-kit/domains-concepts/clinical-judgement

Doherty, C. D. (2022). *Med-surg success: NCLEX-style Q&A review* (4th ed.). F. A. Davis Company.

Irland, N. (2022). *Maternal and newborn success: NCLEX-style Q&A review* (4th ed.). F. A. Davis Company.

NCSBN. (2019). Clinical judgment measurement model. *Next Generation NCLEX News.* https://www.ncsbn.org/publications/NGN-News-Winter-2019

Nugent, P. M., & Vitale B.A. (2023). *Test Success: Clinical Judgment and Test-Taking Strategies* (10th ed.). F. A. Davis Company.

Venes, D. (Ed.). (2021). *Taber's cyclopedic medical dictionary* (24th ed.). F. A. Davis Company.

Basic Concepts in Psychiatric Mental Health Nursing

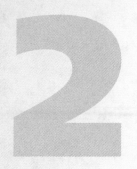

Mental Health/Mental Illness: Theoretical Concepts

KEYWORDS

The following words include English vocabulary, nursing/medical terminology, concepts, principles, or information relevant to content specifically addressed in this chapter or associated with topics presented in it. English dictionaries, your nursing textbooks, and medical dictionaries such as *Taber's Cyclopedic Medical Dictionary* are resources that can be used to expand your knowledge and understanding of these words and related information.

Assertiveness

Beck/Ellis's cognitive behavioral model

Cognitive theory

Cultural norms

Defense mechanisms

Diagnostic and Statistical Manual of Mental Disorders, Fifth Edition, Text Revision (*DSM-5-TR*)

Erickson, Tomlin, and Swain's modeling and role modeling theory of nursing

Erikson's psychosocial theory

Freud's psychoanalytic theory

Glasser's reality theory

Global Assessment of Functioning (GAF)

Leininger's cultural care diversity and universality

Mahler's object relations theory

Maslow's hierarchy of needs

Mental health/mental illness

Neuman's systems model of nursing

Nursing process

Orem's self-care deficit theory of nursing

Outcome

Parse's theory of human becoming

Peplau's nursing theory

Piaget's cognitive development

Rogers's science of unitary human beings

Roy's adaptation model

Selye/Lazarus's stress theory

Sullivan's interpersonal theory

Watson's caring theory

QUESTIONS

Major Theoretical Models

1. Considering the many criteria for good mental health, the nursing student has been instructed to list four of these criteria. The student's list consists of the following: (1) an appropriate perception of reality, (2) the ability to accept oneself, (3) the ability to establish relationships, and (4) a need for detachment and the desire for privacy. How would the nurse evaluate the nursing student's list?
   1. Excellent. All the student's criteria are correct.
   2. Good. Three of the four criteria are correct.
   3. Mediocre. Two of the four criteria are correct.
   4. Poor. All four of the criteria are incorrect.

2. Which assessment is most important when evaluating signs and symptoms of mental illness?
   1. The decreased amount of creativity a client exhibits.
   2. The inability to face problems within one's life.
   3. The intensity of an emotional reaction.
   4. The client's social and cultural norms.

3. Which is an example of an interpersonal intervention for a client on an inpatient psychiatric unit?
   1. Assist the client to note common defense mechanisms and coping skills that are being used.
   2. Discuss acting-out behaviors and assist the client in understanding why they occur.
   3. Ask the client to record thoughts they are having before acting-out behaviors occur.
   4. Ask the client to acknowledge one positive person in their life to assist the client after discharge.

4. Which is an example of appropriate psychosexual development?
   1. An 18-month-old relieves anxiety by the use of a pacifier.
   2. A 5-year-old boy focuses on relationships with other boys.
   3. A 7-year-old girl identifies with her mother.
   4. A 12-month-old begins learning about independence and control.

5. Which client situation is an example of normal ego development?
   1. A client continuously calls out to get their needs met.
   2. A client complains of poor self-esteem because of punishments from their past.
   3. A client exhibits the ability to assert themself without anger or aggression.
   4. A client feels guilty about wanting to have sexual relations outside of marriage.

6. After studying the concepts of personality development, the nursing student understands that Freud is to psychoanalytic theory as Peplau is to:
   1. Psychosocial theory.
   2. Nursing theory.
   3. Interpersonal theory.
   4. Object relations theory.

7. Nursing theorists identify the nurse–client relationship as central to nursing practice. After studying these concepts, the nursing student understands that Peplau is to the phases of the nurse–client relationship as Watson is to:
   1. Seven assumptions about the science of caring.
   2. Cultural care diversity and universality.
   3. Modeling and role modeling.
   4. Human energy fields.

8. After studying nursing interventions in the context of nursing theory, the nursing student understands that Neuman is to primary, secondary, and tertiary prevention as Roy is to:
   1. Activities needed to meet self-care demands and solve self-care deficits.
   2. Assisting the client to examine and understand the meaning of life experiences.
   3. Interventions that alter or manage stimuli so that adaptive responses can occur.
   4. Interactions *with* versus *for* the client to achieve maximum potential.

9. Which is the goal of the cognitive-behavioral theory model according to Beck and Ellis?
   1. Developing satisfactory relationships, maturity, and relative freedom from anxiety.
   2. Substituting rational for irrational beliefs and eliminating self-defeating behaviors.
   3. Facing reality and developing standards for behaving responsibly.
   4. Reducing bodily tensions and managing stress by biofeedback and relaxation training.

10. Which interaction is an example of dialogue that would be used in the context of reality therapy?
    1. *Client:* "I'm so anxious I can't sleep." *Nurse:* "I have a relaxation exercise I can show you."
    2. *Client:* "I was punished frequently by my parent, and now I can't do anything right." *Nurse:* "Tell me about your feelings of anger."
    3. *Client:* "I can't sit still; I'm too anxious and jittery." *Nurse:* "Let's sit for a while and discuss your anxiety."
    4. *Client:* "The stupid doctor revoked my pass for tomorrow." *Nurse:* "What did you do that showed that you were not ready for a pass?"

11. A 4-year-old child is unable to consider another child's ideas about playing house. This situation is an example of which concept of Piaget's theory of cognitive development?
    1. Object permanence.
    2. Reversibility and spatiality.
    3. Egocentrism.
    4. Formal operations.

12. The statement "Growth involves resolution of critical tasks through the eight stages of the life cycle" is a concept of which therapeutic model?
    1. Interpersonal.
    2. Cognitive-behavioral.
    3. Intrapersonal.
    4. Psychoanalytic.

13. A 25-year-old client diagnosed with major depressive disorder remains in their room and avoids others. According to Erikson, what describes this client's developmental task assessment?
    1. Stagnation.
    2. Despair.
    3. Isolation.
    4. Role confusion.

14. A 7-year-old child is active in sports and has received a most improved player award at their baseball tournament. According to Erikson, what describes this client's developmental task assessment?
    1. Autonomy.
    2. Identity.
    3. Industry.
    4. Initiative.

15. Which scenario describes an individual in Erikson's developmental stage of old age exhibiting a negative outcome of despair?
    1. A 60-year-old woman having difficulty taking care of her aged mother.
    2. A 50-year-old man reviewing the positive and negative aspects of his life.
    3. A 65-year-old man openly discussing his life's accomplishments and failures.
    4. A 70-year-old woman angry about where her life has ended up.

16. Which is an example of an individual successfully completing Erikson's school age stage of development?
    1. A 14-year-old verbalizes that they resisted peer pressure to drink alcohol at a party.
    2. A 5-year-old is able to ask others in their class to play hide-and-seek.
    3. A 3-year-old is able to play by themself while other family members play games.
    4. An 11-year-old is trying out for cheerleading.

17. Which initial information gathered by the nurse is most important when assessing Erikson's stages of development?
    1. The chronological age of the individual.
    2. The developmental age exhibited through behaviors.
    3. The time frame needed to complete a successful outcome at a previous stage.
    4. The implementation of interventions based on developmental age.

18. According to Maslow's hierarchy of needs, which of the following client actions would be considered most basic? **Select all that apply.**
    1. A client discusses the need for order in their life and freedom from fear.
    2. A client feels lonely and is seeking to share life experiences.
    3. A client begins to realize their full potential.
    4. A client is role-playing a situation with a nurse to practice assertiveness skills.
    5. A client seeks shelter at a center for domestic violence.

19. According to Maslow's hierarchy of needs, which client action would be an example of a highly evolved, mature client?
    1. A client discusses the need for avoiding harm and maintaining comfort.
    2. A client states the need for giving and receiving support from others.
    3. A client begins to discuss feelings of self-fulfillment.
    4. A client discusses the need to achieve success and recognition in work.

20. According to Maslow's hierarchy of needs, which situation on an inpatient psychiatric unit would require priority intervention?
    1. A client is disturbed that family can be seen only during visiting hours.
    2. A client exhibits hostile and angry behaviors toward another client.
    3. A client states, "I have no one who cares about me."
    4. A client states, "I have never met my career goals."

21. Rank the following statements using Maslow's hierarchy of needs, starting with the basic level of attainment and progressing toward self-actualization.
    1. _____ "I am glad I can now be assertive in controversial situations."
    2. _____ "My spouse and I are planning a second honeymoon for our 20th anniversary."
    3. _____ "Using my CPAP machine consistently has eliminated my sleep apnea."
    4. _____ "I change my smoke alarm batteries every year on New Year's Day."
    5. _____ "Getting my graduate degree was a wonderful 50th birthday gift to myself."

22. A client is developing a sense of identity and learning to form relationships with persons of the opposite sex. According to Sullivan's theory, this client would be assessed at which stage of development?
    1. Childhood (18 months to 6 years)
    2. Juvenile (6 to 9 years)
    3. Preadolescence (9 to 12 years)
    4. Early adolescence (12 to 14 years)

23. Which of the following client statements are correctly matched with the personality structure, as described by Freud, that they exemplify? **Select all that apply.**
    1. "I'll return the purse I found. It's never right to steal."—Superego
    2. "Coming on to my friend's boyfriend is just plain wrong."—Ego
    3. "I might get pregnant if I have sex, so I won't do it."—Id
    4. "I need that car. No one will miss it."—Id
    5. "Cheating on a test could get me expelled, so I won't do it."—Ego

24. According to Maslow's hierarchy of needs, which situation demonstrates the lowest level of attainment?
1. An individual demonstrates an ability to discuss objectively all points of view and possesses a strong sense of ethics.
2. An individual avoids harm while maintaining comfort, order, and physical safety.
3. An individual establishes meaningful interpersonal relationships and can identify himself or herself within a group.
4. An individual desires prestige from personal accomplishments.

Biological Implications

25. Which of the following statements are true as they relate to the history of psychopharmacology? **Select all that apply.**
1. Before 1950, only sedatives and amphetamines were available as psychotropics.
2. Phenothiazines were initially used in pain management for their sedative effect.
3. Atypical antipsychotics were the first medications used to treat the positive symptoms of schizophrenia.
4. Psychotropic medications have assisted health-care providers in their efforts to cure mental illness.
5. Newly developed atypical psychotropics have shown much promise in controlling the negative symptoms of schizophrenia.

26. Which of the following are true statements about neurotransmitters? **Select all that apply.**
1. Neurotransmitters are responsible for essential functions in human emotions and behaviors.
2. Neurotransmitters are targets for the mechanism of action of many psychotropic medications.
3. Neurotransmitters are only studied for their effect related to psychiatric disease processes.
4. Neurotransmitters are nerve cells that generate and transmit the body's electrochemical impulses.
5. Neurotransmitters are cholinergics, such as serotonin, norepinephrine, dopamine, and histamine.

27. Which functions does the limbic system regulate?
1. Perceptions and interpretations of most sensory information.
2. Auditory functions and short-term memory.
3. Emotional experiences.
4. Visual reception and interpretation.

28. Regarding the etiology of schizophrenia spectrum disorders, which of the following support(s) a biological theory? **Select all that apply.**
1. Dopamine hypothesis.
2. Prenatal exposure to influenza.
3. Ventricular and sulci atrophy.
4. Downward drift hypothesis.
5. Increased levels of serotonin.

29. A client is hearing voices saying, "Kill mother soon." The client states, "I am a prophet." The nurse understands that these symptoms are exhibited because of which brain alteration?
1. A decrease in dopamine in the mesocortical dopamine pathway.
2. An increase in dopamine in the mesolimbic dopamine pathway.
3. An increase in dopamine in the nigrostriatal dopamine pathway.
4. A decrease in dopamine in the tuberoinfundibular dopamine pathway.

30. Which situation supports the biological theory of the development of bipolar affective disorder?
    1. A client is prescribed a selective serotonin reuptake inhibitor and then exhibits impulsive behaviors, expansive mood, and flight of ideas.
    2. A client has three jobs, which require increased amounts of energy and the ability to multitask.
    3. A client experiences thoughts of negative self-image and then expresses grandiosity when discussing abilities at work.
    4. A client has been raised in a very chaotic household where there was a lack of impulse control related to excessive spending.

31. Which of the following medications can cause confusion, depression, and increased anxiety? **Select all that apply.**
    1. Meperidine.
    2. Dextromethorphan.
    3. Loratadine.
    4. Levodopa.
    5. Pseudoephedrine.

32. A physician has ordered genetic testing for a client who is experiencing difficulty metabolizing prescribed medications. To answer the client's questions regarding this new order, which of the following nursing statements should be included? The genetic testing will: **Select all that apply.**
    1. Identify which medications will or will not cause significant side effects.
    2. Identify a specific gene that impacts the ability to convert folic acid into active form L-methylfolate.
    3. Require the client to fast for 12 hours prior to having a blood sample drawn.
    4. Work exclusively for clients experiencing depression, anxiety, and attention deficit-hyperactivity disorders.
    5. Identify one specific medication to be prescribed for the symptoms experienced.

Diagnostic and Statistical Manual of Mental Disorders, Fifth Edition, Text Revision (DSM-5-TR)

33. A student nurse asks the instructor about the *Diagnostic and Statistical Manual of Mental Disorders*, Fifth Edition, Text Revision (*DSM-5-TR*). Which of the following instructor statements are correct? **Select all that apply.**
    1. "The *DSM-5-TR* lists all psychiatric and general medical diagnoses."
    2. "The *DSM-5-TR* allows clinicians to rate disorders along a continuum of severity."
    3. "Conditions that do not meet *DSM-5-TR* criteria are termed *not elsewhere defined (NED)*."
    4. "Dimensional assessment tools are included in the *DSM-5-TR*."
    5. "Global Assessment of Functioning (GAF) is included in the *DSM-5-TR*."

34. Which of the following are reasons for the utilization of the *DSM-5-TR* in the mental health-care system? **Select all that apply.**
    1. It is a convenient format for organizing and communicating clinical data.
    2. It is a means for considering the complexity of clinical situations.
    3. It is a means for describing the unique symptoms of psychiatric clients.
    4. It is a format for evaluating clients based on a regulated approach.
    5. It is a means to better understand the etiology of many psychiatric disorders.

35. How is the *DSM-5-TR* helpful to mental health providers? **Select all that apply.**
    1. The *DSM-5-TR* provides a common language related to the diagnoses of mental illness.
    2. The *DSM-5-TR* lists medications that are appropriate for the treatment of mental disorders.
    3. The *DSM-5-TR* presents standard criteria for the classification of mental disorders.
    4. The *DSM-5-TR* provides an axis system to evaluate clients holistically.
    5. The *DSM-5-TR* presents a comprehensive list of community resources.

The correct answer number and rationale for why it is the correct answer are given in boldface blue type. Rationales for why the other answer options are incorrect are given as well, but they are not in boldface type.

Major Theoretical Models

1. 1. **Excellent. All the student's criteria are correct. There are numerous descriptors depicting the concept of good mental health. The student's list is not comprehensive, but all four criteria listed are correct reflections of good mental health. A mentally healthy individual views reality with a realistic perception based on objective data. Accepting oneself, including strengths and weaknesses, is indicative of good mental health. The ability to establish relationships by use of communication skills is essential for good mental health. Mentally healthy individuals seek time to be alone and appreciate periods of privacy.**
   2. Four of four, not three of four, criteria are correct.
   3. Four of four, not two of four, criteria are correct.
   4. All four of the criteria are correct, not incorrect.

   TEST-TAKING HINT: To answer this question correctly, the test taker should review criteria for good mental health as they relate to the concept of self, relationships with others, and interactions with the environment. Recognizing that detachment and a need for privacy are healthy helps the test taker to include these criteria as an indication of good mental health.

2. 1. The amount of creativity a client exhibits is not reflective of mental health or illness. Some individuals are innately more creative than others.
   2. The inability to face a problem is not specific to mental illness. Many individuals not diagnosed with a mental illness have difficulty facing problems, such as a person with diabetes refusing to adhere to an American Diabetes Association diet.
   3. Intensity of emotional reactions is not indicative of mental illness. Grief, an expected response to a perceived loss, can

vary in intensity from person to person and be affected by cultural norms.
   4. **It is important when assessing for mental illness that social and cultural norms be evaluated. The context of cultural norms determines whether behaviors are considered acceptable or aberrant. Belief in reincarnation can be acceptable in one culture and considered delusional in another.**

   TEST-TAKING HINT: To answer this question correctly, the test taker must understand that culture is a particular society's entire way of living, encompassing shared patterns of belief, feelings, and knowledge that guide people's conduct and are passed down from generation to generation.

3. 1. Intrapersonal, not interpersonal, theory deals with conflicts within the individual. Assisting clients in noting defense mechanisms used would be an example of an intervention that reflects the use of intrapersonal theory.
   2. Discussing acting-out behaviors and why they occur is an intervention reflective of behavioral, not interpersonal, theory. A major concept of this theory is that all behavior has meaning.
   3. Discussion of thoughts is an intervention reflective of cognitive, not interpersonal, theory. Cognitive theory is based on the principle that thoughts affect feelings and behaviors.
   4. **Interpersonal theory states that individual behavior and personality development are the direct result of interpersonal relationships. The identification of a positive relationship is an intervention that reflects interpersonal theory.**

   TEST-TAKING HINT: Understanding the basic concepts of interpersonal theory assists the test taker in answering this question correctly. Remember interpersonal theory by thinking "inter" and "personal," or "between people." It often gets confused with intrapersonal theory. Think "intra" and "personal," meaning "within oneself."

4. 1. **From birth to 18 months of age, a child is in the oral stage of Freud's psychosexual development. During this stage, an infant would attempt to decrease anxiety by finding relief using oral gratification.**

2. From age 3 to 6 years, the child is in the phallic stage of Freud's psychosexual development. During this stage, the child is looking to identify with the parent of the same sex and developing their own sexual identity by focusing on genital organs. Focusing on relationships with same-sex peers occurs during the latency stage, which occurs from 6 to 12 years of age.

3. From 6 to 12 years of age, the child is in the latency stage of Freud's psychosexual development. During this stage, the child is suppressing sexuality and focusing on relationships with same-sex peers. Identifying with the parent of the same sex occurs in the phallic stage, which occurs from 3 to 6 years of age.

4. Learning about independence and control occurs in Freud's anal phase of psychosexual development, which occurs from 18 months to 3 years of age.

TEST-TAKING HINT: To answer this question correctly, the test taker must be familiar with the basic concepts of psychosexual development according to Freud. Freud placed much emphasis on the first 5 years of life and believed that characteristics developed during these early years bore heavily on one's adaptation patterns and personality traits in adulthood.

5. 1. The *id* is the locus of instinctual drives— the *pleasure principle*. It endows an infant with drives that seek to satisfy needs and achieve immediate gratification. Id-driven behaviors are impulsive and may be irrational. The answer presented is an example of *id*, not *ego*, development.

2. Between 3 and 6 years of age, the child begins to develop their superego by being rewarded or punished for good and bad behavior. The superego internalizes values and morals set forth by the primary caregivers. This is considered the *perfection principle*. The superego is important in that it assists the ego in controlling the impulses of the id. When the superego becomes penalizing, self-esteem issues can arise. The answer presented is an example of *superego*, not *ego*, development.

3. **The ego is considered the *reality principle* and begins to develop between 4 and 6 months of age. The ego experiences the outside world and then adapts and responds to it. The ego's main goal is to maintain harmony between the id and the superego. The ability to assert**

oneself without anger or aggression is an example of healthy ego development.

4. As children grow and are rewarded for good and bad behavior, they begin to develop their superego. This is considered the *perfection principle*. Not only do parents assist in the development of the superego by a reward-and-punishment system, but also societal norms play a role in superego development. The answer presented is an example of *superego*, not *ego*, development.

TEST-TAKING HINT: To answer this question correctly, the test taker must understand that Freud organized the structure of the personality into three major components: id, ego, and superego. They are distinguished by their unique functions and different characteristics.

6. Freud, known as the father of psychiatry, developed and organized the structure of the personality into three components: the id, ego, and superego. He also described the formation of personality through five stages of psychosexual development: oral, anal, phallic, latency, and genital.

1. Erikson, not Peplau, developed psychosocial theory as a further expansion of Freud's psychoanalytic theory. Erikson's theory is based on developmental task completion during eight stages of personality development throughout the life cycle: trust versus mistrust, autonomy versus shame and doubt, initiative versus guilt, industry versus inferiority, identity versus role confusion, intimacy versus isolation, generativity versus stagnation, and ego integrity versus despair.

2. **Peplau developed the nursing theory that promotes the nurse–client relationship by applying interpersonal theory to nursing practice. Key concepts include the nurse as a resource person, a counselor, a teacher, a leader, a technical expert, and a surrogate.**

3. Sullivan, not Peplau, developed interpersonal theory based on the belief that individual behavior and personality development are the direct results of interpersonal relationships. According to Sullivan, there are six stages of development: infancy, childhood, juvenile, preadolescence, early adolescence, and late adolescence.

4. Mahler, not Peplau, developed the object relations theory (birth to 36 months), which describes the separation-individuation process of the infant from the maternal figure. Using three phases, Mahler described the autistic phase, the symbiotic phase, and the

separation-individuation phase. Mahler's theory of object relations aids the nurse in assessing the client's level of individuation from primary caregivers.

TEST-TAKING HINT: The test taker must have a basic knowledge of human personality development and be able to distinguish among the various theorists who authored these theories to answer this question correctly.

7. Peplau developed the nursing theory that promotes the nurse–client relationship by applying interpersonal theory to nursing practice. Key concepts include the nurse as a resource person, a counselor, a teacher, a leader, a technical expert, and a surrogate.
   1. **The basis of Watson's theory is the belief that curing disease is the domain of medicine, whereas caring is the domain of nursing. Watson developed seven assumptions about the science of caring, which allows the nurse to deliver integrated holistic care.**
   2. The basis of Leininger's, not Watson's, theory of cultural care diversity and universality is the belief that across cultures there are health-care practices and beliefs that are diverse and similar. The nurse must understand the client's culture to provide care.
   3. Erickson, Tomlin, and Swain, not Watson, developed theories that included modeling and role modeling by the use of interpersonal and interactive skills.
   4. A variety of nursing theorists based their theories on the concept of a human energy field. These theories share a common view of the individual as an irreducible whole, comprising a physical body surrounded by an aura.

TEST-TAKING HINT: The focus of this question is the basic concepts of the theoretical models presented. The concept of the nurse–client relationship is the basis of Peplau's nursing theory model. Assumptions of caring are underlying concepts of Watson's theoretical model.

8. Neuman's systems model is based on concepts related to stress and reaction to stress. Nursing interventions are classified as primary prevention (occurs before stressors invade the normal line of defense), secondary prevention (occurs after the system has reacted to the invasion of a stressor), and tertiary prevention (occurs after secondary prevention and focuses on rehabilitation).
   1. Orem, not Roy, developed a general self-care deficit theory of nursing composed of three interrelated concepts: self-care,

self-care deficit, and nursing systems. Nursing interventions described in this theory consist of activities needed to meet self-care demands and solve self-care deficits.
   2. Rizzo Parse, not Roy, developed the theory of human becoming from existential theory. Parse believes that people create reality for themselves through the choices they make at many levels, and nurses intervene by assisting the client to examine and understand the meaning of life experiences.
   3. **Roy developed the Roy adaptation model, which consists of four essential elements: humans as adaptive systems, environment, health, and the goal of nursing. Roy describes nursing actions as interventions that seek to alter or manage stimuli so that adaptive responses can occur.**
   4. Rogers, not Roy, believed that the science of nursing is the "science of unitary human beings." Rogers believed humans are in constant interaction with the environment and described interactions *with* versus *for* the client to achieve maximum potential.

TEST-TAKING HINT: The test taker must note that the focus of this question relates to the nursing interventions that are included in the theoretical models presented. Primary, secondary, or tertiary prevention is Neuman's language to describe nursing interventions. Interventions that seek to alter or manage stimuli so that adaptive responses can occur are Roy's language to describe nursing interventions.

9. 1. Developing satisfactory relationships, maturity, and relative freedom from anxiety is a goal of interpersonal theory subscribed to by Sullivan and Peplau, not Beck and Ellis.
   2. **Substituting rational beliefs for irrational beliefs and eliminating self-defeating behaviors are goals of cognitive-behavioral theory subscribed to by Beck and Ellis.**
   3. Facing reality and developing standards for behaving responsibly are goals of reality theory subscribed to by Glasser, not Beck and Ellis.
   4. Reducing bodily tensions and managing stress by biofeedback and relaxation training are goals of stress theory subscribed to by Selye and Lazarus, not Beck and Ellis.

TEST-TAKING HINT: To answer this question correctly, the test taker must note that the focus of this question is on the goals that are established in the theoretical model presented.

10. 1. Behavioral, not reality, therapy includes advocating for relaxation training as an intervention to deal with stressors.
2. Intrapersonal, not reality, therapy includes understanding how situations during developmental stages affect current emotions.
3. Interpersonal, not reality, therapy deals with faulty patterns of relating to others and encourages interactions with others to develop the self-system.
4. Reality therapy, based on cognitive theory, is a type of therapy in which the client is taught to control thought distortions that are considered to be a factor in the development and maintenance of emotional disorders. The response described focuses the client on the reality of the impact that behaviors have on the consequences of actions.

TEST-TAKING HINT: Sometimes it is helpful for the test taker to determine which theoretical model each answer represents. Note the theory next to the dialogue presented and choose the answer that reflects reality theory.

11. 1. During Piaget's stage one of cognitive development (birth to 2 years), object permanence is developed. With this ability, the infant/toddler comes to recognize that an object will continue to exist when it is no longer visible. The 4-year-old presented in the question has moved beyond this cognitive stage of development.
2. During Piaget's stage three of cognitive development (6 to 12 years), reversibility and spatiality are developed. With this ability, the child recognizes that changes in the shape of objects do not necessarily change the amount, weight, volume, or ability of the object to return to its original form. The 4-year-old presented in the question has not reached this cognitive stage of development.
3. According to Piaget, egocentrism occurs during the stage of preoperational thought (2 to 6 years). Personal experiences are thought to be universal, and the child is unable to accept the differing viewpoints of others.
4. Formal operations (12 to 15 years) is the fourth stage of Piaget's theory of cognitive development. At this stage, the individual is able to think and reason in abstract terms. The 4-year-old presented in the question has not reached this cognitive stage of development.

TEST-TAKING HINT: Developmental theories are based on chronological age. In the question, the test taker must note the client's age to be able to choose the correct answer.

12. 1. Interpersonal theories assume that development occurs in stages related to experiencing different types of relationships.
2. Cognitive-behavioral theories assume that individuals have the potential for rational and irrational thinking, which alters behaviors.
3. Erikson's developmental theory assumes that intrapersonal growth involves resolution of critical tasks throughout eight stages of the life cycle. Erikson's theory is classified as an intrapersonal theory.
4. Psychoanalytic theories assume that individuals are motivated by unconscious desires and conflicts.

TEST-TAKING HINT: The test taker first must determine which theory is being addressed in the question. When a determination has been made that the statement reflects Erikson's theory, the test taker must recognize that this theory is classified as intrapersonal in nature. Erikson described the eight stages of man as a further development of Freud's intrapersonal theory.

13. 1. Stagnation is the negative outcome of Erikson's adulthood stage of development, generativity versus stagnation. Adulthood's stage ranges from 30 to 65 years of age. The major developmental task for the adulthood stage is to achieve the life goals established for oneself while considering the welfare of future generations. The client described does not fall within the age range of the adulthood stage.
2. Despair is the negative outcome of Erikson's old age stage of development, ego integrity versus despair. This stage ranges from age 65 years until death. The major developmental task for this stage is to review one's life and derive meaning from positive and negative events. Through this process, one needs to achieve a positive sense of self-worth. The client described does not fall within the age range of the old age stage.
3. Isolation is the negative outcome of Erikson's young adulthood stage of development, intimacy versus isolation. This stage ranges from 20 to 30 years of age. The major developmental task for young adulthood is to form an intense, lasting relationship or a commitment

to another person, cause, institution, or creative effort. The 25-year-old client falls within the age range for young adulthood and is exhibiting behaviors associated with isolation.

4. Role confusion is the negative outcome of Erikson's adolescence stage of development, identity versus role confusion. This stage ranges from 12 to 20 years of age. The major developmental task for this stage is to integrate the tasks mastered in the previous stages into a secure sense of self. The client described does not fall within the age range of adolescence.

TEST-TAKING HINT: To answer this question correctly, the test taker must understand that Erikson described the eight stages of the life cycle during which individuals struggle with developmental challenges. Being able to recognize these developmental conflicts assists the test taker in recognizing isolation as a negative outcome. The test taker must always remember that Erikson developed his psychosocial theory to be based on chronological age, which is significant information needed to answer this question correctly.

14. 1. Autonomy is the positive outcome of Erikson's early childhood stage of development: autonomy versus shame and doubt. This stage ranges from 18 months through 3 years of age. The major developmental task for early childhood is to gain some self-control and independence within the environment. The client described does not fall within the age range of early childhood.

2. Identity is the positive outcome of Erikson's adolescence stage of development: identity versus role confusion. This stage ranges from 12 to 20 years of age. The major developmental task for adolescence is to develop a sense of confidence, emotional stability, and a view of oneself as a unique individual. The client described does not fall within the age range of adolescence.

3. Industry is the positive outcome of Erikson's school age stage of development: industry versus inferiority. This stage ranges from 6 to 12 years of age. The major developmental task for school age is to achieve a sense of self-confidence by learning, competing, performing successfully, and receiving recognition from significant others, peers, and acquaintances.

The 7-year-old described falls within the age range of school age and is exhibiting behaviors reflective of a positive outcome of industry.

4. Initiative is the positive outcome of Erikson's late childhood stage of development: initiative versus guilt. This stage ranges from 3 to 6 years of age. The major developmental task for late childhood is to develop a sense of purpose and the ability to initiate and direct one's own activities. The client described does not fall within the age range of late childhood.

TEST-TAKING HINT: When assessing for industry, the test taker must look for the development of social, physical, and school skills that generate competence and pride in achievements. The age of the client presented in the question should alert the test taker to the developmental task conflict experienced.

15. 1. A 60-year-old would be in Erikson's developmental stage of adulthood (30 to 65 years old), not old age (65 years old to death). The developmental task conflict of this stage is generativity versus stagnation. The example given presents someone exhibiting behaviors reflective of stagnation, the negative outcome of this stage.

2. A 50-year-old would be in Erikson's developmental stage of adulthood (30 to 65 years old), not old age (65 years old to death). The developmental task conflict of this stage is generativity versus stagnation. The example is of someone exhibiting behaviors reflective of stagnation, the negative outcome of this stage.

3. A 65-year-old would be in Erikson's developmental stage of old age (65 years old to death). The developmental task conflict of this stage is ego integrity versus despair. The example reflects someone who is exhibiting the desire to discuss all aspects of life events and is experiencing the positive, not negative, outcome of ego integrity.

4. A 70-year-old would be in Erikson's developmental stage of old age (65 years old to death). The developmental task conflict of this stage is ego integrity versus despair. The major developmental task in old age is for an individual to review one's life and derive meaning from positive and negative events. The 70-year-old woman presented is exhibiting behaviors reflecting the negative outcome of despair.

TEST-TAKING HINT: When assessing for despair, the test taker must look for feelings of worthlessness and helplessness. Anger, depression, and loneliness are evident. The age of the client presented in the question should alert the test taker to the developmental task conflict experienced.

16. 1. Erikson's developmental stage for a 14-year-old is adolescence: identity versus role confusion. The major developmental task for this stage is to develop a sense of confidence, emotional stability, and a view of oneself as a unique individual. The situation presented is not reflective of the school-age stage of development.
    2. Erikson's developmental stage for a 5-year-old is late childhood: initiative versus guilt. The major developmental task for this stage is to develop a sense of purpose and the ability to initiate and direct one's own activities. The situation presented is not reflective of the school-age stage of development.
    3. Erikson's developmental stage for a 3-year-old is early childhood: autonomy versus shame and doubt. The major developmental task for this stage is to gain some self-control and independence within the environment. The situation presented is not reflective of the school-age stage of development.
    4. **Erikson's developmental stage for an 11-year-old is school age: industry versus inferiority. The major developmental task for this stage is to achieve a sense of self-confidence by learning, competing, performing successfully, and receiving recognition from significant others, peers, and acquaintances. The 11-year-old presented is exhibiting behaviors reflecting a positive outcome of industry.**

TEST-TAKING HINT: Achievement of the task of industry results in a sense of satisfaction and pleasure in interaction and involvement with others. The age of the client presented in the question should alert the test taker to the developmental-task conflict experienced.

17. 1. **Erikson based his psychosocial theory on an individual's chronological age. Although individuals may have some unresolved issues from previous stages, the individual is assessed in a stage based on chronological age.**
    2. Individuals may have unresolved issues from past stages that affect their developmental age; however, they are assessed in Erikson's psychosocial stages based initially on their chronological age.
    3. A time frame of successful completion of any developmental stage is not needed to assess an individual's stage of development. Because progression through any stage is individualized, a time frame would not help assess an individual's stage of development. Erikson placed developmental task conflicts at chronological ages at which successful accomplishment would be anticipated. Failure at a previous stage does not preclude, but may impair, progression to successful future task completion.
    4. Although it is crucial for the nurse to implement interventions to assist clients in meeting their developmental tasks, the question asks for assessment versus implementation data.

TEST-TAKING HINT: Note the word *initial* in the question. When assessing a client's developmental stage, chronological age is used to decide which developmental task a client should be accomplishing. After this developmental assessment, the nurse would look at any deficits that may have occurred in previous stages.

18. 1. **Discussing order in one's life and freedom from fear relates to Maslow's need hierarchy of safety and security, which is the second most basic need after the client has met physiological needs.**
    2. Looking for someone to share experiences relates to Maslow's need hierarchy of love and belonging, which occurs after the client has met safety and security and physiological needs.
    3. When someone begins to realize their full potential, they are in Maslow's need hierarchy of self-actualization. This need occurs last, after the client has met physiological, safety and security, love and belonging, and self-esteem/esteem-of-others needs.
    4. Someone discussing the need for assertiveness skills is an example of Maslow's need hierarchy of self-esteem/esteem-of-others needs. These needs occur after the client has met physiological, safety and security, and love and belonging needs.
    5. **Seeking shelter relates to Maslow's need hierarchy of safety and security, which is the second most basic need after the client has met physiological needs.**

TEST-TAKING HINT: To answer this question correctly, the test taker must understand the principles of Maslow's theory to prioritize client needs. According to Maslow, the order of an individual's needs is prioritized from most basic to highest attainment. The hierarchy begins with physiological needs and moves toward safety and security, love and belonging, self-esteem/esteem-of-others, and finally self-actualization.

19. 1. Discussing the need for avoiding harm and maintaining comfort relates to Maslow's need hierarchy of safety and security, which occurs on a lower level than self-actualization. Being highly evolved and mature indicates reaching Maslow's highest level of development, self-actualization.
    2. Stating the need for giving and receiving support from others relates to Maslow's need hierarchy of love and belonging, which occurs on a lower level than self-actualization. Being highly evolved and mature indicates reaching Maslow's highest level of development, self-actualization.
    3. **When someone begins to realize their full potential, they have reached Maslow's highest level of development, self-actualization. This occurs last, after the client has met physiological, safety and security, love and belonging, and self-esteem/esteem-of-others needs. It is an indication of a highly evolved and mature client.**
    4. Someone discussing the need for achieving success and recognition in work is an example of Maslow's need hierarchy of self-esteem/esteem-of-others, which occurs on a lower level than self-actualization. Being highly evolved and mature indicates reaching Maslow's highest level of development, self-actualization.

TEST-TAKING HINT: Understanding of Maslow's hierarchy of needs assists the test taker in prioritizing client needs, moving from stabilizing physiological needs toward self-actualization.

20. 1. Being disturbed about not being able to see family members relates to Maslow's need hierarchy of love and belonging needs, which occur after the client has met safety and security and physiological needs.
    2. **Maintaining a safe environment is a priority intervention because, according to Maslow, safety and security needs must be met before any other needs, with the exception of physiological ones. When a**

client exhibits hostile and angry behaviors toward another client, interventions must be focused on safety.
    3. Expressing that "no one cares" relates to Maslow's hierarchy of love and belonging needs, which occur after the client has met safety and security, and physiological needs.
    4. Concern about not meeting life goals relates to Maslow's need hierarchy of self-actualization. This occurs last, after the client has met physiological, safety and security, love and belonging, and self-esteem/esteem-of-others needs.

TEST-TAKING HINT: A practical approach in remembering the prioritization of Maslow's hierarchy of needs is to memorize and list the order as a reference to use when answering related test questions.

21. In order of attainment: 4, 3, 1, 2, 5.
    1. Sleeping is one of many basic physiological needs, which should be attained first under Maslow's hierarchy of needs.
    2. Smoke alarms are an assistive device to maintain safety and security, which should be attained second under Maslow's hierarchy of needs.
    3. An intimate relationship shows attainment of love and belonging, which should be attained third under Maslow's hierarchy of needs.
    4. To assert oneself is a behavior that exemplifies self-esteem, which should be attained fourth under Maslow's hierarchy of needs.
    5. A sense of self-fulfillment and accomplishment is an example of self-actualization, which should be attained fifth under Maslow's hierarchy of needs.

TEST-TAKING HINT: On a paper-and-pencil test or on the paper provided during the National Council Licensure Examination (NCLEX®), it might be helpful, when examples are given, to note the need that is reflected in the example. This should assist the test taker in distinguishing the correct order of need assessment.

22. 1. During Sullivan's childhood stage, an individual learns to experience a delay in personal gratification without undue anxiety. The information presented in the question does not reflect this stage.
    2. During Sullivan's juvenile stage, an individual learns to form satisfactory peer relationships. The information presented in the question does not reflect this stage.

3. During Sullivan's preadolescence stage, an individual learns to form satisfactory relationships with persons of the same sex, initiating feelings of affection for another person. The information presented in the question does not reflect this stage.

4. During Sullivan's early adolescence stage, an individual develops a sense of identity and learns to form relationships with persons of the opposite sex. The information presented in the question correctly reflects this stage.

TEST-TAKING HINT: To answer this question correctly, the test taker must review the descriptions of Sullivan's stages of personality development. Noting the opposite sex relationship development should lead you to choose an older age stage.

23. 1. The behavioral example of "I'll return the purse I found. It's never right to steal" is correctly matched with the superego structure of the personality as described by Freud. The superego internalizes the values and morals set forth by primary caregivers.

2. "Coming on to my friend's boyfriend is just plain wrong" is a behavioral example of the superego, not the ego structure of the personality as described by Freud. The ego experiences the reality of the external world, adapts to it, and responds to it. The superego internalizes the values and morals set forth by primary caregivers.

3. "I might get pregnant if I have sex, so I won't do it" is a behavioral example of the ego, not the id structure of the personality as described by Freud. The ego experiences the reality of the external world, adapts to it, and responds to it. The id reflects instinctual drives that seek to satisfy needs and achieve immediate gratification.

4. The behavioral example of "I need that car. No one will miss it" is correctly matched with the id structure of the personality as described by Freud. The id reflects instinctual drives that seek to satisfy needs and achieve immediate gratification.

5. The behavioral example of "Cheating on a test could get me expelled, so I won't do it" is correctly matched with the ego structure of the personality as described by Freud. The ego experiences the reality of the external world, adapts to it, and responds to it.

TEST-TAKING HINT: To answer this question correctly, the test taker must review Freud's organization of personality structure.

24. 1. Demonstrating an ability to discuss objectively all points of view and possessing a strong sense of ethics relates to Maslow's need hierarchy of self-actualization, the fifth and highest level of attainment. This occurs after the client has met physiological, safety and security, love and belonging, and self-esteem/esteem-of-others needs.

2. Avoiding harm while maintaining comfort, order, and physical safety relates to Maslow's need hierarchy of safety and security, which is the lowest level of attainment after the client has met physiological needs.

3. Establishing meaningful interpersonal relationships and identifying oneself within a group relate to Maslow's need hierarchy of love and belonging, the third level of attainment. This occurs after the client has met physiological and safety and security needs.

4. Desiring prestige from personal accomplishments relates to Maslow's need hierarchy of self-esteem/esteem-of-others, the fourth level of attainment. This occurs after the client has met physiological, safety and security, and love and belonging needs.

TEST-TAKING HINT: To answer this question correctly, the test taker must recall the hierarchy of needs as described by Maslow.

Biological Implications

25. 1. Sedatives and amphetamines were the only medications available before 1950, and they were used sparingly because of their toxicity and addictive properties.

2. Phenothiazines were not used for pain management but were used initially to prepare clients for anxiety related to postoperative recovery.

3. Phenothiazines, not atypical antipsychotics, were the first medications that attempted to assist clients with positive symptoms of schizophrenia spectrum disorders.

4. Although psychotropic medications assist with symptoms of mental illness, currently there is no cure.

5. Newly developed atypical psychotropics have shown much promise in controlling the negative symptoms of schizophrenia. Historically, these

negative symptoms tend to be resistant to responding to psychotropic medications.

TEST-TAKING HINT: To answer this question correctly, the test taker must review the history of psychiatry and its impact on client care. Phenothiazine is a chemical classification that includes many typical antipsychotic medications, such as chlorpromazine (Thorazine), perphenazine (Trilafon), and thioridazine (Mellaril). By understanding that these medications are not used for pain, the test taker can eliminate answer 2.

26. Neurotransmitters are released from the presynaptic neuron and are considered the first messengers. They then connect to the postsynaptic neuron to provide a message.
    1. The message sent through a neurotransmitter plays a role in human emotions and behaviors.
    2. Because neurotransmitters send messages specific to emotions and behaviors, they have been found to be useful targets of psychotropic medications.
    3. Neurotransmitters are not limited to psychiatric disease processes alone and are useful in the study and treatment of many disease processes.
    4. Neurons are nerve cells that generate and transmit the body's electrochemical impulses. Neurotransmitters assist the neurons in transmitting their message from one neuron to the next.
    5. There are many different groups of neurotransmitters, such as cholinergics, monoamines, amino acids, and neuropeptides. Those listed in this answer choice are all monoamines, not cholinergics.

TEST-TAKING HINT: The test taker needs to understand the role of a neurotransmitter in psychopharmacology to answer this question correctly. A review of the different chemical classifications of neurotransmitters would assist with this understanding.

27. 1. The parietal lobes, not the limbic system, control perceptions and interpretation of most sensory information.
    2. The temporal lobes, not the limbic system, control auditory functions and short-term memory.
    3. The limbic system, which has some connection with the frontal lobe, plays a role in emotional experiences, as evidenced by changes in mood and character after damage to this area. These

alterations include, but are not limited to, fear, rage, aggressiveness, apathy, irritability, and euphoria.
    4. The occipital lobes, not the limbic system, control visual reception and interpretation.

TEST-TAKING HINT: Understanding regulatory functions of different areas of the brain assists the test taker in answering this question correctly.

28. 1. The dopamine hypothesis suggests that an excess of the neurochemical dopamine in the brain causes schizophrenia spectrum disorders. An alteration in neurochemicals is an example of a biological theory.
    2. There are studies to suggest that exposure to a viral infection is most significant if it occurs during the second trimester of pregnancy. Further research is required to better understand this biological theory, called *psychoimmunology*.
    3. Although changes in the ventricular and sulci areas of the brain fall under a biological theory of etiology, enlargement, not atrophy, is found in clients diagnosed with schizophrenia spectrum disorders.
    4. The downward drift hypothesis holds that individuals diagnosed with schizophrenia spectrum disorders are more likely to live in low socioeconomic areas and tend to be socially isolated. This is an example of sociocultural, not biological, theory.
    5. It has been found that individuals diagnosed with schizophrenia spectrum disorders have increased levels of serotonin.

TEST-TAKING HINT: The test taker must recognize that the question is asking for biological theory; the downward drift hypothesis (answer 4) can be eliminated immediately because it is a sociocultural theory.

29. The client is exhibiting auditory hallucinations and delusions, which are positive symptoms of schizophrenia.
    1. A decrease in dopamine in the mesocortical dopamine pathway may be one of the potential causes of negative, not positive, symptoms of schizophrenia, such as affective flattening, alogia, avolition, anhedonia, and social isolation. There also is debate about whether antipsychotic medications are a causative factor in the worsening of negative symptoms of schizophrenia because they decrease the amount of dopamine in the mesocortical dopamine pathway.

2. An increase in dopamine in the meso-limbic dopamine pathway is thought to have an important role in emotional behaviors, especially auditory hallucinations, delusions, and altered thoughts. Medications prescribed for these symptoms decrease the amount of dopamine in the mesolimbic pathway and decrease positive symptoms.

3. An increase in dopamine in the nigrostriatal dopamine pathway is thought to be the underlying cause of movement disorders, such as hyperkinetic movement, dyskinesias, and tics, and not the cause of the positive symptoms described in the question. A decrease, not increase, in dopamine in this pathway causes movement disorders, such as Parkinson's disease. When clients are prescribed antipsychotic medications, which decrease dopamine in this pathway, pseudoparkinsonian symptoms, such as tremor, shuffling gait, drooling, and rigidity, can occur.

4. A decrease in dopamine in the tuberoinfundibular dopamine pathway results in inhibition of prolactin release, a side effect of antipsychotic medications and not the cause of the positive symptoms described in the question. In the postpartum state, neuronal activity is decreased, and prolactin levels can increase for breastfeeding. Antipsychotic medications decrease the dopamine level in all dopamine pathways, and a side effect of the decrease in the tuberoinfundibular dopamine pathway could be galactorrhea (breast secretions, which can occur in men and women), amenorrhea, and potentially some sexual dysfunction.

TEST-TAKING HINT: The test taker must recognize the symptoms presented in the question as positive symptoms of schizophrenia. To answer this question correctly, the test taker must be familiar with brain chemistry and its effects on the symptoms of schizophrenia.

30. 1. When a client diagnosed with bipolar affective disorder (BPAD) is prescribed a selective serotonin reuptake inhibitor, there is potential for alterations in neurochemicals that could generate a manic episode. Alterations in neurochemicals support biological theory in the development of BPAD.

2. Multiple jobs and the ability to multitask are not related to being diagnosed with BPAD. It has been found that an increased number of individuals diagnosed with BPAD come from upper socioeconomic backgrounds; however, the specific reason behind this is unknown. There are thoughts that the higher incidence may be because of increased education, creativity, and type A personality. This would be an example of a psychosocial, not biological, theory.

3. A negative self-image would relate to a cognitive, not biological, theory, and at this time there are no specific data to support cognitive theory in the development of BPAD.

4. Being raised in a chaotic family with poor impulse control would relate to psychosocial, not biological, theory, and at this time no specific data support this.

TEST-TAKING HINT: The test taker must note the keywords *biological theory* to answer this question correctly. Information about other theories may be correct but would not support a biological theory perspective.

31. Aside from those noted here, other medications can cause confusion, depression, and increased anxiety, such as propoxyphene.
1. **Meperidine can cause confusion, depression, mania, nightmares, and increased anxiety.**
2. Dextromethorphan can cause confusion, delusions, hallucinations, or paranoia, but not anxiety.
3. Loratadine can cause confusion, delusions, hallucinations, or paranoia, but not anxiety.
4. **Levodopa can cause confusion, depression, mania, nightmares, psychosis, or anxiety.**
5. Pseudoephedrine can cause confusion, delusions, hallucinations, paranoia, and psychosis, but not anxiety.

TEST-TAKING HINT: Certain medications, including over-the-counter drugs, can cause symptoms associated with mental illness. The test taker must review these medications and their specific side effects. The test taker must also choose the answer that addresses all, not part, of the symptoms presented in the question.

32. When psychiatric medications are affecting a client in ways that are unexpected or ineffective, a test to analyze the client's genetic makeup may assist the physician to pinpoint better medications, adjust dosages, or even

recognize the need for complementary medications.

1. **This test will analyze the client's genetic makeup in order to determine which medications may or may not cause significant side effects.**

2. **Genetic testing will pinpoint the *MTHFR* gene and determine whether the client's genetic makeup affects the client's ability to convert folic acid into its active form of L-methylfolate. This conversion is integral to the production of the neurotransmitters dopamine, serotonin, and norepinephrine, which impact mental health disorders.**

3. Collecting a DNA sample requires swabbing of the client's cheek, not drawing blood. Fasting is not a prerequisite for this procedure.

4. Genetic testing can help clients experiencing depression, anxiety, and attention deficit-hyperactivity disorder, as well as acute/chronic pain and folate deficiencies. The word *exclusively* in the answer choice makes this answer incorrect.

5. Based on the client's genetic makeup, this test can analyze a medication's effectiveness, absorption and excretion rates, and side-effect potential. This test cannot determine what medication the physician should prescribe for any specific symptom.

TEST-TAKING HINT: Review psychiatric genetic testing and its role in prescribing mental health medications for better and more accurate medication assimilation.

Diagnostic and Statistical Manual of Mental Disorders, Fifth Edition, Text Revision (*DSM-5-TR*)

33. The *Diagnostic and Statistical Manual of Mental Disorders*, Fifth Edition, Text Revision (*DSM-5-TR*) is published by the American Psychiatric Association and provides a common language and standard criteria for the classification of mental disorders.

   1. **The *DSM-5-TR* lists all psychiatric and general medical diagnoses.**

   2. **The *DSM-5-TR* allows clinicians to rate disorders along a continuum of severity.**

   3. **Conditions that do not meet *DSM-5-TR* criteria are termed *not elsewhere defined* (NED).**

   4. **Dimensional assessment tools are included in the *DSM-5-TR*.**

5. Global Assessment of Functioning (GAF) was included in the *DSM-IV*'s multi-axial system. This system is no longer included in the *DSM-5-TR*. Dimensional assessment tools included in the *DSM-5* help to assess a client's functional level.

TEST-TAKING HINT: To answer this question correctly, the test taker must review the components of the *DSM-5-TR*.

34. 1. **The *DSM-5-TR* is a convenient format for organizing and communicating clinical data. It includes a list of psychiatric and medical conditions and facilitates a comprehensive and systematic evaluation.**

   2. **The *DSM-5-TR* is a means for considering the complexity of clinical situations. It addresses behavioral and physical symptoms, long-term problems, stressors, and functioning.**

   3. The *DSM-5-TR* describes the commonalities versus uniqueness of individuals presenting with the same diagnosis.

   4. The *DSM-5-TR* is a format for evaluating clients based on common symptoms of psychiatric disorders, not a regulated approach to the diagnosis of mental illness.

   5. The *DSM-5-TR* is not used to better understand the etiology of different psychiatric disorders because it does not address etiology.

TEST-TAKING HINT: To answer this question correctly, the test taker must understand that the *DSM-5-TR* helps the mental health provider appropriately evaluate clients.

35. 1. **The *DSM-5-TR* provides a common language that facilitates a comprehensive and systematic client evaluation.**

   2. The *DSM-5-TR* does not list medications that are appropriate for the treatment of clients diagnosed with mental illness.

   3. **The *DSM-5-TR* presents standard criteria for the classification of mental disorders. These criteria facilitate consistency of care.**

   4. The previous edition of the *DSM* was structured as a five-axis system. The *DSM-5-TR* does not incorporate a multi-axis system.

   5. The *DSM-5-TR* is not used to provide community resources. It is a reference book used in the diagnosis and treatment of mental disorders.

TEST-TAKING HINT: To answer this question correctly, the test taker must review the purpose of the *DSM-5-TR*.

Psychiatric Nursing

3

KEYWORDS

The following words include English vocabulary, nursing/medical terminology, concepts, principles, or information relevant to content specifically addressed in this chapter or associated with topics presented in it. English dictionaries, your nursing textbooks, and medical dictionaries such as *Taber's Cyclopedic Medical Dictionary* are resources that can be used to expand your knowledge and understanding of these words and related information.

Acceptance

Advocate

Analogy

Beck Depression Inventory

Biases

CAGE Assessment

Cheeking

Clinical Institute Withdrawal Assessment (CIWA)

Clock face assessment

Collaborate

Comorbid

Confidentiality

Congruency

Contract

Counselor

Countertransference

Deinstitutionalization

Diagnostic and Statistical Manual of Mental Disorders, Fifth Edition, Text Revision (*DSM-5-TR*)

Dysfunctional

Empathy

Genuineness

Geriatric Depression Rating Scale (GDS)

Goal

Insight

Intelligence quotient (IQ)

Intervention

Medication manager

Milieu manager

Nurse–client relationship

Nursing diagnosis

Nursing process

Objective data

Occupational therapist

Orientation (introductory) phase

Pre-interaction phase

Primary prevention

Priority

Professionalism

Rapport

Resistant behavior

Resource person

Respect

Role player

Scope of practice

Secondary prevention

Self-assessment

Self-perception

Short Michigan Alcohol Screening Test (SMAST)

Stereotype belief

Subjective data

Surrogate

Sympathy

Teacher

Termination phase

Tertiary prevention

Transference

Working phase

QUESTIONS

Mental Health Nursing

1. Which qualifications are appropriate to the scope of practice of the psychiatric/mental health registered nurse generalist?
   1. The nurse generalist is qualified by meeting a minimum of a master's degree in nursing.
   2. The nurse generalist is qualified to order client medications based on tests and laboratory values.
   3. The nurse generalist is qualified to implement crisis intervention.
   4. The nurse generalist is qualified to assess, designate, and document a client's medical diagnosis.

2. Which is the overall priority goal of inpatient psychiatric treatment?
   1. Maintenance of stability in the community.
   2. Medication adherence.
   3. Stabilization and return to the community.
   4. Better communication skills.

3. When the nurse creates an environment to facilitate healing, the nurse's actions are based on which of the following assumptions? **Select all that apply.**
   1. A therapeutic relationship can be a healing experience.
   2. A healthy relationship cannot be transferred to other relationships.
   3. Group settings can support ego strengths.
   4. Treatment plans can be formulated by observing social behaviors.
   5. Countertransference eases the establishment of the nurse–client relationship.

4. Which of the following was the reason for the establishment of large hospitals or asylums that addressed the care of persons with mental illness? **Select all that apply.**
   1. Mental illness was perceived as incurable.
   2. Clients with mental illness were perceived as a threat to self and others.
   3. Dorothea Dix saw a need for humane care for clients with mental illness.
   4. Federal funding initially was available.
   5. They were mandated by the National Institute of Mental Health.

5. Which of the following are examples of primary prevention in a community mental health setting? **Select all that apply.**
   1. Providing ongoing assessment of individuals at high risk for illness exacerbation.
   2. Teaching physical and psychosocial effects of stress to elementary school students.
   3. Referring for treatment those individuals in whom illness symptoms have been assessed.
   4. Monitoring effectiveness of aftercare services.
   5. Teaching a class on child-rearing skills for a group of new parents.

6. Which nursing intervention within the community is aimed at reducing the residual defects that are associated with severe or chronic mental illness?
   1. Referring clients for various aftercare services such as day treatment programs.
   2. Providing care for individuals in whom mental illness symptoms have been assessed.
   3. Providing education and support to women entering the workforce.
   4. Teaching concepts of mental health to various groups within the community.

7. In the emergency department, the nurse assesses a client who is aggressive and experiencing auditory hallucinations. The client states, "The CIA is plotting to kill me." To which mental health setting would the nurse expect this client to be admitted?
   1. Long-term, inpatient facility.
   2. Day treatment.
   3. Short-term, inpatient, locked unit.
   4. Psychiatric case management.

8. Which action of a mental health nurse case manager reflects the activity of service planning?
   1. Identifying a client who is missing appointments and seeking other community resources to ensure correct treatment.
   2. Calling a client when the client misses an appointment to determine the cause of the absence.
   3. Making an appointment for a client with a nutritionist for dietary counseling.
   4. Holding a care conference for a client who is having difficulty returning to school.

Role of the Nurse

9. A client with a long history of alcohol use disorder has been diagnosed with Wernicke-Korsakoff syndrome. With which member of the mental-health-care team would the nurse collaborate to meet this client's described need?
   1. The psychiatrist to obtain an order for neurocognitive disorder medications.
   2. The psychologist to set up counseling sessions to explore stressors.
   3. The dietitian to help the client increase consumption of thiamine-rich foods.
   4. The social worker to plan transportation to Alcoholics Anonymous.

10. A client on an inpatient psychiatric unit has a nursing diagnosis of nonadherence R/T antipsychotic medications. In which role is the nurse functioning when checking for cheeking?
   1. Advocate.
   2. Educator.
   3. Medication manager.
   4. Counselor.

11. On an inpatient psychiatric unit, which of the following actions exemplify the nurse's role of teacher? **Select all that apply.**
   1. The nurse assesses potentially stressful characteristics of the environment and develops strategies to eliminate or decrease stressors.
   2. The nurse orients new clients to the unit and helps them to fit comfortably into the environment.
   3. The nurse presents information to help the client and family members to understand the effects of mental illness.
   4. The nurse is the guardian of the therapeutic environment.
   5. The nurse holds a group to discuss medication side effects.

12. Which of the following actions reflect the nurse's role of advocate in an inpatient psychiatric setting? **Select all that apply.**
   1. The nurse speaks on behalf of a mentally ill client to ensure adequate access to needed mental health services.
   2. The nurse focuses on improving the mentally ill client's and family members' self-care knowledge and skills.
   3. The nurse explains unit rules and ensures that new clients fit comfortably into the therapeutic environment.
   4. The nurse continually monitors the client in the milieu for side effects of a new psychotropic medication.
   5. The nurse talks with the treatment team to support a shy client's request for less-sedating medications.

13. A resource person's function is to give specific answers to specific questions, as a counselor's function is to:
   1. Identify learning needs and provide information required by the client.
   2. Encourage the client to be an active participant in designing a nursing plan of care.
   3. Serve as a substitute figure for another person.
   4. Listen as a client reviews feelings related to difficulties experienced in life.

14. On an inpatient psychiatric unit, a client diagnosed with borderline personality disorder is challenging other clients and splitting staff. Which response by the nurse reflects the nurse's role of milieu manager?
    1. Setting strict limits and communicating these limits to all staff members.
    2. Using role-play to demonstrate ways of dealing with frustration.
    3. Seeking orders from the physician to force medications.
    4. Holding a group session on relationship skills.

15. On an inpatient psychiatric unit, a client who is anxious and distressed states, "God has abandoned me." Which nursing action would initiate collaboration with the member of the mental-health-care team who can assist this client with this assessed problem?
    1. Notify the psychiatrist to get an order for an antianxiety medication prn.
    2. Consult the social worker to provide community resources.
    3. Notify the psychologist that testing is necessary.
    4. Consult with the chaplain and describe the client's concerns.

16. A client on an inpatient psychiatric unit exhibits traits of borderline personality disorder. Which action by the nurse would initiate collaboration with the member of the mental-health-care team who can best confirm this diagnosis?
    1. Request an order from the psychiatrist for personality disorder medication.
    2. Collaborate with the occupational therapist to meet this client's retraining needs.
    3. Collaborate with the clinical psychologist to prepare the client for personality testing.
    4. Meet with the recreational therapist to plan activities to relieve the client's anxiety.

17. A client with a long history of alcohol use disorder comes to the outpatient clinic after losing a job and driver's license because of a driving under the influence infraction. With which member of the mental-health-care team would the nurse collaborate to meet this client's described need?
    1. The psychiatrist to obtain an order for an antianxiety medication.
    2. The psychologist to set up counseling sessions to explore stressors.
    3. The occupational therapist for retraining and job placement.
    4. The social worker to plan housing.

Nursing Process

18. A client states, "My spouse is unfaithful. I think I am not worth anything." Which of the following describes this assessment information? **Select all that apply.**
    1. This is subjective information or a chief complaint.
    2. This information must be validated by significant others.
    3. This objective information must be verified by individuals other than the client.
    4. This information needs objective measurement by a mood rating scale.
    5. This information indicates the use of defense mechanisms.

19. Which of the following assessment information would be evaluated as objective data? **Select all that apply.**
    1. Clinical Institute Withdrawal Assessment score of 10.
    2. Client's statements of generalized anxiety.
    3. Complaints of anorexia.
    4. Client states, "I can't keep my thoughts together."
    5. Client's mood rating of 5 on a 10-point scale.

20. The nurse is interviewing a client admitted to an inpatient psychiatric unit with a diagnosis of depressive disorder. Which is the primary goal in the assessment phase of the nursing process for this client?
    1. To build trust and rapport.
    2. To identify goals and outcomes.
    3. To collect and organize information.
    4. To identify and validate the medical diagnosis.

21. The nurse uses the clock face assessment test to obtain which assessment data?
    1. Early signs of neurocognitive disorder.
    2. Assessment rating of overall functioning.
    3. Evidence of alcohol/substance use disorders.
    4. Signs and symptoms of depression.

22. A welder who recently lost a leg in a work-related accident is being admitted to an inpatient psychiatric unit. The client states, "I'm worried because I can't support my family anymore!" Which nursing diagnosis is most reflective of this client's presenting problem?
    1. Ineffective coping R/T poor self-esteem.
    2. Ineffective role performance R/T loss of job.
    3. Impaired social interaction R/T altered body image.
    4. Knowledge deficit R/T wound and skin care.

23. An 85-year-old client has become agitated and physically aggressive after having a stroke resulting in right-sided weakness. The client is started on risperidone PO 0.5 mg qhs. Which is a priority nursing diagnosis for this client?
    1. Risk for falls R/T right-sided weakness and sedation from risperidone.
    2. Activity intolerance R/T right-sided weakness.
    3. Disturbed thought processes R/T acting-out behaviors.
    4. Anxiety R/T change in health status and dependence on others.

24. Which nursing intervention would establish trust with a client who is experiencing concrete thinking?
    1. Being consistent in adhering to unit guidelines.
    2. Calling the client by name.
    3. Sharing what the client is feeling.
    4. Teaching the meaning of any idioms used.

25. An inpatient psychiatric client recently diagnosed with bipolar disorder has been prescribed lithium carbonate. When the nurse is functioning in the role of teacher, which of the following nursing interventions are appropriate? **Select all that apply.**
    1. Teaching the neurochemical action of this medication.
    2. Teaching the benefits of taking this medication as prescribed.
    3. Teaching signs and symptoms of lithium toxicity.
    4. Teaching dietary and fluid intake considerations.
    5. Teaching reportable side effects.

26. A client diagnosed with schizophrenia is about to be discharged and is facing the stressor of acquiring independent employment. Using a behavioral approach, which nursing intervention is most appropriate in meeting this client's needs?
    1. Teaching the client to "thought block" auditory hallucinations.
    2. Role-playing a job interview with the client.
    3. Advocating with the discharge planner to provide adequate housing.
    4. Discussing the use of prn medications to decrease stress before the interview.

27. A client diagnosed with bipolar disorder has a nursing diagnosis of sleep pattern disturbance. Which intervention should the nurse implement initially?
    1. Assess normal sleep patterns.
    2. Discourage napping during the day.
    3. Discourage the use of caffeine and nicotine.
    4. Teach relaxation exercises.

28. A nurse in an inpatient setting formulates an outcome for a client who has a nursing diagnosis of altered social interaction R/T paranoid thinking AEB aggressive behaviors. Which initial, correctly written outcome would the nurse expect the client to achieve?
    1. The client will socialize with other clients in the milieu.
    2. The client will use adaptive coping strategies to control impulses.
    3. The client will list two triggers to angry outbursts by day 2 of hospitalization.
    4. The client will walk away from confrontation by discharge.

29. A client diagnosed with a personality disorder has a nursing diagnosis of impaired social interaction. Which is a correctly written, short-term outcome related to this diagnosis?
    1. The client will interact appropriately with others in social and therapeutic settings.
    2. The client will discuss with the nurse behaviors that would impede the development of satisfactory interpersonal relationships by day 2 of hospitalization.
    3. The client will display no evidence of splitting, clinging, or distancing behaviors in relationships by day three of hospitalization.
    4. The client will demonstrate the use of relaxation techniques to maintain anxiety at a manageable level.

Nurse–Client Relationship

30. A nursing student has a special feeling toward a client that is based on acceptance, warmth, and a nonjudgmental attitude. The student is experiencing which characteristic that enhances the achievement of the nurse–client relationship?
    1. Rapport.
    2. Trust.
    3. Respect.
    4. Professionalism.

31. Which is a nursing intervention that would promote the development of trust in the nurse–client relationship?
    1. Simply and clearly providing reasons for policies and procedures.
    2. Calling the client by name and title such as "Mr. Hawkins."
    3. Striving to understand the motivations behind the client's behavior.
    4. Taking the client's ideas into consideration when planning care.

32. In a psychiatric inpatient setting, the nurse observes an adolescent client's peers calling the client names. In this context, which statement by the nurse exemplifies the concept of empathy?
    1. "I can see that you are upset. Tell me how you feel."
    2. "Your peers are being insensitive. I would be upset also."
    3. "I used to be called names as a child. I know it can hurt feelings."
    4. "I get angry when people are treated cruelly."

33. Which statement by the nurse expresses respect for the client?
    1. "Mr. Hawkins, because of your aggressive behavior you cannot attend the outing."
    2. "I assure you that what we discuss will stay within the health-care team."
    3. "I became angry when that other client pushed your buttons and made you mad."
    4. "Everyone loses it sometimes. You might just have a low boiling point."

34. Which is the goal for the orientation phase of the nurse–client relationship?
    1. Explore self-perceptions.
    2. Establish trust.
    3. Promote change.
    4. Evaluate goal attainment.

35. Number the following nursing interventions as they would proceed through the phases of the nurse–client relationship.
    1. _____ Plan for continued care.
    2. _____ Promote client's insight.
    3. _____ Examine personal biases.
    4. _____ Formulate nursing diagnoses.

36. On an inpatient psychiatric unit, a client states, "I want to learn better ways to handle my anger." This interaction is most likely to occur in which phase of the nurse–client relationship?
    1. Pre-interaction phase.
    2. Orientation (introductory) phase.
    3. Working phase.
    4. Termination phase.

37. The nurse helps a client practice various techniques of assertive communication by giving positive feedback for improvement of passive-aggressive interactions. This intervention would occur in which phase of the nurse–client relationship?
    1. Pre-interaction phase.
    2. Orientation (introductory) phase.
    3. Working phase.
    4. Termination phase.

38. On an inpatient psychiatric unit, the goals of therapy have been met, but the client cries and states, "I have to keep coming back to therapy to handle my anger better." This interaction occurs in which phase of the nurse–client relationship?
    1. Pre-interaction phase.
    2. Orientation (introductory) phase.
    3. Working phase.
    4. Termination phase.

39. On an inpatient psychiatric unit, the nurse explores feelings about potentially working with a client whose spouse has abused them and their children physically and verbally. This interaction would occur in which phase of the nurse–client relationship?
    1. Pre-interaction phase.
    2. Orientation (introductory) phase.
    3. Working phase.
    4. Termination phase.

40. The nurse reviews a client's record in preparation for client care. This action is one of the tasks that occur in a phase of the nurse–client relationship. What is the purpose of this phase?
    1. Getting to know each other and establishing trust.
    2. Implementing nursing interventions to achieve outcomes.
    3. Achievement of independence and maintenance of health without nursing care.
    4. Understanding the client's diagnosis and evaluating the nurse's attitudes.

41. The nurse explores any personal misconceptions or prejudices before caring for a client. This action is one of the tasks that occur in a phase of the nurse–client relationship. What is the nurse's major task in this phase?
    1. Determining why the client sought help.
    2. Exploring self.
    3. Assisting the patient in behavioral change.
    4. Establishing and preparing the client for the reality of separation.

42. Which elements are included in the nurse–client contract?
    1. During the pre-interaction phase, the roles are established.
    2. During the orientation phase, the purpose of the interaction is established.
    3. During the working phase, the conditions for termination are established.
    4. During the termination phase, the criteria for discharge are established.

43. A nursing student is experiencing fears related to the first clinical experience in a psychiatric setting. This is most likely to occur in which phase of the nurse–client relationship?
    1. In the pre-interaction phase, because the student is likely to be suspicious of psychiatric clients.
    2. In the orientation phase, because the psychiatric client may threaten the student's role identity.
    3. In the working phase, because the student may feel emotionally vulnerable to past experiences.
    4. In the termination phase, because the student may be uncertain about their ability to make a difference.

44. Number, in a logical series, the skills that the nurse needs to interact therapeutically with clients.
    1. _____ Ability to communicate.
    2. _____ Ability to problem-solve.
    3. _____ Ability to recognize signs and symptoms.
    4. _____ Ability to self-assess.

45. The nursing student is experiencing a severe family crisis. In what way might this situation affect the student's performance in a psychiatric rotation?
    1. The student might overidentify with clients and meet the students own needs.
    2. The student might fear clients and avoid them.
    3. The student might feel inadequate and fear emotionally harming clients.
    4. The student might doubt their value in assisting clients due to lack of knowledge.

46. Which can be described as an example of an oversimplified or undifferentiated belief?
    1. Alcoholism is a disease.
    2. A 12-step program may assist with recovery from alcohol use disorder.
    3. Belief in higher power assists clients diagnosed with alcohol use disorder.
    4. All alcoholics are skid-row bums.

Transference/Countertransference

47. Which of the following behaviors exemplifies the concept of countertransference? **Select all that apply.**
    1. The nurse defends the client's inappropriate behavior to the psychiatrist.
    2. The nurse empathizes with the client's loss.
    3. The nurse subjectively appreciates the client's feelings.
    4. The nurse is uneasy when interacting with the client.
    5. The nurse recognizes that the client is emotionally attached to the social worker.

48. During a recent counseling session with a depressed client, the psychiatric nurse observes signs of transference. Which statement by the client would indicate that the nurse is correct?
    1. "Thanks for taking my side against the staff."
    2. "You sure do remind me of my mom."
    3. "Working on problem-solving together makes sense."
    4. "I won't stop drinking just to please my whole family."

49. The staff observes a new nurse expressing anger and distrust while treating a client with a long history of alcohol use disorder. The staff suspects that the nurse is experiencing countertransference. Which statement by the new nurse validates the staff's suspicions?
    1. "My parent misused alcohol and neglected the family."
    2. "The client said I had the same disposition as their cranky spouse."
    3. "Maybe the client and I can sit down and work out a plan."
    4. "The client refuses to accept responsibility for their alcohol misuse."

50. While talking about an abusive childhood, a client addicted to heroin suddenly blurts out, "I hate my doctor." Which client statement would indicate that transference is taking place?
    1. "The doctor has told me that their child recovered, and I will also."
    2. "I don't care what anyone says; I don't have a problem I can't handle."
    3. "I'd bet my doctor beat and locked their child in a closet when they were young."
    4. "I'm going to stop fighting and start working together with my doctor."

51. A client states, "They're putting rat poison in my food." Which intervention would assist this client to be medication adherent while on the inpatient psychiatric unit?
    1. Remind the client that the psychiatrist ordered the medication for them.
    2. Maintain the same routine for medication administration.
    3. Use liquid medication to avoid cheeking.
    4. Keep medications in sealed packages and open them in front of the client.

52. Which nursing intervention would assist the client who is experiencing bothersome hallucinations in adhering to prescribed medications?
    1. Using liquid or IM injection to avoid cheeking of medications.
    2. Teaching the client about potential side effects from prescribed medications.
    3. Reminding the client that the medication decreases the bothersome hallucinations.
    4. Notifying the client of the action, peak, and duration of the medication.

The correct answer number and rationale for why it is the correct answer are given in **boldface blue type**. Rationales for why the other answer options are incorrect are given as well, but they are not in boldface type.

Mental Health Nursing

1. 1. A psychiatric/mental health registered nurse generalist should be educationally prepared in nursing and licensed to practice in their state. Educational preparation can be at the associate, baccalaureate, or higher level, but a minimum of a master's degree is not required.
   2. A psychiatric/mental health registered nurse generalist cannot order medications. This is the scope of practice for the psychiatric/mental health advanced practice registered nurse.
   3. **Part of the professional responsibilities of the psychiatric/mental health registered nurse generalist is crisis intervention.**
   4. A psychiatric/mental health registered nurse generalist cannot designate a client's medical diagnosis. This is the scope of practice for the psychiatrist or the psychiatric/mental health advanced practice registered nurse.

TEST-TAKING HINT: To answer this question correctly, the test taker must be familiar with the scope of practice of various educational levels of the registered nurse and the roles and responsibilities within this scope.

2. 1. Maintenance of stability in the community is the goal of community mental health care versus inpatient psychiatric treatment.
   2. Medication adherence is important to encourage, but it is not the overall priority goal of inpatient psychiatric treatment.
   3. **Stabilization and return to the community are the overall priority goals of inpatient psychiatric treatment.**
   4. Better communication skills are important to encourage, but this is not the overall priority goal of inpatient psychiatric treatment.

TEST-TAKING HINT: Understanding the current trends in the delivery of mental health care in the community and inpatient settings assists the test taker in answering this question correctly. Note the keywords *priority* and *inpatient*, which determine the correct answer to this question.

3. 1. **A therapeutic relationship is characterized by rapport, genuineness, and respect and can be a healing experience.**
   2. **A healthy relationship can be a prototype for other healthy relationships.**
   3. **Group processes provide learning experiences and support a client's ego strengths.**
   4. **During group processes and interactions, staff members can observe social behaviors, and this can determine client needs. Treatment plans can be customized to meet these needs.**
   5. Countertransference refers to the nurse's behavioral and emotional response to the client. Unresolved feelings toward significant others from the nurse's past may be projected to the client. Countertransference is a hindrance to the establishment of the nurse–client relationship.

TEST-TAKING HINT: Reviewing the nurse's actions that assist in creating an environment that facilitates healing assists the test taker in determining the correct answer to this question. Understanding the meaning of countertransference eliminates answer 5.

4. 1. **Because there was no treatment for mental illness before 1840, it was perceived as incurable, and there was a need to provide continuous supervision in hospitals or asylums.**
   2. **Clients with mental illness were thought to be violent toward themselves and others, and what was at the time considered a reasonable solution to care was to remove them from contact with the general population and observe them continuously in hospitals or asylums.**
   3. **Dorothea Dix advocated for humane treatment for clients with mental illness, and this led to the establishment of many hospitals devoted to their care.**
   4. Federal funding for mental health care was not available until the 1940s with the passing of the National Mental Health Act, which provided funds to develop mental health programs outside of state hospitals.
   5. The National Institute of Mental Health was charged with the responsibility of mental health care in the United States but did not mandate the establishment of large hospitals or asylums.

TEST-TAKING HINT: Reviewing the history of mental health care assists the test taker in understanding how care was delivered in the past.

5. 1. This is an example of secondary, not primary, prevention, which is aimed at reducing the prevalence of psychiatric illness by shortening the duration of the illness.
   2. **This is an example of primary prevention, which is focused on educational programs to help prevent the incidence of mental illness.**
   3. This is an example of secondary, not primary, prevention.
   4. This is an example of tertiary, not primary, prevention, which is focused on reducing the residual defects that are associated with severe or chronic mental illness.
   5. **This is an example of primary prevention, which is focused on educational programs to help prevent the incidence of mental illness.**

TEST-TAKING HINT: Understanding the public health model that describes primary, secondary, and tertiary prevention assists the test taker in answering this question correctly.

6. 1. **Tertiary prevention is aimed at reducing the residual defects that are associated with severe or chronic mental illness. Providing aftercare services, such as day treatment programs, is one way to accomplish this.**
   2. This is an example of a nursing intervention at the secondary prevention level, which is focused on reducing the prevalence of psychiatric illness by shortening the duration of the illness.
   3. This is an example of a nursing intervention at the primary prevention level, which is focused on targeting groups at risk and providing educational programs.
   4. This is an example of a nursing intervention at the primary prevention level, which is focused on targeting groups at risk and providing educational programs.

TEST-TAKING HINT: Reviewing the functions of the nurse at all levels of community mental health prevention helps the test taker to distinguish interventions in each prevention category.

7. 1. Short-term stabilization should be attempted before long-term treatment is initiated. If this client cannot be stabilized in a short-term setting, a long-term setting may be appropriate in the future.
   2. Clients in day treatment do not require 24-hour nursing care, and admissions are voluntary. This client needs closer observation and probably would not consent to voluntary admission because of paranoid thinking.
   3. **A short-term, inpatient, locked unit would be most appropriate for this client. This setting provides containment and structure for clients who are at risk for harming themselves or others.**
   4. Although psychiatric case management may be implemented in the future, this client needs stabilization in an acute-care, short-term setting.

TEST-TAKING HINT: Understanding the types of care available to mentally ill clients and the types of clients these various settings serve assists the test taker in answering this question correctly.

8. 1. Identifying a client who is missing appointments and seeking other community resources to ensure correct treatment reflects the activity of identification and outreach, not service planning.
   2. Calling a client when they miss an appointment to determine the cause of the absence reflects the activity of assessment, not service planning.
   3. Making an appointment for a client with a nutritionist for dietary counseling reflects the activity of linkage with needed services, not service planning.
   4. **Holding a care conference for a client who is having difficulty returning to school reflects the activity of service planning. A service care plan is devised with client participation and should include mutually agreed-on goals, specific actions directed toward goal achievement, and selection of essential resources and services.**

TEST-TAKING HINT: Reviewing examples of case management activities, such as identification and outreach, assessment, service planning, linkage with needed services, monitoring service delivery, and advocacy, assists the test taker in recognizing nursing actions that reflect these activities.

Role of the Nurse

9. 1. The psychiatrist is a physician who prescribes medications for mental illness. Other than supplemental thiamine, there is no

medication specific to Wernicke-Korsakoff syndrome. Neurocognitive disorder medications would not be helpful for a client with Wernicke-Korsakoff syndrome.

2. A client experiencing Wernicke-Korsakoff syndrome has deficits in short-term and long-term memory and uses confabulation. This impairment affects communication, and counseling sessions would not be helpful.

3. The dietitian can help the client to increase the intake of thiamine-rich foods. Thiamine deficiency is the cause of Wernicke-Korsakoff syndrome.

4. The social worker helps clients and their families cope more effectively, identifies community resources, and can function as the discharge planner. A client with Wernicke-Korsakoff syndrome, because of a deficit in cognitive functioning, is an inappropriate candidate for Alcoholics Anonymous meetings.

TEST-TAKING HINT: To answer this question correctly, the test taker needs to recognize the signs, symptoms, and cause of Wernicke-Korsakoff syndrome.

10. *Cheeking* means that the client hides medication between the cheek and gum. Complete inspection of the mouth, with potential use of a tongue blade, is necessary to discover cheeking. Another way to ensure that the client has swallowed medications is to talk to the client for a few minutes after medication administration. During this time, the medication would begin to dissolve if cheeking has occurred.

1. The nurse can advocate for the client's right to refuse medications, but when checking for cheeking medications, the nurse is functioning as a medication manager, not an advocate.

2. Teaching about the importance of medication adherence, correct dosage, and reportable side effects is critical to effective client care but is not reflected in the question. Checking for cheeking medications is an action performed by the nurse in the role of medication manager, not educator.

3. In the role of medication manager, the nurse has the responsibility of ensuring that clients are given the correct medication, in the correct dosage, by the correct route, and at the correct time, and that correct documentation occurs. By checking for cheeking, the nurse is fulfilling this role.

4. A nurse might use therapeutic communication techniques to counsel a client about the importance of taking their medications, but this nursing action is not reflected in the question and does not relate to checking for cheeking.

TEST-TAKING HINT: The test taker must look at the nursing action presented in the question. In what role is the nurse functioning when performing this action?

11. 1. Environmental assessment is within the nurse's role as milieu manager, not the role of teacher.

2. One of the roles of the milieu manager, not the teacher, is to orient new clients and assist them in fitting comfortably into the milieu.

3. In the role of teacher, the nurse assists the client and family members in coping with the effects of mental illness. Helping the client to understand their illness, its signs and symptoms, the medications and potential side effects, and various coping techniques all are interventions of the nurse functioning in the role of teacher.

4. The guardian of the therapeutic environment is the psychiatric nurse in the role of milieu manager, not teacher.

5. In the role of the teacher, the nurse assists the client to understand treatments, including medication actions and their side effects. Holding this teaching group is an intervention that reflects the nurse's role of teacher.

TEST-TAKING HINT: To assist the test taker in distinguishing the various roles of the nurse, they should consider clinical examples that reflect these roles.

12. 1. Advocacy is an essential role of the psychiatric nurse. Often, mentally ill clients cannot identify their personal problems or communicate their needs effectively. A nurse advocate stands alongside clients and empowers them to have a voice when they are weak and vulnerable.

2. In the role of teacher, not advocate, the nurse assists the client and family members in attaining a greater ability to live with the effects of mental illness within the community.

3. Ensuring that new clients fit comfortably into the therapeutic environment is one of the many roles of the milieu manager, not the role of advocate.

4. When the nurse monitors the client in the milieu for side effects of psychotropic medications, the nurse is functioning in the role of medication manager, not advocate.

5. Advocacy is an essential role for the psychiatric nurse. A nurse advocate stands alongside of clients and empowers them to have a voice when they are weak and vulnerable.

TEST-TAKING HINT: Understanding the interventions used by the nurse in a psychiatric setting when assuming various roles assists the test taker in categorizing the behaviors presented in the question correctly.

13. The nurse functioning in the role of a resource person provides specific information that the client can understand and use to benefit health and well-being.
    1. The nurse functioning as a teacher, not a counselor, identifies learning needs and provides information required by the client to improve health situations.
    2. The nurse functioning as a leader, not a counselor, encourages the client to be an active participant in designing a nursing plan of care.
    3. The nurse functioning as a surrogate, not a counselor, serves as a substitute figure for another person. The nurse may be perceived by the client as a parent figure, sibling, teacher, or someone who has provided care in the past. The nurse has the responsibility for exercising professional skill in aiding the relationship to move forward.
    4. **The nurse functioning as a counselor uses interpersonal communication techniques to assist clients in learning to adapt to difficulties or changes in life experiences. These techniques allow the experiences to be integrated with, rather than dissociated from, other experiences in life.**

TEST-TAKING HINT: An analogy is a comparison. Test takers should look at what is being compared and choose an answer that provides information that reflects a similar comparison.

14. Ongoing assessment, diagnosis, outcome identification, planning, implementation, and evaluation of the environment are necessary for the successful management of a therapeutic milieu.
    1. **By setting strict limits on inappropriate or unacceptable behaviors, the nurse functions in the role of the milieu manager. The safety of the milieu is**

always the highest priority. The environment of the milieu should be constructed to provide many opportunities for personal growth and social interaction to build interpersonal skills.

    2. This nurse is functioning in the role of a role player, not a milieu manager, although this is a wonderful way to practice interpersonal skills with the client. It gives the client a sense of security because behaviors in stressful situations can be practiced before the event.
    3. Chemical restraints and forced medications can be administered only if the client is an imminent threat to self or others. There is no indication in the question that the client is an imminent threat.
    4. By holding a group teaching session on relationship skills, the nurse is functioning in the role of teacher, not milieu manager.

TEST-TAKING HINT: To assist in correctly choosing the actions of the nurse that reflect the role of milieu manager, the test taker should review this role and its components.

15. This client is exhibiting spiritual distress and is in need of spiritual counseling.
    1. The psychiatrist is a physician whose specialty is the diagnosis and treatment of clients with mental disorders. A chaplain would best address this client's stated needs.
    2. The social worker helps clients and their families to cope more effectively, identifies community resources, and can function as the discharge planner. A chaplain would best address this client's stated needs.
    3. The psychologist in the inpatient setting selects, administers, and interprets psychological tests such as intelligence quotient tests and personality inventories. A chaplain would best address this client's stated needs.
    4. **The chaplain provides spiritual counseling. Experiencing anger at God or a higher power can indicate spiritual distress that can be addressed by the chaplain.**

TEST-TAKING HINT: To answer this question correctly, the test taker should review the roles of the members of the health-care team in a psychiatric setting and how the nurse would collaborate with each team member.

16. Personality testing must be done initially to diagnose a client with a personality disorder. This testing is administered by a psychologist.
    1. The psychiatrist is a physician whose specialty is the diagnosis and treatment of

clients with mental disorders. No medications are specifically targeted for personality disorders.

2. The occupational therapist uses manual and creative techniques to elicit desired interpersonal and intrapsychic responses and helps the client with job training and placement. The occupational therapist does not administer personality testing.

3. The clinical psychologist selects, administers, and interprets psychological tests. Clients with personality disorder traits need personality testing such as the Minnesota Multiphasic Personality Inventory to confirm a personality disorder diagnosis.

4. The recreational therapist plans recreational activities to provide opportunities for socialization, healthful recreation, and interpersonal experiences. The recreational therapist does not administer personality testing.

TEST-TAKING HINT: To answer this question correctly, the test taker must know that the primary function of the psychologist in an inpatient setting is testing. The psychologist performs personality inventories and intelligence quotient testing.

17. 1. The psychiatrist is a physician whose specialty is the diagnosis and treatment of clients with mental disorders. The psychiatrist can help with alcohol detoxification and prescribe deterrent and anticraving drugs to assist the client with recovery. However, this client's described need relates to job and transportation loss.

2. Counseling sessions with the psychologist may help the client explore causes and effects of alcohol abuse, but this does not directly meet this client's described need related to job and transportation loss.

3. The occupational therapist in a mental health setting focuses on rehabilitation and vocational training to assist clients in becoming productive. The occupational therapist uses manual and creative techniques to elicit desired interpersonal and intrapsychic responses. The occupational therapist helps the client with job training and employment placement, which is the direct problem described in the question.

4. The social worker helps clients and their families cope more effectively, identifies community resources, and can function

as the discharge planner. However, these functions do not directly meet this client's described need related to job and transportation loss. There is no information provided in the question that indicates a housing need.

TEST-TAKING HINT: To answer this question correctly, the test taker should review the roles of the members of the health-care team in a psychiatric setting and how the nurse would collaborate with each team member.

Nursing Process

18. Statements by clients are considered subjective data.

1. Subjective data are reported by the client and significant others in their own words. An example is the chief complaint, which is expressed by the client during the intake interview.

2. Subjective data do not need to be validated. Subjective data are from an individual's perspective.

3. Objective data, which must be verified by individuals other than the client and family, include physical examination findings, results of psychometric tests, rating scale scores, and laboratory tests, not the client's or family's expressed feelings.

4. Subjective data are data expressed in the client's own words and can be made objective by the use of a mood scale measurement tool. Mood or anxiety scales are similar to pain scales. These scales objectively measure subjective data.

5. It is a premature assumption on the part of the evaluator to determine that this client is using defense mechanisms.

TEST-TAKING HINT: To answer this question correctly, the test taker must understand that subjective data consist of the client's perception of their health problems. Objective data are observations or measurements made by the data collector.

19. 1. Objective data include scores of rating scales developed to quantify data. A clinical withdrawal institute score rates symptoms of alcohol withdrawal.

2. Generalized anxiety is a subjective symptom. Objective symptoms, such as elevated blood pressure and pulse rate, may be assessed, but the statement of anxiety is a subjective symptom.

3. Anorexia, or loss of appetite, is a subjective symptom. You may be able to measure the amount of food that a client consumes, but the feeling of appetite loss is subjective.

4. "I can't keep my thoughts together" is a subjective symptom expressed by the client.

5. Objective data include scores of rating scales developed to quantify data. A mood scale has a client objectively rate their mood from 0 to 10 on a 10-point scale. These scales take the subjective data of mood and present it as objective data.

TEST-TAKING HINT: To answer this question correctly, the test taker must understand that the measurement of objective data is based on an accepted standard or scale and may require the use of a measurement tool.

20. 1. Trust and rapport are needed to build a nurse–client relationship, but this is not the primary purpose of the assessment phase.

2. Identification of goals and outcomes occurs during the planning, not assessment, phase of the nursing process.

3. The primary goal in the assessment phase of the interview is to collect and organize data, which is then used to identify and prioritize the client's problems.

4. The identification and validation of the medical diagnosis is not within the scope of practice for the registered nurse.

TEST-TAKING HINT: To assist in answering this question, the test taker should write the steps of the nursing process next to the goals presented. Which goal reflects the assessment phase?

21. 1. The clock face assessment is a sensitive way to assess early signs of neurocognitive disorder. The client is asked to place numbers appropriately on a clock face.

2. Overall functioning is not assessed through a clock face assessment test.

3. Various assessment tools can be used to provide evidence of alcohol/substance use disorder, including the CAGE assessment, Substance History and Assessment Tool, and Short Michigan Alcohol Screening Test. The clock face assessment is not one of these tools.

4. Various tools are used to assess signs and symptoms of depression. The Beck Depression Inventory and the Geriatric Depression Rating Scale are two examples.

The clock face assessment test does not reflect signs and symptoms of depression.

TEST-TAKING HINT: To answer this question correctly, the test taker should be aware of the purpose of various assessment tools, including the clock face assessment test.

22. 1. There is nothing presented in the question that reflects any altered coping behaviors being exhibited by this client.

2. A defining characteristic of the nursing diagnosis of ineffective role performance is a change in physical capacity to resume a role. The client presented has had a change in body and body image that affects their ability to perform their role as welder and provider for the family.

3. There is nothing presented in the question that reflects any impaired social interaction behaviors being exhibited by this client.

4. There is nothing presented in the question that reflects any knowledge deficits being exhibited by this client.

TEST-TAKING HINT: Test takers must use only the situation and client data presented in the question to formulate an appropriate nursing diagnosis and must not read into the question any data that are not presented.

23. 1. Risk for falls R/T right-sided weakness and sedation from risperidone is the priority diagnosis for this client. A fall would endanger this client, and safety issues always take priority.

2. Activity intolerance R/T right-sided weakness may be an appropriate diagnosis for this client because of the client's history of stroke, but it is not the priority diagnosis.

3. There is no behavioral evidence of disturbed thought in this question. Risperidone has been prescribed for the agitation and aggression experienced by this client.

4. Because of the client's agitation, anxiety R/T change in health status and dependence on others can be an appropriate diagnosis, but it is not the priority diagnosis.

TEST-TAKING HINT: When evaluating what is being asked for in the question, the test taker should factor in common side effects of medications that the client is receiving. Safety is always prioritized.

24. 1. Concrete thinking focuses thought processes on specifics rather than generalities and immediate issues rather than eventual outcomes. Being consistent in

adhering to unit guidelines is one way to establish trust with a client who is experiencing concrete thinking.
2. Calling the client by name is a way to establish trust by showing respect but does not address concrete thinking.
3. When the nurse shares what the client is feeling, the nurse is experiencing sympathy. This does not assist the client who is experiencing concrete thinking.
4. A concrete thinker has an inability to perceive abstractions. Knowledge of the meaning of an idiom like "the grass is always greener on the other side of the fence" may not assist the client with the ability to perceive abstractions, leading to frustration and potential anger. Attempts to educate in this area may decrease the client's trust in the nurse.

TEST-TAKING HINT: Test takers must consider the client's problem (concrete thinking) and the establishment of trust when answering this question.

25. 1. Teaching the neurochemical action of this medication would be impractical and less beneficial to the client than more appropriate and useful information such as the importance of adherence, side effects, signs of toxicity, and dietary and fluid requirements.
2. Teaching the benefits of taking this medication and the importance of adherence is an appropriate teaching intervention by the nurse. Knowledge deficit with regard to medication effects and adherence would affect the course of the client's recovery. Affective motivation should be promoted during teaching sessions.
3. Teaching signs and symptoms of lithium toxicity is important so that the client will know when to report these potentially life-threatening side effects.
4. Teaching dietary and fluid intake information is important to prevent imbalances in lithium levels.
5. Teaching reportable side effects is important for the client to avoid adverse effects of the medication.

TEST-TAKING HINT: The test taker should recognize that teaching the neurochemical action of a medication to a client is not beneficial and may confuse the recently diagnosed client. It is more important to teach practical information concerning the client's medications.

26. 1. Teaching thought-blocking techniques is a cognitive, not behavioral, approach.
2. **A client with a thought disorder would need assistance in practicing what to say and do during a job interview. The nurse is functioning in the role of role player as assistance is given to this client to meet immediate needs. Role-playing is a behavioral technique.**
3. Advocating with the discharge planner to provide adequate housing is not related to the need described in the question.
4. The use of prn medications is an example of a biological, not behavioral, intervention.

TEST-TAKING HINT: When answering questions related to the role of the nurse, the test taker should ensure that examples chosen reflect the role that is most appropriate in meeting described client needs. The phrase *behavioral approach* also should be considered when deciding on an answer choice.

27. 1. Assessment of normal sleep patterns is what the nurse does initially so that a comparison can be made with current sleep patterns and an accurate assessment leading to appropriate interventions can be determined.
2. Discouraging napping during the day is a good intervention for a nursing diagnosis of sleep pattern disturbance, but it is not the initial intervention.
3. Discouraging the use of caffeine and nicotine, both stimulants, is a good intervention for a nursing diagnosis of sleep pattern disturbance, but it is not the initial intervention.
4. Teaching relaxation exercises is a good intervention for a nursing diagnosis of sleep pattern disturbance, but it is not the initial intervention.

TEST-TAKING HINT: Note the word *initially* in the question, which determines the correct answer. When answering questions that require an initial response, it is helpful for the test taker to consider the steps of the nursing process. Assessment is the first step of the nursing process.

28. 1. "The client will socialize with other clients in the milieu" is an outcome that is too general and does not contain a time frame, making it impossible to measure.
2. "The client will use adaptive coping strategies to control impulses" is an outcome that would apply to a nursing diagnosis of altered coping, not altered social

interaction. The time frame is missing, and this outcome cannot be evaluated.

3. "The client will list two triggers to angry outbursts by day 2 of hospitalization" is the initial outcome that best relates to the nursing diagnosis of altered social interaction R/T paranoid thinking AEB hostile and aggressive behaviors toward fellow clients. The recognition of triggers must come before being able to implement other strategies to help with altered social interactions. Because this outcome includes a time frame and is specific (two triggers), it is measurable.

4. "The client will walk away from confrontation by discharge" is an outcome that does apply to the nursing diagnosis presented but would not be the initial outcome in this situation. This is a long-term outcome.

TEST-TAKING HINT: To answer this question correctly, the test taker must remember that all outcomes must be client centered, be specific to the client problem addressed, and contain a time frame to be measurable. The more specific the outcome, the easier it is to evaluate. The key word *initial* makes answer 3 correct instead of 4.

29. 1. Interacting appropriately with others in social and therapeutic settings is a long-term outcome for impaired social interaction. This outcome is not correctly written. It does not have a time frame and therefore cannot be measured.

2. Discussing with the nurse behaviors that would impede the development of satisfactory interpersonal relationships is a short-term goal for impaired social interaction. This outcome is correctly written, is measurable, and has a time frame.

3. Displaying no evidence of splitting, clinging, or distancing behaviors in relationships is a long-term, not short-term, outcome for impaired social interaction.

4. Demonstrating the use of relaxation techniques to maintain anxiety at a manageable level is an outcome for the nursing diagnosis of anxiety, not impaired social interaction.

TEST-TAKING HINT: Test takers must ensure that the outcome is related to the nursing diagnosis presented in the question. When choosing a short-term outcome, the test taker should look for something that is realistic to expect the client to achieve during hospitalization. Test takers also must ensure that any outcome is written so that it has a time frame and is measurable.

Nurse–Client Relationship

30. 1. Rapport is the primary task in relationship development. Rapport implies special feelings on the part of the nurse and the client. All other conditions necessary to establish the nurse–client relationship are based on the ability to connect and establish rapport.

2. Confidence is established when the nurse and client have a trusting relationship. Because rapport is necessary to establish this trust, rapport, not trust, is the primary task of nurse–client relationship development.

3. Respect is the ability to believe in the dignity and worth of an individual. After rapport is established, the nurse is called on to establish unconditional positive regard for the client.

4. Professionalism refers to the fact that it is important for the nurse to project an image that is acceptable to the client and sends a message of knowledge and expertise. It is not a specific condition, however, essential to the establishment of the nurse–client relationship.

TEST-TAKING HINT: To facilitate answering this question correctly, the test taker should review the characteristics that enhance the establishment of the nurse–client relationship: rapport, trust, respect, genuineness, and empathy.

31. 1. By being given simple and clear reasons for policies and procedures, the client can count on consistency from the nurse in the implementation of these policies and procedures. This consistency promotes the development of trust in the nurse–client relationship.

2. Calling the client by name and title ("Mr. Hawkins") shows respect but does not directly promote trust.

3. Striving to understand the motivations behind the client's behavior is an empathetic intervention but does not directly promote trust.

4. Taking the client's ideas into consideration when planning care shows that the nurse respects the client's wishes, but this intervention does not directly promote trust.

TEST-TAKING HINT: Although all of these answers are positive interventions toward clients, not all relate directly to the development of trust. Trust is the ability to feel confidence toward a person and must be earned.

32. 1. This empathetic statement appreciates the client's feelings and objectively communicates concern for the client.

2. This statement focuses on the situation versus the client's feelings about the situation and sympathetically rather than empathically communicates the nurse's versus the client's feelings.

3. This is a sympathetic rather than empathetic statement that focuses on the nurse's, not the client's, feelings.

4. Because the nurse's statement represents past personal problems, this can be considered a sympathetic statement in which the nurse overidentifies with the client.

TEST-TAKING HINT: To answer this question correctly, the test taker must distinguish between empathy and sympathy. Empathy is an objective process wherein an individual is able to see beyond outward behavior and sense accurately another's inner experience. Sympathy is a subjective process wherein an individual actually experiences the emotions felt by the client.

33. 1. The nurse conveys a respectful attitude toward this client by focusing on the client's dysfunctional behaviors and not labeling the client as dysfunctional. The nurse also addresses the client by name and title ("Mr. Hawkins").

2. This statement relates to confidentiality, which conveys the specific concept of trust, not respect.

3. The nurse overidentifies with the client's feelings because the client reminds the nurse of past problems. This subjectivity reflects a sympathetic reaction.

4. This statement belittles the feelings of the client by devaluing the client's feelings.

TEST-TAKING HINT: To answer this question correctly, the test taker needs to understand that to show respect is to believe in the dignity and worth of an individual regardless of their unacceptable behavior.

34. 1. Exploring self-perceptions is necessary for the therapeutic use of self and is the goal of the pre-interaction phase, not orientation phase, of the nurse–client relationship.

2. The establishment of trust is the goal of the orientation phase. During this phase, a contract is established with the client.

3. Promoting client change is the goal of the working phase, not orientation phase, of the nurse–client relationship. During this phase, effective interventions and problem-solving occur.

4. Evaluating goal attainment and therapeutic closure is the goal of the termination phase, not orientation phase, of the nurse–client relationship.

TEST-TAKING HINT: To answer this question correctly, the test taker must recognize that creating an environment for the establishment of trust and rapport is the first task and goal of the orientation phase of the nurse–client relationship. Reviewing the phases of the nurse–client relationship—pre-orientation, orientation, working, and termination—assists in answering this question.

35. The correct order is 4, 3, 1, 2.
First, in the pre-orientation phase of the nurse–client relationship, the nurse would examine any personal biases. Second, in the orientation phase, the nurse would formulate nursing diagnostic statements. Third, in the working phase, the nurse would attempt to promote client insight. Fourth, in the termination phase, the nurse would plan for continued client care.

TEST-TAKING HINT: To answer this question correctly, the test taker must be aware of the nursing actions that occur in the various phases of the nurse–client relationship.

36. 1. The pre-interaction phase involves preparation for the first encounter with the client, such as reading previous medical records and exploring feelings regarding working with that particular client. *Goal:* Explore self-perception.

2. The orientation (introductory) phase involves creating an environment that establishes trust and rapport. Another task of this phase includes establishing a contract for interventions that details the expectations and responsibilities of the nurse and the client. In this example, the client has built the needed trust and rapport with the nurse. The client now feels comfortable and ready to acknowledge the problem and contract for intervention. *Goal:* Establish trust and formulate contract for intervention.

3. The working phase includes promoting the client's insight and perception of reality, problem-solving, overcoming resistant behaviors, and continuously evaluating progress toward goal attainment. *Goal:* Promote client change.

4. The termination phase occurs when progress has been made toward attainment of mutually set goals, a plan for continuing care is mutually established, and feelings about termination are recognized and explored. *Goal:* Evaluate goal attainment and ensure therapeutic closure.

TEST-TAKING HINT: Test takers must read this question completely. What makes this answer "orientation (introductory) phase" is that the question presents a client who is willing to work with the nurse. If the question described the actual intervention of teaching adaptive ways to handle the client's aggression, the answer would be "working phase."

37. 1. The pre-interaction phase involves preparation for the first encounter with the client, such as reading previous medical records and exploring feelings regarding working with that particular client. *Goal:* Explore self-perception.
    2. The orientation (introductory) phase involves creating an environment that establishes trust and rapport. Another task of this phase includes establishing a contract for interventions that details the expectations and responsibilities of the nurse and the client. *Goal:* Establish trust and formulate contract for intervention.
    3. The working phase includes promoting the client's insight and perception of reality, problem-solving, overcoming resistant behaviors, and continuously evaluating progress toward goal attainment. In this example, the client works toward better communication and is guided and encouraged with positive feedback from the nurse. *Goal:* Promote client change.
    4. The termination phase occurs when progress has been made toward attainment of mutually set goals, a plan for continuing care is mutually established, and feelings about termination are recognized and explored. *Goal:* Evaluate goal attainment and ensure therapeutic closure.

TEST-TAKING HINT: To assist the test taker in answering this question correctly, the test taker should review the phases of the nurse–client relationship and think of examples of behaviors and interactions that occur in each phase.

38. 1. The pre-interaction phase involves preparation for the first encounter with the client, such as reading previous medical records and exploring feelings regarding working with that particular client. *Goal:* Explore self-perception.
    2. The orientation (introductory) phase involves creating an environment that establishes trust and rapport. Another task of this phase includes establishing a contract for interventions that details the expectations and responsibilities of the nurse and the client. *Goal:* Establish trust and formulate contract for intervention.
    3. The working phase includes promoting the client's insight and perception of reality, problem-solving, overcoming resistant behaviors, and continuously evaluating progress toward goal attainment. *Goal:* Promote client change.
    4. The termination phase occurs when progress has been made toward attainment of mutually set goals, a plan for continuing care is mutually established, and feelings about termination are recognized and explored. In this example, the nurse must establish the reality of separation and resist repeated delays by the client because of dependency needs. *Goal:* Evaluate goal attainment and ensure therapeutic closure.

TEST-TAKING HINT: The question states that the goals of therapy have been met. This information indicates a description of the termination phase of the nurse–client relationship. The test taker also should recognize the client statement as indicative of feelings experienced during termination.

39. When the nurse reviews the client's previous medical record before meeting the client, the nurse–client relationship is in the pre-interaction phase.
    1. The pre-interaction phase involves preparation for the first encounter with the client, such as reading previous medical records and exploring feelings regarding working with that particular client. In this example, the nurse obtains information about the client for initial assessment. This also allows the nurse to become aware of any personal biases about the client. *Goal:* Explore self-perception.
    2. The orientation phase involves creating an environment that establishes trust and rapport. Another task of this phase includes establishing a contract for interventions that details the expectations and responsibilities of the nurse and the client. *Goal:* Establish trust and formulate contract for intervention.

3. The working phase includes promoting the client's insight and perception of reality, problem-solving, overcoming resistant behaviors, and continuously evaluating progress toward goal attainment. *Goal:* Promote client change.

4. The termination phase occurs when progress has been made toward attainment of mutually set goals, a plan for continuing care is mutually established, and feelings about termination are recognized and explored. *Goal:* Evaluate goal attainment and ensure therapeutic closure.

TEST-TAKING HINT: To answer this question correctly, the test taker must understand that self-assessment is a major intervention that occurs in the pre-interaction phase of the nurse–client relationship. The nurse must be self-aware of any feelings or personal history that might affect the nurse's feelings toward the client.

40. When the nurse reviews the client's chart before meeting the client, the nurse–client relationship is in the pre-interaction phase.
    1. Getting to know each other and establishing trust are the purposes of the orientation phase of the nurse–client relationship. Reviewing a client's record in preparation for client care does not occur in the orientation phase.
    2. Implementing nursing interventions to achieve outcomes is the purpose of the working phase of the nurse–client relationship. Reviewing a client's record in preparation for client care does not occur in the working phase.
    3. Achievement of independence and maintenance of health without nursing care is the purpose of the termination phase of the nurse–client relationship. Reviewing a client's record in preparation for client care does not occur in the termination phase.
    4. Understanding the signs and symptoms of the client's diagnosis and evaluating the nurse's attitudes toward the client are the purposes of the pre-orientation phase of the nurse–client relationship.

TEST-TAKING HINT: To answer this question correctly, the test taker first must determine the stage of the nurse–client relationship in which the nurse reviews a client's record in preparation for client care. When the test taker has determined the stage, the next step is to remember the purpose of this stage.

41. The nurse explores any misconceptions or prejudices experienced before caring for a client in the pre-interaction phase.
    1. The task of the nurse during the orientation phase of the nurse–client relationship is to determine why the client sought help.
    2. **The task of the nurse during the pre-interaction phase of the nurse–client relationship is to explore self.**
    3. The task of the nurse during the working phase of the nurse–client relationship is to assist the client in behavioral change.
    4. The task of the nurse during the termination phase of the nurse–client relationship is to establish and prepare the client for separation.

TEST-TAKING HINT: The test taker should first note the action of the nurse to determine the appropriate phase of the nurse–client relationship, then answer the question. There is no nurse–client contact during the pre-interaction phase. This eliminates answers 1, 3, and 4.

42. 1. Roles cannot be established in the pre-interaction phase because the nurse and the client have not met.
    2. **During the orientation phase, the purpose of the interaction is established, and this is a component of the nurse–client contract.**
    3. The conditions for termination are established in the orientation, not working, phase of the nurse–client relationship.
    4. Criteria for discharge are not established in the termination phase. Discharge criteria are determined by the entire treatment team.

TEST-TAKING HINT: To answer this question correctly, the test taker must remember the elements of the nurse–client contract that are established in the orientation phase of the nurse–client relationship.

43. A nursing student is most likely to experience fears related to the first clinical experience in a psychiatric setting in the pre-interaction phase of the nurse–client relationship.
    1. **Students may experience numerous fears related to working with psychiatric clients. Self-analysis in the pre-interaction phase of the nurse–client relationship may make the student aware of these fears. The student may be suspicious of psychiatric clients, feel inadequate about their ability to be therapeutic, or believe that there is a possibility of being harmed.**

2. Threats to a student's role identity usually occur in the pre-orientation, not orientation, phase.
3. The student may feel emotionally vulnerable to past experiences, and this is usually recognized in the pre-orientation, not working, phase.
4. The student's uncertainty about their ability to make a difference occurs in the pre-orientation, not termination, phase.

TEST-TAKING HINT: To answer this question correctly, the test taker must remember that students bring preconceived ideas about clients diagnosed with mental illness to the clinical setting. After exposure to these clients, students are more likely to appreciate client problems and empathize with their situations. The fears described in the question are to be expected in an initial experience in a psychiatric setting. The phase of the nurse–client relationship in which these fears are likely to occur makes answer 1 correct.

44. The logical sequence is 2, 4, 3, 1.
    1. Self-assessment occurs in the pre-interaction stage of the nurse–client relationship. Self-assessment must be completed for the nurse to understand potential preconceived thoughts and feelings about mentally ill clients and how these feelings would affect the development of a relationship.
    2. The ability to communicate therapeutically is essential for any intervention that occurs in a psychiatric setting. Effective communication skills allow the nurse to assess a client's thoughts, feelings, and symptoms and move toward effective interventions.
    3. After self-assessment and the development of effective communication skills, the nurse must have knowledge of the disease processes that a client may be experiencing and how the signs and symptoms exhibited relate to the disease.
    4. The nurse would be unable to intervene effectively and problem-solve if there is a deficit in the nurse's knowledge of the disorder.

TEST-TAKING HINT: It is easy for the test taker to put interventions in order by recognizing the interventions that occur in the phase of the nurse–client relationship.

45. 1. A nursing student who is experiencing a crisis situation may overidentify with clients and communicate or deal with

their own personal problems rather than focus on the clients' problems and concerns. Instead of meeting the client's needs, the student may make their own needs the priority.
2. The novice nurse may fear clients and tend to avoid client interactions, but this is not directly related to the student's current crisis situation.
3. Feeling inadequate and fearing that clients will be harmed by an insensitive remark is a typical fear of the novice nurse in a psychiatric setting. This is not related to the student's experience of personal crisis.
4. Doubting their value in assisting clients because of lack of knowledge is a typical fear of the novice nurse in a psychiatric setting. This fear is not directly related to the student's experience of a family crisis.

TEST-TAKING HINT: To answer this question correctly, the test taker should review self-assessment and the concept of countertransference.

46. 1. This is a rational belief based on objective evidence, not a belief that describes a concept in an oversimplified or undifferentiated manner.
2. This is a rational belief based on the concept of peer support, acceptance, and understanding from others who have experienced the same problems in their lives. This is not a belief that describes a concept in an oversimplified or undifferentiated manner.
3. This is faith, which is held to be true even though no objective evidence exists, not a belief that describes a concept in an oversimplified or undifferentiated manner.
4. A stereotypical belief, such as this characterization of alcoholics, describes a concept in an oversimplified or undifferentiated manner. When a belief is generalized to encompass *all*, the belief becomes oversimplified and undifferentiated.

TEST-TAKING HINT: To answer this question correctly, the test taker must understand the definition of the words *oversimplified* and *undifferentiated*.

Transference/Countertransference

47. Countertransference refers to the emotional and behavioral reactions of the nurse toward clients under the nurse's care. Unresolved

positive and negative feelings from the nurse's past may initiate projection of these feelings toward clients. Countertransference interferes with the establishment of therapeutic relationships by negating professional objectivity.

1. **Defending the client's inappropriate behavior reflects an underlying subjective connection with the client, which is an example of countertransference.**
2. The expression of empathy toward a client's loss is therapeutic and does not reflect the concept of countertransference.
3. **Appreciation of the client's feelings must be from an objective, not subjective, point of view. This subjective appreciation reflects the concept of countertransference.**
4. **The uneasiness that the nurse experiences reflects an underlying subjective connection with the client, which is an example of countertransference.**
5. Emotional attachment by the client toward a health-care team member is an example of transference, not countertransference.

TEST-TAKING HINT: To answer this question correctly, the test taker must understand the concept of countertransference. Countertransference refers to the nurse's behavioral and emotional subjective responses to the client. Test takers must understand that countertransference commonly occurs in a nurse–client relationship. It is the nurse's responsibility to be aware of and deal with these feelings to be objectively therapeutic.

48. 1. In this example, there is the potential that countertransference, and not transference, has occurred. Countertransference refers to the nurse's behavioral and emotional response to the staff on behalf of the client. These feelings may be related to unresolved feelings toward significant others from the nurse's past.
    2. This example of transference occurs when the client unconsciously displaces (or transfers) to the nurse feelings formed toward a person from their past. Transference also can take the form of overwhelming affection with unrealistic expectations of the nurse by the client. When the nurse does not meet the expectations, the client may become angry and hostile.

Intervention: The nurse should work with the client in sorting out the past from the present, identifying the transference, and reassigning a more appropriate meaning to the nurse–client relationship.

3. This example of collaboration embraces the nurse and client's working together and becoming involved in the client's plan of care. Collaboration has great relevance in psychiatric nursing and encourages clients to recognize their own problems and needs; it has nothing to do with transference.
4. This example of resistance is often caused by the client's unwillingness to change when the need for change is recognized. It involves the client's inability to face and deal with various negative aspects of their life and has nothing to do with transference.

TEST-TAKING HINT: To answer this question correctly, the test taker must understand that the communication process involves perception, evaluation, and transmission. The test taker should study structural and transactional analysis models to understand the communication process and identify common problems, such as transference and countertransference.

49. 1. In this example, countertransference refers to the nurse's behavioral and emotional response to the client's diagnosis of alcohol use disorder. These feelings may be related to unresolved feelings toward significant others from the nurse's past, or they may be generated in response to transference feelings on the part of the client. The nurse's statement revealing that their parent misused alcohol and neglected the family is evidence of countertransference. *Intervention:* Have evaluative sessions with the nurse after an encounter with the client, in which the nurse and staff members discuss and compare the exhibited behaviors in the nurse–client relationship. The relationship usually should not be terminated in the face of countertransference.
    2. The client's statement comparing the nurse to their cranky spouse is an example of transference. Transference occurs when the client unconsciously displaces (or transfers) to the nurse feelings formed toward a person from their past. Transference also

can take the form of overwhelming affection with unrealistic expectations of the nurse by the client. When the nurse does not meet the expectations, the client may become angry and hostile.

3. This example of collaboration embraces the nurse and client's working together and becoming involved in the client's plan of care. Collaboration has great relevance in psychiatric nursing and encourages clients to recognize their own problems and needs. This is not evidence of either countertransference or transference.

4. This example of resistance is often caused by the client's unwillingness to change when the need for change is recognized. It also involves the client's reluctance or avoidance of verbalizing or experiencing troubling aspects of the client's life. This is not evidence of either countertransference or transference.

TEST-TAKING HINT: To answer this question correctly, the test taker must understand the concepts of both transference and countertransference and be able to recognize their differences.

50. 1. This is an example of countertransference, because the physician identifies their child's behavior with that of the client. These feelings may be related to unresolved feelings toward significant others from the physician's past.

2. This is an example of resistance, which is often caused by the client's unwillingness to change when the need for change is recognized. It also involves the client's reluctance to verbalize or experience troubling aspects of their life, or avoidance of these aspects.

3. This is an example of transference, which occurs when the client unconsciously displaces (or transfers) to the physician feelings formed toward a person from their past. Transference also can take the form of overwhelming affection with unrealistic expectations of the physician by the client. By accusing the doctor of abusing their own son, the client is transferring strong negative feelings from the client's parent to the doctor. *Intervention:* The physician should work with the client to sort out the past from the present, identify the transference, and reassign a more appropriate meaning to the physician–client relationship.

4. Because this client previously has expressed hostility toward the physician, the client's statement may indicate that they are experiencing the defense mechanism of "undoing." This is not indicative of transference.

TEST-TAKING HINT: To answer this question correctly, the test taker should look for examples of transference in the communication situations presented in the answer choices.

51. *Paranoia* is a term that implies extreme suspiciousness.
1. Telling a client that the psychiatrist ordered a medication for the client does not assist the client in understanding the benefits of taking the medication.

2. When working with a client experiencing paranoia, it is important to keep a routine; however, routine by itself would not help the client to understand why it is important to take the medication.

3. If staff members believed that the client was cheeking the medication, a liquid form would be helpful; however, there is nothing in the stem of the question indicating that the client is doing this. The nurse should not assume that all clients exhibiting paranoia are cheeking their medications; however, the nurse should watch for signs of this behavior.

4. When a client is exhibiting paranoia, it is important for the nurse to take further actions to encourage adherence. Presenting the client with medication that is labeled and sealed shows that no one has tampered with the medication and may assist with medication adherence.

TEST-TAKING HINT: To answer this question correctly, the test taker first must recognize the symptoms of paranoia presented in the question. Then the test taker must understand how this thinking affects nursing interventions related to medication adherence.

52. 1. There is nothing in the question stating that the client is cheeking medications, and liquid or IM injections are not indicated.

2. Although it is important for the nurse to ensure that the client understands potential side effects of medications, this intervention alone would not increase the client's medication adherence.

3. When the nurse is able to link the medication prescribed to specific bothersome

symptoms experienced by the client, the client is more likely to understand why the medication is needed.

4. It is important for the nurse to understand these concepts; however, teaching this technical information to the client would not increase adherence.

TEST-TAKING HINT: When answering the question, the test taker should avoid adding information to the situation. There is no information in the question regarding the client's cheeking medications; by choosing answer 1, an incorrect assumption is made that all psychiatric clients cheek their medications.

Communication

4

KEYWORDS

The following words include English vocabulary, nursing/medical terminology, concepts, principles, or information relevant to content specifically addressed in this chapter or associated with topics presented in it. English dictionaries, your nursing textbooks, and medical dictionaries such as *Taber's Cyclopedic Medical Dictionary* are resources that can be used to expand your knowledge and understanding of these words and related information.

Accepting
Active listening
Aphasia
Attempting to translate words into feelings
Belittling
Broad opening
Challenging
Clarification
Confrontation
Cultural group
Culture
Defending
Density
Disapproving
Dysarthria
Empathy
Encouraging comparison
Evil eye
Exploring
Focusing
Folk practitioner
Genuineness
Ghost sickness
Giving advice
Giving false reassurance
Giving information
Giving recognition
Halal diet
Indicating the existence of an external source
Informing
Interpreting
Introducing an unrelated topic
Kosher diet

Listening
Magical healing
Making an observation
Making stereotyped/superficial comments
Nonthreatening feedback
Nonverbal
Offering general leads
Offering self
Paraphrasing
Personal space
Placing the event in time or sequence
Probing
Reflection
Requesting an explanation
Respect
Restating
Seeking consensual validation
Silence
Specific syndromes
Suggesting
Suggesting collaboration
Sympathy
Territoriality
Testing
Therapeutic communication technique
Therapeutic touch
Touch
Verbalizing the implied
Voicing doubt
Volume
Voodoo
Witchcraft

QUESTIONS

Therapeutic Communication Facilitators

1. A client states, "I don't know what the pills are for or why I am taking them, so I don't want them." Which is an example of the therapeutic communication technique of giving information?
   1. "You must take your medication to get better."
   2. "The doctor wouldn't prescribe these pills if they were harmful."
   3. "Do you feel this way about all your medications?"
   4. "This medication will help to improve your mood."

2. A client diagnosed with depression is discussing marital problems with the nurse and says, "What will I do if my spouse asks me for a divorce?" Which response by the nurse is an example of therapeutic communication?
   1. "Why do you think that your spouse will ask you for a divorce?"
   2. "You seem to be worrying over nothing. I'm sure everything will be fine."
   3. "What has happened to make you think that your spouse will ask for a divorce?"
   4. "Talking about this will only make you more anxious and increase your depression."

3. A client states to the nurse, "I'm thinking about ending it all." Which response by the nurse is an example of therapeutic communication?
   1. "Your attitude will hamper your recovery."
   2. "Wasn't your spouse just here during visiting hours?"
   3. "Why would you want to do something like that?"
   4. "You must be feeling very sad right now."

4. Which of the following statements are examples of the therapeutic communication technique of focusing? **Select all that apply.**
   1. "You say you're angry, but I notice that you're smiling."
   2. "Are you saying that you want to drive to Hawaii?"
   3. "Tell me again about your experiences in the armed services and your feelings after you were wounded during a conflict."
   4. "I see you staring out the window. Tell me what you're thinking."
   5. "Yesterday you described your relationship with your mom. Let's continue that topic."

5. Which of the following therapeutic communication exchanges are examples of reflection? **Select all that apply.**
   1. *Client:* "I get sad because I know I'm going to fail in school." *Nurse:* "So you start feeling down every time a new semester begins?"
   2. *Client:* "I forgot to get my prescription refilled." *Nurse:* "It is important for you to take your medication as prescribed."
   3. *Client:* "I hate my recent weight gain." *Nurse:* "Have you considered Overeaters Anonymous?"
   4. *Client:* "I'm happy that I poisoned my spouse." *Nurse:* "You're happy to have poisoned your spouse?"
   5. *Client:* "I really don't know why I'm here. My stupid spouse is behind this." *Nurse:* "You seem angry at your spouse for bringing you to the hospital."

6. The nurse states to a client on an inpatient unit, "Tell me what's been on your mind." Which describes the purpose of this therapeutic communication technique?
   1. To have the client choose the topic of the conversation.
   2. To present new ideas for consideration.
   3. To convey interest in what the client is saying.
   4. To provide time for the nurse and client to gather thoughts and reflect.

7. The nurse states to the client, "You say that you are sad, but you are smiling and laughing." Which describes the purpose of this therapeutic communication technique?
   1. To provide suggestions for coping strategies.
   2. To redirect the client to an idea of importance.
   3. To bring incongruences or inconsistencies into awareness.
   4. To provide feedback to the client.

8. Which of the following are examples of the therapeutic communication technique of clarification? **Select all that apply.**
   1. "Can we talk more about how you feel about your parent?"
   2. "I'm not sure what you mean when you use the word *fragile*."
   3. "I notice that you seem angry today."
   4. "How does your mood today compare with yesterday?"
   5. "Can you help me understand what you mean by a 'difficult childhood'?"

9. The client states, "I'm not sure that the doctor has prescribed the correct medication for my sadness." Which is a therapeutic nursing response?
   1. "A lot of clients are nervous about new medications. I'll get you some information about it."
   2. "So, you think that this medication is not right for you?"
   3. "Why do you think that this medication won't help your mood?"
   4. "Your doctor has been prescribing this medication for years, and it really does help people."

10. A client admitted for alcohol detoxification states, "I don't think my drinking has anything to do with why I am here in the hospital. I think I have problems with depression." Which statement by the nurse is the most therapeutic response?
    1. "I think you really need to look at the amount you are drinking and consider the effect on your family."
    2. "That's wrong. I disagree with that. Your admission is because of your alcohol abuse and not for any other reason."
    3. "I'm sure you don't mean that. You have to realize that alcohol is the root of your problems."
    4. "I find it hard to believe that alcohol is not a problem because you have recently lost your job and your driver's license."

11. Delving further into a subject, idea, experience, or relationship is to *exploring* as taking notice of a single idea, or even a single word is to:
    1. Broad opening.
    2. Offering general leads.
    3. Focusing.
    4. Accepting.

12. Allowing the client to take the initiative in introducing the topic is to *broad opening* as the nurse's making self available and presenting emotional support is to:
    1. Focusing.
    2. Offering self.
    3. Restating.
    4. Giving recognition.

13. The nurse's lack of verbal communication for therapeutic reasons is to *silence* as the nurse's ability to process information and examine reactions to the messages received is to:
    1. Focusing.
    2. Offering self.
    3. Restating.
    4. Listening.

14. A client asks the evening shift nurse, "How do you feel about my refusing to attend group therapy this morning?" The nurse responds, "How did your refusing to attend group make you feel?" This nurse is using which communication technique?
    1. Therapeutic use of restatement.
    2. Nontherapeutic use of probing.
    3. Therapeutic use of reflection.
    4. Nontherapeutic use of interpreting.

15. A client on an inpatient psychiatric unit states, "My mother hates me. My father is a drunk. Right now, I have nowhere to live." The nurse responds, "Let's talk more about your feelings toward your mother." Which is a description of the technique used by the nurse?
    1. The nurse uses questions or statements to help a client expand on a topic of importance.
    2. The nurse encourages a client to select a topic for discussion.
    3. The nurse delves further into a subject or idea.
    4. The nurse is persistent with the questioning of a client.

16. Which of the following are examples of therapeutic communication techniques? **Select all that apply.**
    1. "Tell me about your impaired driving record."
    2. "How does this compare with the time you were sober?"
    3. "That's good. I'm glad that you think you can stop drinking."
    4. "I think we need to talk more about your previous coping mechanisms."
    5. "What led up to your taking that first drink after 5 years of sobriety?"

17. Which is an example of the therapeutic communication technique of voicing doubt?
    1. "What I heard you say was. . . ."
    2. "I find that hard to believe."
    3. "Are you feeling that no one understands?"
    4. "Let's see if we can find the answer."

Blocks to Therapeutic Communication

18. Indicating that there is no cause for anxiety is to *reassuring* as sanctioning or denouncing the client's ideas or behaviors is to:
    1. Approving/disapproving.
    2. Rejecting.
    3. Interpreting.
    4. Probing.

19. Which of the following are examples of nontherapeutic communication blocks? **Select all that apply.**
    1. "You acted out in group. It made the other clients uncomfortable."
    2. "Why did you refuse your medication this afternoon?"
    3. "I'm so sorry you feel that way. It is a feeling typical of hospitalized clients."
    4. "You just think that you are not getting better. You'll see. Everything will work out."
    5. "What I am hearing you say is that everyone is out to get you."

20. Demanding proof from the client is to *challenging* as persistent questioning of the client and pushing for answers the client does not wish to discuss is to:
    1. Advising.
    2. Defending.
    3. Rejecting.
    4. Probing.

21. Which of the following are examples of the nontherapeutic block to communication of giving reassurance? **Select all that apply.**
    1. "That's good. I'm glad that you. . . ."
    2. "Hang in there, every dog has its day."
    3. "Don't worry, everything will work out."
    4. "I think you should. . . ."
    5. "I'm sure you can beat this addiction."

22. Which is an example of the nontherapeutic block to communication of requesting an explanation?
    1. "Who made you so angry last night?"
    2. "Do you still have the idea that . . . ?"
    3. "How could you be dead when you're still breathing?"
    4. "Why do you feel this way?"

Therapeutic Communication Interventions

23. A client on a psychiatric unit says, "It's a waste of time to be here. I can't talk to you or anyone." Which is an appropriate therapeutic nursing response?
    1. "I find that hard to believe."
    2. "Are you feeling that no one understands?"
    3. "I think you should calm down and look on the positive side."
    4. "Our staff here is excellent, and you are in good hands."

24. Which nurse–client communication-centered skill implies respect?
    1. The nurse communicates regard for the client as a person of worth who is valued and accepted without qualification.
    2. The nurse communicates an understanding of the client's world from the client's internal frame of reference, with sensitivity to the client's feelings.
    3. The nurse communicates that the nurse is an open person who is self-congruent, authentic, and transparent.
    4. The nurse communicates specific terminology rather than abstractions in the discussion of the client's feelings, experiences, and behaviors.

25. A client on a psychiatric unit tells the nurse, "I'm all alone in the world now, and I have no reason to live." Which response by the nurse would encourage further communication by the client?
    1. "You sound like you're feeling lonely and frightened."
    2. "Why do you think that suicide is the answer to your loneliness?"
    3. "I live by myself and know it can be very lonely and frightening."
    4. "Just hang in there and, you'll see, things will work out."

26. The nurse is attempting to establish a therapeutic relationship with an angry, depressed client on a psychiatric unit. Which is the most appropriate nursing intervention?
    1. Work on establishing a friendship with the client.
    2. Use humor to defuse emotionally charged topics of discussion.
    3. Show respect that is not based on the client's behavior.
    4. Sympathize with the client when the client shares sad feelings.

27. On a substance abuse unit, a client diagnosed with cirrhosis of the liver tells the nurse, "I really don't believe that drinking a couple of cocktails every night has anything to do with my liver problems." Which is the best nursing response?
    1. "You find it hard to believe that drinking alcohol can damage the liver?"
    2. "How long have you been drinking a couple of cocktails a night?"
    3. "If not by alcohol, explain how your liver became damaged."
    4. "Everyone knows that increased alcohol consumption can damage your liver."

28. In dealing therapeutically with a variety of psychiatric clients, the nurse knows that incorporating humor into the communication process should be used for which purpose?
    1. To diminish feelings of anger.
    2. To refocus the client's attention.
    3. To maintain a balanced perspective.
    4. To delay dealing with the inevitable.

29. A client on an inpatient psychiatric unit has pressured speech and flight of ideas and is extremely irritable. During an intake assessment, which is the most appropriate nursing response?
    1. "I think you need to know more about your medications."
    2. "What have you been thinking about lately?"
    3. "I think we should talk more about what brought you into the hospital."
    4. "Yes, I see. And go on please."

30. A client in an outpatient clinic states, "I am so tired of these medications." Which nursing response would encourage the client to elaborate further?
    1. "I see you have been taking your medications."
    2. "Tired of taking your medications?"
    3. "Let's discuss different ways to deal with your problems."
    4. "How would your family feel about your stopping your medications?"

31. When a nurse communicates openly and is self-congruent, authentic, and transparent, the nurse is exhibiting which communication-centered skill?
    1. Respect.
    2. Empathy.
    3. Genuineness.
    4. Correctness.

32. A client experienced a stroke resulting in aphasia and dysarthria. Which communication adaptation technique by the nurse would be most helpful to this client?
    1. Using simple sentences and avoiding long explanations.
    2. Speaking to the client as though the client could hear.
    3. Listening attentively, allowing time, and not interrupting.
    4. Providing an interpreter (translator) as needed.

33. A client who has been scheduled for electroconvulsive therapy (ECT) in the morning tells the nurse, "I'm really nervous about having ECT tomorrow." Which is the best nursing response?
    1. "I'll ask the provider for a little medication to help you relax."
    2. "It's okay to be nervous. What are your concerns about the procedure?"
    3. "Clients who have had ECT say there's nothing to it."
    4. "Your doctor is excellent and has done hundreds of these procedures."

34. An instructor overhears the nursing student ask a client, "This is your third admission. Why did you stop taking your medications?" Which is the most appropriate instructor response?
    1. "Your question implied criticism and could have the effect of making the client feel defensive."
    2. "Your question invited the client to share thoughts and feelings regarding their nonadherence."
    3. "Your question recognized and acknowledged the client's reasons for their actions."
    4. "Your question focused the client on the topic in order to gain further specific information."

35. Nonthreatening feedback focuses on client behavior rather than on the client themselves. Which of the following are descriptive characteristics of nonthreatening feedback? **Select all that apply.**
    1. Nonthreatening feedback gives information to clients about how they are perceived by others.
    2. Nonthreatening feedback evaluates individual client characteristics and behaviors.
    3. Nonthreatening feedback should be general rather than specific to preserve self-esteem.
    4. Nonthreatening feedback should be directed toward behavior that the client can modify.
    5. Nonthreatening feedback should be given at the earliest appropriate opportunity following the specific behavior.

36. When the nurse focuses on a client's specific behavior rather than on the individuality of the client, the nurse is using a strategy of nonthreatening feedback. Which of the following nursing statements are examples of this strategy? **Select all that apply.**
    1. "It's okay to be angry, but throwing the book was unacceptable behavior."
    2. "I can't believe that you are always this manipulative."
    3. "You are an irresponsible person regarding your life choices."
    4. "Asking for medications every 2 hours proves that you are drug seeking."
    5. "You belittled your roommate. Let's look at some reasons for this behavior."

37. The nurse understands that one of the many strategies of nonthreatening feedback is to limit the feedback to an appropriate time and place. While in the milieu, which nursing statement is an example of this strategy?
    1. "Let's talk about your marital concerns in the conference room after visiting hours."
    2. "I know your parent is visiting you, but I need answers to these questions."
    3. "Why don't we talk about your childhood sexual abuse?"
    4. "Let's talk about your grievance with your provider during group."

Nonverbal Communication

38. To understand and participate in therapeutic communication, the nurse must understand which of the following? **Select all that apply.**
    1. More than half of all messages communicated are nonverbal.
    2. All communication is best accomplished in a "social" space context.
    3. Touch is always a positive form of communication to convey warmth and caring.
    4. Physical space between two individuals can affect the communication process.
    5. The use of silence never varies across cultures.

39. A nurse is communicating with a client on an inpatient psychiatric unit. The client moves closer and invades the nurse's personal space, making the nurse uncomfortable. Which is an appropriate nursing intervention?
    1. The nurse ignores this behavior because it shows the client is progressing.
    2. The nurse expresses a sense of discomfort and limits behaviors.
    3. The nurse understands that clients require various amounts of personal space and accepts the behavior.
    4. The nurse confronts the client and states that the client will be secluded if this behavior continues.

40. A client on a psychiatric unit is telling the nurse about anger toward the airline after losing an only child in a plane crash. In which situation is the nurse demonstrating active listening?
    1. Agreeing with the client.
    2. Repeating everything that the client says to clarify.
    3. Assuming a relaxed posture and leaning toward the client.
    4. Expressing sorrow and sadness regarding the client's loss.

41. The place where communication occurs influences the outcome of the interaction. Which of the following are aspects of the environment that communicate messages? **Select all that apply.**
   1. Dimension.
   2. Distance.
   3. Territoriality.
   4. Volume.
   5. Density.

Cultural Considerations

42. A client with signs and symptoms of double pneumonia states, "I will not agree to hospital admission unless my shaman is allowed to continue helping me." Which is an appropriate nursing intervention?
   1. Tell the client that the shaman is not allowed in the emergency department.
   2. Have the shaman meet the attending physician at the hospital.
   3. Have the family talk the client into admission without the shaman.
   4. Explain to the client that the shaman is responsible for the client's condition.

43. On an inpatient psychiatric unit, a client, who follows a traditional Taoist philosophy, states, "I must have warm ginger root tea for my migraine headache." The nurse, understanding the effects of cultural influences, attaches which meaning to this statement?
   1. The client is being obstinate and wants control over their care.
   2. The client believes that ginger root has magical qualities.
   3. The client believes that health restoration involves the balance of yin and yang.
   4. The client refuses to take traditional medication for pain.

44. A client who has a 10 a.m. appointment at an outpatient psychiatric clinic arrives at noon, stating, "I was visiting with my mother." How should the nurse interpret the client's failure to arrive on time?
   1. The client is a member of a cultural group that is present oriented.
   2. The client is being passive-aggressive by arriving late.
   3. The client is a member of a cultural group that rejects traditional medicine.
   4. This is the client's way of defying authority.

45. A kosher diet is to the Jewish client as a halal diet is to the:
   1. Mormon (the Church of Jesus Christ of Latter-day Saints) client.
   2. Muslim client.
   3. Christian client.
   4. Buddhist client.

46. A nurse, client, and family meet to discuss the client's discharge. During the meeting, the client speaks and makes eye contact only with family. From a cultural perspective, how might the nurse interpret this behavior?
   1. The client has a lack of understanding of the disease process.
   2. The client is experiencing denial related to their condition.
   3. The client is experiencing paranoid thoughts toward authority figures.
   4. The client has respect for members of the health-care team.

47. A client on a psychiatric unit who practices Orthodox Judaism declines to eat any of their ham, rice, and vegetable entrée. Which information about Jewish culture would the nurse attribute to this behavior?
   1. The client is allergic to the rice.
   2. The client is a vegetarian.
   3. The client is following kosher dietary laws.
   4. The client is following the dietary laws of Islam.

48. A client who practices Orthodox Judaism is upset. The client's child has recently committed suicide. The client tearfully tells the nurse that the child may not be able to be buried in a Jewish cemetery. Which intervention should the nurse implement?
    1. Ask the client why the child won't be buried with honors.
    2. Accept that the client is upset and just needs time alone.
    3. Call the psychiatrist for an antianxiety medication.
    4. Sit with the client and allow expression of loss and sorrow.

49. In some cultures, therapeutic touch can be perceived as uncomfortable. What nursing interventions should the nurse implement when caring for a client who may have aversions to touch?
    1. The nurse should avoid touching during initial interactions.
    2. The nurse should teach the client to incorporate touch in the communication process.
    3. The nurse should avoid talking to the client about feelings related to touch.
    4. The nurse should wear gloves during all client interactions.

The correct answer number and rationale for why it is the correct answer are given in **boldface blue type.** Rationales for why the other answer options are incorrect are given as well, but they are not in boldface type.

Therapeutic Communication Facilitators

1. 1. This is an example of giving advice, which is nontherapeutic because the statement does not allow the client to make personal decisions.
    2. This is an example of defending, which is nontherapeutic because this statement would put the client on the defensive.
    3. This is an example of exploring, which is incorrect because the client has provided information by stating, "I don't know what the pills are for."
    4. **The nurse is giving information about the therapeutic effect of the client's medication because the nurse has assessed from the client's statement that information is needed.**

TEST-TAKING HINT: Students often confuse giving information and giving advice. To answer this question correctly, the test taker must be able to distinguish the difference between giving information, which is therapeutic, and giving advice, which is nontherapeutic.

2. 1. This is an example of requesting an explanation, which requests the client to provide the reasons for thoughts, feeling, and behaviors, which can be an unrealistic expectation. It also may put the client on the defensive.
    2. This is an example of giving false reassurance by indicating to the client that there is no cause for fear or anxiety. This blocks any further interaction and expression of feelings by the client.
    3. **The therapeutic technique of exploring, along with reflective listening, draws out the client and can help the client feel valued, understood, and supported. Exploring also gives the nurse the necessary assessment information to intervene appropriately.**
    4. This is an example of rejection, which shows contempt for the client's need to voice and express fears and anxiety.

TEST-TAKING HINT: To answer this question correctly, the test taker must distinguish between therapeutic and nontherapeutic communication facilitators. In this question, answers 1, 2, and 4 all are nontherapeutic communication blocks and can be eliminated immediately.

3. 1. The nurse, when "disapproving" of the client's attitude, denounces the client's ideas and/or behaviors. This implies that the nurse has the right to pass judgment.
    2. Introducing an unrelated topic is nontherapeutic and puts the nurse, instead of the client, in control of the direction of the conversation. This may occur when the nurse is feeling uncomfortable with the topic being discussed.
    3. Requesting an explanation, by asking the client to provide reasons for thoughts, feelings, behaviors, and events, can be intimidating and implies that the client must defend their behavior or feelings.
    4. **This is the therapeutic technique of attempting to translate words into feelings, by which the nurse tries to find clues to the underlying true feelings and at the same time validates the client's statement. The nurse might then explore and delve more deeply by responding, "Can you tell me more about this sadness you feel?"**

TEST-TAKING HINT: The test taker first must become familiar with therapeutic communication techniques and blocks to communication. Then the test taker can distinguish between the many techniques to answer the question correctly.

4. 1. Here the nurse uses a therapeutic technique of confrontation to bring incongruence or inconsistencies into awareness.
    2. This therapeutic technique of clarification is an attempt by the nurse to check the understanding of what has been said by the client and helps the client make their thoughts or feelings more explicit.
    3. **This is an example of the therapeutic communication technique of focusing. The nurse uses focusing to direct the conversation to a particular topic of importance or relevance to the client.**
    4. The nurse is making an observation and using the therapeutic communication

technique of broad opening, which helps the client initiate the conversation and puts the client in control of the content.

5. **This is an example of the therapeutic communication technique of focusing. The nurse uses focusing to direct the conversation to a particular topic of importance or relevance to the client.**

TEST-TAKING HINT: To answer this question correctly, the test taker must be familiar with the therapeutic communication technique of focusing.

5. 1. **Reflection is used when directing back what the nurse understands in regard to the client's ideas, feelings, questions, and content. Reflection is used to put the client's feelings in the context of when or where they occur.**

2. When the nurse gives valuable information to the client, the nurse is using the therapeutic technique of informing, not reflection.

3. Providing suggestions for coping strategies is a way that the nurse helps the client to consider alternative options. This is the therapeutic technique of suggesting, not reflection.

4. By restating what the client has said, the nurse has the opportunity to verify the nurse's understanding of the client's message. The therapeutic technique of restating also lets the client know that the nurse is listening and wants to understand what the client is saying. This is not an example of reflection.

5. **Reflection is used when directing back what the nurse understands in regard to the client's ideas, feelings, questions, and content. Reflection is used to put the client's feelings in the context of when or where they occur.**

TEST-TAKING HINT: To answer this question correctly, the test taker must review therapeutic communication techniques and note the differences between restating and reflection.

6. Here the nurse is using the therapeutic communication technique of broad opening.
   1. **A broad opening helps the client to choose the topic of the conversation and puts the client in control of the content.**
   2. Presenting new ideas for consideration is the purpose of the therapeutic technique of suggesting. *Example:* "Have you considered the possibility of attending AA meetings?"

3. Conveying interest in what the client is saying is the purpose of the therapeutic technique of listening. *Example:* Being fully present and listening while maintaining eye contact.

4. Providing time for the nurse and client to gather thoughts and reflect is the purpose of the therapeutic technique of silence. The quiet is not broken, providing time for the nurse and the client to reflect.

TEST-TAKING HINT: To answer this question correctly, the test taker must be able to recognize the use of the therapeutic communication technique of broad opening.

7. Here the nurse is using the therapeutic communication technique of confronting.
   1. Here the nurse uses the therapeutic technique of suggesting to provide the client with suggestions for coping strategies and to assist the client in considering alternative options. This is not an example of confronting.
   2. The nurse uses the therapeutic technique of focusing to redirect the client to an idea of importance. This is not an example of confronting.
   3. **The nurse uses the therapeutic technique of confronting to bring incongruences or inconsistencies into awareness.**
   4. The nurse uses the therapeutic technique of restating to provide feedback to the client. Restating lets the client know that the nurse is attentive and that the message is understood. This is not an example of confronting.

TEST-TAKING HINT: To answer this question correctly, the test taker must be able to recognize the use of the therapeutic communication technique of confronting.

8. 1. This is an example of the therapeutic communication technique of focusing, not clarification. The nurse uses focusing to direct the conversation to a particular topic of importance or relevance to the client.
   2. **This example of clarification is an attempt by the nurse to check the nurse's understanding of what has been said by the client and helps the client to make their thoughts or feelings more explicit.**
   3. This is an example of the therapeutic communication technique of making observations, not clarification. This technique lets the client know that the nurse is attentive and aware of the client's situation, actions, and emotional expressions. It is the verbalization of what is perceived.

4. This is an example of the therapeutic communication technique of encouraging comparison, not clarification. This technique helps the client to note similarities and differences.

5. **This example of clarification is an attempt by the nurse to check the nurse's understanding of what has been said by the client and helps the client to make their thoughts or feelings more explicit.**

TEST-TAKING HINT: To answer this question correctly, the test taker must review therapeutic communication techniques to pair the technique presented in the question with the examples presented in the answer choices.

9. 1. In this statement, the nurse is lumping the client with "a lot of clients" and has belittled this individual client's feelings. Belittling is a nontherapeutic block to communication.

2. **By verbalizing the implication that the client thinks the medication is not good for the client's problem, the nurse puts into words what the nurse thinks that the client is saying. If the implication is incorrect, it gives the client an opportunity to clarify the statement further.**

3. By asking a "why" question, the nurse is requesting an explanation, which the client may not be able to give and which may put the client on the defensive in the process. Being asked for reasons for thoughts, feelings, or behaviors can be frustrating for the client and detrimental to the establishment of the nurse–client relationship. Requesting an explanation is a nontherapeutic block to communication.

4. This statement defends the physician. Defending, a nontherapeutic block to communication, is an attempt to protect someone or something from verbal attack and devalues the concerns of the client. Defending hampers the establishment of trust in the nurse–client relationship.

TEST-TAKING HINT: To answer this question correctly, the test taker must review the names and definitions of therapeutic communication techniques and be able to use them in situations.

10. 1. Giving advice is a nontherapeutic block to communication. By telling the client what to do, the nurse takes away the client's ability to sort out options and determine the pros and cons of various choices.

2. By indicating opposition to the client's ideas or opinions, the nurse is using the communication block of disagreeing.

3. Interpreting is a block to communication by telling the client the meaning of the client's experiences. This puts the control of the communication process in the hands of the nurse, rather than exploring and assessing the client's true meaning of what is being communicated.

4. **When using the therapeutic communication technique of voicing doubt, the nurse expresses uncertainty as to the reality of what is being communicated. Because denial is common in clients experiencing addiction, voicing doubt can be a useful tool to help the client face the reality of their situation.**

TEST-TAKING HINT: The test taker should review definitions and purposes of therapeutic communication techniques to answer this question correctly.

11. Exploring by the nurse helps the client to feel free to talk and examine issues in more depth. *Example:* "Tell me about what happened before your admission."

1. Broad opening by the nurse allows the client to take the initiative in introducing the topic and emphasizes the importance of the client's role in the interaction. *Example:* "Tell me what you're thinking."

2. Offering general leads by the nurse encourages the client to continue. *Example:* "Yes, I understand." "Go on." "And after that?"

3. **Focusing by the nurse allows the client to stay with specifics and analyze problems without jumping from subject to subject. *Example:* "Could we continue talking about your infidelity right now?"**

4. Accepting conveys to the client that the nurse comprehends the client's thoughts and feelings. This also is one of the ways that the nurse can express empathy. *Example:* "It sounds like a troubling time for you."

TEST-TAKING HINT: When answering an analogy, it is important to recognize the relationships between the subject matter within the question. In this question, delving further into a subject, idea, experience, or relationship is the definition of exploring.

12. By giving a broad opening, the nurse encourages the client to select topics for discussion. *Example:* "What are you thinking about?"

1. Focusing by the nurse allows a client to stay with specifics and analyze problems

without jumping from subject to subject. *Example:* "Could we continue talking about your infidelity right now?"

2. **Offering self** by the nurse offers the client availability and emotional support. *Example:* "I'll stay with you awhile."

3. Restating by the nurse repeats to the client the main thought that the client has expressed. *Example:* "You say that your mother abandoned you when you were 6 years old."

4. Giving recognition by the nurse is acknowledging something that is occurring at the present moment for the client. *Example:* "I see you've made your bed."

TEST-TAKING HINT: When answering an analogy, the test taker must be able to recognize the relationships between the subject matter within the question. In this question, allowing the client to take the initiative in introducing the topic is the definition of broad opening.

13. Silence by the nurse gives the client an opportunity to collect and organize thoughts, think through a point, or consider reprioritizing subject matter. *Example:* Sitting with a client and nonverbally communicating interest and involvement.

1. Focusing by the nurse allows a client to stay with specifics and analyze problems without jumping from subject to subject. *Example:* "Could we continue talking about your concerns with your family?"

2. Offering self by the nurse offers the client availability and emotional support. *Example:* "I'm right here with you."

3. Restating by the nurse repeats to the client the main thought expressed. *Example:* "You say that you're angry at your spouse?"

4. **Listening** by the nurse is the active process of receiving information and examining one's reaction to the messages received. *Example:* Maintaining eye contact, open posture, and receptive nonverbal communication.

TEST-TAKING HINT: When answering an analogy, it is important to recognize the relationships between the subject matter within the question. In this question, the nurse's lack of verbal communication for therapeutic reasons is the definition of silence.

14. 1. This exchange is not an example of the therapeutic communication technique of restatement. An example of restatement is, "You want to know how I feel about your refusing to attend group?"

2. Probing, a nontherapeutic block to communication, is the persistent questioning of the client and pushing for answers that the client does not wish to discuss. This exchange is not reflective of probing.

3. **Reflection** therapeutically directs back to the client their ideas, feelings, questions, and content. Reflection also is a good technique to use when the client asks the nurse for advice. This exchange is reflective of the therapeutic communication technique of reflection.

4. This exchange is not reflective of the nontherapeutic block to communication of interpreting. Interpreting seeks to make conscious that which is unconscious by telling the client the meaning of their experiences. An example of interpreting is, "What you're really asking is if I approve of your not attending group therapy." Nurses are not trained to use this technique. It is employed by therapists and psychiatrists.

TEST-TAKING HINT: To answer this question correctly, the test taker must be able to note the difference between reflection and restatement. If the same or similar words are repeated to the client, the nurse is using restatement. If the communication directs the statement or feeling back to the client, it is reflection.

15. 1. **This is a description of focusing, which is the therapeutic technique presented in the question. Focusing can be helpful when clients have scattered thoughts, flight of ideas, or tangential thinking.**

2. This is a description of the therapeutic technique of broad opening.

3. This is a description of the therapeutic technique of exploring.

4. This is a description of the nontherapeutic block to communication of probing, which pushes for answers the client may or may not wish to discuss.

TEST-TAKING HINT: To answer this question correctly, the test taker must be able to note the difference between focusing and exploring. When the nurse explores, the nurse is gathering information about the client's thoughts and feelings. Focusing is used to assist the nurse in gathering further information on a particular subject.

16. 1. This is an example of the nontherapeutic block to communication of probing. This

approach may put the client on the defensive and block further interaction. It would be better to say, "Tell me how your drinking is affecting your life."

2. **This is an example of the therapeutic technique of encouraging comparisons, which asks that similarities and differences be noted.**

3. This is an example of the nontherapeutic block to communication of approving/disapproving, which sanctions or denounces the client's ideas or behaviors. It would be better to say, "Let's explore ways that you can use to successfully stop drinking."

4. **This is an example of the therapeutic technique of focusing, which poses a statement that helps the client expand on a particular topic of importance.**

5. **This is an example of the therapeutic technique of placing the event in time or sequence, which clarifies the relationship of events in time so that the nurse and client can view them in perspective.**

TEST-TAKING HINT: To answer this question correctly, the test taker must review therapeutic and nontherapeutic communication techniques.

17. 1. This is an example of the therapeutic communication technique of seeking consensual validation, which searches for mutual understanding in the meaning of words.

2. **This is an example of the therapeutic communication technique of voicing doubt. Voicing doubt expresses uncertainty as to the reality of the client's perceptions and is often used with clients experiencing delusional thinking. Although it may feel uncomfortable, this is a necessary technique to present reality.**

3. This is an example of the therapeutic communication technique of verbalizing the implied. By using this technique, the nurse voices what the client has directly hinted at or suggested.

4. This is an example of the therapeutic communication technique of suggesting collaboration. The nurse uses this technique to attempt to work together with the client for the client's benefit.

TEST-TAKING HINT: To answer this question correctly, the test taker must recognize voicing doubt as a therapeutic communication technique.

Blocks to Therapeutic Communication

18. Reassuring and approving/disapproving are blocks to therapeutic communication. Reassurance by the nurse indicates to the client that there is no cause for anxiety. Devaluing the client's feelings may discourage the client from further expression of feelings. *Example:* "I wouldn't worry about that if I were you."

1. **Approving/disapproving is a nontherapeutic block to communication. It implies that the nurse has the right to pass judgment on whether the client's ideas or behaviors are good or bad. *Example:* "That's good. I'm glad that you . . ." or "That's bad. I'd rather you wouldn't . . ."**

2. Rejecting is a nontherapeutic block to communication. It occurs if the nurse refuses to consider or shows contempt for the client's ideas or behavior. *Example:* "Let's not discuss . . ." or "I don't want to hear about . . ."

3. Interpreting is a nontherapeutic block to communication. It involves seeking to make conscious that which is unconscious by telling the client the meaning of their experiences. *Example:* "What you really mean is . . ." or "On an unconscious level you really want to . . ."

4. Probing is a nontherapeutic block to communication. It involves persistently questioning the client and pushing for answers the client does not wish to reveal. *Example:* "Tell me how you feel about your mother now that she's dead."

TEST-TAKING HINT: When answering an analogy, it is important for the test taker to recognize the relationships between the subject matter within the question. In this question, indicating that there is no cause for anxiety is an example of reassuring so look for an example of approving/disapproving.

19. 1. This is an example of nonthreatening feedback. Nonthreatening feedback is therapeutic because it is descriptive rather than evaluative and focuses on the client's behavior, rather than personal characteristics of the client.

2. **This is an example of the nontherapeutic block to communication of requesting an explanation. It involves asking the client to provide reasons for thoughts, feelings, behaviors, and events. Asking why a client did something or feels a certain way can be intimidating and implies that the client must defend their behavior or feelings.**

3. This is an example of the nontherapeutic block to communication of belittling. Belittling minimizes the client's concerns and causes the client to feel insignificant or unimportant. When one is experiencing discomfort, it is no relief to hear that others are or have been in similar situations.

4. This is an example of the nontherapeutic block to communication of giving reassurance. Reassurance by the nurse indicates to the client that there is no cause for anxiety. By devaluing the client's feelings, the client may be discouraged from further expression of feelings.

5. This is an example of the therapeutic communication technique of reflection. Reflection is used when directing back what the nurse understands in regard to the client's ideas, feelings, questions, and content. Reflection is used to put the client's feelings in the context of when or where they occur.

TEST-TAKING HINT: To answer this question correctly, the test taker must review therapeutic and nontherapeutic communication techniques.

20. Challenging and probing are blocks to therapeutic communication. Challenging by the nurse puts the client on the defensive by calling into question the client's feelings and demanding proof of the client's statements. *Example:* "If you are dead, why is your heart still beating?"
    1. Advising by the nurse assumes that the "nurse knows best" and the client cannot think for themselves. *Example:* "I think you should . . ." or "Why don't you . . . ?"
    2. Defending by the nurse attempts to protect someone or something from verbal attack. It implies that the client has no right to express ideas, opinions, or feelings. *Example:* "I'm sure that your psychiatrist has only your best interests in mind."
    3. Rejecting occurs if the nurse refuses to consider or shows contempt for the client's ideas or behavior. *Example:* "Let's not discuss . . ." or "I don't want to hear about . . ."
    4. **Probing by the nurse involves persistently questioning the client and pushing for answers that the client does not wish to reveal.** *Example:* "Give me the details about your sexual abuse."

TEST-TAKING HINT: The test taker must understand that because probing causes the client to feel used and valued only for what is shared with the nurse, it is considered a block to therapeutic communication.

21. 1. This is an example of the nontherapeutic block to communication of approving/disapproving, which sanctions or denounces the client's ideas or behaviors.
    2. This is an example of the nontherapeutic block to communication of making stereotyped/superficial comments, which offers meaningless clichés or trite expressions.
    3. **This is an example of the nontherapeutic block to communication of giving reassurance. The use of this block indicates to the client that there is no cause for anxiety. This block involves giving the client a false sense of confidence and devaluing the client's feelings. It also may discourage the client from further expression of feelings if the client believes those feelings would only be downplayed or ridiculed.**
    4. When the nurse uses the nontherapeutic block to communication of giving advice, the nurse tells the client what to do. This implies that the nurse knows what is best and that the client is incapable of any self-direction.
    5. **This is an example of the nontherapeutic block to communication of giving reassurance. The use of this block indicates to the client that there is no cause for anxiety. This block involves giving the client a false sense of confidence and devaluing the client's feelings. It also may discourage the client from further expression of feelings if the client believes those feelings would only be downplayed or ridiculed.**

TEST-TAKING HINT: To answer this question correctly, the test taker must be familiar with the many blocks to therapeutic communication and be able to recognize the nontherapeutic block of giving reassurance.

22. 1. The nontherapeutic block to communication of indicating the existence of an external source attributes thoughts, feelings, and behavior to others or outside influences.
    2. The nontherapeutic block to communication of testing involves appraising the client's degree of insight. Testing the client is considered nontherapeutic except when conducting a mental status examination.

3. The nontherapeutic block to communication of challenging demands proof and may put the client on the defensive.

4. **Requesting an explanation is a nontherapeutic block to communication that involves asking the client to provide reasons for thoughts, feelings, behaviors, and events. Asking why a client did something or feels a certain way can be intimidating and implies that the client must defend their behavior or feelings.**

TEST-TAKING HINT: To answer this question correctly, the test taker must be familiar with the many blocks to therapeutic communication and be able to recognize the nontherapeutic block of requesting an explanation.

Therapeutic Communication Interventions

23. 1. Expressing uncertainty as to the reality of the client's perceptions is the therapeutic communication technique of voicing doubt. This technique is used most often when a client is experiencing delusional thinking, not frustration (as presented in the question).

2. **Putting into words what the client has only implied or said indirectly is the therapeutic communication technique of verbalizing the implied. This clarifies that which is implicit rather than explicit by giving the client the opportunity to agree or disagree with the implication.**

3. The nontherapeutic communication block of giving advice tells the client what to do or how to behave and implies that the nurse knows what is best. It also reinforces that the client is incapable of any self-direction. It nurtures the client in the dependent role by discouraging independent thinking.

4. The nontherapeutic communication block of defending attempts to protect someone or something from verbal attack. Defending does not change the client's feelings and may cause the client to think that the nurse is taking sides against the client.

TEST-TAKING HINT: To answer this question correctly, the test taker must be able to distinguish the use of therapeutic techniques and nontherapeutic communication blocks. The question is asking for a therapeutic

technique, so answers 3 and 4 can be eliminated immediately.

24. 1. **Respect is the responsive dimension that is presented in this example. Respect suggests that the client is regarded as a person of worth who is valued and accepted without qualifications.**

2. Empathetic understanding, not respect, is the responsive dimension that is presented in this example.

3. Genuineness, not respect, is the responsive dimension that is presented in this example.

4. Correctness, not respect, is the responsive dimension that is presented in this example.

TEST-TAKING HINT: To answer this question correctly, the test taker first must understand the nurse–client, communication-centered skill respect and then be able to choose the answer that exemplifies this term.

25. 1. **By understanding the client's point of view, the nurse communicates empathy with regard to the client's feelings. An empathic response communicates that the nurse is listening and cares and encourages the client to continue communicating thoughts and feelings.**

2. Asking "why" demands an answer to something that the client may not understand or know. "Why" questions can cause resentment, insecurity, and mistrust.

3. Sympathy is concern, sorrow, or pity felt for the client generated by the nurse's personal identification with the client's needs. Sympathy focuses on the nurse's feelings instead of the client's.

4. Offering reassurances not supported by facts or based in reality can do more harm than good. Although it may be intended kindly, it is often used to help the nurse avoid the client's personal distress.

TEST-TAKING HINT: The test taker first must review therapeutic communication techniques and nontherapeutic blocks to communication. The question is asking for a therapeutic statement that would "encourage further communication." Answers 2, 3, and 4 all are nontherapeutic communication blocks and can be eliminated.

26. 1. The nurse should maintain a professional relationship with the client. Although being friendly toward a client is appropriate, establishing a friendship is unprofessional.

2. When emotionally charged issues are dealt with by using humor, the response

may be viewed as minimizing the client's concerns and creating a barrier to further communication.

3. Emotionally charged topics should be approached with respectful, sincere interactions. Therapeutic communication techniques are specific responses that encourage the expression of feeling or ideas and convey the nurse's acceptance and respect. This acceptance and respect should not be negatively affected by maladaptive behaviors such as expressions of inappropriate anger.

4. Sympathy is a subjective look at another person's world that prevents a clear perspective of the issues confronting that person. Sympathy denotes pity, which should be avoided. The nurse should empathize, not sympathize, with the client.

TEST-TAKING HINT: To answer this question correctly, the test taker must understand how to address an angry and depressed client appropriately. The use of humor may minimize concern, and therefore answer 2 can be eliminated.

27. 1. Paraphrasing is briefly restating another's message using one's own words. Through paraphrasing, the nurse sends feedback that lets the client know that the nurse is actively involved in the search for understanding.

2. This response does not address the content of the client's statement. In addition, this probing question may be a barrier to further communication.

3. This confronting, judgmental response may put the client on the defensive, cutting off further communication.

4. This response is condescending, judgmental, and confrontational, putting the client on the defensive. It does not encourage further interactions.

TEST-TAKING HINT: To answer this question correctly, the test taker might want to look first at all the possible choices. Answer choice 4 is confrontational and can be eliminated first.

28. 1. Humor has a high potential for being misinterpreted as uncaring by individuals not involved in the situation. Humor used inappropriately can increase, suppress, or repress anger.

2. Humor is a distraction and is not effectively used to refocus a client's attention.

3. **Humor is an interpersonal tool, is a healing strategy, and assists in**

maintaining a balanced perspective. The nurse's goal in using humor is to bring hope and joy to the situation and to enhance the client's well-being and the therapeutic relationship.

4. Humor should not be used to delay dealing with the inevitable because procrastination increases stress and anxiety and prolongs the healing process.

TEST-TAKING HINT: The test taker must review the appropriate uses of humor to answer this question correctly.

29. The client in the question is exhibiting signs and symptoms of a manic episode associated with bipolar affective disorder.

1. It is important to note that the question is asking what the nurse is supposed to do during an intake assessment. Teaching during an intake assessment and when the client is exhibiting signs of mania and is unable to learn would be inappropriate.

2. Asking a broad opening question about what the client has been thinking about would not assist the nurse in gathering information specific to an intake assessment and is inappropriate for a client experiencing flight of ideas.

3. The nurse in this example is using the therapeutic communication technique of focusing. Focusing is an important facilitator when doing an assessment and when dealing with a client exhibiting flight of ideas.

4. The nurse in this example is using the therapeutic communication technique of general leads. Although this is a therapeutic communication technique, it is inappropriate to use when dealing with a client exhibiting signs of mania. It encourages the client to continue their scattered thought pattern and does not allow the nurse to gather the needed information for the intake assessment.

TEST-TAKING HINT: It is important when using therapeutic communication techniques that the test taker understands the circumstances in which they are used most effectively. Offering general leads may be used best in situations in which a client is less likely to talk, such as with a client diagnosed with major depression, and focusing would help when working with a client exhibiting flight of ideas.

30. 1. This is an example of giving recognition and does not encourage the client to elaborate further but reinforces to the client that the nurse notices the work that the client is doing.

2. **This is an example of restating and encourages the client to continue to talk about the topic being discussed. Restating lets the client know that the nurse has understood the expressed statement.**

3. This is an example of formulating a plan and does not encourage the client to elaborate further but does encourage the client to begin planning for discharge.

4. This is an example of encouraging evaluation. Although it can encourage the client to think about all aspects of a situation, it does not encourage the client to talk further about why the client is tired of taking the medication.

TEST-TAKING HINT: The test taker must review therapeutic communication skills and understand how the different techniques can assist the nurse in different situations.

31. 1. When a nurse communicates regard for the client as a person of worth who is valued and accepted without qualification, the nurse is using the communication-centered skill of respect. The characteristics presented in the question do not reflect the communication-centered skill of respect.

2. When a nurse communicates an understanding of the client's world from the client's internal frame of reference, with sensitivity to the client's feelings, the nurse is using the communication-centered skill of empathy. The characteristics presented in the question do not reflect the communication-centered skill of empathy.

3. **When a nurse communicates as an open person and is self-congruent, authentic, and transparent, the nurse is using the communication-centered skill of genuineness.**

4. When a nurse communicates specific terminology rather than abstractions in the discussion of client feelings, experiences, and behaviors, the nurse is using the communication-centered skill of correctness. The characteristics presented in the question do not reflect the communication-centered skill of correctness.

TEST-TAKING HINT: To answer this question correctly, the test taker must review responsive and action dimensions for therapeutic nurse–client relationships.

32. Aphasia is defined as the absence or the impairment of the ability to communicate through speech. Dysarthria is defined as difficult and defective speech because of impairment of the tongue or other muscles essential to speech.

1. Using simple sentences and avoiding long explanations is appropriate when the client is cognitively impaired. This client has difficulty with expression, not understanding.

2. Speaking to the client as though the client could hear is appropriate when trying to communicate with a client who is unresponsive but is inappropriate in this situation.

3. **Clients who cannot speak clearly require special thought and sensitivity. When a client has aphasia and dysarthria, the nurse needs to listen intently, allow time, and not interrupt the client. Effective communication is critical to nursing practice.**

4. Providing an interpreter or translator is appropriate when trying to communicate with a client who does not speak the same language as the nurse, but is inappropriate in this situation.

TEST-TAKING HINT: To answer this question correctly, the test taker first must understand the meaning of the medical terms *aphasia* and *dysarthria* in order to implement an appropriate intervention.

33. 1. This response avoids the client's feelings and may put the client on the defensive.

2. **This response recognizes the client's feelings of nervousness and encourages more communication with regard to the electroconvulsive therapy (ECT) procedure itself.**

3. This is a generalization that minimizes the client's concern and should be avoided.

4. This response offers false reassurance, which indicates that there is no need for anxiety, and discourages further discussions of thoughts and fears.

TEST-TAKING HINT: To answer this question correctly, the test taker must review communication techniques that encourage a client's expressions of anxiety.

34. The nursing student's question illustrates the nontherapeutic communication block of requesting an explanation.

1. **"Why" questions put the nurse in the role of an interrogator and can make the client defensive by demanding information without respect for the client's readiness or willingness to respond. It would be better to say, "Tell me about your concerns regarding your medications."**

2. The student's question did not invite the client to share personal experiences and feelings.

3. Recognizing and acknowledging reasons for actions describe the therapeutic technique of empathy. The student's statement was not empathic.
4. Taking notice of a single idea, or even a single word, and pursuing it until its meaning or importance is clear describes the therapeutic technique of focusing. The student did not use the technique of focusing.

TEST-TAKING HINT: To answer this question correctly, the test taker first must note the use of the nontherapeutic communication block of requesting an explanation in the student's statement. Then the test taker must understand the impact that the use of requesting an explanation has on developing a relationship with the client.

35. 1. Nonthreatening feedback gives information to clients about how they are being perceived by others. It should be presented in a manner that discourages defensiveness on the part of the client.
2. Nonthreatening feedback should be descriptive rather than evaluative and focused on client behaviors, not characteristics.
3. Nonthreatening feedback should be specific rather than general. Information that gives details about client behavior, rather than a generalized description, can be more effective in helping to modify behavior.
4. **Nonthreatening feedback should be directed toward behavior that the client has the capacity to modify. To provide feedback about a characteristic or situation that the client cannot change will only provoke frustration.**
5. Nonthreatening feedback should be well timed. Feedback is most useful when given at the earliest appropriate opportunity following the specific behavior.

TEST-TAKING HINT: To answer this question correctly, the test taker must understand the characteristics of nonthreatening feedback.

36. 1. **When the nurse focuses on the client's behavior rather than making assumptions about the client, the nurse is using nonthreatening feedback to facilitate the communication process.**
2. In this interchange, the nurse is labeling the client as manipulative. To provide nonthreatening feedback, manipulative behaviors should be addressed separately

from the individuality of the client. A better response would be, "I feel manipulated when you. . . ."
3. In this interchange, the nurse is focusing on the client's irresponsibility rather than separating the irresponsible behaviors from the individuality of the client. A better response would be, "Let's look at how your choices have affected your life. . . ."
4. In this interchange, the nurse is focusing on the client's drug-seeking behavior rather than separating the behavior from the individuality of the client. A better response would be, "Let's explore your need for medications every 2 hours. . . ."
5. **When the nurse focuses on the client's behavior rather than making assumptions about the client, the nurse is using nonthreatening feedback to facilitate the communication process.**

TEST-TAKING HINT: To answer this question correctly, the test taker must understand the reasoning behind addressing a client's inappropriate behaviors versus making value judgments about the individuality of the client.

37. 1. **Providing a private place and adequate time for successful interactions is essential to nonthreatening feedback.**
2. Inappropriate timing is not conducive to successful, open, complete, and accurate exchange of ideas.
3. Because this exchange occurs in the milieu, and there is no mention of providing privacy, this is an inappropriate place for feedback.
4. Discussion of this topic is inappropriate in a group setting.

TEST-TAKING HINT: To answer this question correctly, the test taker must remember that client security is a priority. To gain appropriate feedback, the nurse must provide privacy and adequate time and ensure client readiness.

Nonverbal Communication

38. 1. *Nonverbal communication* refers to messages sent by other than verbal or written means. It is estimated that more than half of all messages communicated are nonverbal, which include behaviors, cues, and presence.
2. Studies of interactions of people in North America indicate that a person has four zones of interaction defined by the distance between two people. The zones are defined

as public space, 12 feet; social space, 9 to 12 feet; personal space, 4 feet to 18 inches; and intimate space, closer than 18 inches. Some clients may feel that social interactions in a social space context are too invasive and cause discomfort, whereas other clients may interpret an interaction in this space as supportive.

3. Touch can convey warmth and positive regard but also may be interpreted in many other ways depending on the client's perception of the intended message.

4. **The physical space between two individuals has great meaning in the communication process. Space between two individuals gives a sense of their relationship and is linked to cultural norms and values.**

5. The use of silence varies across cultures; for instance, among some cultures, one stops talking when another starts, but in other cultures one does not stop speaking before the other begins. And in even other cultures, there may be a momentary pause between responses.

TEST-TAKING HINT: The test taker must note words such as *always, never, none,* and *all*. When superlatives such as these are used as part of an answer, the test taker should consider that this answer may be incorrect.

39. 1. When a nurse becomes uncomfortable by a client's invasion of personal space, the nurse should communicate this discomfort to the client in order to assist the client to recognize inappropriate spatial boundaries.

2. **The nurse should express feelings of discomfort and ask the client to move back. If the nurse allows the client to invade the nurse's personal space, the nurse has missed the opportunity to role-play appropriate interpersonal boundaries.**

3. Although different circumstances allow for different spatial boundaries, communication in a professional setting should be at a distance that provides comfort for the client and the nurse.

4. Although the nurse should set limits on inappropriate behaviors, threatening the client with seclusion would cause resentment and hostility. This action is inappropriate because the nurse must implement the least restrictive measure prior to initiating seclusion.

TEST-TAKING HINT: To answer this question correctly, the test taker must understand the appropriate interventions for clients who invade one's personal space. The nurse must

use the least restrictive measures first, so answer 4 can be eliminated.

40. 1. Agreeing or disagreeing sends the subtle message that the nurse has the right to make value judgments about client feelings. This is not an example of active listening.

2. Repeating everything that the client says is called "parroting." This is considered an automatic response and is not an example of active listening.

3. **Active listening does not always require a response by the nurse. Body posture and facial expression may be all that are required for the client to know that the nurse is listening and interested in what is going on with the client.**

4. Sympathy is a subjective look at another person's world that prevents a clear perspective of the issues confronting that person. This is not an example of active listening.

TEST-TAKING HINT: It is important for the test taker to understand that being attentive to what the client is saying verbally and nonverbally is the foundation for active listening.

41. 1. A measurement of length, width, and depth is the definition of *dimension* according to *Webster's Dictionary* and has nothing to do with the effect of environment on communication.

2. *Distance* is the means by which various cultures use space to communicate. The following are four kinds of distances: intimate distance, personal distance, social distance, and public distance.

3. *Territoriality* influences communication when an interaction occurs in the territory "owned" by one or the other. For example, a nurse may choose to conduct a psychosocial assessment in an interview room rather than the client's room.

4. Increased noise volume in the environment can interfere with receiving accurate incoming verbal messages.

5. *Density* refers to the number of people within a given environmental space and has been shown to influence interactions. Some studies show that high density is associated with aggression, stress, criminal activity, and hostility toward others.

TEST-TAKING HINT: To answer this question correctly, the test taker must note important words in the question, such as *environment*. Because dimension has nothing to do with the environment in which communication takes place, answer 1 can be eliminated.

Cultural Considerations

Cultural beliefs, customs, and behaviors vary from individual to individual within any given culture. The nurse must understand the effects of various cultural influences in order to deliver individualized client care.

42. 1. Religion and health practices are intertwined in some cultures, and the medicine man or woman, called a "shaman," may be part of the belief system. Refusing to allow the shaman to be a part of the client's health care may result in the client's refusing needed treatment.
    2. **Physicians may confer with a shaman regarding the care of hospitalized clients. The nurse should comply with the client's request and make contact with the shaman.**
    3. Acting in this manner shows disrespect for the client's culture and may result in the client's refusing needed treatment.
    4. Blaming the shaman for the client's condition would alienate the client and undermine the client's belief system.

TEST-TAKING HINT: To answer this question correctly, the test taker must analyze, compare, and evaluate worldviews to apply the concepts of culture to psychiatric/mental health nursing assessment and practice.

43. 1. Although any member of any cultural background may become obstinate and controlling, this behavior is not specifically associated with this client's Taoist philosophy.
    2. Magical healing is not traditionally associated with Taoist philosophy. When illness is encountered, traditions from some cultural groups may include massage, diet, rest, indigenous herbs, magic, and supernatural rituals.
    3. **Restoring the balance of yin and yang is a fundamental concept of Taoist philosophy. Yin and yang represent opposite forces of energy, such as hot/cold, dark/light, hard/soft, and masculine/feminine. The balance of these opposite forces restores health. In the question scenario, the client may believe that the warm ginger root tea will bring the forces of hot and cold into balance and relieve the headache symptoms.**
    4. There is no evidence that clients who adhere to a Taoist philosophy have adverse reactions to or show reluctance in taking pain medications.

TEST-TAKING HINT: To answer this question correctly, the test taker must analyze, compare, and evaluate worldviews to apply the concepts of culture to psychiatric/mental health nursing assessment and practice.

44. 1. **All cultures have past, present, and future time dimensions. It is important for a nurse to understand a client's time orientation. This client's concept of being punctual is perceived as less important than present-oriented activities, such as the client's visiting with their mother.**
    2. It is necessary for a nurse to understand that certain cultural groups operate in a present time dimension, and the fact that an individual does not show up at the designated time does not indicate passive-aggressive behavior. This information can be useful in planning a day of care, setting up appointments, and helping the client separate social and business priorities.
    3. There is not enough information given in the question to determine if this client rejects traditional medicine.
    4. This client's tardiness is part of a present time dimension and is not intended to reflect animosity, anger, or defiance.

TEST-TAKING HINT: It is important for the test taker to understand issues related to cultural time orientation to answer this question correctly.

45. *Kosher* refers to a diet that is clean or fit to eat according to Jewish dietary laws (Leviticus 11). The dietary laws forbid eating pork and crustaceans, such as shellfish, lobster, crab, shrimp, or crawfish.
    1. Alcohol, coffee, and tea (which contain caffeine) are considered taboo for members of the Mormon (the Church of Jesus Christ of Latter-day Saints) religion. For some Mormons, this taboo extends to cola and other caffeinated beverages, but usually not to chocolate. Members of the Mormon religion do not typically follow a halal diet.
    2. **In Arabic-speaking countries, the term *halal* refers to anything permissible under Islamic law. In the English language, it most frequently refers to food or dietary laws. Muslims who adhere to these dietary laws eat only meats that have been slaughtered according to traditional guidelines. Similar to Jewish dietary laws, Islamic law also forbids the consumption of pork.**

3. Though some Christian religions have dietary restrictions, Christians do not typically follow a halal diet.
4. Buddhism, in general, fundamentally prohibits *any* and *all* animal meat or intoxicants at all times. Buddhists do not typically follow a halal diet.

TEST-TAKING HINT: To answer this question correctly, the test taker must understand that there are religious dietary restrictions that must be considered when planning client care.

46. 1. Although this client may have a knowledge deficit related to the disease process experienced, this assessment is not from a cultural perspective.
2. Although this client may be experiencing denial related to imminent discharge, this assessment is not from a cultural perspective.
3. If this client is experiencing paranoid thoughts, imminent discharge may not be appropriate. Also, this assessment is not from a cultural perspective.
4. **Nonverbal communication is important among many cultures. Maintaining distance, avoiding direct eye contact, and silence should be evaluated through a cultural perspective in order to provide appropriate client care.**

TEST-TAKING HINT: To answer this question correctly, the test taker must analyze, compare, and evaluate worldviews to apply the concepts of culture to psychiatric/mental health nursing assessment and practice.

47. 1. Information about food allergies would have been presented in the question and provided to the nurse in the intake interview.
2. Information about vegetarianism would have been presented in the question and provided to the nurse in the intake interview.
3. **The practicing Orthodox Jewish client is following kosher dietary law, which forbids the consumption of pork, including ham. Judaism considers swine unclean.**
4. A practicing Orthodox Jewish client would not follow the dietary laws of Islam; however, pork also is forbidden according to Islamic dietary law.

TEST-TAKING HINT: It is important for the test taker to understand which foods and drinks are considered taboo and must be abstained from for religious or cultural reasons.

48. 1. Requesting an explanation by asking this client to provide reasons for this event might put the client on the defensive and close the door to further communication.
2. The nurse cannot assume that when a client is upset, they benefit from being alone. Although this sometimes may be the case, most distressed clients appreciate being listened to and allowed to verbalize their concerns.
3. Treating the client's symptoms with medications instead of exploring the underlying problem is of no value to the client and should be considered a counterproductive method of treatment.
4. **Sitting with a client and nonverbally communicating interest and involvement is a nonthreatening therapeutic technique that allows the client to be comfortably introspective and gives the client the opportunity to collect and organize thoughts.**

TEST-TAKING HINT: To answer this question correctly, the test taker must appreciate cultural diversity and recognize that being present and silent may offer the comfort that is needed.

49. 1. **Avoiding touching during initial interactions is the nurse's best response. This allows the nurse time to accurately evaluate the client's receptivity to touch.**
2. If touch is uncomfortable due to a client's cultural background, teaching this communication skill is inappropriate, as it denies their cultural diversity.
3. Talking about feelings related to touch would assist the client to express personal preferences related to this communication technique.
4. Wearing gloves would not affect a client's cultural response to therapeutic touch and may send a negative message that the nurse is avoiding skin-to-skin contact.

TEST-TAKING HINT: To answer culturally based questions, it is necessary to understand that the response to touch is often culturally defined.

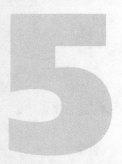

Legal and Ethical Considerations

KEYWORDS

The following words include English vocabulary, nursing/medical terminology, concepts, principles, or information relevant to content specifically addressed in this chapter or associated with topics presented in it. English dictionaries, your nursing textbooks, and medical dictionaries such as *Taber's Cyclopedic Medical Dictionary* are resources that can be used to expand your knowledge and understanding of these words and related information.

Advance directive

Against medical advice (AMA)

Assault

Autonomy

Battery

Beneficence

Breach of confidentiality

Committed

Confidentiality

Defamation of character

Durable power of attorney

Duty to warn

Elopement

Ethical egoism

False imprisonment

Federal law

Four-point restraints

Health-care proxy

Incompetent

Informed consent

Justice

Kantianism

Libel

Malpractice

National Alliance of the Mentally Ill (NAMI)

Nonmaleficence

Restraint

Seclusion

Slander

State law

Tarasoff ruling

Utilitarianism

Veracity

Voluntarily

QUESTIONS

Legal and Ethical Concepts

1. Which determines the scope of practice for a registered nurse employed in a psychiatric inpatient facility?
   1. National Alliance on Mental Illness (NAMI).
   2. State law, which may vary from state to state.
   3. Federal law, which applies nationwide.
   4. National League of Nursing (NLN).

2. The right to determine one's own destiny is to *autonomy* as the duty to benefit or promote the good of others is to:
   1. Nonmaleficence.
   2. Justice.
   3. Veracity.
   4. Beneficence.

3. Which statement reflects the ethical principle of utilitarianism?
   1. "The end justifies the means."
   2. "If you mean well, you will be justified."
   3. "Do unto others as you would have them do unto you."
   4. "What is right is what is best for me."

4. A nursing student observes an incorrect dosage of medication being given to a client receiving electroconvulsive therapy. To implement the ethical principle of veracity, which action would the nursing student take?
   1. Keep the information confidential to avoid harm to others.
   2. Inform the student's instructor and the client's primary nurse and document the situation.
   3. Tell only the client about the incident because the decision about actions would be determined only by the client.
   4. Because the client was not harmed, the incident would not need to be reported.

Safety Issues

5. A nurse is pulled from a medical/surgical floor to the psychiatric unit. Which of the following clients would the nurse manager assign to this nurse? **Select all that apply.**
   1. A chronically depressed client.
   2. An actively psychotic client.
   3. A client experiencing paranoid thinking.
   4. A client diagnosed with cluster B personality disorder traits.
   5. A client diagnosed with generalized anxiety disorder.

6. A nursing student states to the instructor, "I'm afraid of clients with mental illness. They are all violent." Which of the following statements would the instructor use to clarify this perception for the student? **Select all that apply.**
   1. "Even though most clients with a mental illness are violent, there are ways to de-escalate these behaviors."
   2. "A very few clients with mental illness exhibit violent behaviors."
   3. "There are medications that can be given to clients to prevent violent behaviors."
   4. "Only paranoid clients exhibit violent behaviors."
   5. "There is little difference in violence statistics between clients diagnosed with mental illness and the general population."

7. In which situation does a health-care worker have a duty to warn a potential victim?
   1. When clients manipulate and split the staff and are a danger to self.
   2. When clients curse at family members during visiting hours.
   3. When clients exhibit paranoid delusions and auditory or visual hallucinations.
   4. When clients make specific threats toward someone who is identifiable.

8. A client's spouse is visiting the client during visiting hours. A nurse walking by hears them verbally abuse the client. Which nursing response is appropriate?
   1. Ask the client to ask the spouse to leave the unit.
   2. Remind the client's spouse of the unit rules.
   3. Ask the spouse to come to the nurse's station to talk about their feelings.
   4. Sit with the client and the spouse to begin discussing anger issues.

Client Rights

9. On which client would a nurse on an inpatient psychiatric unit appropriately use four-point restraints?
   1. A client who is hostile and threatening the staff and other clients.
   2. A client who is intrusive and demanding and requires added attention.
   3. A client who is nonadherent with medications and treatments.
   4. A client who splits staff and manipulates other clients.

10. A client has been placed in seclusion because the client has been deemed a danger to others. Which is the priority nursing intervention for this client?
    1. Have little contact with the client to decrease stimulation.
    2. Provide the client with privacy to maintain confidentiality.
    3. Maintain contact and assure the client that seclusion will maintain the client's safety.
    4. Teach the client relaxation techniques and effective coping strategies to deal with anger.

11. Which of the following clients retain the right to give informed consent? **Select all that apply.**
    1. A 21-year-old who is hearing and seeing things that others do not.
    2. A 32-year-old who is diagnosed with severe intellectual development disorder.
    3. A 65-year-old declared legally incompetent.
    4. A 14-year-old with attention-deficit/hyperactivity disorder (ADHD).
    5. An 80-year-old who wants to participate in a medical research study.

12. A client has the right to treatment in the least restrictive setting. Number the following restrictive situations in the order of hierarchy from least restrictive to most restrictive.
    1. _____ Restriction of the ability to use money and control resources.
    2. _____ Restriction of emotional or verbal expression (censorship).
    3. _____ Restriction of decisions of daily life (what to eat, when to smoke).
    4. _____ Restriction of body movement (four-point restraints).
    5. _____ Restriction of movement in space (seclusion rooms, restrictions to the unit).

13. The treatment team is recommending disulfiram for a client who has had multiple admissions for alcohol detoxification. Which nursing question directed to the treatment team would protect this client's right to informed consent?
    1. "Does this client have the cognitive ability to be prescribed this medication?"
    2. "Will this client be adherent with this medication?"
    3. "Will the team be liable if this client is harmed by this medication?"
    4. "Is this the least restrictive means of meeting this client's needs?"

14. Which of the following clients does **not** have the ability to refuse medications or treatments? **Select all that apply.**
    1. An involuntarily committed client.
    2. A voluntarily committed client.
    3. A client who has been deemed incompetent by the court.
    4. A client who has a diagnosis of antisocial personality disorder.
    5. A client who is an imminent danger to self.

Voluntary and Involuntary Commitment

15. When a client makes a written application to be admitted to a psychiatric facility, which statement about this client applies?
    1. The client may retain none, some, or all civil rights depending on state law.
    2. The client cannot make discharge decisions. These are initiated by the hospital or court or both.
    3. The client has been determined to be a danger to self or others.
    4. The client makes decisions about discharge, unless they are determined to be a danger to self or others.

16. A client has been involuntarily committed to a psychiatric unit. During the delivery of the evening dinner trays, the client elopes from the unit, gets on a bus, and crosses into a neighboring state. Which nursing intervention is appropriate in this situation?
    1. Call the psychiatric facility located in the neighboring state and attempt to have that facility involuntarily admit the client.
    2. Notify the client's physician, follow facility policy, document the incident, and review elopement precautions.
    3. Send a therapeutic assistant out to relocate the client and bring them back to the facility.
    4. Notify the police in the neighboring state and have them pick the client up and readmit the client to the facility.

17. On an inpatient locked psychiatric unit, a newly admitted client requests to leave against medical advice (AMA). What should be the initial nursing action for this client?
    1. Tell the client that, because they are on a locked unit, they cannot leave AMA.
    2. Check the client's admission status and discuss the client's reasons for wanting to leave.
    3. In a matter-of-fact way, initiate room restrictions.
    4. Place the client on one-to-one observation.

Confidentiality

18. A nursing student uses a client's full name on an interpersonal process recording submitted to the student's instructor. What is the instructor's priority intervention?
    1. Reinforce the importance of accurate documentation, including the client's full name.
    2. Correct and remind the student of the importance of maintaining client confidentiality.
    3. Tell the student that because the client has been deemed incompetent, confidentiality is not an issue.
    4. Tell the student that because the client is involuntarily committed, confidentiality is not an issue.

19. The nurse is having a therapeutic conversation with a client in a locked inpatient psychiatric unit. The client states, "Please don't tell anyone about my sexual abuse." Which is the appropriate nursing response?
    1. "Yes, I will keep this information confidential."
    2. "All of the health-care team are focused on helping you. I will bring information to the team members that can assist them in planning your treatment."
    3. "Why don't you want the team to know about your sexual abuse? It is significant information."
    4. "Let's talk about your feelings about your history of sexual abuse."

20. Walking down the aisle of a local grocery store, a nurse encounters a client the nurse has recently cared for on an inpatient psychiatric setting. Which is the appropriate reaction by the nurse?
    1. Inquire how the former client is doing since discharge.
    2. Ignore the client to protect confidentiality.
    3. Talk to the client but refrain from using names.
    4. Make eye contact with the client, and if the client responds, respond back.

21. The phone rings at the nurse's station of an inpatient psychiatric facility. The caller asks to speak with Mr. Hawkins, a client in room 200. Which nursing response protects this client's right to autonomy and confidentiality?
    1. "I am sorry; you cannot talk to Mr. Hawkins."
    2. "I cannot confirm or deny that Mr. Hawkins is a client admitted here."
    3. "I'll see if Mr. Hawkins wants to talk with you."
    4. "I'm sorry; Mr. Hawkins is not taking any calls."

Potential Liability

22. Which of the following situations may put a nurse on an inpatient unit in legal jeopardy for battery? **Select all that apply.**
    1. A nurse threatens a client with bodily harm if the client refuses medications.
    2. A client is injured while being forcibly placed in four-point restraints because of low staffing.
    3. A nurse gives three times the ordered medication dosage because of a calculation error and does not report the incident, resulting in harm to the client.
    4. A client is held against their will because of medication nonadherence.
    5. A frustrated nurse pushes a client who refuses to take ordered medication.

23. A psychiatric nurse documents in a client's chart: "Seems to have no regard for legal or ethical standards. A problem client who needs constant limit setting." Which response by the nurse manager reflects the potential liability related to this entry?
    1. "Documenting this breaches the client's right to confidentiality."
    2. "Documenting this puts you at risk for malpractice."
    3. "Documenting this puts you at risk for defamation of character."
    4. "Documenting this breaches the client's right to informed consent."

24. Which of the following are examples of a situation that may lead to a nurse being sued for slander? **Select all that apply.**
    1. Documentation in the client's record that the client "has no moral or ethical principles and is probably stealing company material."
    2. Discussion with the client's family members, who are unaware of the information, about a DUI that the client has recently received.
    3. Talking about the client's behaviors in a crowded elevator on the way to lunch.
    4. Threatening a calm client with seclusion if the client does not take medications.
    5. Telling a reporter about a client's history of aggressive behavior.

Advance Directives

25. In which situation is there the potential for an advance directive not to be honored? **Select all that apply.**
    1. In an emergency situation in which the advance directive document is not readily available.
    2. When the advance directive states that there "will be no heroic measures used."
    3. When the health-care proxy is unsure of the client's wishes.
    4. When a client can no longer make rational decisions about their health care.
    5. When a state does not recognize the advance directive or durable power of attorney.

26. An unconscious client with a self-inflicted gunshot wound to the head is admitted. Family members allude to the existence of a living will in which the client mandates no implementation of life support. What is the legal obligation of the health-care team?
    1. Follow the family's wishes because of the family's knowledge of the living will.
    2. Follow the directions given in the living will because of mandates by state law.
    3. Follow the ethical concept of nonmaleficence and place the client on life support.
    4. Follow the ethical concept of beneficence, implementing lifesaving measures.

The correct answer number and rationale for why it is the correct answer are given in **boldface blue type**. Rationales for why the other answer options are incorrect are given as well, but they are not in boldface type.

Legal and Ethical Concepts

1. 1. National Alliance on Mental Illness (NAMI) is a group that advocates for clients experiencing mental illness. NAMI does not determine the scope of practice for a registered nurse employed in a psychiatric inpatient facility.
   2. **The legal parameters of professional nursing are defined within each state by the state's nurse practice act.**
   3. There is no federal law that determines the scope of practice for registered nurses even though the National Council of Licensure Examinations (NCLEX®) is a national standardized test that determines safety standards of nursing practice.
   4. National League of Nursing (NLN) accredits schools of nursing but does not determine the scope of practice for the nurse.

TEST-TAKING HINT: To answer this question correctly, the test taker should study and understand the legal parameters of a nurse's scope of practice as they are defined in each state's nurse practice act.

2. *Autonomy* respects individuals as rational agents able to determine their own destiny.
   1. *Nonmaleficence* is the requirement that health-care providers do no harm to their clients.
   2. *Justice* deals with the right of the individual to be treated equally regardless of race, sex, marital status, medical diagnosis, social standing, economic level, or religious belief.
   3. *Veracity* is the requirement that health-care providers always be truthful and not mislead.
   4. ***Beneficence* is the duty to benefit or promote the good of others.**

TEST-TAKING HINT: To answer this question correctly, the test taker must distinguish among the ethical principles of autonomy, beneficence, nonmaleficence, veracity, and justice.

3. 1. Utilitarianism is the theoretical perspective that bases decisions on the viewpoint that looks at the results of the decision. Action is taken on the basis of the results that produce the most good (happiness) for the most people, or in other words, "the end justifies the means."
   2. Kantianism holds that it is not the consequences or end results that make an action right or wrong; rather, it is the principle or motivation on which the action is based, or in other words, "if you mean well, you will be justified."
   3. Christian ethics treats others as moral equals. This is also known as the Golden Rule, or in other words, "do unto others as you would have them do unto you."
   4. Ethical egoism holds that what is right and good is what is best for the individual making the decision, or in other words, "what is right is what is best for me."

TEST-TAKING HINT: To answer this question correctly, the test taker must understand and be able to distinguish among various theories related to ethical behavior.

4. 1. Confidentiality of personal information is a client's right, but in this situation the ethical principle of veracity (truthfulness) should be applied.
   2. **By applying the ethical principle of veracity, the student should tell the truth and report and document the incident. The only limitation to the ethical principle of veracity is when telling the truth would knowingly produce harm. Veracity must be in the context of hospital policy and procedures and within the chain of command.**
   3. Autonomy is the ethical principle that presumes that an individual is capable of making independent choices for themself. In this situation, the nursing student autonomously takes responsibility for informing the client directly. The student should truthfully follow hospital protocol and maintain the chain of command.
   4. This action would violate the ethical principle of veracity and potentially violate the ethical principle of nonmaleficence, which requires that no harm be done to the client.

TEST-TAKING HINT: Understanding ethical principles and relating them to clinical situations assist the test taker in answering this question correctly.

Safety Issues

5. 1. Because there is no indication that this client is suicidal, of the five clients presented, this client is most appropriate to assign to the medical/surgical nurse.
   2. Special skill is needed to assess, empathize with, and redirect a client who is actively psychotic. This client would require a more experienced psychiatric nurse.
   3. Clients experiencing paranoid thinking may become aggressive, thinking that they need to defend themselves against attack. This client would require a more experienced psychiatric nurse and preferably a nurse with whom the client is familiar.
   4. Clients diagnosed with cluster B personality disorder traits can be manipulative and tend to split staff. These clients require a more experienced psychiatric nurse.
   5. Clients diagnosed with generalized anxiety disorder are typically not a danger to themselves or others and tend not to be manipulative. Of the five clients presented, this client is most appropriate to assign to the medical/surgical nurse.

TEST-TAKING HINT: In this question, the test taker should look for the client exhibiting the least complicated signs and symptoms or behaviors and consider safety.

6. 1. Only a few psychiatric clients are violent. The instructor's statement is based on false information.
   2. **It is true that a very few clients with mental illness exhibit violent behaviors.**
   3. There are medications that can be given to decrease anxiety and slow the central nervous system to calm a hostile and aggressive client. However, the instructor's statement does not clarify the student's misperception about violence and mental illness.
   4. Clients experiencing paranoid thinking can become violent because they think others may be hostile toward them, and they strike defensively. Clients with other diagnoses also may exhibit violent behaviors in certain circumstances. The instructor's statement does not clarify the student's misperception about violence and mental illness.
   5. **It is true that there is little difference in violence statistics between clients**

diagnosed with mental illness and the general population.

TEST-TAKING HINT: To answer this question correctly, the test taker must understand that most mentally ill clients are not violent.

7. Duty to warn was established by a landmark court case, *Tarasoff v. University of California* (usually called the Tarasoff ruling). This ruling established the responsibility of a treating mental health professional to notify an intended, identifiable victim.
   1. The nurse should set limits on clients who manipulate and split staff, and place clients who are a danger to themselves on suicide precautions. Duty to warn is not required in this situation.
   2. Limits should be set on inappropriate behaviors, but duty to warn is not required in this situation.
   3. The nurse should empathize and present reality to clients experiencing delusions or auditory or visual hallucinations. Duty to warn is not required in this situation.
   4. **When a client makes specific threats toward someone who is identifiable, it is the duty of the health-care worker to warn the potential victim. The nurse should bring this information to the treatment team and document the report.**

TEST-TAKING HINT: To choose the correct answer, the test taker must understand that a threat must be specific and an intended victim must be identifiable to implement duty to warn accurately.

8. 1. Placing the client in this situation is inappropriate. The nurse needs to ensure the milieu is safe for all clients and to act as the client's immediate advocate.
   2. **Reminding the client's spouse of the rules of the unit addresses the inappropriate behavior. If the spouse's behavior continues, it is the nurse's responsibility to ask the visitor to leave. The incident should be documented, and the treatment team should be notified.**
   3. The spouse is not the client, and it is not the nurse's responsibility to discuss their feelings at this time. If the client and spouse were in family therapy during the time of the incident, feelings would be discussed.
   4. To sit with the client and spouse to discuss angry feelings is inappropriate during visiting hours. Couples therapy would need to be approved by the client, and a release would need to be in place before the therapy session.

TEST-TAKING HINT: The test taker needs to recognize that it is the duty of the nurse to maintain a safe environment. Other interventions may be appropriate, but interventions related to safety must be prioritized.

Client Rights

9. All clients have the right to the least restrictive treatment. Restraints generally refer to a set of leather straps that are used to restrain the extremities of an individual whose behavior is out of control and who poses an inherent risk to the physical safety and psychological well-being of the individual, other clients, and staff.
   1. **When a client is hostile and threatening the staff and other clients, that client is a danger to others and, after attempts at de-escalation have failed, should be secluded and restrained.**
   2. A client can be intrusive and demanding, and require added attention without being a danger to self and others, which would require seclusion and restraint.
   3. Clients have the right to refuse treatments and medications. It would be unnecessary to seclude or restrain this client.
   4. A client can split staff and manipulate other clients without being a danger to self and others, which would require seclusion and restraint.

   TEST-TAKING HINT: To answer this question correctly, the test taker must understand that all attempts should be made to de-escalate hostile and threatening behaviors before secluding or restraining a client.

10. The nurse should focus on the client's behavior and seek interventions to assist the client in controlling the behavior in the future. Seclusion is a type of physical restraint in which the client is confined alone in a room from which they are unable to leave.
    1. This client has been put in seclusion because the client is a danger to others. The client needs constant monitoring, even in seclusion, to ensure their safety and the safety of others.
    2. Providing privacy in this situation is inappropriate. Because the client is a danger to others, the client needs constant observation. Confidentiality can be maintained without avoiding the client.
    3. **It is important to maintain contact with the client and assure the client that seclusion is a way to maintain the client's safety. Seclusion, when**

appropriate, should be implemented in a matter-of-fact manner, focusing on the client's behavior and the consequences of the behavior.
    4. When a client is in seclusion, the client is not in a readiness state to learn. When the hostility and threatening behavior are under control, this would be an appropriate intervention.

TEST-TAKING HINT: Answers 1 and 2 describe minimal nurse–client contact. The test taker should question any answer that avoids client contact. Because teaching is hampered by stress, answer 4 also can be eliminated.

11. A client's consent must be informed, competent, and voluntary. The goal of informed consent is to help clients make better decisions.
    1. **A diagnosis of psychosis does not mean that a client is unable to consent to treatment.**
    2. A client diagnosed with severe intellectual developmental disorder does not have the ability to give informed consent because of decreased cognitive abilities.
    3. When a client has been declared legally incompetent, the client cannot give informed consent. Informed consent could be obtained from a substitute decision maker.
    4. Minors cannot give informed consent. Informed consent could be obtained from a substitute decision maker, such as a parent or guardian.
    5. **Advanced age does not affect a client's ability to give informed consent.**

TEST-TAKING HINT: To answer this question correctly, the test taker must recognize that the diagnosis of intellectual developmental disorder, minor status, and incompetency determine a client's ability to give informed consent.

12. The order of hierarchy from least restrictive to most restrictive is 2, 1, 3, 5, 4.
    1. **The least restrictive situation would be the censorship of emotional or verbal expression.**
    2. **The next highest restrictive situation would be limitations on the ability to use money and control resources.**
    3. **The next highest restrictive situation would be limitations of the ability to make decisions of daily life such as what to eat and when to smoke.**
    4. **The next highest restrictive situation would include room seclusion, restriction to the unit, or both.**

5. The highest restrictive situation would involve the limitation of body movement by the application of four-point restraints.

TEST-TAKING HINT: To answer this question correctly, the test taker must recognize that clients have the right to the least amount of restriction necessary in any given situation. Restrictions are ordered on the basis of what rights the client forfeits because of the restriction.

13. 1. The ability to take disulfiram safely depends on a client's understanding of the effects of ingesting alcohol while taking disulfiram. If the client does not have the cognitive ability to understand the teaching related to disulfiram, the client could be placed at high risk for injury.
    2. Medication adherence is important to encourage, but this answer does not relate to informed consent.
    3. This statement does not relate to informed consent and is focused on the team rather than the client.
    4. There is nothing either physically or chemically restrictive related to the use of disulfiram.

TEST-TAKING HINT: To choose the correct answer, the test taker must determine which answer deals with the concept of informed consent.

14. 1. Involuntary commitment results in substantial restriction of the rights of the individual, but protection against loss of liberty and due process is retained. Involuntarily committed clients can refuse medications unless they are an imminent danger to themselves or others.
    2. A voluntarily committed client makes direct application to an institution for services and may stay as long as treatment is deemed necessary. Voluntarily committed clients can refuse medications.
    3. When a client is declared incompetent, the client has a mental disorder resulting in a defect in judgment, and this defect makes the client incapable of handling personal affairs. A guardian is appointed. The guardian makes decisions for the client, and the client loses the right to refuse medications.
    4. Although clients diagnosed with antisocial personality disorder often need limit setting, unless they are an imminent danger to self or others, they can refuse their medications.

5. When a client is declared an imminent danger to self or others, they lose the ability to refuse medications or treatments.

TEST-TAKING HINT: To answer this question correctly, the test taker must understand that the ability to refuse medications or treatments does not depend on voluntary or involuntary admission status.

Voluntary and Involuntary Commitment

15. Because this client's admission is based on the client's making a written application for admission, this client's admission status is voluntary.
    1. When a client is involuntarily committed, the client may retain none, some, or all of their civil rights, depending on state law. With a voluntary admission, all rights are retained.
    2. Discharge decisions are initiated by the hospital or court, or both, but not by the client when a client is involuntarily admitted. With voluntary admission, however, discharge is initiated by the client unless the client has been deemed by the treatment team as a danger to self or others.
    3. If the client has been determined to be a danger to self or others, the client would be admitted involuntarily.
    4. A voluntarily admitted client can make decisions about discharge unless the client has been determined to be a danger to self or others. If the treatment team determines that a voluntarily admitted client is a danger to self or others, the client is held for a court hearing, and the client's admission status is changed to involuntary.

TEST-TAKING HINT: Understanding that the criterion for involuntary admission or commitment is danger to self or others assists the test taker in eliminating answer 3.

16. When a state court rules that a client be involuntarily committed to psychiatric care, the ruling applies only to the state in which the court ruling occurred. If a client crosses state lines, the court ruling does not apply in a different state.
    1. Because the court ruling applies only in the original state that issued the ruling, this would not be an appropriate intervention.
    2. Elopement occurs when a client leaves the hospital without permission. In this situation, all the nurse can do is notify

the client's physician, follow facility policy, and document the incident. Elopement precautions should be reviewed and actions taken to prevent a future occurrence.
3. It is not within the scope of practice of the therapeutic assistant to search for the missing client and bring the client back to the facility.
4. Because the court ruling applies only in the original state that issued the ruling, this would not be an appropriate intervention.

TEST-TAKING HINT: To answer this question correctly, the test taker must understand that the court ruling applies only in the original state that issued the ruling.

17. 1. Unless the client is a danger to self or others, the client may leave a locked unit against medical advice (AMA).
    2. It is important for the nurse to know the admission status of this client. If the client is involuntarily admitted, the client is unable to leave the facility. If the client is voluntarily admitted, the client may leave AMA unless the treatment team has determined that the client is a danger to self or others.
    3. Initiation of room restrictions may be appropriate, depending on the client's behavior and admission status, but it would not be the initial action of the nurse.
    4. A client is placed on one-to-one observation when the client is considered a danger to self or others. This has not been established.

TEST-TAKING HINT: The test taker must understand that the nurse needs information about a client's admission status to determine appropriate interventions and actions. The keyword *initial* determines the answer to this question. Because assessment is the first step in the nursing process, initial actions of the nurse often refer to nursing assessments.

Confidentiality

18. A student's clinical paperwork is taken outside of the clinical setting and submitted to instructors. The student's family members and others could see the client's name on this paperwork. This is a breach of confidentiality.
    1. Accurate documentation is important, but the priority intervention of the instructor here is to make the student aware of the student's breach of confidentiality.

2. It is the priority intervention of the instructor to correct and remind the student of the importance of maintaining client confidentiality. The instructor should advise the student to use only client initials on any student paperwork.
3. Clients who have been deemed incompetent by the courts still have the right to confidentiality.
4. Clients who have been involuntarily committed by the courts still have the right to confidentiality.

TEST-TAKING HINT: To answer this question correctly, the test taker must realize that confidentiality can be breached unintentionally by the use of client names on student clinical paperwork or any other documentation taken home from the clinical facility (e.g., laboratory value lists or medication lists).

19. 1. The nurse, as a member of the client's treatment team, is obligated to bring any significant client information to the team. The nurse cannot promise to keep this important information secret.
    2. The nurse is being honest and open with the client and giving information about the client focus of the treatment team. This builds trust and sets limits on potentially manipulative behavior by the client.
    3. By requesting an explanation from the client, the nurse may put the client on the defensive. This hinders the building of a trusting relationship.
    4. Although talking about feelings is a positive intervention, in this situation, the nurse needs to deal with the concerns of the client and give information about the function of the treatment team.

TEST-TAKING HINT: To answer this question correctly, the test taker must understand that confidentiality does not apply within the context of the client's treatment team. The sharing of information within the treatment team benefits the client.

20. Client confidentiality can be easily and unconsciously breached in social and professional settings. Although public understanding of mental illness has evolved over the years, there continues to be stigmatization of the mentally ill. Consequently, it is critical to maintain client confidentiality.
    1. By inquiring how the former client is doing, the nurse has potentially breached confidentiality. If someone in the store knows that the nurse works in a psychiatric

setting, that person could make this connection and assume that the client has required psychiatric care.

2. By ignoring the client, the nurse may block any communication in which the client may wish to engage.

3. By talking with the client, recognition is established, and a potential breach of confidentiality has occurred.

4. **By making eye contact and waiting for a response from the client, the nurse has placed the control of the encounter with the client. The client then decides whether any communication should occur, and the client decides confidentiality issues.**

TEST-TAKING HINT: When confidentiality is addressed in a question, the test taker should choose the most conservative approach presented in the answer choices. In this case, any recognition of the client by the nurse could breach confidentiality.

21. 1. By stating that the caller could not speak to Mr. Hawkins, the nurse has indirectly informed the caller that Mr. Hawkins is on the unit.

2. **This statement gives no information related to the presence of the client at the facility. This statement maintains the client's right to confidentiality.**

3. This statement directly gives the caller information about the client's presence at an inpatient facility and breaches confidentiality.

4. This statement directly gives the caller information about the client's presence at an inpatient facility and breaches confidentiality.

TEST-TAKING HINT: To answer this question correctly, the test taker should consider how the nurse can directly and indirectly provide confidential information about a client.

Potential Liability

22. 1. This is an example of assault. Assault is an act that results in a person's genuine fear and apprehension that they will be touched without consent.

2. **This is an example of battery. Battery is the touching of another person without consent.**

3. This is an example of malpractice. Malpractice is conduct that falls below the legal standard established to protect others against unreasonable risk of harm.

4. This is an example of false imprisonment. False imprisonment is the deliberate and unauthorized confinement of a person within fixed limits by the use of verbal or physical means.

5. **This is an example of battery. Battery is the touching of another person without consent.**

TEST-TAKING HINT: Assault and battery are commonly confused. Assault is a threat, and battery is actual contact.

23. 1. This charting entry is not related to a potential breach-of-confidentiality issue.

2. Malpractice is negligence or incompetence on the part of a professional that causes harm to the client. Malpractice is not addressed in this charting entry.

3. **When information is shared that could be detrimental to a client's reputation, the nurse may be at risk for defamation of character. Information documented in a chart should reflect objective findings, not the nurse's perception of a client.**

4. Informed consent is related to the preservation and protection of individual autonomy in determining what will and will not happen to the person's body. This charting entry does not relate to informed consent.

TEST-TAKING HINT: To answer this question correctly, the test taker first must recognize the charting entry as inappropriate, subjective data and then understand the legal ramification of defamation of character as it relates to documenting client information.

24. 1. **This is an example of libel. Libel is the sharing of information in writing that could be detrimental to the client's reputation.**

2. **This is an example of slander. Slander is sharing of information orally that could be detrimental to the client's reputation.**

3. This is an example of a breach of confidentiality.

4. This is an example of assault. Assault is an act that results in a person's genuine fear and apprehension that they will be touched without consent.

5. **This is an example of slander. Slander is sharing of information orally that could be detrimental to the client's reputation.**

TEST-TAKING HINT: Libel and slander are commonly confused. Libel is the sharing of information in writing, whereas slander is the sharing of information orally.

Advance Directives

25. An advance directive refers to either a living will or a durable power of attorney for health care. Clients who have chronic mental illness can use advance directives. The client's wishes for health-care treatment are documented when the client's thought processes are under control and implemented when the client is having an exacerbation of their illness and does not have the insight needed to make rational decisions related to treatment.
    1. **If the advance directive document is not readily available, it may not be honored by the health-care team caring for the client.**
    2. **Advance directives must be specific in the directions related to care. Stating that there "will be no heroic measures used" is vague and may be challenged by the health-care team caring for the client.**
    3. **If the health-care proxy (the individual assigned by the client to carry out the client's wishes) is unsure of the client's wishes, the advance directive can be challenged.**
    4. An advance directive is implemented when the client no longer can make rational decisions about health care.
    5. Every state has enacted legislation that allows individuals to execute living wills or durable powers of attorney for health care.

    TEST-TAKING HINT: To choose the correct answer, the test taker needs to understand the criteria that must be met for an advance directive to be honored.

26. 1. Because there is no legal document to which the health-care team can refer, it is the legal obligation of the health-care team to benefit or promote the good of this client by placing the client on life support. If a legal document can be produced, and the family members agree, a decision may be made later to remove life support.
    2. There is not a living will to refer to in this situation. If there was, state law would mandate adherence to the client's wishes, legally recorded in the document.
    3. The ethical principle of nonmaleficence requires that health-care workers do no harm to their clients, either intentionally or unintentionally. Because there is nothing in the question that indicates that the health-care team is considering actions that potentially may harm the client, this does not apply.
    4. **Beneficence is the duty to benefit or promote the good of others. Because no legal document has been produced that would indicate the client's wishes to the contrary, it is the legal responsibility of the health-care team to initiate life-support measures.**

    TEST-TAKING HINT: To answer this question correctly, the test taker must understand that if documentation of an advance directive cannot be produced, the health-care team should default to the ethical principle of beneficence and maintain life support.

Management of Care for Individuals With Psychiatric Disorders

Stress Adaptation, Trauma, and Related Disorders

6

KEYWORDS

The following words include English vocabulary, nursing/medical terminology, concepts, principles, or information relevant to content specifically addressed in this chapter or associated with topics presented in it. English dictionaries, your nursing textbooks, and medical dictionaries such as *Taber's Cyclopedic Medical Dictionary* are resources that can be used to expand your knowledge and understanding of these words and related information.

Adaptive

Adjustment disorders

Compensation

Conscious

Coping

Defense mechanism

Denial

Displacement

Ego

Ego defense

Erikson's stages of development

Id

Identification

Intellectualization

Introjection

Isolation

Maladaptive

Posttraumatic stress disorder (PTSD)

Prodromal syndrome

Projection

Rationalization

Reaction formation

Regression

Repression

Stress adaptation

Sublimation

Superego

Suppression

Survivor's guilt

Symbolization

Temperament

Unconscious

Undoing

QUESTIONS

Theory

1. A client on an inpatient psychiatric unit has impulse control issues and at times can be irritable and hostile with little regard for others. Using psychoanalytic theory, which describes this behavior?
   1. The behavior is id driven.
   2. The behavior is ego driven.
   3. The behavior is superego driven.
   4. The behavior is ego-ideal driven.

2. A client on an inpatient psychiatric unit is exhibiting extreme agitation. Using a biological approach, which nursing intervention should be implemented?
   1. The nurse should discuss emotional triggers that precipitate angry outbursts.
   2. The nurse should encourage the client to use exercise to deal with increased agitation.
   3. The nurse should give ordered prn medications to decrease anxiety and agitation.
   4. The nurse should develop a plan to address tension during family therapy.

3. A client on an inpatient psychiatric unit is exhibiting extreme agitation. Using a behavioral approach, which nursing intervention should be implemented?
   1. The nurse should role-play stressful situations to promote adaptive coping.
   2. The nurse should develop a plan to deal with stressors during a family meeting.
   3. The nurse should give ordered prn medications to decrease agitation.
   4. The nurse should discuss emotional triggers that precipitate angry outbursts.

4. Which client statement indicates that the client understands the term *temperament?*
   1. "I understand that my behaviors have affected my development, so I need to work hard now to fix the problem."
   2. "I was born 'cranky,' and this continues to affect how I relate to others."
   3. "The way I perceive, relate to others, and think of myself in social and personal situations makes up my temperament."
   4. "My childhood really affected my ability to develop an appropriate temperament."

5. An 88-year-old client on an inpatient psychiatric unit states, "My children are refusing to visit me. I feel like giving up." This client has a deficit in which of Erikson's stages of development?
   1. Initiative versus guilt.
   2. Industry versus inferiority.
   3. Identity versus role confusion.
   4. Integrity versus despair.

6. A client exhibits a pattern of terminating relationships with significant others and poor self-esteem. Using Sullivan's interpersonal theory, what major developmental state is this client struggling to master?
   1. Late adolescence.
   2. Early adolescence.
   3. Preadolescence.
   4. Juvenile.

7. A client diagnosed with posttraumatic stress disorder (PTSD) is close to discharge. Which client statement would indicate that teaching about the psychosocial cause of PTSD was effective?
1. "My experience, how I deal with it, and my support system all affect my disease process."
2. "I have learned to try and avoid stressful situations as a way to decrease my emotional pain."
3. "So, natural opioid released during the trauma caused my body to become 'addicted.'"
4. "Because of the trauma, I have a negative perception of the world and feel hopeless."

8. Counselors have been sent to a location that has experienced a natural disaster to assist the population in dealing with the devastation. This is an example of _____ prevention.

Ego Defense Mechanisms

9. A client has been fired from work because of downsizing. Although clearly upset, when explaining the situation to a friend, the client states, "Imagine what I can do with this extra time." Which defense mechanism is this client using?
1. Denial.
2. Intellectualization.
3. Rationalization.
4. Suppression.

10. Which best exemplifies a client's use of the defense mechanism of reaction formation?
1. A client feels rage at being raped at a young age, which later is expressed by joining law enforcement.
2. A client is unhappy about being a parent, although others notice how much attention the client gives their child.
3. A client is drinking six to eight beers a day while still attending Alcoholics Anonymous and functioning as a group leader.
4. A client is angry that the call bell is not answered and decides to call the nurse when it is unnecessary.

11. Which best exemplifies an individual's use of the defense mechanism of compensation?
1. A person feels unattractive but decides to pursue fashion design as a career.
2. A shy person who abuses alcohol tells others that alcohol helps them overcome their shyness.
3. A poorly paid employee consistently yells at their assistant for minimal mistakes.
4. A teenager injures an ankle playing basketball and curls into a fetal position to deal with the pain.

12. Which best exemplifies the use of the defense mechanism of sublimation?
1. A child who has been told by parents that stealing is wrong reminds a friend not to steal.
2. A person who loves sports but is unable to play decides to become an athletic trainer.
3. Having chronic asthma with frequent hospitalizations, a young child admires their nurses. That child later chooses nursing as a career.
4. A child who feels angry and hostile decides to become a mental health therapist to help others.

13. A nursing instructor is teaching about defense mechanisms. Which of the following student statements indicate that learning has occurred? **Select all that apply.**
    1. "Defense mechanisms are used when anxiety increases and the strength of the ego is tested."
    2. "All individuals who use defense mechanisms as a means of stress adaptation exhibit healthy egos."
    3. "When defense mechanisms are overused or maladaptive, unhealthy ego development may result."
    4. "Defense mechanisms are used only by individuals with mental illness to assist them in coping with the stressors of life."
    5. "At times of mild to moderate anxiety, defense mechanisms are used adaptively to deal with stress."

14. A client is admitted to the emergency department after a car accident but does not remember anything about it. The client is unconsciously using which defense mechanism?
    1. Undoing.
    2. Rationalization.
    3. Suppression.
    4. Repression.

15. A client in the emergency department was violently attacked and raped. When discussing the incident with the nurse, the client shows no emotion related to the event. Which defense mechanism is the client exhibiting?
    1. Isolation.
    2. Displacement.
    3. Compensation.
    4. Regression.

16. After failing an examination, a physician in their psychiatric residency begins smoking a pipe and growing a beard to look like Sigmund Freud. The nurse manager, realizing the physician's insecurities, recognizes the use of which defense mechanism?
    1. Identification.
    2. Repression.
    3. Regression.
    4. Reaction formation.

17. Which situation reflects the defense mechanism of projection?
    1. A person has an extramarital affair, then buys their spouse a diamond anniversary bracelet.
    2. A promiscuous spouse accuses the other spouse of having an affair.
    3. A spouse who is unable to become pregnant works harder at becoming teacher of the year.
    4. A person who was sexually assaulted as a child remembers nothing of the event.

18. Which situation reflects the defense mechanism of denial?
    1. When a client's twin sibling excels in golf, the client begins lessons with a golf pro.
    2. After a parent spanks their child for misbehaving, the child pulls the cat's tail.
    3. After years of excessive drinking, the client fails to acknowledge a problem.
    4. The client who has been given a diagnosis tells their family that 50% of people with that diagnosis survive.

19. During visiting hours, a client who is angry at their ex-spouse's charges of child neglect expresses this anger by lashing out at their sister-in-law. The nurse understands that the client is demonstrating the use of which defense mechanism?
    1. Denial.
    2. Projection.
    3. Displacement.
    4. Rationalization.

Nursing Process—Assessment

20. A person who expected a scholarship is jealous of their best friend for winning the same scholarship. The person agrees to meet their friend for lunch and then arrives 1 hour late, apologizing, and begging forgiveness. The person is displaying which behavior?
1. Self-assertion.
2. Passive-aggressiveness.
3. Splitting.
4. Omnipotence.

21. Which of the following are examples of cognitive responses to mild levels of anxiety? **Select all that apply.**
1. Increased respirations.
2. Feelings of horror or dread.
3. Pacing the hall.
4. Increased concentration.
5. Heightened alertness.

22. Which is an example of a behavioral response to a moderate level of anxiety?
1. Narrowing perception.
2. Heart palpitations.
3. Limited attention span.
4. Restlessness.

23. Which is an example of a physiological response to a panic level of anxiety?
1. Inability to focus.
2. Loss of consciousness.
3. Dilated pupils.
4. Possible psychosis.

24. A nurse on an inpatient psychiatric unit is assessing a client at risk for acting-out behaviors. Which of the following behavioral symptoms would the nurse expect to be exhibited? **Select all that apply.**
1. Invasion of personal space.
2. Flushed face.
3. Increased anxiety.
4. Misinterpretation of stimuli.
5. Pacing the halls.

25. Which of the following medical diagnoses can be affected by psychological factors? **Select all that apply.**
1. Cancer.
2. Asthma.
3. Coronary artery disease.
4. Upper respiratory tract infection.
5. Sepsis.

26. Which would the nurse expect to assess in a client with long-term maladaptation to stressful events?
1. Diarrhea.
2. Pulse 100, blood pressure 150/94 mm Hg.
3. Profuse diaphoresis.
4. Ulcerative colitis.

27. At an outpatient obstetric clinic, a pregnant client receiving public assistance exhibits extreme anxiety when discussing a failure in school. This is an example of which type of crisis?
1. Dispositional crisis.
2. Crisis of anticipated life transition.
3. Maturational/developmental crisis.
4. Crisis reflecting psychopathology.

28. The nurse should assess which of the following client behaviors when completing a risk assessment? **Select all that apply.**
    1. Past history of violence.
    2. Disturbed thought process.
    3. Invasion of personal space.
    4. Flushed face.
    5. Self-mutilation.

29. On an inpatient psychiatric unit, a nurse is completing a risk assessment on a newly admitted agitated client. Which expressed client symptom would the nurse categorize as cognitive?
    1. Incarceration for fighting.
    2. Paranoid delusions.
    3. History of throwing objects on the unit.
    4. Reddened face.

30. A client diagnosed with posttraumatic stress disorder (PTSD) states to the nurse, "All those wonderful people died, and yet I was allowed to live." Which is the client experiencing?
    1. Denial.
    2. Social isolation.
    3. Anger.
    4. Survivor's guilt.

31. Which of the following would the nurse expect to assess in a client diagnosed with posttraumatic stress disorder (PTSD)? **Select all that apply.**
    1. Dissociative events.
    2. Intense fear and helplessness.
    3. Excessive attachment and dependence toward others.
    4. Full range of affect.
    5. Avoidance of activities that are associated with the trauma.

32. When treating individuals with posttraumatic stress disorder (PTSD), which variable is included in the recovery environment?
    1. Degree of ego strength.
    2. Availability of social supports.
    3. Severity and duration of the stressor.
    4. Amount of control over recurrence.

33. A newly admitted client is diagnosed with posttraumatic stress disorder (PTSD). Which behavioral symptom would the nurse expect to assess?
    1. Recurrent, distressing flashbacks.
    2. Intense fear, helplessness, and horror.
    3. Diminished participation in significant activities.
    4. Detachment or estrangement from others.

Nursing Process—Diagnosis

34. A client is experiencing a high level of occupational stress and has a history of migraine headaches. Which nursing diagnosis takes priority?
    1. Pain.
    2. Anxiety.
    3. Activity intolerance.
    4. Ineffective role performance.

35. Which nursing diagnosis takes priority when a client experiences an acute asthma attack precipitated by the death of the client's parent?
    1. Anxiety R/T loss AEB increased respirations.
    2. Impaired gas exchange R/T stress AEB decreased O_2 saturation levels.
    3. Risk for suicide R/T grief.
    4. Ineffective coping R/T grief AEB psychosomatic complaints.

36. A client has a nursing diagnosis of knowledge deficit R/T relationship of anxiety to hypertension. Which intervention addresses this client's problem?
    1. Assess the client for suicidal or homicidal ideations.
    2. Encourage the client to verbalize feelings about anxiety.
    3. Role-play situations in which anxiety is experienced.
    4. Teach the client about the mind-body connection.

37. A client with rigid posture and raised voice uses profanity while demanding to use the phone. Which correctly written nursing diagnosis is a priority?
    1. Risk for injury toward others R/T anxiety AEB rigid posture and profanity.
    2. Ineffective coping R/T inability to express feelings AEB aggressive demeanor.
    3. Disturbed thought process R/T altered perception AEB demanding behaviors.
    4. Social isolation R/T anger AEB inability to get along with staff.

38. In group therapy, an angry client becomes increasingly restless and irritable and shouts at the facilitator. Which nursing diagnosis takes priority?
    1. Risk for violence toward others R/T inability to deal with frustration.
    2. Ineffective coping R/T inability to express feelings AEB raised voice.
    3. Anxiety R/T topic at hand AEB restlessness in group therapy.
    4. Social isolation R/T intimidation of others AEB solitary activities.

39. A newly admitted client diagnosed with posttraumatic stress disorder (PTSD) is exhibiting recurrent flashbacks, nightmares, sleep deprivation, and isolation from others. Which nursing diagnosis takes priority?
    1. Posttrauma syndrome R/T a distressing event AEB flashbacks and nightmares.
    2. Social isolation R/T anxiety AEB isolating because of fear of flashbacks.
    3. Ineffective coping R/T flashbacks AEB inappropriate use of alcohol.
    4. Risk for injury R/T exhaustion because of sustained levels of anxiety.

Nursing Process—Planning

40. On an inpatient unit, a client is isolating self in a room and refusing to attend group therapy. Which is an appropriate, correctly written short-term outcome for this client?
    1. Client participation will be expected in one group session.
    2. Provide opportunities for the client to increase self-esteem by discharge.
    3. The client will interact with staff by the end of the 3 to 11 shift.
    4. The client will demonstrate socialization skills when in the milieu.

41. A hospitalized client diagnosed with posttraumatic stress disorder (PTSD) has a nursing diagnosis of ineffective coping R/T history of rape AEB abusing alcohol. Which is the expected short-term outcome for this client problem?
    1. The client will recognize triggers that precipitate alcohol abuse by day 2.
    2. The client will attend follow-up weekly therapy sessions after discharge.
    3. The client will refrain from self-blame regarding the rape by day 2.
    4. The client will be free from injury to self throughout the shift.

42. A client on an inpatient psychiatric unit is sarcastic to staff and avoids discussions in group therapy. Which correctly written short-term outcome is appropriate for this client?
    1. The client will not injure self or anyone else.
    2. The client will express feelings of anger in group therapy by end of shift.
    3. The client will take responsibility for their own feelings.
    4. The client will participate in outpatient group therapy after discharge.

Nursing Process—Implementation

43. Which of the following interventions should the nurse include when caring for a client experiencing migraine headaches? **Select all that apply.**
    1. Monitor pain level using a pain scale.
    2. Explore with the client how stress may trigger this disorder.
    3. Encourage the client to note patterns of exacerbation triggers by journaling.
    4. Assess for suicidal ideations.
    5. Administer divalproex sodium as prescribed.

44. A client has been diagnosed with an exacerbation of tension headaches. Which of the following behavioral interventions would assist the client during active symptoms? **Select all that apply.**
    1. Help the client to decrease stress by teaching assertiveness skills.
    2. Help the client to acknowledge and address the source of anger.
    3. Administer medications, such as propranolol.
    4. Discuss how personality type may affect exacerbations of tension headaches.
    5. Teach the client progressive relaxation.

45. A severely anxious client experiencing headaches, palpitations, and inability to concentrate is admitted to a medical floor. Which nursing intervention would take priority?
    1. Encourage the client to express feelings.
    2. Discuss alternative coping strategies with the client.
    3. Use a distraction, such as having the client attend group.
    4. Sit with the client and use a calm but directive approach.

46. A client is exhibiting tension and needs direction to solve problems. Which of the following interventions would the nurse implement using a behavioral approach? **Select all that apply.**
    1. Assess the client's family history for anxiety disorders.
    2. Encourage the client to use deep breathing techniques.
    3. Ask the client to think of a time in the past when anxiety was manageable.
    4. Encourage journal writing to express feelings.
    5. Educate the client on aromatherapy.

47. The nursing student is developing a plan of care for a client experiencing a crisis situation. Number the following in priority order for implementation of this plan.
    1. _____ Assess for suicidal and homicidal ideation.
    2. _____ Discuss coping skills used in the past and note if they were effective.
    3. _____ Establish a working relationship by active listening.
    4. _____ Develop a plan of action for dealing with future stressors.
    5. _____ Evaluate the developed plan's effectiveness.

48. The nurse is assessing clients on an inpatient psychiatric unit. Which client would require immediate intervention?
    1. A client experiencing rapid, pressured speech and poor personal boundaries.
    2. A client expressing homicidal ideations toward the neighborhood butcher.
    3. A client who has slept only 1 to 2 hours per night for the past 2 nights.
    4. A client secluding self from others and refusing to attend groups in the milieu.

49. A 17-year-old client whose partner has recently broken their engagement is brought into the emergency department after taking a handful of lorazepam. Which nursing intervention would take priority during this psychiatric crisis?
    1. Discuss the client's feelings about the breakup with their partner.
    2. Monitor vital signs and note any signs of central nervous system depression.
    3. Allow the client time to rest because lorazepam is sedating.
    4. Decrease fluids and place the client on close observation.

50. An agency nurse is coming to an inpatient psychiatric unit for the first time. The charge nurse of the unit would assign which client to this nurse?
    1. A client newly admitted for suicidal ideations with a plan to jump off a bridge.
    2. A client admitted 2 days ago for alcohol detoxification with a history of seizures.
    3. A client grimacing and pacing the halls with a grim, defiant affect.
    4. A client starting clozapine therapy to treat auditory hallucinations.

51. The nurse is using an intrapersonal approach to assist a client in dealing with survivor's guilt. Which nursing intervention is appropriate?
    1. Encourage the client to attend a survivors group for peer support.
    2. Facilitate expression of feelings during one-to-one interactions with the nurse.
    3. Ask the client to challenge the irrational beliefs associated with the event.
    4. Administer scheduled paroxetine to deal with depressive symptoms.

52. A client on an inpatient psychiatric unit is experiencing a flashback. Which intervention takes priority?
    1. Maintain and reassure the client of their safety and security.
    2. Encourage the client to express feelings.
    3. Decrease extraneous external stimuli.
    4. Use a nonjudgmental and matter-of-fact approach.

53. A person whose spouse has died is diagnosed with adjustment disorder with depressed mood. Symptoms include chronic migraines, feelings of hopelessness, social isolation, and self-care deficit. Which nursing intervention is most appropriate?
    1. Present the reality of the consequences of impulsive behaviors.
    2. Encourage independent completion of activities of daily living.
    3. Discuss the effects of behaviors that guarantee immediate gratification.
    4. Teach techniques to improve positive body image.

Nursing Process—Evaluation

54. The nursing student is reviewing information about crisis. Which of the following student statements indicates that learning has occurred? **Select all that apply.**
    1. "A crisis is associated with psychopathology."
    2. "A crisis is precipitated by a specific identifiable event."
    3. "A crisis is chronic in nature and needs multiple interventions over time."
    4. "A crisis is specific to an individual, and the cause may vary."
    5. "A crisis contains the potential for psychological growth or deterioration."

55. A student is learning about prodromal syndrome. Which student statement indicates that learning has occurred?
    1. "Behaviors associated with prodromal syndrome necessitate immediate action by the nurse."
    2. "Prodromal syndrome occurs after a client's outburst."
    3. "Staff cannot assist clients who are experiencing prodromal syndrome in gaining control."
    4. "Very few symptoms are associated with prodromal syndrome."

56. A client diagnosed with posttraumatic stress disorder (PTSD) has a nursing diagnosis of disturbed sleep patterns R/T nightmares. Which evaluation would indicate that the stated nursing diagnosis was resolved?
    1. The client expresses feelings about the nightmares during group.
    2. The client asks for prn trazodone before bed to fall asleep.
    3. The client states, "My nightmares have stopped, and I feel rested."
    4. The client avoids napping during the day to help enhance sleep.

57. The nurse teaches an anxious client diagnosed with posttraumatic stress disorder (PTSD) a breathing technique. Which client action would indicate that the teaching was successful?
    1. The client eliminates anxiety by using the breathing technique.
    2. The client performs activities of daily living independently by discharge.
    3. The client recognizes signs and symptoms of escalating anxiety.
    4. The client maintains a 3/10 anxiety level without medications.

58. A nursing instructor is teaching about clients diagnosed with an adjustment disorder. Which student statement indicates that learning has occurred?
    1. "A client with this disorder should exhibit symptoms within 1 year of the precipitating event."
    2. "A client with this disorder should exhibit symptoms within 3 months of the precipitating event."
    3. "A client with this disorder should exhibit symptoms within 6 months of the precipitating event."
    4. "A client with this disorder should exhibit symptoms within 9 months of the precipitating event."

Psychopharmacology

59. A client diagnosed with posttraumatic stress disorder (PTSD) is prescribed paroxetine 30 mg qhs. Paroxetine is supplied as a 20 mg tablet. The nurse would administer _____ tablets.

60. A client rates anxiety at 8 out of 10 on a scale of 1 to 10, is restless, and has narrowed perceptions. Which of the following medications could be appropriately prescribed to address these symptoms? **Select all that apply.**
    1. Chlordiazepoxide.
    2. Clonazepam.
    3. Lithium carbonate.
    4. Clozapine.
    5. Oxazepam.

The correct answer number and rationale for why it is the correct answer are given in **boldface blue type.** Rationales for why the other answer options are incorrect are given as well, but they are not in boldface type.

Theory

1. 1. **The id is the locus of instinctual drives, or the *pleasure principle*. The client is exhibiting id-driven behaviors that are impulsive and egocentric, and may be irrational.**
   2. The ego also is called the rational self, or *reality principle*. The ego experiences the reality of the external world, adapts to it, and responds to it. A primary function of the ego is one of mediator between the id and the superego. A cooperative and pleasant client, unlike the one presented in the question, who responds well to others has a well-developed ego.
   3. The superego is referred to as the *perfection principle*. Derived from a system of rewards and punishments, the superego is composed of two major components: the ego-ideal and the conscience. When a child is continually rewarded for "good" behavior, self-esteem is increased. When corrected for "bad" behavior, the child learns what is morally right and wrong in society and culture. A client who considers the rights of others and recognizes the difference between right and wrong, unlike the client presented in the question, has a well-developed superego.
   4. The ego-ideal is part of the superego. When "good" behavior is consistently rewarded, self-esteem is enhanced and becomes part of the ego-ideal. This is internalized as part of the individual's value system. A client who is medication compliant because the client values continued mental health, unlike the client presented in the question, has a well-developed ego-ideal.

TEST-TAKING HINT: To answer this question correctly, the test taker must understand the differences between the id, ego, and superego, and that id-driven behaviors may be impulsive and irrational.

2. 1. Discussing emotional triggers that precipitate angry outbursts is an intrapersonal, not a biological, approach to dealing with agitation.
   2. Encouraging the client to use exercise to deal with increased agitation is a behavioral, not biological, approach to dealing with agitation.
   3. **Administering ordered prn medications when the client is experiencing extreme anxiety and tension is a biological approach to dealing with the client's agitation.**
   4. When the nurse develops a plan to deal with client agitation during family therapy, the nurse is using an interpersonal, not a biological, approach.

TEST-TAKING HINT: In this question, the test taker must note keywords such as *biological*. Only answer 3 describes a biological intervention.

3. 1. **Role-playing a stressful situation to assist the client in coping is an example of a behavioral intervention.**
   2. Developing a plan for dealing with stressors during a family meeting is an example of an interpersonal, not a behavioral, intervention.
   3. Using ordered prn medications to decrease anxiety and agitation is an example of a biological, not behavioral, intervention.
   4. Discussing emotional triggers that precipitate angry outbursts is an example of an intrapersonal, not a behavioral, intervention.

TEST-TAKING HINT: The test taker needs to review the different theories related to anxiety and examine interventions that support these theories. In this scenario, answer 1 is the only approach that is behavioral.

4. 1. This is the definition of life-cycle development, not temperament. Specialists in life-cycle development believe that people continue to develop and change throughout life, suggesting the possibility for renewal and growth in adults.
   2. **The client is describing temperament. Temperament is defined as the inborn personality characteristics that influence an individual's manner of reacting to the environment and ultimately their developmental progress.**

3. This is a definition of personality, not of temperament.

4. Temperament refers to inborn personality characteristics and not characteristics learned in childhood.

TEST-TAKING HINT: To answer this question correctly, the test taker needs to have a basic knowledge of human personality development and understand the meaning of the term *temperament.*

5. 1. During initiative versus guilt, late childhood (3 to 6 years of age), an individual is working to develop a sense of purpose and the ability to initiate and direct one's own activities. A negative outcome of this stage hampers the development of initiative, independence, and assertiveness. This client does not fall within the age range for this developmental conflict.

2. During industry versus inferiority, school age (6 to 12 years of age), an individual is working to achieve a sense of self-confidence by learning, competing, performing, and receiving recognition from significant others, peers, and acquaintances. A negative outcome of this stage hampers the development of distinguishing between the world of home and the world of peers, leading to feelings of inferiority. This client does not fall within the age range for this developmental conflict.

3. During identity versus role confusion, adolescence (12 to 20 years of age), an individual is working to integrate the tasks mastered in the previous stages into a secure sense of self. A negative outcome of this stage leads to indecision regarding vocation, social relationships, and life in general. This client does not fall within the age range for this developmental conflict.

4. **During integrity versus despair, late adulthood (65 years of age to death), an individual reviews life accomplishments, deals with loss, and prepares for death. A negative outcome of this stage is despair and fear of death. This client falls within the age range for this developmental conflict and is lacking feelings of accomplishment, fulfillment, and completeness.**

TEST-TAKING HINT: To answer this question correctly, the test taker must understand that the assessment of Erikson's stages of development is based on a client's chronological age.

6. 1. **During the stage of late adolescence, the major developmental task is to establish self-identity; experience satisfying**

relationships; and work to develop a lasting, intimate, relationship with another person. The client in the question is struggling to master the developmental stage of late adolescence.

2. During the stage of early adolescence, the major developmental task is to learn to form satisfactory relationships with other individuals and to develop a sense of identity. The client's struggle in the question does not reflect this stage of development.

3. During the stage of preadolescence, the major developmental task is to learn to form satisfactory peer relationships and initiate feelings of affection for another individual. The client's struggle in the question does not reflect this stage of development.

4. During the juvenile stage, the major developmental task is to learn to form satisfactory peer relationships. The client's struggle in the question does not reflect this stage of development.

TEST-TAKING HINT: To answer this question correctly, the test taker needs to be familiar with how Sullivan categorizes developmental stages.

7. 1. **When the client verbalizes understanding of how the experienced event, individual traits, and available support systems affect their diagnosis, the client demonstrates a good understanding of the psychosocial cause of posttraumatic stress disorder (PTSD).**

2. Avoiding situations as a way to decrease emotional pain is an example of a learned, not psychosocial, cause of PTSD.

3. The release of natural opioids during a traumatic event is an example of a biological, not psychosocial, cause of PTSD.

4. Having a negative perception of the world because of a traumatic event is an example of a cognitive, not psychosocial, cause of PTSD.

TEST-TAKING HINT: To answer this question correctly, the test taker should review the different theories as they relate to the causes of including PTSD. Only answer 1 describes a psychosocial etiology of this disorder.

8. Sending counselors to a natural disaster site to assist individuals in dealing with the devastation is an example of *primary* prevention. Primary prevention reduces the incidence of mental disorders, such as posttraumatic stress disorder (PTSD), within the population by helping individuals to cope more effectively with stress early in the grieving process.

Primary prevention is extremely important for individuals who experience any traumatic event, such as a rape, war, hurricane, tornado, or school shootings.

TEST-TAKING HINT: To answer this question correctly, it is necessary to understand the differences among primary, secondary, and tertiary prevention.

Ego Defense Mechanisms

9. Some ego defenses are more adaptive than others, but all are used either consciously or unconsciously as a protective device for the ego in an effort to relieve mild to moderate anxiety. Until an individual is able to deal with stressful situations, ego defense mechanisms are commonly used.
    1. Denial occurs when an individual refuses to acknowledge the existence of a real situation or the feelings associated with it. The client in the question is not exhibiting denial.
    2. **Intellectualization occurs when an individual attempts to avoid expressing actual emotions associated with a stressful situation by using the intellectual processes of logic, reasoning, and analysis. The individual in the question is using reasoning to avoid dealing with feelings about being fired.**
    3. Rationalization occurs when an individual attempts to make excuses or formulate logical reasons to justify unacceptable feelings or behaviors. The client in the question is not exhibiting rationalization.
    4. Suppression occurs when an individual voluntarily blocks unpleasant feelings and experiences from awareness. The client in the question is not exhibiting suppression.

TEST-TAKING HINT: To answer this question correctly, the test taker needs to differentiate among defense mechanisms and recognize behaviors that reflect the use of these defenses.

10. 1. Feelings of rage at being raped at a young age, which later are expressed by joining law enforcement, is an example of the defense mechanism of sublimation, not reaction formation. Sublimation is a method of rechanneling drives or impulses that are personally or socially unacceptable into activities that are constructive.
    2. **Giving excessive attention to the child publicly, while privately being unhappy with parenthood, is an example of the defense mechanism of reaction**

formation. Reaction formation assists in preventing unacceptable or undesirable thoughts or behaviors from being expressed by exaggerating opposite thoughts or types of behavior.
    3. Drinking six to eight beers a day while still attending Alcoholics Anonymous as a group leader is an example of the defense mechanism of denial, not reaction formation. Denial assists the client in ignoring the existence of a real situation or the feelings associated with it.
    4. When a client is angry that the call bell is not answered and then decides to use the call bell when it is unnecessary, the client is expressing passive-aggressive behavior, not reaction formation. Passive-aggressive behavior occurs when an individual's behavior is expressed in sly, devious, and undermining actions that convey the opposite of what the client is really feeling.

TEST-TAKING HINT: To answer this question correctly, the test taker needs to understand that reaction formation prevents thoughts or behaviors from being expressed by expressing opposite thoughts or feelings. In the correct answer choice, publicly treasuring the client's child camouflages the client's parental misgiving.

11. 1. **When a person feels unattractive and pursues a career in fashion design, that person is using the defense mechanism of compensation. Compensation is a method of hiding a real or perceived deficit by emphasizing a strength. The person feels unattractive, a perceived deficit, but pursues a career in fashion to compensate for this feeling.**
    2. A person who abuses alcohol and excuses it by claiming a need to use alcohol for socialization is using the defense mechanism of rationalization, not compensation. Rationalization is a method of attempting to make excuses or formulating logical reasons to justify unacceptable feelings or behaviors.
    3. A poorly paid employee who consistently yells at their assistant for minimal mistakes is using the defense mechanism of displacement, not compensation. Displacement is a method of transferring feelings from one threatening target to another target that is considered less threatening or neutral.
    4. Curling into a fetal position after injuring an ankle is an example of the use of the defense mechanism of regression, not compensation. Regression is a method of responding to stress by retreating to an

earlier level of development. This allows the individual to embrace the comfort measures associated with this earlier level of functioning.

TEST-TAKING HINT: To answer this question correctly, the test taker needs to understand that compensation covers up a perceived weakness by emphasizing a more desirable trait. An example is a parent who is ineffective working to become teacher of the year.

12. 1. A child telling a friend not to steal after being told it is wrong is an example of the defense mechanism of introjection, not sublimation. Introjection is a method of integrating the beliefs and values of another individual into one's own ego structure.
   2. A person becoming an athletic trainer because of their inability to play sports is an example of the defense mechanism of compensation, not sublimation. Compensation is the method of covering up a real or perceived weakness by emphasizing a trait one considers more desirable.
   3. By choosing a nursing career as the result of admiring nurses who have provided care, this young child is implementing the defense mechanism of identification, not sublimation. Identification is a method of attempting to increase self-worth by acquiring certain attributes and characteristics of an admired individual.
   4. **Directing hostile feelings into productive activities, such as becoming a therapist to help others, is an example of the defense mechanism of sublimation. Sublimation is the method of rechanneling drives or impulses that are personally or socially unacceptable into activities that are constructive.**

TEST-TAKING HINT: To answer this question correctly, the test taker must review and understand the differences between similar defense mechanisms, such as sublimation and compensation.

13. 1. Ego defense mechanisms are used when anxiety increases and the individual's ego is being tested.
   2. Defense mechanisms can be used adaptively to deal with stress and protect the ego. Unhealthy ego development may result from the overuse or maladaptive use of defense mechanisms. Not all individuals who use defense mechanisms as a means of stress adaptation exhibit healthy egos. The word *all* in this statement makes it incorrect.

3. When defense mechanisms are used excessively and interfere with an individual's ability to cope, they are considered maladaptive and may result in unhealthy ego development.
4. Defense mechanisms are used by all individuals, not just individuals diagnosed with mental illness. Whether defense mechanisms are used adaptively or maladaptively contributes to the individual's healthy ego development.
5. **Defense mechanisms are used adaptively during times of mild to moderate anxiety to decrease stress and assist with coping.**

TEST-TAKING HINT: To answer this question correctly, the test taker needs to note important words in the answers, such as *all* in answer 2. The use of the words *never, only,* and *always* should alert the test taker to reconsider the answer choice.

14. 1. Undoing is an act of atonement for one's unacceptable acts or thoughts. An example is a client accusing their spouse of infidelity and then buying the spouse a diamond bracelet. The situation in the question is not reflective of undoing.
   2. Rationalization is an attempt to make excuses or formulate logical reasons to justify unacceptable feelings or behaviors. An example is a client stating, "I drink because it's the only way I can deal with my bad marriage and my job." The situation in the question is not reflective of rationalization.
   3. Suppression is the voluntary blocking of unpleasant feelings and experiences from one's awareness. An example is a client stating, "I don't want to think about it now; I will think about that tomorrow." The situation in the question is not reflective of suppression.
   4. **The client in the question is using the defense mechanism of repression. Repression is the unconscious, involuntary blocking of unpleasant feelings and experiences from one's own awareness.**

TEST-TAKING HINT: To answer this question correctly, the test taker must pair the situation presented in the question with the appropriate defense mechanism.

15. 1. **Isolation is the separation of thought or memory from the feeling, tone, or emotion associated with the memory or event. The client in the question showing no emotion related to the rape is using the defense mechanism of isolation.**

2. Displacement is the transferring of feelings from one target to another target that is considered less threatening or neutral. An example is when a client is angry with the physician but directs this anger toward the nurse. The situation in the question is not reflective of displacement.

3. Compensation occurs when a person covers up a real or perceived weakness by emphasizing a trait considered more desirable. An example is when a child with a physical disability who is unable to participate in football compensates by becoming a great scholar. The situation in the question is not reflective of compensation.

4. Regression occurs when a person responding to stress retreats to an earlier level of development and the comfort measures associated with that level of functioning. An example is when a hospitalized 2-year-old child drinks only from a bottle, although the parent states the child has been drinking from a cup for the past 4 months. The situation in the question is not reflective of regression.

TEST-TAKING HINT: The test taker needs to understand that the defense mechanism of isolation does not refer to physical seclusion, but rather to an emotional isolation of feelings.

16. **1. Identification is an attempt to increase self-esteem by acquiring certain attributes of an admired individual. This psychiatric resident is identifying with Sigmund Freud.**

2. Repression is the unconscious blocking of material that is threatening or painful. *Example:* "I know I took the MCAT, but I can't remember anything about the test." The situation in the question is not reflective of repression.

3. Regression is used to respond to stress by retreating to an earlier, more comfortable level of development. *Example:* "It's not fair, the instructor's inept, and I'm quitting if things don't change." The situation in the question is not reflective of regression.

4. Reaction formation prevents unacceptable thoughts or feelings from being expressed by exaggerating the opposite thoughts or feelings. *Example:* "Even though I failed the course, I'm writing a letter of academic appreciation to the medical school faculty." The situation in the question is not reflective of reaction formation.

TEST-TAKING HINT: To answer this question correctly, the test taker must pair the situation presented in the question with the appropriate defense mechanism. Although *repression* and *regression* may sound and be spelled similarly, there is a major difference in their meaning. Repression is an involuntary thought-blocking defense, whereas regression is an abnormal return to an earlier level of development.

17. 1. This is an example of the defense mechanism of undoing, not projection, which is an act of atonement for one's unacceptable acts or thoughts.

2. **This is an example of the defense mechanism of projection, in which a person attributes unacceptable impulses and feelings to another.**

3. This is an example of the defense mechanism of compensation, not projection, in which a person counterbalances a deficiency in one area by excelling in another.

4. This is an example of the defense mechanism of repression, not projection, which is the involuntary blocking of unacceptable ideas or impulses from one's awareness.

TEST-TAKING HINT: To answer this question correctly, the test taker needs to understand that projection is a defense mechanism in which the individual "passes the blame," or attributes undesirable feelings or impulses to another, providing relief from associated anxiety.

18. 1. This is an example of the defense mechanism of identification, not denial, which enables a person to manage anxiety by imitating the behavior of someone respected or feared.

2. This is an example of the defense mechanism of displacement, not denial, which enables a person to discharge emotional reactions from one object or person to another object or person.

3. **This is an example of the defense mechanism of denial, which enables a person to ignore unacceptable realities by refusing to acknowledge them.**

4. This is an example of the defense mechanism of intellectualization, not denial, which enables a person to use logic and reasoning to control or minimize painful situations or feelings.

TEST-TAKING HINT: To answer this question correctly, the test taker needs to recognize a situation in which the defense mechanism enables the person to ignore a stressful situation and the feelings associated with it.

19. 1. The client would use denial to negate their unacceptable guilt related to child neglect. *Example:* "I don't know where my spouse gets the idea that I have neglected our children." The situation in the question is not reflective of denial.
2. Projection involves behaviors that are personally unacceptable. These behaviors are then attributed to others. *Example:* "My spouse is a workaholic, and that is who has neglected the children." The situation in the question is not reflective of projection.
3. **Displacement transfers feelings that are unacceptable to express to one person (their spouse) to a less threatening person (their sister-in-law).**
4. Rationalization is the attempt to make excuses or formulate logical reasons to justify unacceptable feelings or behaviors. *Example:* "My job is so demanding, I have little time to devote to the children." The situation in the question is not reflective of rationalization.

TEST-TAKING HINT: To answer this question correctly, the test taker needs to understand that projection is often confused with displacement. Projection occurs when a person's unacceptable feelings or impulses are attributed to others. Displacement occurs when feelings are transferred from one target to a less threatening or neutral target.

Nursing Process—Assessment

20. 1. Self-assertion is the ability to express one's thoughts and feelings in direct ways that are not intimidating or manipulative. The behavior in the question does not reflect self-assertion.
2. **Passive-aggressiveness is a covert way of expressing aggression toward others indirectly and nonassertively. By making the friend wait, the person is indirectly expressing their hostility.**
3. Splitting is the failure to integrate positive and negative aspects of self or others. This polarized image results in seeing self and others as all good or all bad. Splitting turns people against each other and generates hostilities. The behavior in the question does not reflect splitting.
4. Omnipotence occurs when a person depicts themself in actions or feelings that convey superiority, unlimited power, and authority. The behavior in the question does not reflect omnipotence.

TEST-TAKING HINT: The test taker needs to study different maladaptive behaviors to understand that a person displaying passive-aggressive behaviors exhibits on the surface an appearance of compliance that masks covert resistance, resentment, and hostility.

21. A mild level of anxiety is positive and adaptive. Mild anxiety prepares people for action.
1. Increased respirations are a physiological, not cognitive, response to a moderate, not mild, level of anxiety.
2. Feelings of horror or dread are cognitive responses to severe or panic levels, not mild levels, of anxiety.
3. Pacing the hall is a behavioral, not cognitive, response to moderate or severe, not mild, levels of anxiety.
4. **An increase in the ability to concentrate is a cognitive response to a mild level of anxiety.**
5. **A heightened alertness is a cognitive response to a mild level of anxiety.**

TEST-TAKING HINT: To answer this question correctly, the test taker needs to understand that mild anxiety sharpens the senses, increases motivation for productivity, increases the perceptual field, and heightens awareness in the environment.

22. When a person is experiencing moderate levels of anxiety, the perceptual field diminishes. Attention span and the ability to concentrate decrease; however, with direction, an individual may be able to complete a task. Assistance would be required. Increased muscle tension and restlessness are evident.
1. Narrowing perception is a cognitive, not behavioral, response to a moderate to severe level of anxiety.
2. Heart palpitations are a physiological, not behavioral, response to a severe, not moderate, level of anxiety.
3. Limited attention span is a cognitive, not behavioral, response to a moderate level of anxiety.
4. **Restlessness is a behavioral response to a moderate level of anxiety.**

TEST-TAKING HINT: To answer this question correctly, the test taker needs to note that the two keywords in this question are *behavioral* and *moderate* and look for a behavioral response to moderate anxiety.

23. During panic levels of anxiety, the individual is unable to focus on even one detail in the environment. Misperceptions are common, and a loss of contact with reality may occur.

Behaviors are characterized as wild and desperate or extreme withdrawal. Prolonged panic levels of anxiety can lead to physical and emotional exhaustion and can be life threatening.

1. Inability to focus is a cognitive, not physiological, response to a moderate, not panic, level of anxiety.
2. Loss of consciousness does not typically occur as a result of an increased level of anxiety.
3. **Dilated pupils are a physiological response to panic levels of anxiety. Pupil dilation occurs because of the predominance of the sympathetic nervous system reaction in panic responses.**
4. Possible psychosis is a perceptual, not physiological, response to panic levels of anxiety.

TEST-TAKING HINT: To answer this question correctly, the test taker must know the physiological responses to all four levels of anxiety. When considering the state of panic, the test taker must understand that a client would be unable to sustain significant levels of anxiety without getting exhausted physically, emotionally, and psychologically.

24. 1. **Invasion of personal space is a behavioral symptom exhibited by clients at risk for acting-out behaviors.**
2. Flushed face is a physical, not behavioral, symptom exhibited by a client at risk for acting-out behaviors.
3. Increased anxiety is an emotional, not behavioral, symptom exhibited by a client at risk for acting-out behaviors.
4. Misinterpretation of stimuli is a cognitive, not behavioral, symptom exhibited by a client at risk for acting-out behaviors.
5. **Pacing the halls is a behavioral symptom exhibited by clients at risk for acting-out behaviors.**

TEST-TAKING HINT: To answer this question correctly, the test taker must understand the difference between cognitive, physical, and behavioral symptoms. The keyword *behavioral* determines the correct answer.

25. Psychological factors can contribute to the initiation or exacerbation of a physical condition.
1. **Research shows that certain personality types (type C personality) are associated with the development of cancer. These clients tend to suppress rather than express anxiety. Cancer can be affected by psychological factors.**

2. **Research shows that individuals diagnosed with asthma are characterized as having excessive dependency needs, although no specific personality type has been identified. These individuals share the personality characteristics of fear, emotional lability, increased anxiety, and depression. Asthma can be affected by psychological factors.**
3. **Research shows that certain personality types (type A personality) are associated with the development of coronary artery disease. These clients tend to have an excessive competitive drive and a chronic, continuous sense of time urgency. Coronary artery disease can be affected by psychological factors.**
4. Viruses, bacteria, fungi, parasites, and the inhalation of foreign bodies directly cause an upper respiratory tract infection. An upper respiratory tract infection is not affected by psychological factors.
5. Sepsis is the spread of an infection from its initial site to the bloodstream, initiating a systemic response. Infection is directly caused by viruses, bacteria, fungi, or parasites. Sepsis is not affected by psychological factors.

TEST-TAKING HINT: To answer this question correctly, the test taker must understand what medical diagnoses are affected by psychological factors.

26. 1. Diarrhea is a symptom exhibited during short-term, not long-term, maladaptation to stress.
2. Increased pulse and blood pressure are symptoms exhibited during short-term, not long-term, maladaptation to stress.
3. Profuse diaphoresis is a symptom exhibited during short-term, not long-term, maladaptation to stress.
4. **Ulcerative colitis, which is defined as an ulceration of the mucosa of the colon, can lead to hemorrhage and perforation. This medical diagnosis may occur when a client experiences maladaptation to long-term stress.**

TEST-TAKING HINT: To answer this question correctly, the test taker should note the keyword *long-term*. All the other answers are short-term physical effects of maladaptation to stress.

27. 1. A dispositional crisis is an acute response to an external situational stressor, for example, a spouse who has experienced intimate partner violence (IPV). The situation in the question does not reflect a dispositional crisis.

2. Crisis of anticipated life transitions occurs when a normal life-cycle transition may be anticipated, and the individual experiences a lack of control over these events. The student in the question is receiving public assistance, failing in school, and anticipating the birth of a child. An already stressful situation will be complicated further by the life-changing event of childbirth.

3. Maturational/developmental crisis occurs in response to situations that trigger emotions related to unresolved conflicts in one's life. An example is a middle-aged individual who has been passed over for a promotion for the fourth time. The situation in the question does not reflect a maturational/developmental crisis.

4. A crisis reflecting psychopathology occurs when a pre-existing psychopathology has been instrumental in precipitating a crisis or when psychopathology significantly impairs or complicates adaptive resolution. An example is a client diagnosed with borderline personality disorder who is having problems with interpersonal relationships. The situation in the question is not a crisis reflecting psychopathology.

TEST-TAKING HINT: To answer this question correctly, the test taker needs to know that stressful situations are a part of everyday life. Any stressful situation can precipitate a crisis. In this case, the anticipated birth event leaves the client feeling out of control and extremely anxious.

28. 1. It is important for the nurse to assess for a past history of violent behavior when completing a risk assessment. Clients who have been violent in the past have an increased risk for repeated violence.

2. Although it is important for the nurse to assess for disturbed thought processes while completing a risk assessment, the question is asking for a behavior the client is exhibiting. A disturbed thought process is a cognitive, not behavioral, impairment.

3. When a client invades personal space, there is increased potential for violent behavior from the client and others, who may interpret this behavior as aggressive.

4. A flushed face may be a sign of frustration or anger, which can lead to increased risk for altercation; however, it is a physiological, not behavioral, sign.

5. Self-mutilation is a behavior that needs to be noted during a risk assessment. Clients who self-mutilate are at

increased risk for serious injury and need to be monitored closely.

TEST-TAKING HINT: To answer this question correctly, the test taker needs to note the keyword *behaviors*. Completing a risk assessment includes assessment for cognitive, behavioral, and physiological signs that place the client at increased risk. In this question, the test taker is asked to focus on behavioral signs.

29. 1. Incarceration for fighting is important to note and document during a risk assessment, but this is categorized as a behavioral, not cognitive, symptom.

2. A paranoid delusion is categorized as a cognitive symptom, and it is important to note and document it on a risk assessment.

3. A history of throwing objects on the unit is important to note and document during a risk assessment, but this is categorized as a behavioral, not cognitive, symptom.

4. Reddened face is important to note and document during a risk assessment, but this is categorized as a physical, not cognitive, symptom.

TEST-TAKING HINT: The test taker needs to note that the keywords in the question are *cognitive symptom*. All symptoms presented need to be noted and documented, but only the paranoid delusion is categorized as a cognitive symptom.

30. 1. Denial is defined as refusing to acknowledge the existence of a situation or the feelings associated with it. No information is presented in the question that indicates the use of denial.

2. Social isolation is defined as aloneness experienced by the individual and perceived as imposed by others and as a negative or threatening statement. No information is presented in the question that indicates the client is experiencing social isolation.

3. Anger is broadly applicable to feelings of resentful or revengeful displeasure. No information is presented in the question that indicates the client is experiencing anger.

4. The client in the question is experiencing survivor's guilt. Survivor's guilt is a common situation that occurs when an individual experiences a traumatic event in which others died and the individual survived.

TEST-TAKING HINT: To answer this question correctly, the test taker needs to understand common phenomena experienced by individuals diagnosed with posttraumatic stress disorder and relate this understanding to the client statement presented in the question.

31. 1. A client diagnosed with posttraumatic stress disorder (PTSD) may have dissociative events in which the client feels detached from the situation or feelings.
    2. A client diagnosed with PTSD may have intense fear and feelings of helplessness.
    3. A client diagnosed with PTSD has feelings of detachment or estrangement toward others, not excessive attachment and dependence.
    4. A client diagnosed with PTSD has restricted, not full, range of affect.
    5. A client diagnosed with PTSD avoids activities associated with the traumatic event.

TEST-TAKING HINT: To answer this question correctly, the test taker must be aware of the different symptoms associated with the diagnosis of PTSD.

32. 1. The degree of ego strength is a part of individual variables, not part of the recovery environment. Other variables of the individual include effectiveness of coping resources, presence of pre-existing psychopathology, outcomes of previous experiences with stress and trauma, behavioral tendencies (e.g., temperament), current psychosocial developmental stage, and demographic factors (socioeconomic status and education).
    2. **Availability of social supports is part of environmental variables. Others include cohesiveness and protectiveness of family and friends, attitudes of society regarding the experience, and cultural and subcultural influences.**
    3. Severity and duration of the stressor is a variable of the traumatic experience, not part of the recovery environment. Other variables of the traumatic experience include amount of control over the recurrence, extent of anticipatory preparation, exposure to death, the number affected by the life-threatening situation, and location where the traumatic event was experienced.
    4. Amount of control over the recurrence is a variable of the traumatic experience, not part of the recovery environment.

TEST-TAKING HINT: To answer this question correctly, the test taker needs to understand the following three significant elements in the development of posttraumatic stress disorder: traumatic experience, individual variables, and environmental variables.

33. 1. Recurrent, distressing flashbacks are emotional, not behavioral, symptoms of posttraumatic stress disorder (PTSD).
    2. Intense fear, helplessness, and horror are cognitive, not behavioral, symptoms of PTSD.
    3. **Diminished participation in significant activities is a behavioral symptom of PTSD.**
    4. Detachment or estrangement from others is an interpersonal, not behavioral, symptom of PTSD.

TEST-TAKING HINT: To answer this question correctly, the test taker should take note of the keyword *behavioral*, which determines the correct answer. All symptoms may be exhibited in PTSD, but only answer choice 3 is a behavioral symptom.

Nursing Process—Diagnosis

34. 1. Pain is an appropriate nursing diagnosis for a client currently experiencing a migraine headache. Although the client has a history of migraine headaches, there is nothing presented in this question to indicate that this client is currently experiencing migraine headache pain.
    2. **The client in the question currently is experiencing anxiety as a result of high levels of occupational stress. Anxiety is a priority nursing diagnosis, and if anxiety is not addressed, it may lead to a migraine headache episode.**
    3. Activity intolerance may be an appropriate nursing diagnosis for clients experiencing the acute pain of migraine headaches; however, this client is not currently experiencing migraine headache pain. No evidence is presented in the question to indicate activity intolerance.
    4. Although this client is experiencing a high level of occupational stress, nothing in the question suggests that this client is experiencing ineffective role performance.

TEST-TAKING HINT: The test taker must read this question carefully to discern the current symptoms experienced by the client. A history of a problem takes a lower priority than a current problem.

35. 1. Anxiety often triggers acute asthma attacks and is an appropriate diagnosis for this client; however, it is not the priority diagnosis.
    2. **Impaired gas exchange is the priority diagnosis for this client. Meeting the client's oxygen need is critical to maintaining viability. This life-threatening**

situation needs to be resolved before any other client need is met.

3. No information in the question suggests that the client is suicidal, and so this is an inappropriate nursing diagnosis.

4. This client has reacted to the parent's death by experiencing increased levels of anxiety triggering an acute asthma attack. Because asthma is an autonomic response to stress, this client's physiological reaction is not reflective of ineffective coping.

TEST-TAKING HINT: When prioritizing nursing diagnoses, it is important for the test taker to consider physiological needs first. The test taker can draw from knowledge of the ABCs (airway, breathing, and circulation) to determine priorities.

36. 1. No indication for the assessment of suicidal or homicidal ideations is presented in the question. Also, this intervention does not relate to the nursing diagnosis of knowledge deficit.

2. Encouraging the client to verbalize feelings regarding anxiety would relate to the nursing diagnosis of anxiety, not knowledge deficit.

3. Role-playing situations in which the client experiences anxiety do not address a nursing diagnosis of knowledge deficit.

4. **Teaching the client about the mind–body connection is an intervention that directly supports the nursing diagnosis of knowledge deficit R/T relationship of anxiety to hypertension.**

TEST-TAKING HINT: When answering this question, the test taker needs to choose the intervention linked to the presented nursing diagnosis of knowledge deficit.

37. 1. Although risk for injury toward others is a priority diagnosis, the nursing diagnostic statement is incorrectly formulated. When using a "risk for" nursing diagnosis, there is no "as evidenced by" statement because the problem has yet to occur.

2. **Ineffective coping R/T inability to express feelings AEB aggressive demeanor is a correctly worded diagnostic statement. This diagnosis takes priority because altered or ineffective coping can lead to aggressive behaviors that may result in injury.**

3. There is no evidence presented in the question that indicates the client is exhibiting disturbed thought process.

4. There is no evidence presented in the question that indicates the client is exhibiting social isolation.

TEST-TAKING HINT: When developing nursing diagnoses, it is necessary to formulate the nursing diagnostic statement correctly and prioritize based on client needs.

38. 1. **Because safety is always a priority, risk for violence toward others should be prioritized. The behaviors presented in the question indicate that the client may be in a prodromal state of crisis and may present an immediate threat.**

2. Ineffective coping is an appropriate nursing diagnosis; however, it is not the priority diagnosis.

3. Anxiety is an appropriate nursing diagnosis; however, it is not the priority nursing diagnosis.

4. There is not enough evidence presented in the question to determine that this is an appropriate nursing diagnosis.

TEST-TAKING HINT: When prioritizing client problems, the first consideration should be safety. Using Maslow's hierarchy of needs assists the test taker with this prioritization.

39. 1. Although posttraumatic stress disorder (PTSD) is an appropriate nursing diagnosis for this client, it is not the priority nursing diagnosis at this time.

2. Although social isolation is an appropriate nursing diagnosis for this client, it is not the priority nursing diagnosis at this time.

3. Although ineffective coping may be an appropriate nursing diagnosis for clients diagnosed with PTSD, there is no information in the question to suggest alcohol use.

4. **Risk for injury is the priority nursing diagnosis for this client. In the question, the client is exhibiting recurrent flashbacks, nightmares, and sleep deprivation that can cause exhaustion and lead to injury. It is important for the nurse to prioritize the nursing diagnosis that addresses safety.**

TEST-TAKING HINT: When the question asks for a priority, it is important for the test taker to understand that all answer choices may be appropriate statements. Client safety always should be prioritized.

Nursing Process—Planning

40. Client outcomes need to be realistic, specific, and client centered, and they must have a time frame to be measurable. This client is exhibiting signs and symptoms of social isolation.

1. Client participation in group therapy is an appropriate outcome for this client, but

because this outcome does not have a time frame, it is not measurable.
2. This statement is focused on the nurse's interventions, not the expected client outcome. This statement is not client focused.
3. This outcome is correctly written because it is client-centered, short-term, realistic, and measurable.
4. It is important for the client to socialize while in the milieu to counteract social isolation; however, this outcome does not have a time frame and is not measurable.

TEST-TAKING HINT: The test taker needs to understand that client outcomes must be realistic, specific, and client-centered and have a time frame to be measurable. Without any one component, the answer choice is incorrect.

41. 1. It is a realistic expectation for a client who copes with previous trauma by abusing alcohol to recognize the triggers that precipitate this behavior. This outcome should be developed early in treatment.
2. Attending follow-up weekly therapy sessions after discharge is a long-term, not short-term, outcome.
3. Expecting the client to refrain from self-blame regarding the rape by day 2 is an unrealistic outcome. Clients who experience traumatic events need extensive outpatient therapy.
4. Being free from injury does not relate to the nursing diagnosis of ineffective coping.

TEST-TAKING HINT: It is important to relate outcomes to the stated nursing diagnosis. In this question, the test taker should choose an answer that relates to the nursing diagnosis of ineffective coping. Answer 4 can be eliminated immediately because it does not assist the client in coping more effectively. Also, the test taker must note important words, such as *short-term*. Answer 2 can be eliminated immediately because it is a long-term outcome.

42. 1. Although the staff does not want the client to injure self or anyone else, there is no time frame presented in this short-term outcome, and it is not measurable.
2. It is important for the client to be able to discuss feelings of anger with staff in order to work through these feelings. This is a short-term outcome.
3. Although it is important for the client to take responsibility for their feelings, there is no time frame presented in this outcome, and it is not measurable.

4. Expecting the client to participate actively in outpatient follow-up group therapy sessions is a long-term, not short-term, outcome.

TEST-TAKING HINT: A properly written outcome must be specific to the client's need, be realistic, be measurable, and contain a reasonable time frame. If any of these characteristics is missing in an outcome, the outcome is incorrectly written. The test taker should note the word *short-term* in the question. Short-term outcomes are expectations for clients during hospitalization, and long-term outcomes focus on what the client can accomplish after discharge.

Nursing Process—Implementation

43. 1. When working with a client diagnosed with migraine headaches, the nurse should include an assessment of pain by using a pain scale. A pain scale objectifies the subjective symptom of pain and assists the nurse in the evaluation of this symptom.
2. When working with a client diagnosed with migraine headaches, the nurse should explore with the client how stress may trigger this disorder. This awareness may encourage the client to avoid stressful situations and use stress-reducing techniques.
3. Encouraging the client to keep a journal documenting patterns of exacerbation triggers assists the client in recognizing the effects that stressful stimuli have on the incidence of migraine headaches.
4. Assessing for suicidal ideations is an inappropriate intervention when working with this client because nothing is presented in the question that would suggest this client is at risk for self-violence.
5. When working with a client diagnosed with migraine headaches, administering divalproex sodium, as prescribed, is an appropriate intervention. Divalproex sodium is a vascular headache suppressant. Other preventive medications include propranolol, amitriptyline, fluoxetine, verapamil, and venlafaxine.

TEST-TAKING HINT: To answer this question correctly, the test taker must understand how anxiety affects psychophysiological disorders, such as migraine headaches, and then recognize appropriate ways to intervene.

44. Behavioral interventions are focused on helping the client gain the tools needed to change behaviors.

    1. Helping the client to decrease stress by teaching assertiveness skills is an example of a behavioral approach. The ability to assert self can lead to decreased anxiety and a decrease in stress-related illnesses.
    2. Helping the client to acknowledge and address the source of anger is an intrapersonal, not behavioral, approach to decreasing anxiety.
    3. Propranolol blocks beta-adrenergic receptor sites and is administered to prevent vascular headaches. This intervention is an example of a biological, not behavioral, approach to decreasing anxiety.
    4. Discussing how personality type may affect exacerbations of tension headaches is an example of an intrapersonal, not behavioral, approach to decreasing anxiety.
    5. Teaching progressive relaxation to decrease physical and emotional tension is an example of a behavioral approach. Physically releasing tension can decrease stress-related illness.

    TEST-TAKING HINT: Numerous interventions can assist clients in decreasing the exacerbations of anxiety-related illnesses. The keyword *behavioral* determines the intervention choice. The test taker must recognize that although teaching is cognitive in nature, when the nurse teaches techniques to change behaviors, the nurse is using a behavioral approach.

45. The symptoms noted in the question reflect a severe level of anxiety. Interventions for anxiety do not differ from one area of nursing to another.

    1. During severe levels of anxiety, it is inappropriate for the nurse to encourage the client to express feelings. After the client's anxiety has been reduced to a mild to moderate level, the nurse can explore the client's feelings.
    2. It is never appropriate to discuss alternative coping strategies during severe levels of anxiety. The client is unable to concentrate, and learning cannot occur.
    3. An important intervention during severe levels of anxiety is to decrease stimulation in the environment. Group therapy may increase external stimuli and increase the client's anxiety further.
    4. The nurse must be present at all times for the client experiencing severe levels of anxiety. During this time, decision making is impaired, necessitating direction from the nurse until client anxiety has decreased.

    TEST-TAKING HINT: To answer this question correctly, the test taker needs to review the different symptoms exhibited in mild, moderate, severe, and panic levels of anxiety and understand that interventions should be appropriate, client-centered, and timely during different levels of anxiety.

46. The client in the question is experiencing a moderate level of anxiety.

    1. Assessing the client's family history for anxiety disorders is an example of a biological, not behavioral, intervention. Genetic predisposition falls under biological theory.
    2. Encouraging the client to use deep breathing techniques is an example of a behavioral intervention.
    3. Asking the client to think about a time in the past when anxiety was manageable is an example of a cognitive, not behavioral, intervention.
    4. Encouraging the client to use journal writing as a means to express feelings is an example of an intrapersonal, not behavioral, intervention.
    5. Educating the client about aromatherapy is an example of a behavioral intervention. Inhaling the scent of basil, anise, and chamomile can decrease tension and increase mental alertness.

    TEST-TAKING HINT: To answer this question correctly, the test taker needs to review the different theories of etiology for anxiety. The keyword *behavioral* determines the correct answer choice.

47. The priority order of implementation is 1, 3, 2, 4, 5.

    1. First, the nurse must assess for safety, such as assessing for suicidal and homicidal ideations. Safety is always the primary priority.
    2. Next, the nurse needs to build a therapeutic relationship with the client. Without a trusting, therapeutic relationship, a plan of action cannot be implemented successfully.
    3. Next, the nurse must assess previously used coping skills. To help a client build a plan of action, the nurse needs to assess what has worked for the client in the past.
    4. The nurse then assists the client in developing a plan of action for dealing with future stressors.

5. Finally, the nurse evaluates the developed plan to determine its effectiveness and viability.

TEST-TAKING HINT: To assist the test taker in answering priority questions appropriately, the test taker should use the nursing process: assessment, nursing diagnosis/analysis, planning, implementation, and evaluation, remembering that safety always takes priority.

48. 1. Clients experiencing rapid, pressured speech and poor personal boundaries are at increased risk for violence. The nurse needs to monitor clients exhibiting these behaviors closely to ensure that the individual and the milieu remain safe.
2. Although it is important to monitor for homicidal ideations, this client's anger is directed toward the neighborhood butcher and not toward anyone in the milieu and therefore is not a priority concern. As compared with the other situations presented, this situation does not require immediate intervention.
3. Although it is important to note altered sleep patterns, this deficit does not place the client or others at risk. As compared with the other situations presented, this situation does not require immediate intervention.
4. Although it is important for clients to attend groups and socialize, this deficit does not place the client or others at risk. As compared with the other situations presented, this situation does not require immediate intervention.

TEST-TAKING HINT: To answer this question correctly, the test taker must consider all behaviors and signs and symptoms before deciding on the priority problem. The test taker should always prioritize safety within the milieu.

49. 1. At some future time, it would be appropriate to discuss the client's feelings, but during a crisis situation this discussion would be inappropriate.
2. It is important when a client has overdosed to ensure that the client is physiologically safe. Monitoring vital signs is an important intervention to determine which medical interventions may be needed.
3. Lorazepam is a central nervous system depressant. In this situation, to detect any alterations of the central nervous system the nurse needs to continuously monitor

vital signs during periods of both activity and rest.
4. Fluids should be increased, not decreased, in this situation to dilute the effects of the lorazepam. It is important to observe this client closely, but before any intervention, assessment data should be obtained.

TEST-TAKING HINT: The test taker needs to understand that just because a client is being seen for a mental health disorder does not eliminate the need to prioritize physical safety concerns. It is helpful to refer to Maslow's hierarchy of needs when prioritization is required.

50. 1. The charge nurse would assign the agency nurse this client. Although this suicidal client is extremely ill, the client does not have access to the means to carry out the suicide plan and can be monitored every 15 minutes by the agency nurse safely and effectively.
2. During days 2 to 3 of detoxification from alcohol, the client is at the highest risk for alcohol-induced withdrawal. The agency nurse may be unfamiliar with the critical complications and signs and symptoms of detoxification. The agency nurse's knowledge deficit might place this client at high risk for injury. This client would be in need of a more experienced psychiatric nurse.
3. Pacing the halls with a grim, defiant affect is a sign of prodromal syndrome, a predictor of potential violent behavior. The agency nurse may not be aware of these symptoms or the importance of proactive intervention. This client would be in need of a more experienced psychiatric nurse.
4. The agency nurse may not be familiar with this medication. Clients starting clozapine have failed many other trials with antipsychotic medications and are extremely ill. The client may have specific questions regarding clozapine, and it would be best for a nurse familiar with the treatment and side effects to manage the client's care.

TEST-TAKING HINT: When delegating, the test taker needs to match the experience of the health-care worker with the acuity of the client. In this question, the test taker should compare the clients presented and look for the client with a safety risk level that can be managed by a nurse unfamiliar with psychiatric client behaviors.

51. 1. Encouraging a client to attend a group for peer support is an interpersonal, not intrapersonal, approach to treating survivor's guilt.

2. Facilitating expression of feelings during one-to-one interactions with the nurse is an intrapersonal approach to interventions that treat survivor's guilt.
3. Asking the client to challenge the irrational beliefs associated with the event is a cognitive, not intrapersonal, intervention to treat survivor's guilt.
4. Administering regularly scheduled paroxetine is a biological, not intrapersonal, intervention to treat survivor's guilt.

TEST-TAKING HINT: To answer this question correctly, the test taker needs to differentiate among various theoretical approaches and select interventions that support these theories.

52. 1. **During a flashback, the client is experiencing severe to panic levels of anxiety; the priority nursing intervention is to maintain and reassure the client of their safety and security. The client's anxiety needs to decrease before other interventions are attempted.**
2. Encouraging the client to express feelings during a flashback would only increase the client's level of anxiety. The client's anxiety level needs to decrease to a mild or moderate level before the nurse encourages the client to express feelings.
3. Although the nurse may want to decrease external stimuli in an attempt to reduce the client's anxiety, ensuring safety and security takes priority.
4. It is important for the nurse to be nonjudgmental and use a matter-of-fact approach when dealing with a client experiencing a flashback. However, because this client is experiencing a severe to panic level of anxiety, safety is the priority.

TEST-TAKING HINT: It is important to understand timewise interventions when dealing with individuals experiencing anxiety. When the client experiences severe to panic levels of anxiety during flashbacks, the nurse needs to maintain safety and security until the client's level of anxiety has decreased.

53. 1. Impulsive behaviors are symptoms of impulse control, not adjustment disorders.
2. **Encouraging the independent completion of activities of daily living provides client success experiences that serve to decrease feelings of hopelessness, social isolation, and self-care deficit.**
3. The inability to delay gratification is a symptom of impulse control, not adjustment disorder.

4. There is no evidence presented in the question that indicates that the client has a body image distortion.

TEST-TAKING HINT: To answer this question correctly, the test taker must have knowledge of various symptoms associated with adjustment disorders and the nursing interventions that would address these problems.

Nursing Process—Evaluation

54. 1. A crisis is not associated with psychopathology. Anyone can experience a crisis. This student statement is incorrect.
2. **A crisis is precipitated by a specific identifiable event. This student statement is correct.**
3. A crisis is acute, not chronic, in nature. This student statement is incorrect.
4. **A crisis is specific to an individual, and the cause of the crisis may vary. This student statement is correct.**
5. **A crisis contains the potential for psychological growth or deterioration. This student statement is correct.**

TEST-TAKING HINT: To answer this question correctly, the test taker must understand and recognize the concepts of crisis.

55. *Prodromal syndrome* is a group of symptoms that a client exhibits before acting out and becoming aggressive. Some of these symptoms include, but are not limited to, anxiety, tension, verbal abuse, profanity, and increased hyperactivity.
1. **Prodromal syndrome is associated with behaviors that occur before the client begins acting out aggressively, and these behaviors need to be addressed immediately by staff members. Successful management of aggressive behavior depends on the ability to predict which clients are most likely to become violent.**
2. Prodromal syndrome occurs before, not after, acting-out behaviors are exhibited.
3. During a prodromal syndrome, staff members must assist clients in gaining control. It is important for staff members to assess consistently for prodromal syndrome to maintain safety.
4. Many behavioral symptoms are associated with prodromal syndrome. Some of these include anxiety, tension, verbal abuse, profanity, increasing hyperactivity, rigid posture, clenched fists and

jaws, grim defiant affect, talking in a rapid and raised voice, threats, arguing, demanding, pacing, pounding, and slamming.

TEST-TAKING HINT: To answer this question correctly, the test taker must understand the meaning of *prodromal syndrome*.

56. 1. Although the nurse would like the client to express feelings about the experienced nightmares, this statement does not relate to the nursing diagnosis of disturbed sleep patterns.
    2. Although the client requests the prescribed trazodone to assist with falling asleep, there is no assessment information to indicate that this medication has resolved the sleep pattern problem.
    3. **The client's statement, "My nightmares have stopped, and I feel rested," is the evaluation data needed to support the fact that the nursing diagnosis of disturbed sleep patterns R/T nightmares has been resolved.**
    4. When the client avoids daytime napping, the client has employed a strategy to enhance nighttime sleeping. However, this is not evaluation information that indicates the disturbed sleep problem has been resolved.

TEST-TAKING HINT: To answer this question correctly, the test taker needs to discern evaluation data that indicates problem resolution. Answers 1, 2, and 4 all are interventions to assist in resolving the stated nursing diagnosis, not evaluation data that indicate problem resolution.

57. 1. It is impossible for clients to eliminate anxiety from daily life. Mild anxiety is beneficial and necessary to completing tasks of daily living.
    2. Optimally, a client should be able to perform activities of daily living independently by discharge; however, this client action does not indicate successful teaching about breathing techniques.
    3. It is important that a client recognizes signs and symptoms of escalating anxiety, but this client action does not indicate successful teaching about breathing techniques.
    4. **A client's ability to maintain an anxiety level of 3/10 without medications indicates that the client is using breathing techniques successfully to reduce anxiety.**

TEST-TAKING HINT: To answer this question correctly, the test taker should understand that anxiety cannot be eliminated from life. This understanding eliminates answer 1 immediately.

58. To be diagnosed with adjustment disorder, clients must experience marked distress that is considered excessive given the nature of the stressor or have significant impairment in social or occupational functioning.
    1. Diagnostic criteria for adjustment disorders, the development of emotional and/or behavioral symptoms in response to an identifiable stressor, should occur within 3 months, not 1 year, of the onset of the stressor.
    2. **Diagnostic criteria for adjustment disorders, the development of emotional and/or behavioral symptoms in response to an identifiable stressor, should occur within 3 months of the onset of the stressor.**
    3. Diagnostic criteria for adjustment disorders, the development of emotional and/or behavioral symptoms in response to an identifiable stressor, should occur within 3 months, not 6 months, of the onset of the stressor.
    4. Diagnostic criteria for adjustment disorders, the development of emotional and/or behavioral symptoms in response to an identifiable stressor, should occur within 3 months, not 9 months, of the onset of the stressor.

TEST-TAKING HINT: To answer this question correctly, the test taker must have knowledge of the diagnostic criteria for adjustment disorders.

Psychopharmacology

59. **1.5 tablets.**

    $$\frac{x \text{ tab}}{30 \text{ mg}} = \frac{1 \text{ tab}}{20 \text{ mg}}$$

    $20x = 30 \qquad x = 1.5 \text{ tabs}$

TEST-TAKING HINT: The test taker should set up the ratio and proportion problem based on the number of milligrams contained in one tablet and solve this problem by cross multiplication and solving for *x* by division.

60. An anxiety rating of 8 out of 10, restlessness, and narrowed perceptions all are symptoms of increased levels of anxiety.
    1. Chlordiazepoxide is a benzodiazepine. Benzodiazepines are classified as antianxiety medications and would be appropriately prescribed to address signs and symptoms of anxiety.

2. Clonazepam is a benzodiazepine. Benzodiazepines are classified as antianxiety medications and would be appropriately prescribed to address signs and symptoms of anxiety.

3. Lithium carbonate is a mood stabilizer that treats mania and would not be used to treat signs and symptoms of anxiety.

4. Clozapine is an atypical antipsychotic and would not be used to treat signs and symptoms of anxiety.

5. Oxazepam is a benzodiazepine. Benzodiazepines are classified as antianxiety medications and would be appropriately prescribed to address signs and symptoms of anxiety.

TEST-TAKING HINT: The test taker first must recognize the signs and symptoms presented in the question as an indication of increased levels of anxiety. Next, the test taker must recognize the medications that address these symptoms. Also, it is common to confuse lithium carbonate and Librium and clozapine and clonazepam. To answer this question correctly, the test taker needs to distinguish between medications that are similar in spelling.

Anxiety, Obsessive-Compulsive, and Related Disorders, Issues Related to Sexuality

KEYWORDS

The following words include English vocabulary, nursing/medical terminology, concepts, principles, or information relevant to content specifically addressed in this chapter or associated with topics presented in it. English dictionaries, your nursing textbooks, and medical dictionaries such as *Taber's Cyclopedic Medical Dictionary* are resources that can be used to expand your knowledge and understanding of these words and related information.

Acrophobia

Anxiety

Compulsions

Cynophobia

Delayed ejaculation

Erectile disorder

Exhibitionistic disorder

Female sexual interest/arousal disorder

Fetishistic disorder

Frotteuristic disorder

Generalized anxiety disorder (GAD)

Genito-pelvic pain/penetration disorder

Hoarding

Hypersomnia

Insomnia

Male hypoactive sexual desire disorder

Nightmare disorder

Obsessions

Obsessive-compulsive disorder (OCD)

Panic attack

Paraphilic disorder

Parasomnia

Pedophilic disorder

Premature ejaculation

Pyrophobia

Relaxation therapy

Sexual dysfunction

Sexual masochism disorder

Sexual sadism disorder

Sleep apnea

Sleep patterns

Sleepwalking

Social anxiety disorder

Somnolence

Tertiary syphilis

Transvestic disorder

Trichotillomania (hair-pulling disorder)

Voyeuristic disorder

QUESTIONS

Theory

1. From a cognitive theory perspective, which is a possible cause of panic disorder?
   1. Inability of the ego to intervene when conflict occurs.
   2. Abnormal elevations of blood lactate and increased lactate sensitivity.
   3. Increased involvement of the neurochemical norepinephrine.
   4. Distorted thinking patterns that precede maladaptive behaviors.

2. An overuse or ineffective use of ego defense mechanisms, which results in a maladaptive response to anxiety, is an example of the _____ theory of generalized anxiety disorder (GAD) development.

3. Which statement explains the etiology of obsessive-compulsive disorder (OCD) from a biological theory perspective?
    1. Individuals diagnosed with OCD have weak and underdeveloped egos.
    2. Obsessive and compulsive behaviors are a conditioned response to a traumatic event.
    3. Regression to the pre-Oedipal anal sadistic phase produces the symptoms of OCD.
    4. Abnormalities in various regions of the brain have been implicated in the cause of OCD.

4. After being diagnosed with pyrophobia, the client states, "I believe this started at the age of 7 when I was trapped in a house fire." When examining theories of phobia etiology, this situation would be reflective of _____ theory.

5. A client diagnosed with social anxiety disorder has an outcome that states, "Client will voluntarily participate in group activities by day 3." Which would be an appropriate intrapersonal nursing intervention to assist the client in achieving this outcome?
    1. Offer prn lorazepam 1 hour before group begins.
    2. Attend group with client to assist in decreasing anxiety.
    3. Encourage discussion about fears related to socialization.
    4. Role-play scenarios that may occur in group to decrease anxiety.

6. Using psychodynamic theory, which intervention would be appropriate for a client diagnosed with panic disorder?
    1. Encourage the client to evaluate the power of distorted thinking.
    2. Ask the client to include their family in scheduled therapy sessions.
    3. Discuss the overuse of ego defense mechanisms and their impact on anxiety.
    4. Teach the client regarding blood lactate level as it relates to the client's panic attacks.

7. Which nursing diagnosis reflects the intrapersonal theory of the etiology of obsessive-compulsive disorder (OCD)?
    1. Ineffective coping R/T punitive superego.
    2. Ineffective coping R/T active avoidance.
    3. Ineffective coping R/T alteration in serotonin.
    4. Ineffective coping R/T classic conditioning.

Defense Mechanisms

8. Clients diagnosed with obsessive-compulsive disorder (OCD) commonly use which defense mechanism?
    1. Suppression.
    2. Repression.
    3. Undoing.
    4. Denial.

Nursing Process—Assessment

9. Which charting entry documents a subjective assessment of sleep patterns?
    1. "Reports satisfaction with the quality of sleep since admission."
    2. "Slept 8 hours during night shift."
    3. "Rates quality of sleep as 3/10."
    4. "Woke up three times during the night."

10. Which of the following are important when assessing an individual for a sleep disturbance? **Select all that apply.**
    1. Limit caffeine intake in the evening hours.
    2. Teach the importance of a bedtime routine.
    3. Keep the client's door locked during the day to avoid napping.
    4. Check the chart to note the client's baseline sleeping habits per night.
    5. Monitor the client every 15 minutes through the night and document sleep pattern.

11. A client has been diagnosed with insomnia. Which of the following data would the nurse expect to assess? **Select all that apply.**
    1. Daytime irritability.
    2. Problems with attention and concentration.
    3. Inappropriate use of substances.
    4. Nightmares.
    5. Sleepwalking.

12. What is the most common form of breathing-related sleep disorders?
    1. Parasomnia.
    2. Hypersomnia.
    3. Apnea.
    4. Cataplexy.

13. Which would the nurse expect to assess in a client suspected of having nightmare disorder?
    1. The client, on awakening, is able to explain the nightmare in vivid detail.
    2. The client is easily awakened after the nightmare.
    3. The client experiences an abrupt arousal from sleep with a piercing scream or cry.
    4. The client, when awakening during the nightmare, is alert and oriented.

14. Which assessment data would support the disorder of acrophobia?
    1. A client is fearful of basements because of encountering spiders.
    2. A client refuses to go to Europe because of a fear of flying.
    3. A client is unable to commit to marriage after a 10-year engagement.
    4. A client refuses to leave home during stormy weather.

15. In which situation would the nurse suspect a diagnosis of social anxiety disorder?
    1. A client uses marijuana daily and avoids social situations because of fear of humiliation.
    2. An 8-year-old child isolates from adults because of fear of embarrassment but has good peer relationships in school.
    3. A client diagnosed with Parkinson's disease avoids social situations because of embarrassment regarding tremors and drooling.
    4. A college student avoids taking classes that include an oral presentation because of fear of being scrutinized by others.

16. A client experiencing a panic attack would display which physical symptom?
    1. Fear of dying.
    2. Sweating and palpitations.
    3. Depersonalization.
    4. Restlessness and pacing.

17. A client newly admitted to an inpatient psychiatric unit is diagnosed with obsessive-compulsive disorder (OCD). Which behavioral symptom would the nurse expect to assess?
    1. The client uses excessive hand washing to relieve anxiety.
    2. The client rates anxiety at 8/10.
    3. The client uses breathing techniques to decrease anxiety.
    4. The client exhibits diaphoresis and tachycardia.

18. Anxiety is a symptom that can result from which of the following physiological conditions? **Select all that apply.**
    1. Chronic obstructive pulmonary disease.
    2. Hyperthyroidism.
    3. Hypertension.
    4. Diverticulosis.
    5. Hypoglycemia.

19. Which assessment data would support a physician's diagnosis of an anxiety disorder in a client?
    1. A client experiences severe levels of anxiety in one area of functioning.
    2. A client experiences an increased level of anxiety in one area of functioning for a 6-month period.
    3. A client experiences increased levels of anxiety that affect functioning in more than one area of life over a 6-month period.
    4. A client experiences increased levels of anxiety affecting at least three areas of functioning.

20. Which of the following symptom assessments would validate the diagnosis of generalized anxiety disorder (GAD)? **Select all that apply.**
    1. Excessive worry about items difficult to control.
    2. Muscle tension.
    3. Hypersomnia.
    4. Excessive amounts of energy.
    5. Feeling "keyed up" or "on edge."

21. A client diagnosed with obsessive-compulsive disorder (OCD) is newly admitted to an inpatient psychiatric unit. Which cognitive symptom would the nurse expect to assess?
    1. Compulsive behaviors that occupy more than 4 hours per day.
    2. Excessive worrying about germs and illness.
    3. Comorbid abuse of alcohol to decrease anxiety.
    4. Excessive sweating and an increase in blood pressure and pulse.

22. Which of the following would you expect to assess in a client diagnosed with a hoarding disorder? **Select all that apply.**
    1. The client experienced a brain injury, which initiated the hoarding behaviors.
    2. The client reports the thought of parting with possessions causes symptoms of panic.
    3. The client has been collecting items for the past year, keeping them neatly in a closet.
    4. The landlord has evicted the client because their possessions have become a fire hazard.
    5. The family has to discard possessions because the client is psychologically unable to discard them.

23. Which would the nurse expect to assess in a client diagnosed with fetishistic disorder?
    1. History of exposing genitalia to strangers.
    2. History of sexually arousing fantasies involving nonliving objects.
    3. History of urges to touch and rub against nonconsenting individuals.
    4. History of fantasies involving the act of being humiliated, beaten, or bound.

24. A client is diagnosed with delayed ejaculation disorder. Which of the following assessment data support this diagnosis? **Select all that apply.**
    1. Inability to maintain an erection.
    2. A delay in ejaculation following normal sexual excitement.
    3. Premature ejaculation.
    4. Dyspareunia.
    5. The absence of ejaculation.

25. A 65-year-old client with a history of prostitution is seen in the emergency department experiencing a recent onset of auditory hallucinations and bizarre behaviors. Which diagnosis would the nurse expect to document?
    1. Schizophrenia.
    2. Tertiary syphilis.
    3. Gonorrhea.
    4. Schizotypal personality disorder.

26. Nail biting, scratching, and hair pulling for extended periods of time in a private setting are symptoms associated with the diagnosis of _____.

Nursing Process—Diagnosis

27. A client diagnosed with hypersomnia states, "I can't even function anymore; I feel worthless." Which nursing diagnosis would take priority?
    1. Risk for suicide R/T expressions of hopelessness.
    2. Social isolation R/T sleepiness AEB the statement, "I can't function."
    3. Self-care deficit R/T increased need for sleep AEB being unable to bathe without help.
    4. Chronic low self-esteem R/T inability to function AEB the statement, "I feel worthless."

28. A client leaving home for the first time in a year arrives on the psychiatric inpatient unit wearing a surgical mask and white gloves. The client states, "The germs in here are going to kill me." Which correctly written nursing diagnosis addresses this client's problem?
    1. Social isolation R/T fear of germs AEB continually refusing to leave the home.
    2. Fear of germs R/T obsessive-compulsive disorder.
    3. Ineffective coping AEB dysfunctional isolation R/T unrealistic fear of germs.
    4. Anxiety R/T the inability to leave home, resulting in dysfunctional fear of germs.

29. A client seen in an outpatient clinic for ongoing management of panic attacks states, "I have to make myself come to these appointments. It is hard because I don't know when an attack will occur." Which nursing diagnosis takes priority?
    1. Ineffective breathing patterns R/T hyperventilation.
    2. Impaired spontaneous ventilation R/T panic levels of anxiety.
    3. Social isolation R/T fear of spontaneous panic attacks.
    4. Knowledge deficit R/T triggers for panic attacks.

30. During an assessment, a client diagnosed with generalized anxiety disorder (GAD) rates anxiety as 9/10 and states, "I have thought about suicide because nothing ever seems to work out for me." Based on this information, which nursing diagnosis takes priority?
    1. Hopelessness R/T anxiety AEB the statement, "Nothing ever seems to work out."
    2. Ineffective coping R/T client rating anxiety as 9/10 AEB thoughts of suicide.
    3. Anxiety R/T thoughts about work AEB client rating anxiety as 9/10.
    4. Risk for suicide R/T expressing thoughts of suicide.

Nursing Process—Planning

31. A client has a nursing diagnosis of disturbed sleep patterns R/T increased anxiety AEB inability to fall asleep. Which correctly written short-term outcome is appropriate for this client?
    1. The client will use one coping skill before bedtime to assist in falling asleep.
    2. The client will sleep 6 to 8 hours a night and report a feeling of being rested.
    3. The client will ask for prescribed prn medication to assist with sleep by day 2.
    4. The client will verbalize their level of anxiety as less than 3/10.

32. Which client would the charge nurse assign to an agency nurse who is new to a psychiatric setting?
    1. A client diagnosed with posttraumatic stress disorder currently experiencing flashbacks.
    2. A newly admitted client experiencing anxiety beginning benzodiazepines for the first time.
    3. A client admitted 4 days ago with the diagnosis of algophobia.
    4. A newly admitted client diagnosed with obsessive-compulsive disorder (OCD).

33. A newly admitted client diagnosed with social anxiety disorder has a nursing diagnosis of social isolation R/T fear of ridicule. Which correctly written outcome is appropriate for this client?
    1. The client will participate in two daily group activities by day 4.
    2. The client will use relaxation techniques to decrease anxiety.
    3. The client will verbalize one positive attribute about self by discharge.
    4. The client will request buspirone (BuSpar) prn to attend group by day 2.

34. When a client experiences a panic attack, which correctly written outcome takes priority?
    1. The client will remain safe throughout the duration of the panic attack.
    2. The client will verbalize an anxiety level of less than 2/10.
    3. The client will use learned coping mechanisms to decrease anxiety.
    4. The client will verbalize the positive effects of exercise by day 2.

35. The nurse has received the evening report. Which client would the nurse need to assess first?
    1. A newly admitted client with a history of panic attacks.
    2. A client who slept 2 to 3 hours last night because of nightmares.
    3. A client pacing the halls and stating that his anxiety is an 8/10.
    4. A client diagnosed with generalized anxiety disorder (GAD) awaiting discharge.

36. A client was admitted to an inpatient psychiatric unit 4 days ago for the treatment of obsessive-compulsive disorder (OCD). Which outcome takes priority for this client at this time?
    1. The client will use a thought-stopping technique to eliminate obsessive and/or compulsive behaviors.
    2. The client will stop obsessive and/or compulsive behaviors in order to focus on activities of daily living.
    3. The client will seek assistance from the staff to decrease obsessive and/or compulsive behaviors.
    4. The client will use one relaxation technique to decrease obsessive and/or compulsive behaviors.

37. A client diagnosed with body dysmorphic disorder has a nursing diagnosis of disturbed body image R/T reddened face. Which is a correctly written long-term outcome for this client?
    1. The client will recognize the exaggeration of a reddened face by day 2.
    2. The client will acknowledge the link between anxiety and exaggerated perceptions.
    3. The client will use behavioral modification techniques to begin accepting a reddened face.
    4. The client will verbalize acceptance of a reddened face by 3-month follow-up visit.

Nursing Process—Implementation

38. A 10-year-old client diagnosed with nightmare disorder is admitted to an inpatient psychiatric unit. Which of the following interventions would be appropriate for this client's problem? **Select all that apply.**
    1. Involving the family in therapy to decrease stress within the family.
    2. Using phototherapy to assist the client in adapting to changes in sleep.
    3. Administering medications such as tricyclic antidepressants or low-dose benzodiazepines or both.
    4. Giving central nervous system (CNS) stimulants, such as amphetamines.
    5. Using relaxation therapy, such as meditation and deep breathing techniques, to assist the client in falling asleep.

39. A client experiencing sleepwalking is newly admitted to an inpatient psychiatric unit. Which nursing intervention would take priority?
    1. Equip the bed with an alarm that is activated when the bed is exited.
    2. Discourage strenuous exercise within 1 hour of bedtime.
    3. Limit caffeine-containing substances within 4 hours of bedtime.
    4. Encourage activities that prepare one for sleep, such as soft music.

40. A client diagnosed with panic attacks is being admitted for the fifth time in 1 year because of hopelessness and helplessness. Which precaution would the nurse plan to implement?
    1. Elopement precautions.
    2. Suicide precautions.
    3. Homicide precautions.
    4. Fall precautions.

41. A client diagnosed with obsessive-compulsive disorder (OCD) has been hospitalized for the past 4 days. Which intervention would be a priority at this time?
    1. Notify the client of the expected limitations on compulsive behaviors.
    2. Reinforce the use of learned relaxation techniques.
    3. Allow the client the time needed to complete the compulsive behaviors.
    4. Say "stop" to the client as a thought-stopping technique.

42. The nurse on the inpatient psychiatric unit should include which of the following interventions when working with a newly admitted client diagnosed with obsessive-compulsive disorder (OCD)? **Select all that apply.**
    1. Assess previously used coping mechanisms and their effects on anxiety.
    2. Allow time for the client to complete compulsions.
    3. With the client's input, set limits on ritualistic behaviors.
    4. Present the reality of the impact that the compulsions have on the client's life.
    5. Discuss client feelings surrounding the obsessions and compulsions.

43. During an intake assessment, a client diagnosed with generalized anxiety disorder (GAD) rates mood at 3/10, rates anxiety at 8/10, and states, "I'm thinking about suicide." Which nursing intervention takes priority?
    1. Teach the client relaxation techniques.
    2. Ask the client, "Do you have a plan to commit suicide?"
    3. Call the physician to obtain a prn order for an anxiolytic medication.
    4. Encourage the client to participate in group activities.

44. A client newly admitted to an inpatient psychiatric unit has a diagnosis of pedophilic disorder. When working with this client, which should be the nurse's initial action?
    1. Assess the part of the sexual response cycle in which the disturbance occurs.
    2. Evaluate the nurse's feelings regarding working with the client.
    3. Establish a therapeutic nurse–client relationship.
    4. Explore the developmental alterations associated with pedophilia.

45. A client diagnosed with exhibitionistic disorder is newly admitted to an inpatient psychiatric unit. Which would be an example of a behavioral nursing intervention for this client?
    1. Encourage the client to pair noxious stimuli with sexually deviant impulses.
    2. Help the client to identify unresolved conflicts and traumas from childhood.
    3. Administer prescribed medications that block or decrease circulating androgens.
    4. Administer prescribed progestin derivatives to decrease the client's libido.

Nursing Process—Evaluation

46. The nurse is using a cognitive intervention to decrease anxiety during a client's panic attack. Which client statement would indicate that the intervention has been successful?
    1. "I reminded myself that the panic attack would end soon, and it helped."
    2. "I paced the halls until I felt my anxiety was under control."
    3. "I felt my anxiety increase, so I took lorazepam to decrease it."
    4. "Thank you for staying with me. It helped to know staff was there."

47. The nursing student is learning about paraphilic disorder. Which student statement indicates that learning has occurred?
    1. "The term *paraphilia* is used to identify repetitive or preferred sexual fantasies or behaviors."
    2. "Individuals diagnosed with a paraphilic disorder experience extreme personal distress and frequently seek treatment."
    3. "Binge eating disorder, anorexia nervosa, and bulimia nervosa are currently viewed as paraphilic disorders."
    4. "Most individuals with a paraphilic disorder are women, and more than 50% of these individuals have onset of their paraphilic arousal after age 18."

48. A client is diagnosed with male hypoactive sexual desire disorder. A nursing diagnosis of sexual dysfunction is documented for this client. Which behavior indicates successful resolution of this client's problem?
    1. The client resumes sexual activities at a level satisfactory to self and partner.
    2. The client expresses satisfaction with their own sexual patterns.
    3. The client's deviant sexual behaviors have decreased.
    4. The client accepts the experienced change in sexual functioning.

Psychopharmacology

49. Which of the following medications can be used to treat clients with anxiety disorders? **Select all that apply.**
    1. Clonidine hydrochloride.
    2. Fluvoxamine maleate.
    3. Buspirone.
    4. Alprazolam.
    5. Haloperidol.

50. A client is prescribed alprazolam 2 mg bid and 1.5 mg q6h prn for agitation. The maximum daily dose of alprazolam is 10 mg/d. The client can receive _____ prn doses of alprazolam within a 24-hour period.

51. Which teaching need is important when a client is newly prescribed buspirone 5 mg tid?
    1. Encourage the client to avoid drinking alcohol while taking this medication because of the additive central nervous system (CNS) depressant effects.
    2. Encourage the client to take the medication continuously as prescribed because onset of action is delayed 2 to 3 weeks.
    3. Encourage the client to monitor for signs and symptoms of anxiety to determine the need for additional buspirone prn.
    4. Encourage the client to be compliant with monthly laboratory tests to monitor for medication toxicity.

52. A client is prescribed lorazepam 0.5 mg qid and 1 mg prn q8h. The maximum daily dose of lorazepam should not exceed 4 mg daily. This client would be able to receive _____ prn doses as the maximum number of prn lorazepam doses.

53. A client diagnosed with generalized anxiety disorder (GAD) is placed on clonazepam and buspirone. Which client statement indicates teaching has been effective?
    1. The client verbalizes that the clonazepam is to be used for long-term therapy in conjunction with buspirone.
    2. The client verbalizes that buspirone can cause sedation and should be taken at night.
    3. The client verbalizes that clonazepam is to be used short term until the buspirone takes full effect.
    4. The client verbalizes that tolerance could result with the long-term use of buspirone.

54. In which situation would benzodiazepines be prescribed appropriately?
    1. Long-term treatment of posttraumatic stress disorder, convulsive disorder, and alcohol-induced withdrawal.
    2. Short-term treatment of generalized anxiety disorder (GAD), alcohol-induced withdrawal, and preoperative sedation.
    3. Short-term treatment of obsessive-compulsive disorder (OCD), skeletal muscle spasms, and essential hypertension.
    4. Long-term treatment of panic disorder, alcohol use disorder, and bipolar affective disorder: manic episode.

55. A client recently diagnosed with generalized anxiety disorder (GAD) is prescribed clonazepam, buspirone, and citalopram. Which assessment related to the concurrent use of these medications is most important?
    1. Monitor for signs and symptoms of worsening depression and suicidal ideation.
    2. Monitor for changes in mental status, diaphoresis, tachycardia, tremor, and diarrhea.
    3. Monitor for hyperpyrexia, dystonia, and muscle rigidity.
    4. Monitor for spasms of face, legs, and neck and for bizarre facial movements.

56. Which of the following symptoms are seen when a client abruptly stops taking diazepam? **Select all that apply.**
    1. Insomnia.
    2. Tremor.
    3. Delirium.
    4. Dry mouth.
    5. Lethargy.

57. Risperidone is to *hallucinations* as clonazepam is to:
    1. Anxiety.
    2. Depression.
    3. Mania.
    4. Catatonia.

58. In which situation would the nurse expect an additive central nervous system (CNS) depressant effect?
    1. When the client is prescribed chloral hydrate and thioridazine.
    2. When the client is prescribed temazepam and methylphenidate.
    3. When the client is prescribed zolpidem and buspirone.
    4. When the client is prescribed zaleplon and verapamil.

59. Which of the following clients would have to be monitored closely when prescribed triazolam 0.125 mg qhs? **Select all that apply.**
    1. An 80-year-old client diagnosed with a depressive disorder.
    2. A 45-year-old client diagnosed with alcohol use disorder.
    3. A 25-year-old client admitted to the hospital after a suicide attempt.
    4. A 60-year-old client admitted after a panic attack.
    5. A 50-year-old client who has a diagnosis of Parkinson's disease.

60. A client is prescribed estazolam 1 mg qhs. In which situation would the nurse clarify this order with the physician?

1. A client with a blood urea nitrogen (BUN) of 16 mg/dL and creatinine level of 1.0 mg/dL.
2. A client with an aspartate aminotransferase (AST) of 60 mcg/L and an alanine aminotransferase (ALT) of 70 U/L.
3. A client sleeping 2 to 3 hours per night.
4. A client rating anxiety level at night to be a 5 out of 10.

61. A client complains of poor sleep and loss of appetite. When prescribed trazodone 50 mg qhs, the client states, "Why am I taking an antidepressant? I'm not depressed." Which nursing response is most appropriate?

1. "Sedation is a side effect of this low dose of trazodone. It will help you sleep."
2. "Trazodone is an appetite stimulant used to prevent weight loss."
3. "Trazodone is an antianxiety medication that decreases restlessness at bedtime."
4. "Trazodone is an antipsychotic medication used off-label to treat insomnia."

The correct answer number and rationale for why it is the correct answer are given in **boldface blue type**. Rationales for why the other answer options are incorrect are given as well, but they are not in boldface type.

Theory

1. 1. Inability of the ego to intervene when conflict occurs relates to the psychoanalytic, not cognitive, theory of panic disorder development.
   2. Abnormal elevations of blood lactate and increased lactate sensitivity relate to the biological, not cognitive, theory of panic disorder development.
   3. Increased involvement of the neurochemical norepinephrine relates to the biological, not cognitive, theory of panic disorder development.
   4. **Distorted thinking patterns that precede maladaptive behaviors relate to the cognitive theory perspective of panic disorder development.**

TEST-TAKING HINT: The test taker should note important words in the question, such as *cognitive*. Although all of the answers are potential causes of panic disorder development, only answer 4 is from a cognitive perspective.

2. **An overuse or ineffective use of ego defense mechanisms, which results in a maladaptive response to anxiety, is an example of the *psychodynamic* theory of generalized anxiety disorder (GAD) development.**

TEST-TAKING HINT: To answer this question correctly, the test taker should review the various theories related to the development of GAD.

3. 1. The belief that individuals diagnosed with obsessive-compulsive disorder (OCD) have weak and underdeveloped egos is an explanation of OCD etiology from a psychoanalytic, not biological, theory perspective.
   2. The belief that obsessive and compulsive behaviors are a conditioned response to a traumatic event is an explanation of OCD etiology from a learning theory, not biological theory, perspective.
   3. The belief that regression to the pre-Oedipal anal sadistic phase produces the clinical symptoms of OCD is an explanation of OCD etiology from a psychoanalytic, not biological, theory perspective.
   4. **The belief that abnormalities in various regions of the brain cause OCD is an explanation of OCD etiology from a biological theory perspective.**

TEST-TAKING HINT: To answer this question correctly, the test taker must understand the different theories of OCD etiology. This question calls for a biological theory perspective, making answer 4 the only correct choice.

4. **When examining theories of phobia etiology, this situation would be reflective of *learning* theory. Some learning theorists believe that fears are conditioned responses, and they are learned by imposing rewards for certain behaviors. In the instance of phobias, when the individual avoids the phobic object, they escape fear, which is a powerful reward. This client has learned that avoiding the stimulus of fire eliminates fear.**

TEST-TAKING HINT: To answer this question correctly, the test taker needs to review the different theories of the causation of specific phobias.

5. 1. Offering prn lorazepam before group is an example of a biological, not intrapersonal, nursing intervention.
   2. Attending group with the client is an example of an interpersonal, not intrapersonal, nursing intervention.
   3. **Encouraging discussion about fears is an intrapersonal nursing intervention.**
   4. Role-playing a scenario that may occur is a behavioral, not intrapersonal, nursing intervention.

TEST-TAKING HINT: It is important to understand that interventions are based on theories of causation. In this question, the test taker needs to know that intrapersonal theory relates to feelings or developmental issues. Only answer 3 deals with client feelings.

6. 1. Encouraging the client to evaluate the power of distorted thinking is based on a cognitive, not psychodynamic, perspective.
   2. Asking the client to include their family in scheduled therapy sessions is based on an interpersonal, not psychodynamic, perspective.
   3. **The nurse discussing the overuse of ego defense mechanisms illustrates a**

psychodynamic approach to address the client's behaviors related to panic disorder.

4. Teaching the client the effects of blood lactate on anxiety is based on the biological, not psychodynamic, perspective.

TEST-TAKING HINT: When answering this question, the test taker must be able to differentiate among various theoretical perspectives and their related interventions.

7. 1. **Ineffective coping R/T punitive superego reflects an intrapersonal theory of the etiology of obsessive-compulsive disorder (OCD). The punitive superego is a concept contained in Freud's psychosocial theory of personality development.**
   2. Ineffective coping R/T active avoidance reflects a behavioral, not intrapersonal, theory of the etiology of OCD.
   3. Ineffective coping R/T alteration in serotonin reflects a biological, not intrapersonal, theory of the etiology of OCD.
   4. Ineffective coping R/T classic conditioning reflects a behavioral, not intrapersonal, theory of the etiology of OCD.

TEST-TAKING HINT: To answer this question correctly, the test taker needs to understand the different theories of the etiology of OCD. The keyword *intrapersonal* should make the test taker look for a concept inherent in this theory, such as *punitive superego*.

Defense Mechanisms

8. 1. Suppression, the voluntary blocking from one's awareness of unpleasant feelings and experiences is not a defense mechanism commonly used by individuals diagnosed with obsessive-compulsive disorder (OCD).
   2. Repression, the involuntary blocking of unpleasant feelings and experiences from one's awareness, is not a defense mechanism commonly used by individuals diagnosed with OCD.
   3. **Undoing is a defense mechanism commonly used by individuals diagnosed with OCD. Undoing is used symbolically to negate or cancel out an intolerable previous action or experience. An individual diagnosed with OCD experiencing intolerable anxiety would use the defense mechanism of undoing to undo this anxiety by substituting obsessions or compulsions or both. Other commonly used defense mechanisms are isolation, displacement, and reaction formation.**

4. Denial, the refusal to acknowledge the existence of a real situation or the feelings associated with it or both, is not a defense mechanism commonly used by individuals diagnosed with OCD.

TEST-TAKING HINT: To answer this question correctly, the test taker needs to understand the underlying reasons for the ritualistic behaviors used by individuals diagnosed with OCD.

Nursing Process—Assessment

9. 1. **When the client reports satisfaction with the quality of sleep, the client is providing subjective assessment data. Good sleepers self-define themselves as getting enough sleep and feeling rested. These individuals feel refreshed in the morning, have energy for daily activities, fall asleep quickly, and rarely awaken during the night.**
   2. The number of hours a client has slept during the night is an objective assessment of sleep. Sleep can be observed objectively by noting closed eyes, snoring sounds, and regular breathing patterns.
   3. The use of a sleep scale objectifies the subjective symptom of sleep quality.
   4. The number of midnight awakenings is an objective assessment of sleep. Even though the client reports this assessment, the number of midnight awakenings is objective data.

TEST-TAKING HINT: The test taker must look for an answer choice that meets the criteria of a subjective assessment. Subjective symptoms are symptoms of internal origin, evident only to the client.

10. 1. Limiting caffeine intake may be important for clients experiencing a sleep disturbance, but this is an intervention, not an assessment.
    2. Teaching the importance of a bedtime routine may be important for clients experiencing a sleep disturbance, but this is an intervention, not an assessment.
    3. Keeping the client's door locked during the day to avoid napping may be important for clients experiencing a sleep disturbance, but this is an intervention, not an assessment.
    4. **An important nursing assessment for a client experiencing a sleep disturbance is to note the client's baseline sleep patterns. These data allow the nurse to recognize alterations in normal**

patterns of sleep and to intervene appropriately.

5. It would be important to monitor the client regularly during the night to determine sleep pattern. Frequently, clients report less sleep than what is actually experienced.

TEST-TAKING HINT: To answer this question correctly, it is important to note the word *assessing*. Answers 1, 2, and 3 can be eliminated immediately because they are interventions, not assessments.

11. Primary insomnia may manifest by a combination of difficulty falling asleep and intermittent wakefulness during sleep.
    1. Lack of sleep results in daytime irritability.
    2. Lack of sleep results in problems with attention and concentration.
    3. Individuals diagnosed with insomnia may inappropriately use substances, including hypnotics for sleep and stimulants to counteract fatigue.
    4. Nightmares are frightening dreams that occur during sleep. Because clients diagnosed with insomnia have trouble sleeping, nightmares are not a characteristic of this disorder.
    5. Sleepwalking is characterized by the performance of motor activity during sleep, not wakefulness, in which the individual may leave the bed and walk about, dress, go to the bathroom, talk, scream, and even drive.

TEST-TAKING HINT: The test taker must recognize possible symptoms that insomnia may cause to answer this question correctly.

12. 1. Parasomnia refers to the unusual or undesirable behaviors that occur during sleep (e.g., nightmares, sleep terrors, and sleepwalking). Parasomnias are not classified as breathing-related sleep disorders.
    2. Hypersomnia refers to excessive sleepiness or seeking excessive amounts of sleep. Hypersomnia is not classified as a breathing-related sleep disorder.
    3. Apnea refers to the cessation of breathing during sleep. To be so classified, the apnea must last for at least 10 seconds and occur 30 or more times during a 7-hour period of sleep. Apnea is classified as a breathing-related sleep disorder.
    4. Cataplexy refers to a sudden, brief loss of muscle control brought on by strong emotion or emotional response, such as a hearty laugh, excitement, surprise, or anger.

Cataplexy is not classified as a breathing-related sleep disorder.

TEST-TAKING HINT: To answer this question correctly, the test taker first needs to be familiar with the terminology related to sleep disorders and then to note what affects breathing patterns.

13. The parasomnia of nightmare disorder is closely associated with sleepwalking, and often a night terror episode progresses into a sleepwalking episode. Approximately 1% to 6% of children experience nightmare disorder, and the incidence seems to be more common in boys than in girls. Resolution usually occurs spontaneously during adolescence. If the disorder begins in adulthood, it usually runs a chronic course.
    1. The client, on awakening, is not able to explain the nightmare. On awakening in the morning, the client experiences amnesia about the entire episode.
    2. The client is not easily awakened after the nightmare. The client is often difficult to awaken or comfort following the event.
    3. **During a nightmare, the client does experience an abrupt arousal from sleep with a piercing scream or cry.**
    4. The client, on awakening during a nightmare, is usually disoriented, not alert and oriented. The client expresses a sense of intense fear but cannot recall the dream episode.

TEST-TAKING HINT: To answer this question correctly, the test taker must understand the characteristics associated with a nightmare disorder.

14. 1. A client fearful of spiders is experiencing arachnophobia, not acrophobia.
    2. **Acrophobia is the fear of heights. An individual experiencing acrophobia may be unable to travel by air because of this fear.**
    3. A client fearful of marriage is experiencing gamophobia, not acrophobia.
    4. A client fearful of lightning is experiencing astraphobia, not acrophobia.

TEST-TAKING HINT: To answer this question correctly, the test taker needs to review the definitions of specific commonly diagnosed phobias.

15. 1. A client cannot be diagnosed with social anxiety disorder when under the influence of substances such as marijuana. It would be unclear if the client is experiencing the fear because of the mood-altering substance or a true social phobia.

2. Children can be diagnosed with social anxiety disorder. However, in children, there must be evidence of the capacity for age-appropriate social relationships with familiar people, and the anxiety must occur in peer and adult interactions.

3. If a general medical condition or another mental disorder is present, the social anxiety must be unrelated. If the fear is related to the medical condition, the client cannot be diagnosed with social anxiety disorder.

4. **A student who avoids classes because of the fear of being scrutinized by others meets the criteria for a diagnosis of social anxiety disorder.**

TEST-TAKING HINT: The test taker must understand the diagnostic criteria for social anxiety disorder to answer this question correctly.

16. 1. Fear of dying is an affective, not physical, symptom of a panic attack.
    2. **Sweating and palpitations are physical symptoms of a panic attack.**
    3. Depersonalization is an alteration in the perception or experience of the self so that the feeling of one's own reality is temporarily lost. Depersonalization is a cognitive, not physical, symptom of a panic attack.
    4. Restlessness and pacing are behavioral, not physical, symptoms of a panic attack.

TEST-TAKING HINT: The test taker must note important words and phrases in the question, such as *physical symptoms*. Although all the answers are actual symptoms that a client experiences during a panic attack, only answer 2 is a physical symptom.

17. 1. **Using excessive hand washing to relieve anxiety is a behavioral symptom exhibited by clients diagnosed with obsessive-compulsive disorder (OCD).**
    2. The verbalization of anxiety is not classified as a behavioral symptom of OCD.
    3. Using breathing techniques to decrease anxiety is a behavioral intervention, not a behavioral symptom.
    4. Excessive sweating and increased pulse are biological, not behavioral, symptoms of OCD.

TEST-TAKING HINT: To answer this question correctly, the test taker must be able to differentiate among various classes of symptoms exhibited by clients diagnosed with OCD. The keyword *behavioral* determines the correct answer to this question.

18. 1. **Chronic obstructive pulmonary disease causes shortness of breath. Air**

deprivation causes anxiety, sometimes to the point of panic.

2. **Hyperthyroidism (Graves' disease) involves excess stimulation of the sympathetic nervous system and excessive levels of thyroxine. Anxiety is one of several symptoms brought on by these increases.**

3. Hypertension is often asymptomatic characterized by persistently elevated blood pressure. Hypertension may be caused by anxiety, but normally clients do not experience anxiety due to hypertension.

4. Diverticulosis results from the outpocketing of the colon. Unless these pockets become inflamed, diverticulosis is generally asymptomatic.

5. **Marked irritability and anxiety are some of the many symptoms associated with hypoglycemia.**

TEST-TAKING HINT: To answer this question correctly, the test taker needs to understand that anxiety is manifested by physiological responses.

19. 1. A client cannot be diagnosed with an anxiety disorder if anxiety is experienced in only one area of functioning.
    2. Although anxiety does need to be experienced for a period of time before being diagnosed as an anxiety disorder, this answer states *one* area of functioning and so is incorrect.
    3. For a client to be diagnosed with an anxiety disorder, the client must experience symptoms that interfere in a minimum of two areas, such as social, occupational, or other important functioning. These symptoms must be experienced for durations of 6 months or longer.
    4. **A client needs to experience high levels of anxiety that affect functioning in a minimum of two areas of life, and these must have durations of 6 months or longer.**

TEST-TAKING HINT: To answer this question correctly, the test taker must understand that specific symptoms must be exhibited and specific time frames achieved for clients to be diagnosed with anxiety disorders.

20. 1. **A client diagnosed with generalized anxiety disorder (GAD) would experience excessive worry about items difficult to control.**
    2. **A client diagnosed with GAD would experience muscle tension.**
    3. A client diagnosed with GAD would experience insomnia, not hypersomnia. Sleep disturbances would include difficulty

falling asleep, difficulty staying asleep, and restless sleep.

4. A client diagnosed with GAD would be easily fatigued and not experience excessive amounts of energy.

5. **A client diagnosed with GAD would experience an increased startle reflex and tension, causing feelings of being "keyed up" or being "on edge."**

TEST-TAKING HINT: To answer this question correctly, the test taker would need to recognize the signs and symptoms of GAD.

21. 1. Compulsive behaviors that occupy many hours per day would be a behavioral, not cognitive, symptom experienced by clients diagnosed with obsessive-compulsive disorder (OCD).

2. **Excessive worrying about germs and illness is a cognitive symptom experienced by clients diagnosed with OCD.**

3. Comorbid abuse of alcohol to decrease anxiety would be a behavioral, not cognitive, symptom experienced by clients diagnosed with OCD.

4. Excessive sweating and increased blood pressure and pulse are physiological, not cognitive, symptoms experienced by clients diagnosed with OCD.

TEST-TAKING HINT: To answer this question correctly, the test taker must note the keyword *cognitive*. Only answer 2 is a cognitive symptom.

22. 1. To be diagnosed with hoarding disorder, the hoarding cannot be attributed to another medical condition, such as brain injury, cerebrovascular disease, or Prader-Willi syndrome.

2. **Clients diagnosed with hoarding disorder will report panic levels of anxiety when asked to part with possessions.**

3. In a hoarding disorder, the hoarding causes clinically significant distress or impairment in social, occupational, or other important areas of function, including maintaining a safe environment. A client collecting possessions, which are kept neatly in a closet, would not meet the criteria for the diagnosis of hoarding disorder.

4. **A client being evicted because their possessions have become a safety hazard would meet the criteria for the diagnosis of a hoarding disorder.**

5. **A client needing family to remove possessions because the client is psychologically unable to remove them would meet the criteria for the diagnosis of a hoarding disorder.**

TEST-TAKING HINT: To answer this question correctly, the test taker must recognize the criteria needed to be diagnosed with a hoarding disorder.

23. 1. Exhibitionistic disorder, not fetishistic disorder, is characterized by recurrent, intense sexual urge, behavior, or sexually arousing fantasy, of at least a 6-month duration, involving the exposure of one's genitals to an unsuspecting stranger.

2. **Fetishistic disorder involves recurrent, intense sexual urges or behaviors, of at least 6-months in duration, involving the use of nonliving objects. The sexual focus is commonly on objects intimately associated with the human body (e.g., shoes, gloves, or stockings).**

3. Frotteuristic disorder, not fetishistic disorder, is the recurrent preoccupation with intense sexual urges, behaviors, or fantasies, of at least a 6-month duration, involving touching and rubbing against a nonconsenting person. Almost without exception, the sex of the frotteur is male. The frotteur waits in a crowd until he identifies a victim; he then allows the rush of a crowd to push him against this individual.

4. Masochistic disorder, not fetishistic disorder, is the recurrent, intense sexual urge, behavior, or sexually arousing fantasy, of at least a 6-month duration, involving the act (real, not simulated) of being humiliated, beaten, bound, or otherwise made to suffer.

TEST-TAKING HINT: The test taker must be able to distinguish among the various types of paraphilic disorders to answer this question correctly.

24. 1. Male erectile disorder, not delayed ejaculation disorder, is characterized by persistent or recurrent inability to attain, or to maintain until completion of the sexual activity, an adequate erection.

2. **Delayed ejaculation disorder is characterized by persistent or recurrent delay in achieving orgasm following a normal sexual excitement phase during sexual activity, which the clinician, taking into account the client's age, judges to be adequate in focus, intensity, and duration.**

3. Premature ejaculation is defined as the persistent or recurrent ejaculation with minimal sexual stimulation before, on, or shortly after penetration and before the man wishes it. Premature ejaculation is not a symptom of delayed ejaculation disorder.

4. Genito-pelvic pain/penetration disorder is recurrent or persistent genital pain (dyspareunia) associated with sexual intercourse in a man or a woman. Genito-pelvic pain/penetration disorder is not a symptom of male orgasmic disorder.

5. Delayed ejaculation disorder is characterized by marked infrequency or absence of ejaculation following a normal sexual excitement phase during sexual activity, which the clinician, taking into account the client's age, judges to be adequate in focus, intensity, and duration.

TEST-TAKING HINT: The test taker must differentiate among the types of sexual dysfunction and the accompanying symptoms to answer this question correctly.

25. 1. Because of this client's age, the diagnosis of schizophrenia is unlikely. The typical onset of schizophrenia is late adolescence through early adulthood.

2. **One of the symptoms of the tertiary stage of syphilis is psychosis and bizarre behaviors. The client's symptoms of auditory hallucinations and bizarre behaviors would be reflective of this diagnosis. Although there can be other reasons for these symptoms, the client's history of prostitution and recent onset of symptoms would warrant investigation into the possible diagnosis of tertiary syphilis.**

3. Gonorrhea is initially asymptomatic. The signs and symptoms progress to infection of the cervix, urethra, and fallopian tubes, which may result in infertility and ectopic pregnancy. Auditory hallucinations and bizarre behaviors are not potential complications of gonorrhea.

4. The diagnosis of a personality disorder occurs early in life. Schizotypal personality disorder is characterized by odd and eccentric behavior. Because of this client's age and the recent onset of symptoms, schizotypal personality disorder can be ruled out.

TEST-TAKING HINT: The test taker must carefully note the client's age and recent onset of symptoms, which would lead to the immediate elimination of answers 1 and 4. It is important to understand that there can be physical and psychological symptoms associated with sexually transmitted diseases.

26. Nail biting, scratching, and hair pulling for extended periods of time in a private setting are symptoms associated with the diagnosis of *trichotillomania (hair-pulling disorder)*.

TEST-TAKING HINT: To answer this question correctly, the test taker must have knowledge of various symptoms associated with trichotillomania.

Nursing Process—Diagnosis

27. Hypersomnia, or somnolence, can be defined as excessive sleepiness or seeking excessive amounts of sleep. Excessive sleepiness interferes with attention, concentration, memory, and productivity. It also can lead to disruption in social and family relationships. Depression is a common side effect of hypersomnia, as are substance-related disorders.

1. **Verbalizations of worthlessness may indicate that this client is experiencing suicidal ideations. After assessing suicide risk further, the risk for suicide should be prioritized.**

2. Social isolation R/T sleepiness would be an appropriate nursing diagnosis for a client diagnosed with hypersomnia because of limited contact with others as a result of increased sleep. Compared with the other nursing diagnoses presented, however, this diagnosis would not take priority.

3. Self-care deficit R/T increased need for sleep AEB being unable to bathe without assistance would be an appropriate nursing diagnosis for a client diagnosed with hypersomnia because of the limited energy for bathing related to increased sleepiness. Compared with the other nursing diagnoses presented, however, this diagnosis would not take priority.

4. Chronic low self-esteem R/T inability to function AEB the statement, "I feel worthless," is an appropriate nursing diagnosis for a client diagnosed with hypersomnia. Compared with the other nursing diagnoses presented, however, this diagnosis would not take priority.

TEST-TAKING HINT: All the nursing diagnoses presented document problems associated with hypersomnia. Because the nurse always prioritizes safety, the nursing diagnosis of risk for suicide takes precedence.

28. 1. According to NANDA-I, the nursing diagnosis format must contain three essential components: (1) identification of the health problem, (2) presentation of the etiology (or cause) of the problem, and (3) description of a cluster of signs and symptoms known as *defining characteristics*. The

correct answer, 1, contains all three components in the correct order: health problem/NANDA-I stem (social isolation); etiology/cause, or R/T (fear of germs); and signs and symptoms, or AEB (refusing to leave home for the past year). Because this client has been unable to leave home for a year as a result of fear of germs, the client's behaviors meet the defining characteristics of social isolation.

2. Obsessive-compulsive disorder (OCD) is a medical diagnosis and cannot be used in any component of the nursing diagnosis format. Nursing diagnoses are functional client problems that fall within the scope of nursing practice. Also missing from this nursing diagnosis are the signs and symptoms, or AEB, component of the problem.

3. The etiology (R/T) and signs and symptoms (AEB) are out of order in this nursing diagnostic statement, and, therefore, it is written incorrectly.

4. The inability to leave home is a sign or symptom, which is the third component of the nursing diagnosis format (AEB), not the cause of the problem (R/T statement).

TEST-TAKING HINT: To answer this question correctly, the test taker needs to know the components of a correctly stated nursing diagnosis and the order in which these components are written.

29. 1. Although ineffective breathing patterns would be an appropriate nursing diagnosis during a panic attack, the client in the question is not experiencing a panic attack, so this nursing diagnosis is inappropriate at this time.

2. Although impaired spontaneous ventilation would be an appropriate nursing diagnosis during a panic attack, the client in the question is not experiencing a panic attack, so this nursing diagnosis is inappropriate at this time.

3. Social isolation is seen frequently with individuals diagnosed with panic attacks. The client in the question expresses anticipatory fear of unexpected attacks, which affects the client's ability to interact with others.

4. Nothing in the question indicates that the client has a knowledge deficit related to triggers for panic attacks. The client in the question is expressing fear as it relates to the unpredictability of panic attacks.

TEST-TAKING HINT: To answer this question correctly, the test taker must link the behaviors presented in the question with the nursing diagnosis that is reflective of these behaviors. The test taker must remember the importance of timewise interventions. Nursing interventions differ according to the degree of anxiety the client is experiencing. If the client were currently experiencing a panic attack, other interventions would be appropriate.

30. 1. Although hopelessness can be an appropriate nursing diagnosis for a client diagnosed with generalized anxiety disorder (GAD) and expressing suicidal ideations, it is not the priority nursing diagnosis at this time because it does not directly address the risk for suicide.

2. Although ineffective coping can be an appropriate nursing diagnosis for a client diagnosed with GAD, it is not the priority nursing diagnosis at this time.

3. Although anxiety can be an appropriate nursing diagnosis for a client diagnosed with GAD, it is not the priority nursing diagnosis at this time.

4. Because the client is expressing suicidal ideations, the nursing diagnosis of risk for suicide takes priority at this time. Client safety is prioritized over all other client problems.

TEST-TAKING HINT: When looking for a priority nursing diagnosis, the test taker always must prioritize client safety. Even if other problems exist, client safety must be ensured.

Nursing Process—Planning

31. 1. Although the nurse may want the client to use one coping skill before bedtime to assist in falling asleep, there is no time frame on this outcome, and it is not measurable.

2. The outcome of being able to sleep 6 to 8 hours a night and report a feeling of being rested has no time frame and is not measurable.

3. The client's being able to ask for prescribed prn medication to assist with falling asleep by day 2 is a short-term outcome that is specific, has a time frame, and relates to the stated nursing diagnosis.

4. Although the nurse may want the client to verbalize a decreased level of anxiety, this outcome does not have a time frame and is not measurable.

TEST-TAKING HINT: When given a nursing diagnosis in the question, the test taker should choose the outcome that directly relates to the client's specific problem. If a client had a nursing diagnosis of disturbed sleep patterns R/T frequent naps during the day, the short-term outcome for this client may be "the client will stay in the milieu for all scheduled groups by day 2." Staying in the milieu would assist the client in avoiding napping, which is the cause of this client's problem. Also, when a question asks for an outcome, the outcome must be client centered, specific, realistic, and measurable and must also include a time frame.

32. 1. A client diagnosed with posttraumatic stress disorder experiencing acute flashbacks would need special treatment. An inexperienced agency nurse may find this situation overwhelming.
    2. A client diagnosed with generalized anxiety disorder (GAD) beginning benzodiazepine therapy for the first time may have specific questions about the disease process or the prescribed medication. An inexperienced agency nurse may be unfamiliar with client teaching needs.
    3. A client admitted 4 days ago with a diagnosis of algophobia, fear of pain, would be an appropriate assignment for the agency nurse. Of the clients presented, this client would pose the least challenge to a nurse unfamiliar with psychiatric clients.
    4. A client diagnosed with obsessive-compulsive disorder (OCD) would need to be allowed to use their ritualistic behaviors to control anxiety to a manageable level. An inexperienced agency nurse may not fully understand client behaviors that reflect the diagnosis of OCD and may intervene inappropriately.

TEST-TAKING HINT: To answer this question correctly, the test taker needs to recognize the complexity of psychiatric diagnoses and understand the ramifications of potentially inappropriate nursing interventions by inexperienced staff members.

33. 1. Expecting the client to participate in a set number of group activities by day 4 directly relates to the stated nursing diagnosis of social isolation and is a measurable outcome that includes a time frame.
    2. Although the nurse may want the client to use relaxation techniques to decrease anxiety, this outcome does not have a time frame and is not measurable.

3. Having the client verbalize one positive attribute about self by discharge relates to the nursing diagnosis of low self-esteem, not social isolation.
4. Buspirone is not used on a prn basis, so this is an inappropriate outcome for this client.

TEST-TAKING HINT: To express an appropriate outcome, the statement must be related to the stated problem, be measurable and attainable, and have a time frame. The test taker can eliminate answer 2 immediately because there is no time frame, and then answer 3 because it does not relate to the stated problem.

34. 1. Remaining safe throughout the duration of the panic attack is the priority outcome for the client.
    2. Although a decreased anxiety level is a desired outcome for a client experiencing panic, this outcome is not measurable because it contains no time frame.
    3. Although the use of coping mechanisms to decrease anxiety is a desired outcome, this outcome is not measurable because it contains no time frame.
    4. The verbalization of the positive effects of exercise is a desired outcome, and it contains a time frame that is measurable. This would be an unrealistic outcome, however, for a client experiencing a panic attack.

TEST-TAKING HINT: All outcomes must be appropriate for the situation described in the question. In the question, the client is experiencing a panic attack; having the client verbalize the positive effects of exercise would be inappropriate. All outcomes must be client centered, specific, realistic, positive, and measurable and contain a time frame.

35. 1. A client newly admitted with a panic attack history does not command the immediate attention of the nurse. If the client presents with signs and symptoms of panic, the nurse's priority would then shift to this client.
    2. The nurse would assess a client experiencing flashbacks during the night, but this assessment would not take priority at this time over the other clients described.
    3. A client pacing the halls and experiencing an increase in anxiety commands immediate assessment. If the nurse does not take action on this assessment, there is a potential for client injury to self or others.
    4. A client with generalized anxiety disorder (GAD) awaiting discharge does not

command the immediate attention of the nurse. To meet the criteria for discharge, this client should be in stable mental condition.

TEST-TAKING HINT: When the nurse is prioritizing client assessments, it is important to note which client might be a safety risk. When asked to prioritize, the test taker must review all the situations presented before deciding which one to address first.

36. 1. It is unrealistic to expect the client to use a thought-stopping technique totally to eliminate obsessive and/or compulsive behaviors by day 4 of treatment.
    2. It is unrealistic for clients diagnosed with obsessive-compulsive disorder (OCD) to abruptly stop obsessive and/or compulsive behaviors in order to focus on activities of daily living.
    3. It is desirable for the client to seek assistance from the staff to decrease the amount of obsessive or compulsive behaviors. However, this outcome should be prioritized earlier than day 4 of treatment.
    4. By day 4, it would be realistic to expect the client to use one relaxation technique to decrease obsessive or compulsive behaviors. This would be the current priority outcome.

TEST-TAKING HINT: The test taker must recognize the importance of timewise interventions when establishing outcomes. In the case of clients diagnosed with OCD, expectations on admission vary greatly from outcomes developed closer to discharge.

37. 1. It is important for the client to gain insight into the exaggerated nature of their symptoms. However, expecting the client, by day 2, to recognize that their perception of a reddened face is exaggerated is unrealistic. This is also a short-term, not long-term, outcome.
    2. It is important for the client to acknowledge the link between anxiety and exaggerated perceptions. This outcome does not contain a time frame, however, and so cannot be measured.
    3. Behavioral modification may be effective in helping the client to accept a reddened face. This outcome does not contain a time frame, however, and so cannot be measured.
    4. The long-term outcome of the verbalization of acceptance of a reddened face by the scheduled 3-month follow-up appointment is an outcome that is client specific, measurable, and attainable and has a stated time frame.

TEST-TAKING HINT: It is important to note keywords in the question, such as *long-term*. The test taker can eliminate answer 1 immediately because it is a short-term, not long-term, outcome. To be measurable, an outcome must include a time frame, which eliminates answers 2 and 3.

Nursing Process—Implementation

38. The parasomnia of nightmare disorder is diagnosed when there is a repeated occurrence of frightening dreams that interfere with social or occupational functioning. Nightmares are common between the ages of 3 and 6 years, and most children outgrow the phenomenon. The individual is usually fully alert on awakening from the nightmare and, because of the lingering fear or anxiety, may have difficulty returning to sleep.
    1. **Family stress can occur as the result of repeated client nightmares. This stress within the family may exacerbate the client's problem and hamper any effective treatment. Involving the family in therapy to relieve obvious stress would be an appropriate intervention to assist in the treatment of clients diagnosed with a nightmare disorder.**
    2. Phototherapy to assist clients in adapting to changes in sleep would be an appropriate intervention for clients diagnosed with circadian rhythm sleep disorders, not a nightmare disorder. Phototherapy, or "bright light" therapy, has been shown to be effective in treating the circadian rhythm sleep disorders of delayed sleep phase disorder and jet lag.
    3. **Administering medications such as tricyclic antidepressants or low-dose benzodiazepines or both is an appropriate intervention for clients diagnosed with a parasomnia disorder, such as a nightmare disorder.**
    4. Giving central nervous system (CNS) stimulants, such as amphetamines, would be an appropriate intervention for clients diagnosed with hypersomnia, not a nightmare disorder.
    5. **Relaxation therapy, such as meditation and deep breathing techniques, would be appropriate for clients diagnosed with a nightmare disorder to help them fall back to sleep after the nightmare occurs.**

TEST-TAKING HINT: To answer this question correctly, the test taker must be able first to understand the manifestation of a nightmare disorder and then to choose the interventions that would address these manifestations effectively.

39. Sleepwalking is considered a parasomnia. Sleepwalking is characterized by the performance of motor activity during sleep in which the individual may leave the bed and walk about, dress, go to the bathroom, talk, scream, or even drive.
    1. **Equipping the bed with an alarm that activates when the bed is exited is a priority nursing intervention. During a sleepwalking episode, the client is at increased risk for injury, and interventions must address safety.**
    2. Discouraging strenuous exercise before bedtime is an appropriate intervention to promote sleep; however, this intervention does not take priority over safety.
    3. Limiting caffeine-containing substances within 4 hours of bedtime is an appropriate intervention to promote sleep; however, this intervention does not take priority over safety.
    4. Encouraging activities that prepare one for sleep, such as soft music, is an appropriate intervention to promote sleep; however, this intervention does not take priority over safety.

TEST-TAKING HINT: To answer this question correctly, the test taker must understand that a client experiencing sleepwalking is at increased risk for injury. An intervention that addresses safety concerns must be prioritized.

40. 1. If a client is being admitted for panic attacks because of feeling hopeless and helpless, the client is seeking help; elopement precautions are not yet necessary. If behaviors indicate that the client is a danger to self or others, and the client has intentions of leaving the unit, treatment team discussions of elopement precautions are indicated.
    2. **Any client who is exhibiting hopelessness or helplessness needs to be monitored closely for suicide intentions.**
    3. There is no information in the question that supports the need for homicide precautions.
    4. There is no information in the question that supports the need for fall precautions.

TEST-TAKING HINT: To answer this question correctly, the test taker should note the words *hopelessness* and *helplessness,* which would be indications of suicidal ideations that warrant suicide precautions.

41. 1. The nurse would include, not notify, the client when making decisions to limit compulsive behaviors. To be successful, the client and the treatment team must be involved with the development of the plan of care.
    2. **It is important for the client to learn techniques to reduce overall levels of anxiety to decrease the need for compulsive behaviors. The teaching of these techniques should begin by day 4.**
    3. By day 4, the nurse, with the client's input, should begin setting limits on the compulsive behaviors.
    4. The client, not the nurse, should say the word *stop* as a technique to limit obsessive thoughts and behaviors.

TEST-TAKING HINT: To answer this question correctly, the test taker must understand that nursing interventions should be based on time frames appropriate to the expressed symptoms and severity of the client's disorder.

42. 1. **When a client is newly admitted, it is important for the nurse to assess past coping mechanisms and their effects on anxiety. Assessment is the first step in the nursing process, and this information needs to be gathered to intervene effectively.**
    2. **Allowing time for the client to complete compulsions is important for a client who is newly admitted. If compulsions are limited, anxiety levels increase. If the client had been hospitalized for a while, then, with the client's input, limits would be set on the compulsive behaviors.**
    3. The nurse would set limits on ritualistic behaviors, with the client's input, later in the treatment process, not when a client is newly admitted.
    4. A newly admitted client who is exhibiting compulsions is experiencing a high level of anxiety. To present the impact of these compulsions on daily living would be inappropriate at this time and may lead to further increases in anxiety. Clients diagnosed with obsessive-compulsive disorder (OCD) are aware that their compulsions are "different."
    5. **It is important for the nurse to allow the client to express their feelings about the obsessions and compulsions. This assessment of feelings should begin at admission.**

TEST-TAKING HINT: It is important for the test taker to note the words *newly admitted* in the question. The nursing interventions implemented vary and are based on length of stay on the unit, along with client's insight into their disorder. For clients with OCD, it is important to understand that the compulsions are used to decrease anxiety. If the compulsions are limited, anxiety increases. Also, the test taker must remember that during treatment it is imperative that the treatment team includes the client in decisions related to any limitation of compulsive behaviors.

43. 1. Although it is important to teach the client relaxation techniques, this is not the current priority. The client has expressed suicidal ideations, and the priority is to assess the suicide plan further.
2. **It is important for the nurse to ask the client about a potential plan for suicide in order to evaluate the client's intentions and safety risk. This knowledge would direct appropriate and timely nursing interventions. Clients who have developed suicide plans are at higher risk than clients who may have vague suicidal thoughts.**
3. The nurse may want to call the physician to obtain a prn order for anxiolytic medications; however, a thorough physical evaluation and further assessment of suicidal ideations need to occur before calling the physician.
4. It is important for the client to participate in group activities. However, the nurse's first priority is assessing suicidal ideations and developing a plan to intervene quickly and appropriately to maintain client safety.

TEST-TAKING HINT: To answer this question correctly, the test taker must recognize the importance of assessing the plan for suicide first. Interventions would differ depending on the client's plan. The intervention for a plan to use a gun at home would differ from an intervention for a plan to hang oneself during hospitalization.

44. 1. Sexual dysfunctions, not pedophilic disorder, occur as disturbances in any of the phases of the sexual response cycle. An understanding of anatomy and physiology is a prerequisite to considerations of pathology and treatment for sexual dysfunctions.
2. **When working with clients diagnosed with pedophilic disorder, the nurse's initial action should be to evaluate personal feelings. Personal feelings, attitudes, and values should not interfere with acceptance of the client. The nurse must remain nonjudgmental.**

3. To establish a therapeutic nurse–client relationship, the nurse first must evaluate personal feelings related to working with a client diagnosed with pedophilic disorder. If feelings are negative toward these clients, judgmental attitudes probably would prevail, preventing the establishment of a therapeutic relationship.
4. Although it is important to understand the developmental alterations associated with the diagnosis of pedophilic disorder, compared with the other nursing actions presented, this would not be the nurse's initial action. Awareness of feelings assists the nurse to accept the client compassionately and empathetically while rejecting the client's sexually deviant behaviors.

TEST-TAKING HINT: The test taker should note the keywords *initial action* to choose an action that takes priority. Even if other nursing actions are appropriate, the test taker must look for the intervention that should be implemented first.

45. 1. **Aversion therapy is a behavioral nursing intervention that encourages the pairing of noxious stimuli, such as bad odors, with deviant sexual impulses in an attempt to assist the client in avoiding inappropriate behavior. This behavioral approach is used in the treatment of clients diagnosed with paraphilic disorder such as exhibitionistic disorder.**
2. Helping the client identify unresolved conflicts and traumas from early childhood is an intervention that supports a psychoanalytic, not behavioral, approach in the treatment of clients diagnosed with paraphilic disorders such as exhibitionistic disorder.
3. Administering medications that block or decrease the level of circulating androgens is a nursing intervention that supports a biological, not behavioral, approach in the treatment of clients diagnosed with paraphilic disorder such as exhibitionistic disorder. Various studies have implicated several organic factors in the etiology of paraphilic disorders, including abnormal levels of androgens that may contribute to inappropriate sexual arousal.
4. Administering prescribed progestin derivatives to decrease the client's libido is a nursing intervention that supports a biological, not behavioral, approach in the treatment of clients diagnosed with paraphilic disorders such as exhibitionistic disorder.

TEST-TAKING HINT: To answer this question correctly, the test taker must recognize that exhibitionistic disorder is a type of paraphilic disorder. The keyword in this question is *behavioral*. The test taker must be able to choose the intervention that supports a behavioral approach.

Nursing Process—Evaluation

46. 1. This statement is an indication that the cognitive intervention was successful. By remembering that panic attacks are self-limiting, the client is applying the information gained from the nurse's cognitive intervention.
    2. This statement is an indication that a behavioral, not cognitive, intervention was implemented by the nurse. From a behavioral perspective, the nurse has taught this client that exercise can decrease anxiety.
    3. This statement is an indication that the nurse implemented a biological, not cognitive, intervention. From a biological perspective, the nurse has taught this client that anxiolytic medication can decrease anxiety.
    4. This statement is an indication that the nurse implemented an interpersonal, not cognitive, intervention. From an interpersonal perspective, the nurse has taught this client that a social support system can decrease anxiety.

TEST-TAKING HINT: To answer this question correctly, the test taker needs to understand which interventions support which theories of causation. When looking for a cognitive intervention, the test taker must remember that the theory involves thought processes.

47. 1. The term *paraphilia* is used to identify repetitive or preferred sexual fantasies or behaviors that involve any of the following: the preference for use of non-human objects, repetitive sexual activity with humans that involves real or simulated suffering or humiliation, or repetitive sexual activity with nonconsenting partners.
    2. Most individuals diagnosed with a paraphilic disorder do not experience distress from their behaviors. These individuals come for treatment only because of pressure from their partners or legal authorities. Of clients diagnosed with paraphilic disorders, 45% are diagnosed with pedophilic disorder, 25% with exhibitionistic disorder, and 12% with voyeuristic disorder.
    3. Binge eating disorder, anorexia nervosa, and bulimia nervosa are feeding and eating disorders.
    4. Most individuals with paraphilic disorders are male, not female. Also, more than 50% of these individuals develop the onset of their paraphilic arousal before, not after, age 18.

TEST-TAKING HINT: The test taker must understand the definition and diagnostic criteria of paraphilic disorder to answer this question correctly.

48. Male hypoactive sexual desire disorder is characterized by a persistent or recurrent extreme aversion to, and avoidance of, all genital sexual contact with a sexual partner.
    1. A client's resuming sexual activities at a level satisfactory to self and partner indicates successful resolution of the client's sexual dysfunction problem. Sexual dysfunction is defined as the state in which an individual experiences a change in sexual function that is viewed as unsatisfying, unrewarding, or inadequate.
    2. A client expressing satisfaction with their own sexual patterns is a behavior that reflects successful resolution of the client's problem of altered sexual patterns, not sexual dysfunction. Altered sexual patterns are defined as the state in which an individual expresses concern regarding their sexuality.
    3. Deviant sexual behavior is defined as behavior that is abnormal or socially unacceptable. This client is experiencing extreme aversion to and avoidance of sex, not sexual deviation. Deviant sexual behavior also is not a symptom of male hypoactive sexual desire disorder. Sexual dysfunction is defined as unsatisfying, unrewarding, or inadequate sexual functioning.
    4. Accepting the experienced change in sexual functioning would not exhibit successful resolution of male hypoactive sexual desire disorder.

TEST-TAKING HINT: The test taker must differentiate between the nursing diagnosis of sexual dysfunction and the nursing diagnosis of altered sexual patterns to answer this question correctly.

Psychopharmacology

49. 1. Clonidine hydrochloride, an antihypertensive, is used in the treatment of panic disorders and generalized anxiety disorder (GAD).

2. Fluvoxamine maleate, an antidepressant, is used in the treatment of obsessive-compulsive disorder (OCD).
3. Buspirone, an anxiolytic, is used in the treatment of panic disorder and generalized anxiety disorder (GAD).
4. Alprazolam, a benzodiazepine, is used for the short-term treatment of anxiety disorders.
5. Haloperidol is an antipsychotic used to treat thought disorders, not anxiety disorders.

TEST-TAKING HINT: To answer this question correctly, the test taker needs to understand that many medications are used off-label to treat anxiety disorders.

50. The client can receive *four* prn doses. Medications are given four times in a 24-hour period when the order reads q6h: 1.5 mg × 4 = 6 mg. The test taker must factor in 2 mg bid = 4 mg. These two dosages together add up to 10 mg, the maximum daily dose of alprazolam, so the client can receive all four prn doses.

TEST-TAKING HINT: To answer this question correctly, the test taker must recognize that the timing of standing medication may affect the decision-making process related to administration of prn medications. In this case, the client would be able to receive all possible doses of prn medication because the standing and prn ordered medications together do not exceed the maximum daily dose.

51. Buspirone is an antianxiety medication that does not depress the central nervous system (CNS) the way benzodiazepines do. Although its action is unknown, the drug is believed to produce the desired effects through interactions with serotonin, dopamine, and other neurotransmitter receptors.
   1. Alcohol consumption is contraindicated while taking any psychotropic medication; however, buspirone does not depress the CNS, so there is no additive effect.
   2. It is important to teach the client that the onset of action for buspirone is 2 to 3 weeks. Often the nurse may see a benzodiazepine, such as clonazepam, prescribed because of its quick onset of effect, until the buspirone begins working.
   3. Buspirone is not effective in prn dosing because of the length of time it takes to begin working. Benzodiazepines have a quick onset of effect and are used prn.

4. No current laboratory tests monitor buspirone toxicity.

TEST-TAKING HINT: To answer this question correctly, the test taker must understand that buspirone has a delayed onset of action, which can affect medication adherence. If the effects of the medication are delayed, the client is likely to stop taking the medication. Teaching about delayed onset is an important nursing intervention.

52. This client should receive *two* prn doses. The test taker must recognize that medications are given three times in a 24-hour period when the order reads q8h: 1 mg × 3 = 3 mg. The test taker must factor in the 0.5 mg qid = 2 mg. These two dosages together add up to 5 mg, 1 mg above the maximum daily dose of lorazepam. The client would be able to receive only two of the three prn doses of lorazepam.

TEST-TAKING HINT: To answer this question correctly, the test taker must recognize that the timing of standing medication may affect the decision-making process related to administration of prn medications. In this case, although the prn medication is ordered q8h and could be given three times, the standing medication dosage limits the prn to two doses, each at least 8 hours apart.

53. Clonazepam, a benzodiazepine, is a CNS depressant; buspirone, an antianxiety medication, does not affect the central nervous system (CNS).
   1. Clonazepam is used in the short-term, not long-term, treatment of anxiety, while waiting for buspirone to take effect, which can take 2 to 3 weeks.
   2. Buspirone does not cause sedation because it is not a CNS depressant.
   3. Clonazepam would be used for short-term treatment while waiting for the buspirone to take effect, which can take 2 to 3 weeks.
   4. Tolerance can result with long-term use of clonazepam, but not with buspirone.

TEST-TAKING HINT: To answer this question correctly, the test taker must note appropriate teaching needs for clients prescribed different classifications of antianxiety medications.

54. 1. Benzodiazepines, used to decrease anxiety symptoms, are not intended to be prescribed for long-term treatment. They can be prescribed for short-term treatment for individuals diagnosed with posttraumatic stress disorder, convulsive disorder, and alcohol-induced withdrawal.

2. Benzodiazepines are prescribed for short-term treatment of generalized anxiety disorder (GAD) and alcohol-induced withdrawal and can be prescribed during preoperative sedation.

3. Although benzodiazepines are prescribed for short-term treatment, they are not prescribed for essential hypertension. Benzodiazepines are prescribed for short-term treatment of obsessive-compulsive disorder (OCD) and skeletal muscle spasms.

4. Benzodiazepines are not intended to be prescribed for long-term treatment. They can be prescribed for short-term treatment for individuals diagnosed with panic disorder; for alcohol-induced withdrawal; and for agitation related to a manic episode.

TEST-TAKING HINT: The test taker needs to note the words *long-term* and *short-term* in the answers. Benzodiazepines are prescribed in the short-term because of their addictive properties. The test taker must understand that when taking a test, if one part of the answer is incorrect, the whole answer is incorrect, as in answer choice 3.

55. Clonazepam, a benzodiazepine, acts quickly to assist clients with anxiety symptoms. Buspirone, an antianxiety agent, and citalopram, a selective serotonin reuptake inhibitor, are used in the long-term treatment of anxiety symptoms. Buspirone and citalopram take about 4 to 6 weeks to take full effect, and the quick-acting benzodiazepine would be needed to assist the client with decreasing anxiety symptoms before these other medications take effect. All of these medications affect the neurotransmitter serotonin.

1. Although it is important for all clients to be assessed for depression and suicidal ideation, the question is asking for the nurse to note important information related to concurrent use of these medications. This assessment does not answer the stated question.

2. It is important for the nurse to monitor for serotonin syndrome, which occurs when a client takes multiple medications that affect serotonin levels. Symptoms include change in mental status, restlessness, myoclonus, hyperreflexia, tachycardia, labile blood pressure, diaphoresis, shivering, tremor, and diarrhea.

3. These symptoms are signs of neuroleptic malignant syndrome, a rare but potentially deadly side effect of all antipsychotic medications, such as haloperidol, but not of the medications listed in the question.

4. These symptoms are signs of tardive dyskinesia and dystonia, which are potential side effects of all antipsychotic medications but not of the medications listed in the question.

TEST-TAKING HINT: To answer this question correctly, the test taker must be familiar with the signs and symptoms of serotonin syndrome and which psychotropic medications affect serotonin, potentially leading to this syndrome.

56. Diazepam is a benzodiazepine. Benzodiazepines are physiologically and psychologically addictive. If a benzodiazepine is stopped abruptly, a rebound stimulation of the CNS occurs, and the client may experience insomnia, increased anxiety, abdominal and muscle cramps, tremors, vomiting, sweating, convulsions, and delirium.

1. Insomnia may be experienced if diazepam is abruptly stopped.

2. Tremor may be experienced if diazepam is abruptly stopped.

3. Delirium may be experienced if diazepam is abruptly stopped.

4. Dry mouth is a side effect of taking benzodiazepines and is not related to stopping the medication abruptly.

5. Lethargy is a side effect of taking benzodiazepines and is not related to stopping the medication abruptly.

TEST-TAKING HINT: The test taker must distinguish between benzodiazepine side effects and symptoms of withdrawal to answer this question correctly.

57. Risperidone is an antipsychotic medication that decreases excessive dopamine, a neurotransmitter, and decreases hallucinations.

1. Clonazepam is a benzodiazepine that works quickly to relieve anxiety.

2. Medications prescribed for depression are monoamine oxidase inhibitors, tricyclic antidepressants, or selective serotonin reuptake inhibitors.

3. Medications to assist with manic symptoms are atypical antipsychotics and mood stabilizers (e.g., anticonvulsants).

4. Catatonia is a symptom associated with a thought disorder, and these clients would be prescribed antipsychotic, not antianxiety, medications.

TEST-TAKING HINT: When answering an analogy, it is important for the test taker to recognize the relationships between the subject matter within the question.

58. Chloral hydrate, temazepam, zolpidem, and zaleplon are all sedative/hypnotic medications. Additive central nervous system (CNS) depression can occur when sedative/hypnotic medications are taken concomitantly with alcohol, antihistamines, antidepressants, phenothiazines, or any other CNS depressant.
    1. Chloral hydrate is a sedative/hypnotic, and thioridazine is a phenothiazine. When they are given together, the nurse needs to watch for an additive CNS depressant effect.
    2. Temazepam, a sedative/hypnotic, is a CNS depressant; methylphenidate (Concerta), a medication used to treat attention-deficit hyperactivity disorder, is not a CNS depressant. There would be no additive effects when combining these drugs.
    3. Zolpidem, a sedative/hypnotic, is a CNS depressant; buspirone, an antianxiety medication, does not have a CNS depressant effect. There would be no additive effects when combining these drugs.
    4. Zaleplon, a sedative/hypnotic, is a CNS depressant; verapamil, used to assist individuals having flashbacks from posttraumatic stress disorder, does not have a CNS depressant effect. There would be no additive effects when combining these drugs.

TEST-TAKING HINT: To answer this question correctly, the test taker must review medication actions and recognize potential CNS depressive effects.

59. Triazolam is a benzodiazepine used in the treatment of anxiety or sleep disturbances.
    1. An 80-year-old is at risk for injury, and giving this client a central nervous system (CNS) depressant can increase the risk for falls. This client needs to be monitored closely.
    2. Benzodiazepines such as triazolam can be addictive. Individuals diagnosed with alcohol use disorder may have increased risk of abusing a benzodiazepine and would need to be monitored closely. Alcohol is a CNS depressant and, if taken with a benzodiazepine, could cause the client to experience an additive CNS depressant effect.
    3. CNS depressants such as triazolam increase depressive symptoms. It would be important that the nurse monitor this client closely for suicidal ideations.

4. There are no risk factors in this situation that would warrant close observation.
5. A client who is diagnosed with Parkinson's disease is at increased risk for injury because of altered gait and poor balance, and giving this client a CNS depressant can increase the risk for falls. This client needs to be monitored closely.

TEST-TAKING HINT: To answer this question correctly, the test taker first must understand that triazolam is a CNS depressant. Next, the test taker must choose a client whose situation would be exacerbated by the addition of a sedative/hypnotic.

60. Estazolam is prescribed to assist clients with sleep. Before administering an initial dose of estazolam, the nurse needs to ensure that the client's kidney and liver functions are normal.
    1. A client with a blood urea nitrogen (BUN) of 16 mg/dL (normal range 10 to 26 mg/dL) and a creatine of 1.0 mg/dL (normal range 0.6 to 1.4 mg/dL) is within the normal range for both, and there is no concern related to the use of estazolam.
    2. A nurse would be concerned if a client's aspartate aminotransferase (AST) is 60 mcg/L (normal range 16 to 40 mcg/L) and alanine aminotransferase (ALT) is 70 U/L (normal range 8 to 54 U/L). A client needs to have normal liver function to metabolize estazolam properly, and the nurse would need to check with the physician to clarify the safety of this order.
    3. A client sleeping only 2 to 3 hours a night would be an appropriate candidate for any sedative that would assist with sleep.
    4. A client having an anxiety rating of 5 out of 10 should not deter the nurse from administering estazolam because this agent is being prescribed for sleep.

TEST-TAKING HINT: To answer this question correctly, the test taker first has to understand that sedative/hypnotics are metabolized through the liver and then recognize that AST and ALT are liver function studies; the values presented are outside the normal range.

61. Trazodone is an antidepressant and when prescribed at low dosage, such as 50 mg, can be used as a sleep aid due to its sedating properties. High doses of trazodone are needed for an antidepressant effect, and because this medication is poorly tolerated due to sedation, it is rarely prescribed for depression.

1. Trazodone is an antidepressant and when prescribed at a low dose can be used to improve sleep.
2. Trazodone is not an appetite stimulant.
3. Trazodone is not an antianxiety medication.
4. Trazodone is not an antipsychotic medication.

TEST-TAKING HINT: To answer this question correctly, the test taker first must recognize that this dosage is lower than the normal range for trazodone. The test taker should review the normal dosage range for medications and think critically about potential alternative reasons for prescribing these medications.

Depressive Disorders and the Suicidal Client

8

KEYWORDS

The following words include English vocabulary, nursing/medical terminology, concepts, principles, or information relevant to content specifically addressed in this chapter or associated with topics presented in it. English dictionaries, your nursing textbooks, and medical dictionaries such as *Taber's Cyclopedic Medical Dictionary* are resources that can be used to expand your knowledge and understanding of these words and related information.

Affect

Anhedonia

Dysfunctional grieving

Dysthymic disorder

Electroconvulsive therapy (ECT)

Euthymic mood

Major depressive disorder (MDD)

Monoamine oxidase inhibitor (MAOI)

Mood

Normal grief response

Psychomotor agitation

Psychomotor retardation

Selective serotonin reuptake inhibitor (SSRI)

Serotonin syndrome

Shiva

Stages of grief

Suicidal ideations

Suicide

Tricyclic antidepressant

Transcranial magnetic stimulation (TMS)

Vagus nerve stimulation

QUESTIONS

Theory

1. Which nursing diagnosis supports the psychoanalytic theory of development of a major depressive disorder (MDD)?
   1. Social isolation R/T self-directed anger.
   2. Low self-esteem R/T learned helplessness.
   3. Risk for suicide R/T neurochemical imbalances.
   4. Imbalanced nutrition less than body requirements R/T weakness.

2. Which client statement is evidence of the etiology of a major depressive disorder (MDD) from a genetic perspective?
   1. "My maternal grandmother was diagnosed with bipolar affective disorder."
   2. "My mood is a 7 out of 10, and I won't harm myself or others."
   3. "I am so angry that my father left our family when I was 6."
   4. "I just can't do anything right. I am worthless."

3. During an intake assessment, which client statement is evidence of the etiology of a major depressive disorder (MDD) from an object-loss theory perspective?
   1. "I am so angry all the time and seem to take it out on myself."
   2. "My grandmother and great-grandfather also had depression."
   3. "I just don't think my life is ever going to get better. I keep messing up."
   4. "I don't know about my biological family; I was in foster care as an infant."

Nursing Process—Assessment

4. Which statement describes a major difference between a client diagnosed with a major depressive disorder (MDD) and a client diagnosed with persistent depressive disorder (dysthymia)?
   1. A client diagnosed with persistent depressive disorder is at higher risk for suicide.
   2. A client diagnosed with persistent depressive disorder may experience psychosis and delusions.
   3. A client diagnosed with persistent depressive disorder experiences excessive guilt.
   4. A client diagnosed with persistent depressive disorder has symptoms for at least 2 years.

5. A client plans and follows through with the wake and burial of a child killed in an automobile accident. Using Engel's model of normal grief response, in which stage would this client fall?
   1. Resolution of the loss.
   2. Recovery.
   3. Restitution.
   4. Developing awareness.

6. Which charting entry most accurately documents a client's mood?
   1. "The client expresses an elevation in mood."
   2. "The client appears euthymic and is interacting with others."
   3. "The client isolates self and is tearful most of the day."
   4. "The client rates mood at a two out of ten."

7. Which client is at highest risk for the diagnosis of a major depressive disorder (MDD)?
   1. A 24-year-old married woman.
   2. A 64-year-old single woman.
   3. A 30-year-old single man.
   4. A 70-year-old married man.

8. A client is admitted to an inpatient psychiatric unit with a diagnosis of a major depressive disorder (MDD). Which of the following data would the nurse expect to assess? **Select all that apply.**
   1. Loss of interest in almost all activities and anhedonia.
   2. A change of more than 5% of body weight in 1 month.
   3. Fluctuation between increased energy and loss of energy.
   4. Psychomotor retardation or agitation.
   5. Insomnia or hypersomnia.

9. A client is exhibiting behavioral symptoms of depression. Which of the following charting entries would appropriately document these symptoms? **Select all that apply.**
   1. "Rates mood as 4/10."
   2. "Expresses thoughts of poor self-esteem during group."
   3. "Became irritable and agitated on waking."
   4. "Rates anxiety as 2/10 after receiving lorazepam."
   5. "Stayed in bed when asked to join group."

10. Which of the following symptoms are examples of physiological alterations exhibited by clients diagnosed with moderate depression? **Select all that apply.**
    1. Decreased libido.
    2. Difficulty concentrating.
    3. Slumped posture.
    4. Helplessness.
    5. Muscle aches.

11. A major depressive disorder (MDD) would be most difficult to detect in which of the following clients?
    1. A 5-year-old girl.
    2. A 13-year-old boy.
    3. A 25-year-old woman.
    4. A 75-year-old man.

12. Which exhibited symptom is the key to understanding whether a child or adolescent is experiencing an underlying depressive disorder?
    1. Irritability with authority.
    2. Being uninterested in school.
    3. A change in behaviors over a 2-week period.
    4. Feeling insecure at a social gathering.

13. The nurse in the emergency department is assessing a client suspected of being suicidal. Number the following assessment questions, beginning with the most critical and ending with the least critical.
    1. _____ "Are you currently thinking about suicide?"
    2. _____ "Do you have a gun in your possession?"
    3. _____ "Do you have a plan to commit suicide?"
    4. _____ "Do you live alone? Do you have local friends or family?"

14. A nurse is planning to teach about appropriate coping skills. The nurse would expect which client to be at the highest level of readiness to participate in this instruction?
    1. A newly admitted client with an anxiety level of 8/10 and racing thoughts.
    2. A client admitted 6 days ago for a manic episode refusing to take medications.
    3. A newly admitted client experiencing suicidal ideations with a plan to overdose.
    4. A client admitted 6 days ago for suicidal ideations following a depressive episode.

Nursing Process—Diagnosis

15. A newly admitted client has been diagnosed with a major depressive disorder (MDD). Which nursing diagnosis takes priority?
    1. Social isolation R/T poor mood AEB refusing visits from family.
    2. Self-care deficit R/T hopelessness AEB not taking a bath for 2 weeks.
    3. Anxiety R/T hospitalization AEB anxiety rating of 8/10.
    4. Risk for self-directed violence R/T depressed mood.

16. Which nursing diagnosis takes priority for a client immediately after electroconvulsive therapy (ECT)?
    1. Risk for injury R/T altered mental status.
    2. Impaired social interaction R/T confusion.
    3. Activity intolerance R/T weakness.
    4. Chronic confusion R/T side effect of ECT.

17. A newly admitted client diagnosed with a major depressive disorder (MDD) has a history of two suicide attempts by hanging. Which nursing diagnosis takes priority?
    1. Risk for violence directed at others R/T anger turned outward.
    2. Social isolation R/T depressed mood.
    3. Risk for suicide R/T history of attempts.
    4. Hopelessness R/T multiple suicide attempts.

18. A client's outcome states, "The client will make a plan to take control of one life situation by discharge." Which nursing diagnosis documents the client's problem that this outcome addresses?
    1. Impaired social interaction.
    2. Powerlessness.
    3. Knowledge deficit.
    4. Dysfunctional grieving.

Nursing Process—Planning

19. A client admitted with a major depressive disorder (MDD) has a nursing diagnosis of ineffective sleep pattern R/T aches and pains. Which is an appropriate correctly written short-term outcome for this client?
    1. The client will express feeling rested upon awakening.
    2. The client will rate pain level at or below a 4/10.
    3. The client will sleep 6 to 8 hours at night by day 5.
    4. The client will maintain a steady sleep pattern while hospitalized.

20. Which client would the charge nurse assign to an agency nurse working on the inpatient psychiatric unit for the first time?
    1. A client experiencing passive suicidal ideations with a past history of an attempt.
    2. A client rating mood as 3/10 and attending but not participating in group therapy.
    3. A client lying in bed all day long in a fetal position and refusing all meals.
    4. A client admitted for the first time with a diagnosis of major depression.

21. A client has a nursing diagnosis of risk for suicide R/T a past suicide attempt. Which outcome, based on this diagnosis, would the nurse prioritize?
    1. The client will remain free from injury throughout hospitalization.
    2. The client will set one realistic goal related to relationships by day 3.
    3. The client will verbalize one positive attribute about self by day 4.
    4. The client will be easily redirected when discussion about suicide occurs by day 5.

Nursing Process—Implementation

22. A client who practices Judaism is admitted to an inpatient psychiatric unit 2 days after attempting suicide R/T the death of a parent. Which intervention must the nurse include in the care of this client?
    1. Allow the client time to mourn the loss during this time of shiva.
    2. Distract the client from the loss and encourage participation in unit groups.
    3. Teach the client alternative coping skills to deal with grief.
    4. Discuss positive aspects the client has in their life to build on strengths.

23. A client denying suicidal ideations comes into the emergency department complaining about insomnia, irritability, anorexia, and depressed mood. Which intervention would the nurse implement first?
    1. Request a psychiatric consultation.
    2. Complete a thorough physical assessment including laboratory tests.
    3. Remove all hazardous materials from the environment.
    4. Place the client on a one-to-one observation.

24. A client diagnosed with a major depressive disorder (MDD) has a nursing diagnosis of low self-esteem R/T negative view of self. Which cognitive nursing intervention would be appropriate to deal with this client's problem?
    1. Promote attendance in group therapy to assist the client in socializing.
    2. Teach assertiveness skills by role-playing situations.
    3. Encourage the client to journal to uncover underlying feelings.
    4. Focus on strengths and accomplishments to minimize failures.

25. A newly admitted client diagnosed with a major depressive disorder (MDD) isolates self in room and stares out the window. Which nursing intervention would be the most appropriate to implement when first establishing a nurse–client relationship?
    1. Sit with the client and offer self frequently.
    2. Notify the client of group therapy schedule.
    3. Introduce the client to others on the unit.
    4. Help the client to identify stressors of life that precipitate life crises.

26. A client diagnosed with a major depressive disorder (MDD) is being considered for electroconvulsive therapy (ECT). Which client teaching should the nurse prioritize?
    1. Empathize with the client about fears regarding ECT.
    2. Monitor for any cardiac alterations to prevent possible negative outcomes.
    3. Discuss with the client and family expected short-term memory loss.
    4. Inform the client that injury related to induced seizure commonly occurs.

27. Which nursing intervention takes priority when working with a newly admitted client experiencing suicidal ideations?
    1. Monitor the client at close, but irregular, intervals.
    2. Encourage the client to participate in group therapy.
    3. Enlist friends and family to assist the client in remaining safe after discharge.
    4. Remind the client that it takes 6 to 8 weeks for antidepressants to be fully effective.

Nursing Process—Evaluation

28. A nursing student is studying major depressive disorder (MDD). Which student statement indicates that learning has occurred?
    1. "One percent of the population is affected by depression yearly."
    2. "Two to five percent of women experience depression during their lifetimes."
    3. "One to three percent of men become clinically depressed."
    4. "Major depression is a leading cause of disability in the United States."

29. A client has a nursing diagnosis of dysfunctional grieving R/T loss of a job AEB inability to seek employment because of sad mood. Which would support a resolution of this client's problem?
    1. The client reports an anxiety level of 2 out of 10 and denies suicidal ideations.
    2. The client exhibits trusting behaviors toward the treatment team.
    3. The client is noted to be in the denial stage of the grief process.
    4. The client recognizes and accepts the role they played in the loss of the job.

30. A nursing instructor is presenting statistics regarding suicide. Which student statement indicates that learning has occurred?
    1. "Approximately 10,000 individuals in the United States will commit suicide each year."
    2. "Almost 95% of all individuals who commit or attempt suicide have a diagnosed mental disorder."
    3. "Suicide is the eighth leading cause of death among young Americans 15 to 24 years old."
    4. "Depressive disorders account for one-third of all individuals who commit or attempt suicide."

31. A client diagnosed with a major depressive disorder (MDD) has an outcome that states, "The client will verbalize a measure of hope about the future by day three." Which client statement indicates this outcome was successful?
    1. "I don't want to die because it would hurt my family."
    2. "I need to go to group and get out of this room."
    3. "I think I am going to talk to my boss about conflicts at work."
    4. "I thank you for your compassionate care."

Psychopharmacology

32. Which of the following medications may be administered before electroconvulsive therapy (ECT)? **Select all that apply.**
    1. Glycopyrrolate.
    2. Thiopental sodium.
    3. Succinylcholine chloride.
    4. Lorazepam.
    5. Divalproex sodium.

33. A client diagnosed with a major depressive disorder (MDD) is prescribed phenelzine. Which teaching should the nurse prioritize?
    1. Remind the client that the medication takes 6 to 8 weeks to take full effect.
    2. Instruct the client and family about the many food–drug and drug–drug interactions.
    3. Teach the client about the possible sexual side effects and insomnia that can occur.
    4. Educate the client about taking the medication prescribed even after symptoms improve.

34. A client diagnosed with a major depressive disorder (MDD) is prescribed vortioxetine. Which of the following teaching points would the nurse review with the client? **Select all that apply.**
    1. Ask the client about suicidal ideations related to depressed mood.
    2. Discuss the need to take medications, even when symptoms improve.
    3. Instruct the client about the risks of abruptly stopping the medication.
    4. Alert the client to the risks of dry mouth, sedation, nausea, and sexual side effects.
    5. Remind the client that the medication's full effect may not occur for 6 to 8 weeks.

35. Which symptoms would the nurse expect to assess in a client experiencing serotonin syndrome?
    1. Confusion, restlessness, tachycardia, labile blood pressure, and diaphoresis.
    2. Hypomania, akathisia, cardiac arrhythmias, and panic attacks.
    3. Dizziness, lethargy, headache, and nausea.
    4. Orthostatic hypotension, urinary retention, constipation, and blurred vision.

36. Which of the following medications would be classified as tricyclic antidepressants? **Select all that apply.**
    1. Bupropion.
    2. Mirtazapine.
    3. Citalopram.
    4. Nortriptyline.
    5. Doxepin.

37. Which of the following are examples of anticholinergic side effects from tricyclic antidepressants? **Select all that apply.**
    1. Urinary hesitancy.
    2. Constipation.
    3. Blurred vision.
    4. Sedation.
    5. Weight gain.

38. A client diagnosed with a major depressive disorder (MDD) and experiencing suicidal ideation is showing signs of anxiety. Alprazolam is prescribed. Which assessment should be prioritized?
    1. Monitor for signs and symptoms of physical and psychological withdrawal.
    2. Teach the client about side effects of the medication and how to handle these side effects.
    3. Assess for nausea and give the medication with food if nausea occurs.
    4. Ask the client to rate their mood on a mood scale and monitor for suicidal ideations.

39. Which of the following situations would place a client at high risk for a life-threatening hypertensive crisis? **Select all that apply.**
    1. A client is prescribed tranylcypromine and eats chicken salad.
    2. A client is prescribed isocarboxazid and drinks hot chocolate.
    3. A client is prescribed venlafaxine and drinks wine.
    4. A client is prescribed phenelzine and eats fresh roasted chicken.
    5. A client is prescribed rasagiline and eats smoked pork.

40. A client has been taking bupropion for more than 1 year. The client has been in a car accident with loss of consciousness and is brought to the emergency department (ED). For which reason would the nurse question the continued use of this medication?
    1. The client may have a possible injury to the gastrointestinal system.
    2. The client is at risk for seizures from a potential closed head injury.
    3. The client is at increased risk of bleeding while taking bupropion.
    4. The client may experience sedation from bupropion, making assessment difficult.

41. A client experiencing suicidal ideations with a plan to overdose on medications is admitted to an inpatient psychiatric unit. Vilazodone is prescribed. Which nursing intervention takes priority?
    1. Remind the client that medication effectiveness may take 2 to 3 weeks.
    2. Teach the client to take the medication with food to avoid nausea.
    3. Check the client's blood pressure every shift to monitor for hypertension.
    4. Monitor closely for signs that the client might be "cheeking" medications.

42. A client recently prescribed venlafaxine 37.5 mg bid complains of dry mouth, orthostatic hypotension, and blurred vision. Which nursing intervention is appropriate?
    1. Hold the next dose and document symptoms immediately.
    2. Reassure the client that side effects are transient and teach ways to deal with them.
    3. Call the physician to receive an order for benztropine.
    4. Notify dietary about food restrictions related to monoamine oxidase inhibitors (MAOIs).

43. A client, admitted after experiencing suicidal ideations, is prescribed citalopram. Four days later, the client has pressured speech and is noted wearing heavy makeup. What may be a potential reason for this client's behavior?
    1. The client is in a manic episode caused by the citalopram.
    2. The client is showing improvement and is close to discharge.
    3. The client is masking depression in an attempt to get out of the hospital.
    4. The client has "cheeked" medications and taken them all in an attempt to overdose.

44. A client is prescribed venlafaxine 75 mg qam and 150 mg qhs. Venlafaxine is supplied in a 37.5 mg tablet. How many tablets would the nurse administer a day? _____ tablets.

45. Which of the following medications must be taken with food? **Select all that apply.**
    1. Levomilnacipran.
    2. Lurasidone.
    3. Vilazodone.
    4. Vortioxetine.
    5. Risperidone.

46. A client asks the nurse about nonpharmacological treatments for depression. Which of the following information should the nurse include in client teaching? **Select all that apply.**
    1. "Transcranial magnetic stimulation (TMS) is approved by the Food and Drug Administration (FDA) as a treatment for depression."
    2. "Cognitive-behavioral therapy (CBT) can help clients dealing with mild to moderate depression."
    3. "Research has shown that light therapy can be used for the treatment of all types of depressive disorders."
    4. "Vagus nerve stimulation (VNS) has been shown to be effective for depressed clients who have poor response to medications."
    5. "Electroconvulsive therapy (ECT) affects brain chemistry and decreases depressive symptoms."

47. A client, diagnosed with depression, has been prescribed dextromethorphan HBr and bupropion HCl (Auvelity). Which client statement reflects that teaching was understood?
    1. "Auvelity is the same medication as bupropion HCl, so I can substitute them for each other."
    2. "Auvelity works faster because it is better absorbed in the digestive track."
    3. "Auvelity is different because it works on the N-methyl-D-aspartate (NMDA) receptor, affecting glutamate."
    4. "Auvelity is different because it affects serotonin, norepinephrine and dopamine."

The correct answer number and rationale for why it is the correct answer are given in boldface blue type. Rationales for why the other answer options are incorrect are given as well, but they are not in boldface type.

Theory

1. 1. **Social isolation R/T self-directed anger supports the psychoanalytic theory in the development of major depressive disorder (MDD). Freud defines melancholia as a profoundly painful dejection and cessation of interest in the outside world, which culminates in a delusional expectation of punishment. He observed that melancholia occurs after the loss of a love object. Freud postulated that when the loss has been incorporated into the self (ego), the hostile part of the ambivalence that has been felt for the lost object is turned inward toward the ego. Another way to state this concept is that the client turns anger toward self.**

   2. Low self-esteem R/T learned helplessness supports a learning, not psychoanalytic, theory in the development of MDD. From a learning theory perspective, learned helplessness results from clients experiencing numerous failures, real or perceived.

   3. Risk for suicide R/T neurochemical imbalances supports a biological, not psychoanalytic, theory in the development of MDD. From a neurochemical perspective, it has been hypothesized that depressive illness may be related to a deficiency of the neurotransmitter's norepinephrine, serotonin, and dopamine at functionally important receptor sites in the brain.

   4. Imbalanced nutrition less than body requirements R/T weakness supports a physiological, not psychoanalytic, theory in the development of MDD. From a physiological perspective, it has been hypothesized that deficiencies in vitamin B_1 (thiamine), vitamin B_6 (pyridoxine), vitamin B_{12}, niacin, vitamin C, iron, folic acid, zinc, calcium, and potassium may produce symptoms of depression.

   TEST-TAKING HINT: To answer this question correctly, the test taker must be able to recognize the connection between the underlying cause (R/T) of the client's problem and the theory that is stated in the question.

2. 1. **A family history of a mood disorder indicates a genetic predisposition to the development of an MDD. Twin, family, and adoptive studies further support a genetic link as an etiological influence in the development of mood disorders.**

   2. This statement by the client gives the nurse important assessment data about the client's mood but does not address etiological influences in the development of mood disorders.

   3. The development of mood disorders, from a psychoanalytic, not genetic, perspective, involves anger that is turned inward. The client in the question is experiencing anger from a paternal loss at a young age. The psychoanalytic theorist would postulate that when the loss has been incorporated into the self (ego), the anger felt for the lost father figure is turned inward toward the client's sense of self. This leads to the development of a depressive disorder.

   4. The development of mood disorders, from a cognitive, not genetic, perspective, involves cognitive distortions that result in negative, defeatist attitudes. Cognitive theorists believe that depression is the product of negative thinking.

   TEST-TAKING HINT: The test taker needs to understand the various theories that are associated with the development of mood disorders to answer this question correctly.

3. 1. When the client expresses self-anger, it is a reflection of the psychoanalytic, not object-loss, theory perspective of the etiology of MDD. Freud describes depression as anger turned inward.

   2. When clients indicate a family history of mood disorders, it is a reflection of the genetic, not object-loss, theory perspective of the etiology of MDD. Research has indicated a genetic link in the transmission of mood disorders.

   3. When a client indicates cognitive distortions, it is a reflection of the cognitive, not object-loss, theory perspective of the etiology of MDD. Cognitive theorists believe that depression is a product of negative thinking.

   4. **Object-loss theorists suggest that depressive illness occurs as a result of being abandoned by or otherwise separated from a significant other during the first 6 months of life. The client in the**

question experienced parental abandonment, and according to object-loss theory, this loss has led to the diagnosis of MDD.

TEST-TAKING HINT: The test taker needs to understand the various theories that are associated with the development of mood disorders to answer this question correctly.

Nursing Process—Assessment

4. Characteristics of persistent depressive disorder (dysthymia) are similar to, but milder than, the characteristics ascribed to a major depressive disorder (MDD).
   1. Clients diagnosed with persistent depressive disorder and MDD are at equally high risk for suicide.
   2. A client diagnosed with MDD, not persistent depressive disorder, may experience psychotic features.
   3. A client diagnosed with persistent depressive disorder may experience guilt, but it would not be excessive as noted in MDD.
   4. An individual suspected to have persistent depressive disorder needs to experience symptoms for at least 2 years before a diagnosis can be made. The essential feature is a chronically depressed mood (or possibly an irritable mood in children and adolescents) for most of the day, more days than not, for at least 2 years (1 year for children and adolescents). Clients with a diagnosis of MDD show impaired social and occupational functioning that has existed for at least 2 weeks.

TEST-TAKING HINT: To answer this question correctly, the test taker needs to understand the chronic nature of persistent depressive disorder, which differentiates this diagnosis from MDD.

5. Engel's model consists of five stages of grief, including shock and disbelief, developing awareness, restitution, resolution of the loss, and recovery.
   1. The client in the question is exhibiting signs associated with Engel's stage of restitution, not resolution of the loss. Resolution of the loss is the fourth stage of Engel's model of the normal grief response. This stage is characterized by a preoccupation with the loss in which the deceased is idealized.
   2. The client in the question is exhibiting signs associated with Engel's stage of restitution, not recovery. Recovery is the fifth stage of Engel's model of the normal grief response. This stage is characterized by the individual's ability to continue with life.

3. The client in the question is exhibiting signs associated with Engel's stage of restitution. Restitution is the third stage of Engel's model of the normal grief response. In this stage, the various rituals associated with loss within a culture are performed. Examples include funerals, wakes, special attire, a gathering of friends and family, and religious practices customary to the spiritual beliefs of the bereaved.
4. The client in the question is exhibiting signs associated with the stage of restitution, not developing awareness. Developing awareness is the second stage of Engel's model of the normal grief response. This stage begins within minutes to hours of the loss. Behaviors associated with this stage include excessive crying and regression to the state of helplessness and a childlike manner.

TEST-TAKING HINT: The test taker must be aware of the behaviors exhibited in the stages of Engel's grief model to answer this question correctly.

6. 1. When the nurse documents, "The client expresses an elevation in mood," the nurse is not providing objective, measurable data. Baseline information regarding mood would be needed to compare any verbalization of mood elevation.
   2. Euthymia is a description of a normal range of mood. Mood is a subjective symptom that needs to be assessed from the client's perspective. When the nurse states, "The client appears euthymic," without validation from the client, the nurse has assumed assessment data that may be inaccurate.
   3. It is important for the nurse to document client behaviors that may indicate changes in mood, but because mood is a subjective symptom that needs to be assessed from the client's perspective, the nurse may be misinterpreting observations. For example, tears can represent a range of emotional feelings varying from sadness to extreme happiness.
   4. The use of a mood scale objectifies the subjective symptom of mood as a pain scale objectifies the subjective symptom of pain. The use of scales is the most accurate way to assess subjective data.

TEST-TAKING HINT: In a question that requires a charting entry, the test taker must understand that nursing documentation should avoid assumptions and be based on objective data.

7. 1. **Research indicates that depressive symptoms are highest among young, married women of low socioeconomic background. Compared with the other clients presented, this client is at highest risk for the diagnosis of MDD.**

2. Research indicates that there is a higher rate of depressive disorders diagnosed in young, not older, and married, not single, women. Compared with the other clients presented, this client is at lower risk for the diagnosis of MDD.

3. Although the diagnosis of MDD is higher among single men, this client's young age places him at lower risk compared with the other clients presented. Research indicates that there is a lower rate of depressive disorders diagnosed in younger men.

4. Although the diagnosis of MDD is higher among older men, this client's marital status places him at lower risk compared with the other clients presented. Research indicates that there is a lower rate of depressive disorders diagnosed in married men.

TEST-TAKING HINT: To answer this question correctly, the test taker needs to understand that age and marital status affect the incidence of depression.

8. 1. **Loss of interest in almost all activities and anhedonia, the inability to experience or even imagine any pleasant emotion, are symptoms of MDD.**

2. **Significant weight loss or gain of more than 5% of body weight in 1 month is one of the many diagnostic criteria for MDD.**

3. Fluctuation between increased energy and loss of energy is an indication of mood lability, a classic symptom of bipolar affective disorder, not MDD. Manic episodes experienced by the client would rule out the diagnosis of MDD.

4. **Psychomotor retardation or agitation, occurring nearly every day, is a diagnostic criterion for MDD. These symptoms should be observable by others and not merely subjective feelings of restlessness or lethargy.**

5. **Sleep alterations, such as insomnia or hypersomnia, that occur nearly every day are diagnostic criteria for MDD.**

TEST-TAKING HINT: The test taker needs to recognize the diagnostic criteria for the diagnosis of MDD to answer this question correctly.

9. 1. When the client rates mood as 4 on a 10-point rating scale, the client is exhibiting affective, not behavioral, symptoms of depression.

2. When the client expresses thoughts of poor self-esteem, the client is exhibiting cognitive, not behavioral, symptoms of depression.

3. **When the client becomes irritable and agitated on awakening, the client is exhibiting behavioral symptoms of depression. Other behavioral symptoms include, but are not limited to, tearfulness, restlessness, slumped posture, and withdrawal.**

4. When a client rates anxiety as 2/10 after receiving lorazepam, the client is exhibiting affective, not behavioral, symptoms of depression.

5. **When a client stays in bed instead of going to group, the client is isolating self and exhibiting a behavioral symptom of depression.**

TEST-TAKING HINT: The test taker must be able to identify various categories of symptoms of depression, including affective, behavioral, cognitive, and physiological. This question is asking the test taker to distinguish a behavioral symptom from the other symptoms described.

10. A moderate level of depression represents more problematic disturbances than mild depression.
1. **Decreased libido is a physiological alteration exhibited by clients diagnosed with moderate depression.**

2. Difficulty concentrating is a cognitive, not physiological, alteration exhibited by clients diagnosed with moderate depression.

3. Slumped posture is a behavioral, not physiological, alteration exhibited by clients diagnosed with moderate depression.

4. Helplessness is an affective, not physiological, alteration exhibited by clients diagnosed with moderate depression.

5. **Muscle aches are physiological alterations experienced by clients diagnosed with moderate depression.**

TEST-TAKING HINT: The test taker must be able to identify various categories of depressive symptoms, including affective, behavioral, cognitive, and physiological. This question is asking the test taker to distinguish physiological symptoms from other symptoms described.

11. 1. Assessment of depressive disorders in 5-year-old children would include evaluating the symptoms of being accident prone, experiencing phobias, and expressing excessive self-reproach for minor infractions. Compared with the other age-groups presented, MDD would be less difficult to detect in childhood.

2. Assessment of depressive disorders in a 13-year-old adolescent would include feelings of sadness, loneliness, anxiety, and hopelessness. These symptoms may be perceived as normal emotional stresses of growing up. Many teens whose symptoms are attributed to the normal adjustments of adolescence are not accurately diagnosed and do not get the help they need.

3. A 25-year-old client is no longer faced with the developmental challenges of adolescence. Compared with the other age-groups presented, MDD would be less difficult to detect in adulthood.

4. In elderly individuals, adaptive coping strategies may be seriously challenged by major stressors, such as financial problems, physical illness, changes in body functioning, increasing awareness of approaching death, and numerous losses. Because these situations are expected in this age-group, MDD would be anticipated and more easily diagnosed.

TEST-TAKING HINT: To answer this question correctly, the test taker must be able to recognize that the normal developmental challenges faced during adolescence may mirror symptoms of depression, making diagnostic determinations difficult.

12. 1. A child or adolescent expressing irritability toward authority figures reflects behavior that can be within the parameters of normal emotional development for this age-group.

2. A child or adolescent being uninterested in school reflects behavior that can be within the parameters of normal emotional development for this age-group.

3. Change in behavior is an indicator that differentiates mood disorders from the typical stormy behaviors of adolescence. Depression can be a common manifestation of the stress and independence conflicts associated with the normal maturation process. Assessment of normal baseline behaviors would help the nurse recognize changes in behaviors that may indicate underlying depressive disorders.

4. A child or adolescent feeling insecure at social gatherings reflects behavior that can be within the parameters of normal emotional development for this age-group.

TEST-TAKING HINT: The test taker must recognize normal child and adolescent conduct to choose a behavior that is outside the norm for child and adolescent development.

13. The assessment questions should be numbered as follows: 1, 3, 2, 4.
    1. Assessment of suicidal ideations must occur before any other assessment data are gathered. If the client is not considering suicide, continuing with the suicide assessment is unnecessary.
    2. Assessment of a suicide plan is next. A client's risk for suicide increases if the client has developed a specific plan.
    3. Assessment of the access to the means to commit suicide is next. The ability for the client to access the means to carry out the suicide plan is an important assessment in order for the nurse to intervene appropriately. If a client has a loaded gun available to them at home, the nurse would be responsible to assess this information and initiate actions to decrease the client's access.
    4. Assessment of the client's potential for rescue is next. If a client has an involved support system, even if a suicide attempt occurs, there is a potential for rescue. Without an involved support system, the client is at higher risk.

TEST-TAKING HINT: When placing assessment questions in order, the test taker must take a practical approach by first determining the underlying problem being assessed (thoughts of suicide) and then ordering subsequent questions based on gathered data. The client must have a plan in place before the nurse inquires about the means necessary to implement the plan.

14. 1. High anxiety levels decrease the ability for this client to concentrate, and racing thoughts make focusing and learning difficult. Compared with the other clients described, this client would have a lower level of readiness to participate in instruction.

2. During a manic episode, cognition and perceptions become fragmented. Rapid thinking proceeds to racing and disjointed thoughts, making learning difficult. Because of nonadherence with medications, this client would still be experiencing manic symptoms. Compared with the other clients described, this client would have a lower level of readiness to participate in instruction.

3. Because a newly admitted client experiencing suicidal ideations with a plan to overdose is in a crisis situation, focusing and learning would be difficult to accomplish. Compared with the other clients described, this client would have a lower level of readiness to participate in instruction.

4. A client admitted 6 days ago for suicidal ideations has begun to stabilize because of the treatment received during this time frame. Compared with the other clients described, this client would have the highest level of readiness to participate in instruction.

TEST-TAKING HINT: To answer this question correctly, it is important for the test taker to understand that symptoms of mania, anxiety, and crisis all affect a client's ability to learn.

Nursing Process—Diagnosis

15. 1. Social isolation is defined as aloneness experienced by the individual and perceived as imposed by others and as a negative or threatened state. Although a newly admitted client diagnosed with an MDD may experience social isolation because of withdrawal behaviors, this problem is not life threatening and therefore is not the priority.
    2. Self-care deficit is defined as an impaired ability to perform or complete feeding, bathing/hygiene, dressing/grooming, or toileting activities. Although clients diagnosed with MDD experience self-care deficits related to poor self-esteem and low energy levels, this problem is not life threatening and therefore is not the priority.
    3. Anxiety is defined as a vague uneasy feeling of discomfort or dread, accompanied by an autonomic response. Although clients diagnosed with MDD commonly experience anxiety, this problem is not life threatening and therefore is not the priority.
    4. Risk for self-directed violence is the priority diagnosis for a newly admitted client diagnosed with MDD. Risk for self-directed violence is defined as behaviors in which the individual demonstrates that they can be physically harmful to self. This is a life-threatening problem that requires immediate prioritization by the nurse.

TEST-TAKING HINT: To answer this question correctly, the test taker needs to recognize the importance of prioritizing potentially life-threatening problems associated with the diagnosis of MDD.

16. 1. Immediately after electroconvulsive therapy (ECT), risk for injury R/T altered mental status is the priority nursing diagnosis. The most common side effect of ECT is memory loss and confusion, and these place the client at risk for injury.
    2. Confusion is a side effect of ECT, and this may affect the client's ability to interact socially. However, because safety is a critical concern, this diagnosis is not prioritized.
    3. As consciousness is regained during the postictal period after the seizure generated by ECT, the client is often confused, fatigued, and drowsy. These symptoms may contribute to activity intolerance, but because safety is a critical concern, this diagnosis is not prioritized.
    4. The most common side effects of ECT are memory loss and short-term, not chronic, confusion.

TEST-TAKING HINT: To answer this question correctly, the test taker must note keywords in the question, such as *immediately after*. A nursing diagnosis that would be prioritized during ECT may not be the nursing diagnosis prioritized immediately after the treatment.

17. 1. Risk for violence directed at others is an inappropriate nursing diagnosis for this client because no evidence is presented in the question that would indicate violence toward others.
    2. Although social isolation R/T depressed mood is a common problem for clients diagnosed with major depression, no evidence is presented in the question that would indicate the client is isolating self.
    3. Risk for suicide R/T history of attempts is a priority nursing diagnosis for a client who is diagnosed with major depression and has a history of two suicide attempts by hanging. A history of a suicide attempt increases a client's risk for future attempts. Because various means can be used to hang oneself, the client is at risk for accessing these means, even on an inpatient unit. These factors would cause the nurse to prioritize this safety concern.
    4. Because of this client's history of suicide attempts, hopelessness is a problem for this client. However, compared with the nursing diagnoses presented, hopelessness would be prioritized lower than risk for suicide. After the nurse ensures the client's safety, hopelessness can be addressed.

TEST-TAKING HINT: In choosing a priority diagnosis, the test taker must look for a client problem that needs immediate attention. In this question, if risk for suicide is not prioritized, the client may not live to deal with other problems.

18. 1. Impaired social interaction is defined as the state in which the individual participates in an insufficient or excessive quantity or ineffective quality of social exchange. This nursing diagnosis does not address the outcome presented in the question.
    2. Powerlessness is defined as the perception that one's own action would not significantly affect an outcome—a perceived lack of control over a current situation or immediate happening. Because the client outcome presented in the question addresses the lack of control over life situations, the nursing diagnosis of powerlessness documents this client's problem.
    3. Knowledge deficit is defined as the lack of specific information necessary for the client to make informed choices regarding condition, therapies, and treatment plan. This nursing diagnosis does not address the outcome presented in the question.
    4. Dysfunctional grieving is defined as extended, unsuccessful use of intellectual and emotional responses by which individuals attempt to work through the process of modifying self-concept based on the perceptions of loss. This nursing diagnosis does not address the outcome presented in the question.

TEST-TAKING HINT: To select the correct answer, the test taker must be able to pair the outcome presented in the question with the nursing diagnosis that documents the client problem.

Nursing Process—Planning

19. Any sleep pattern outcome assessment must be based on the client's normal sleep pattern baseline.
    1. The outcome of feeling rested upon awakening is appropriate for the nursing diagnosis of ineffective sleep pattern; however, this outcome cannot be measured because it does not include a time frame.
    2. Because pain is the cause of this client's ineffective sleep pattern, this outcome can be appropriate for this nursing diagnosis; however, this outcome cannot be measured because it does not include a time frame.
    3. **The appropriate short-term outcome for the nursing diagnosis of ineffective sleep pattern R/T aches and pains is to expect the client to sleep 6 to 8 hours a night by day 5. This outcome is client**

specific, realistic, and measurable and includes a time frame.
    4. The problem with this outcome relates to inclusion of the term *steady sleep pattern*. This term is abstract and can be interpreted in various ways and would not be measured consistently.

TEST-TAKING HINT: To answer this question, the test taker must recognize a correctly written outcome for the stated nursing diagnosis. Outcomes must always be client specific, realistic, and measurable and include a time frame.

20. 1. The agency nurse working on an inpatient psychiatric unit for the first time may be unfamiliar with critical assessments related to suicide risk. A client with a history of a suicide attempt is at an increased risk for a future attempt. Compared with the other clients described, this client would require an assignment of a more experienced psychiatric nurse.
    2. **Although this client rates mood low, there is no indication of suicidal ideations, and the client is attending groups in the milieu. Because this client is observable in the milieu by all staff members, assignment to an agency nurse would be appropriate.**
    3. The agency nurse working on an inpatient psychiatric unit for the first time may be unfamiliar with critical assessments needed when the client is isolating self and being nonadherent with meals. This client is at risk for nutritional deficits and needs encouragement to participate actively in the plan of care. Compared with the other clients described, this client would require an assignment of a more experienced psychiatric nurse.
    4. The agency nurse working on an inpatient psychiatric unit for the first time may be unfamiliar with the diagnostic criteria for major depression. Because this client is admitted for the first time, there is no history of past assessments or successful interventions. Therefore, it is critical that the nurse have an understanding of needed assessments and appropriate interventions to evaluate this client initially.

TEST-TAKING HINT: In a question that requires a choice of delegation to inexperienced personnel, the test taker must look for the client who requires the least complicated nursing assessment and intervention and is at a lower safety risk.

21. 1. Remaining free from injury throughout hospitalization is a priority outcome for the nursing diagnosis of risk for suicide R/T a past suicide attempt. Because this outcome addresses client safety, it is prioritized.
    2. Setting one realistic goal related to relationships by day 3 is a positive outcome that addresses an altered social interaction problem, not a problem that deals with a risk for suicide.
    3. Verbalizing one positive attribute about self by day 4 is a positive outcome that addresses a low self-esteem problem, not a problem that deals with a risk for suicide.
    4. It is important to encourage clients to express suicidal ideations so the nurse can evaluate suicide risk. Redirecting the client from discussions about suicide is an inappropriate intervention; the outcome that reflects this intervention also is inappropriate.

TEST-TAKING HINT: To select the correct answer, the test taker must be able to pair the nursing diagnosis with the correct outcome. There always must be a correlation between the stated problem and client expectations documented in the outcome.

Nursing Process—Implementation

22. 1. In the Jewish faith, the 7-day period beginning with the burial is called shiva. During this time, mourners do not work, and no activity is permitted that diverts attention from thinking about the deceased. This practicing Jewish client is grieving the death of a parent who died 2 days ago; the client needs time to participate in this religious ritual.
    2. By encouraging participation in group, the nurse is not addressing the client's need to focus completely on the deceased. This indicates that the nurse is unfamiliar with the religious ritual of shiva practiced by individuals of Jewish faith.
    3. By teaching the client alternative coping skills to deal with grief, the nurse insinuates that the religious ritual of shiva is not a healthy coping mechanism. The nurse needs to recognize and appreciate the spiritual customs of various clients as normal behavior.
    4. By focusing on discussion of the client's positive aspects, the nurse has diverted the client's attention from the deceased. The

Jewish ritual of shiva requires mourners to focus completely on the deceased. The nurse needs to recognize and appreciate the spiritual customs of clients.

TEST-TAKING HINT: To answer this question correctly, the test taker must be familiar with commonly occurring religious rituals that address a client's spiritual needs.

23. 1. It may be appropriate to request a psychiatric consultation for a client experiencing insomnia, irritability, anorexia, and depressed mood, but this determination would be made after ruling out physical problems that may cause these symptoms.
    2. **Numerous physical conditions can contribute to symptoms of insomnia, including irritability, anorexia, and depressed mood. It is important for the nurse to rule out these physical problems before assuming that the symptoms are psychological in nature. The nurse can do this by completing a thorough physical assessment including review of laboratory tests.**
    3. Because the client has denied suicidal ideations, it would be unnecessary at this time to remove all hazardous materials from the environment.
    4. Because the client has denied suicidal ideations, it would be unnecessary at this time to place the client on a one-to-one observation.

TEST-TAKING HINT: Client symptoms presented in the question determine the priority nursing intervention. Because this client has denied suicidal ideations, answers 3 and 4 can be eliminated immediately as priority interventions. Also, the nurse must never make the initial assumption that presented symptoms are psychological in nature before assessing for a physical cause.

24. 1. Promoting attendance in group therapy to assist in socialization would be an interpersonal, not cognitive, nursing intervention. Interpersonal interventions focus on promoting appropriate interactions between individuals.
    2. Teaching assertiveness skills by role-playing would be a behavioral, not cognitive, nursing intervention. Behavioral interventions focus on promoting appropriate behaviors by the use of rewards and deterrents.
    3. Encouraging the client to journal to uncover underlying feelings would be an intrapersonal, not cognitive, nursing

intervention. Intrapersonal interventions focus on discussions of feelings, internal conflicts, and developmental problems.

4. Focusing on strengths and accomplishments to minimize failures is a cognitive nursing intervention. Cognitive interventions focus on altering distortions of thoughts and negative thinking.

TEST-TAKING HINT: To answer this question correctly, the test taker must recognize nursing interventions that use a cognitive approach. All other interventions presented may be appropriate to deal with client problems but are not from a cognitive perspective.

25. 1. Offering self is one technique to generate the establishment of trust with a newly admitted client diagnosed with an MDD. Trust is the basis for the establishment of any nurse–client relationship.

2. It is important for the nurse to promote attendance at group therapy by notifying the client of the group schedule, but this intervention does not assist the nurse in establishing a nurse–client relationship.

3. A newly admitted client with a diagnosis of MDD who is isolating self is not at a point in treatment to be able to socialize with peers. Imposed socialization can be perceived by the client as negative and could strain the nurse–client relationship.

4. A newly admitted client with a diagnosis of MDD who is isolating self is not at a point in treatment to be able to identify stressors. At this time, the client lacks the energy to participate actively in identifying stressors, and this intervention could strain the nurse–client relationship.

TEST-TAKING HINT: The test taker must understand the importance of timewise interventions. Client readiness determines appropriate and effective interventions.

26. 1. It is important to empathize with a client about fears related to ECT; however, this intervention would not be categorized as teaching.

2. It is important to monitor for any cardiac alterations during the ECT procedure to prevent possible cardiac complications; however, this intervention would not be categorized as teaching.

3. An expected and acceptable side effect of ECT is short-term memory loss. It is important for the nurse to teach the client and family members this information to prevent unnecessary anxiety about this symptom.

4. During ECT, the effects of induced seizure are mediated by the administration of muscle relaxant medications. This lowers the client's risk for injury.

TEST-TAKING HINT: To answer this question correctly, the test taker must differentiate a teaching intervention from other interventions presented.

27. 1. Clients who experience suicidal ideations must be monitored closely to prevent suicide attempts. By monitoring at irregular intervals, the nurse would prevent the client from recognizing patterns of observation. If a client recognizes a pattern of observation, the client can use the time in which they are not observed to plan and implement a suicide attempt.

2. It is important for a client experiencing suicidal ideations to attend group therapy to benefit from treatment. However, compared with the other answers to this question, this is not a priority.

3. The focus of nursing interventions with a newly admitted client experiencing suicidal ideations should be on maintaining safety. As the client stabilizes, the nurse can enlist friends and family to assist the client in remaining safe after discharge. Compared with the other answers to this question, this is not a priority.

4. It is important for a client experiencing suicidal ideations to understand that it takes 6 to 8 weeks for antidepressants to be fully effective. However, compared with the other answers to this question, this is not a priority.

TEST-TAKING HINT: The test taker must recognize that the priority nursing interventions, when working with a newly admitted client experiencing suicidal ideations, must focus on client safety.

Nursing Process—Evaluation

28. 1. It is 10%, not 1%, of the population, or 19 million Americans, who are affected by depression yearly.

2. During their lifetimes, 10% to 25%, not 2% to 5%, of women experience depression.

3. During their lifetimes, 5% to 12%, not 1% to 3%, of men become clinically depressed.

4. Major depression is one of the leading causes of disability in the United States. This is not to be confused with an occasional bout of the "blues," a feeling of sadness or downheartedness. Such

feelings are common among healthy individuals and are considered a normal response to everyday disappointments in life.

TEST-TAKING HINT: To answer this question correctly, the test taker must understand the epidemiology of MDD.

29. 1. Grieving clients may experience anxiety; however, the anxiety level described supports evidence of the resolution of client anxiety, not dysfunctional grieving.
    2. It is important for a client to develop trusting relationships; however, the ability to trust is not evidence that supports the resolution of dysfunctional grieving.
    3. A client in the denial stage of the grief response continues to be actively grieving, and therefore grief has not been resolved.
    4. Accepting responsibility for the role played in a loss indicates that the client has moved forward in the grieving process and resolved the problem of dysfunctional grieving.

TEST-TAKING HINT: To select the correct answer, the test taker must be able to pair the nursing diagnosis presented in the question with the correct evidence for resolution of the client problem. There always must be a correlation between the stated problem and the evaluation data.

30. 1. Approximately 30,000, not 10,000, individuals in the United States complete successful death by suicide each year.
    2. Almost 95% of all individuals who complete or attempt suicide have a diagnosed mental disorder. Most suicides are associated with mood disorders.
    3. Suicide is the third, not eighth, leading cause of death among young Americans 15 to 24 years of age. Only accidents and homicides have a higher incidence in this age-group. Suicide is the eighth leading cause of death among adult Americans.
    4. Depressive disorders account for four-fifths, not one-third, of all individuals who complete or attempt suicide.

TEST-TAKING HINT: The test taker must be aware of epidemiological factors about suicide to answer this question correctly.

31. 1. When the client states that the only reason to stay alive is to avoid hurting family, the client is focused on the needs of others rather than valuing self. This lack of self-value indicates continued hopelessness.
    2. Although it is encouraging when clients attend group, this client's statement does

not indicate a successful outcome as it relates to an increase in hope for the future.
    3. When the client begins to plan how to deal with conflicts at work, the client is focusing on a hopeful future. This indicates that the outcome of verbalizing a measure of hope about the future by day 3 has been successful.
    4. Although it is encouraging that the client can recognize and appreciate the compassionate care of the staff, this statement does not indicate a successful outcome as it relates to an increase in hope for the future.

TEST-TAKING HINT: To select the correct answer, the test taker must be able to pair the outcome presented in the question with the client statement that reflects the successful completion of this outcome.

Psychopharmacology

32. 1. Glycopyrrolate is given to decrease secretions and counteract the effects of vagal stimulation induced by ECT.
    2. Thiopental sodium is a short-acting anesthetic medication administered to produce loss of consciousness during ECT.
    3. Succinylcholine chloride is a muscle relaxant administered to prevent severe muscle contractions during the seizure, reducing the risk for fractured or dislocated bones.
    4. Because lorazepam, a central nervous system depressant, interferes with seizure activity, this medication would be inappropriate to administer before ECT.
    5. Because divalproex sodium, an anticonvulsant, interferes with seizure activity, this medication would be inappropriate to administer before ECT.

TEST-TAKING HINT: The test taker must recognize that any medication that inhibits seizure activity would be inappropriate to administer before ECT, which requires the client to experience a seizure.

33. Phenelzine, an antidepressant, is categorized as a monoamine oxidase inhibitor (MAOI).
    1. It is important for the nurse to teach a client who has been prescribed phenelzine that this medication takes 6 to 8 weeks to take full effect. But, compared with the other answer choices, this teaching topic is not prioritized.

2. Because there are numerous food–drug and drug–drug interactions that may precipitate a hypertensive crisis during treatment with MAOIs, it is critical that the nurse prioritize this teaching.

3. It is important for the nurse to teach a client who has been prescribed phenelzine that possible sexual side effects and insomnia can occur with the use of this drug. However, these symptoms are not as severe as a hypertensive crisis, so compared with the other answer choices, this teaching topic is not prioritized.

4. It is important for the nurse to educate the client about consistently taking the prescribed medications, even after improvement of symptoms. However, compared with the other answer choices, this teaching topic is not prioritized.

TEST-TAKING HINT: To answer this question correctly, the test taker must be aware that there are many special considerations related to the use of MAOIs. Understanding these considerations assists the test taker in prioritizing client teaching needs.

34. Vortioxetine, an antidepressant, affects many different serotonin pathways.

1. Because of the numerous suicides associated with mood disorders, it is important to monitor this client for suicidal ideations related to depressed mood. However, this is a client assessment and not a teaching intervention.

2. **Discussing the need for medication adherence, even when symptoms improve, is a teaching point that the nurse would need to review with a client who is prescribed vortioxetine.**

3. **Instructing the client about the risk for discontinuation syndrome is a teaching point that the nurse would need to review with a client prescribed vortioxetine.**

4. **Alerting the client to the risks of dry mouth, sedation, nausea, and sexual side effects is a teaching point that the nurse would need to review with a client prescribed vortioxetine.**

5. **Reminding the client that vortioxetine's full effect may not occur for 6 to 8 weeks is a teaching point that the nurse would need to review with a client prescribed vortioxetine.**

TEST-TAKING HINT: The test taker first must recognize vortioxetine as an antidepressant that affects serotonin. Knowing this would provide general medication information, rather than having to remember specific information about each medication.

35. Serotonin syndrome is a potentially life-threatening drug reaction that causes the body to have too much serotonin, a chemical produced by nerve cells. Most often this occurs when two drugs used concurrently potentiate serotoninergic neurotransmission.

1. **Confusion, restlessness, tachycardia, labile blood pressure, and diaphoresis all are symptoms of serotonin syndrome. Other symptoms include dilated pupils, loss of muscle coordination or twitching, diarrhea, headache, shivering, and goose bumps. If this syndrome were suspected, the offending agent would be discontinued immediately.**

2. Hypomania, akathisia, cardiac arrhythmias, and panic attacks all are symptoms associated with discontinuation syndrome from tricyclic antidepressants, not serotonin syndrome. Discontinuation syndrome occurs with the abrupt discontinuation of any class of antidepressants.

3. Dizziness, lethargy, headache, and nausea are symptoms associated with discontinuation syndrome from selective serotonin reuptake inhibitors (SSRIs), not serotonin syndrome. Discontinuation syndrome occurs with the abrupt discontinuation of any class of antidepressants.

4. Orthostatic hypotension, urinary retention, constipation, and blurred vision are side effects associated with the use of tricyclics and heterocyclics, not symptoms of serotonin syndrome.

TEST-TAKING HINT: The test taker must be able to differentiate among the symptoms of discontinuation syndrome, the symptoms of serotonin syndrome, and the side effects associated with the use of antidepressants to answer this question correctly.

36. 1. Bupropion is a norepinephrine dopamine reuptake inhibitor (NDRI), not tricyclic, antidepressant. This medication is FDA approved to assist with smoking cessation. Among the off-label, nonapproved uses are antidepressant-induced sexual dysfunction, attention-deficit/hyperactivity disorder (ADHD), depression associated with bipolar disorder, and obesity.

2. Mirtazapine is a tetracyclic, not tricyclic, antidepressant.

3. Citalopram is an SSRI, not a tricyclic antidepressant.

4. Nortriptyline is classified as a tricyclic antidepressant. Other tricyclic antidepressants include amitriptyline, doxepin, and imipramine.
5. Doxepin is classified as a tricyclic antidepressant.

TEST-TAKING HINT: To answer this question correctly, the test taker must be familiar with the various classes of antidepressant medications and the drugs within these classes.

37. Anticholinergic side effects include urinary hesitancy, constipation, blurred vision, and dry mouth.
   1. Urinary hesitancy is an anticholinergic side effect of tricyclic antidepressant.
   2. Constipation is an anticholinergic side effect of tricyclic antidepressant.
   3. Blurred vision is an anticholinergic side effect of tricyclic antidepressant.
   4. Sedation is a histamine effect of tricyclic antidepressant.
   5. Weight gain is a histamine effect of tricyclic antidepressant.

TEST-TAKING HINT: A way for the test taker to remember anticholinergic effects is to remember that they dry the system. When the system is dry, the client exhibits urinary hesitancy, constipation, blurred vision, and dry mouth.

38. Alprazolam is a benzodiazepine used to treat symptoms of anxiety. Benzodiazepines depress the central nervous system, and clients can exhibit increased depressive symptoms.
   1. Although physical withdrawal can occur when clients abruptly stop their benzodiazepine, this is not a priority intervention when the medication is first prescribed.
   2. Although the nurse would need to teach the client about the newly prescribed medication and ways of handling any side effects, the question is asking for an assessment, not the intervention of teaching.
   3. A side effect of alprazolam may be nausea, and to decrease this side effect, clients can take the medication with food; however, this is not the nurse's priority assessment in this situation.
   4. Alprazolam is a central nervous system depressant, and it is important for the nurse in this situation to monitor for worsening depressive symptoms and possible worsening of suicidal ideations.

TEST-TAKING HINT: The test taker needs to note important words in the question, such as *assessment* and *priority*, to choose the correct answer. Although some of the answers may be correct statements, as in answer 2, they do not meet the criteria of assessment.

39. Monoamine oxidase inhibitors (MAOIs) are used to treat depression. A nurse working with a client prescribed one of these medications must provide thorough instruction regarding interactions with other medications and foods. While taking MAOIs, clients cannot consume a long list of foods, which include, but are not limited to, the following: aged cheese, wine (especially Chianti), beer, chocolate, colas, coffee, tea, sour cream, beef/chicken livers, canned figs, soy sauce, overripe and fermented foods, pickled herring, preserved sausages, yogurt, yeast products, smoked and processed meats, cold remedies, and diet pills. Clients must be reminded that they must talk with their physician before taking any medication, including over-the-counter medications, to avoid a life-threatening hypertensive crisis. If a client consumes these foods or other medications during, or within 2 weeks after stopping, treatment with MAOIs, a life-threatening hypertensive crisis could occur.
   1. Chicken salad is safe to eat with MAOIs such as tranylcypromine.
   2. Isocarboxazid is an MAOI, and the intake of chocolate would likely cause a life-threatening hypertensive crisis.
   3. Venlafaxine is a serotonin norepinephrine reuptake inhibitor (SNRI). Although it should not be taken with wine, concurrent use would not cause a hypertensive crisis.
   4. Fresh roasted chicken is safe to eat with MAOIs such as phenelzine.
   5. Rasagiline is an MAOI. Eating smoked pork while taking rasagiline would likely cause a life-threatening hypertensive crisis.

TEST-TAKING HINT: To answer this question correctly, the test taker must take special note of medications, such as MAOIs, that have potentially serious side effects when drug–drug or drug–food interactions occur.

40. Bupropion is an antidepressant that has a side effect of lowering the seizure threshold.
   1. There is not a concern with injury to the gastrointestinal system while taking bupropion.
   2. Bupropion lowers the seizure threshold. Bupropion is contraindicated for clients who have increased potential for seizures, such as a client with a closed head trauma injury.
   3. Bupropion does not place a client at risk for increased bleeding.
   4. Bupropion has a mild stimulant effect and would not cause sedation.

TEST-TAKING HINT: The test taker must understand that bupropion lowers the seizure threshold and that clients with a head injury are at high risk for seizure activity. The combination of these two facts would lead the nurse to question the use of this medication.

41. Vilazodone is an SSRI used to treat depressive symptoms. When a client has decided not to take the medications and chooses not to share this decision with the team, the client may choose to "cheek," or hide medications in the mouth. This allows the client either to discard the medication or hoard the medication to implement a plan to overdose.
    1. Although the medication may take 2 to 3 weeks to begin taking effect, the question is asking for a priority intervention. The priority in this situation is to ensure the client is not cheeking the medication to follow through with their suicide plan.
    2. A nurse must teach a client to take vilazodone with food to help with absorption of the drug, not to prevent nausea.
    3. Although it is always important to monitor blood pressure, vilazodone does not cause hypertension, so this statement is incorrect.
    4. **If a client comes into the inpatient psychiatric unit with a plan to overdose, it is critical that the nurse monitor for cheeking and hoarding of medications. Clients may cheek and hoard medications to take, as an overdose, at another time.**

TEST-TAKING HINT: The test taker needs to note important words in the question, such as *priority*. Although answer 1 is a correct statement, when a client is initially admitted to an inpatient psychiatric unit with a plan to overdose, the nurse's priority is to monitor for cheeking and hoarding of medications to prevent a future suicide attempt.

42. Venlafaxine is a serotonin norepinephrine reuptake inhibitor (SNRI) prescribed for the treatment of depressive symptoms.
    1. Dry mouth, orthostatic hypotension, and blurred vision all are transient symptoms and usually dissipate after 1 or 2 weeks. These symptoms are not life threatening, so it is not necessary for the medications to be held.
    2. **The nurse needs to teach the client about acceptable side effects and what the client can do to deal with them. The nurse can suggest that the client use**
       ice chips, sip small amounts of water, or chew sugar-free gum or candy to moisten the dry mouth. For orthostatic hypotension, the nurse may encourage the client to change positions slowly. For blurred vision, the nurse may encourage the use of moisturizing eyedrops.
    3. Benztropine is an antiparkinsonian medication used to treat extrapyramidal symptoms (EPS) caused by antipsychotic medications, not antidepressants.
    4. Venlafaxine is not an MAOI, and dietary restrictions are not indicated.

TEST-TAKING HINT: To answer this question correctly, the test taker needs to distinguish the difference between life-threatening side effects and side effects that may be transient and acceptable.

43. Citalopram is an SSRI prescribed for depressive disorders. Frequently, clients are admitted to an inpatient psychiatric unit complaining of depressive symptoms and are not asked about possible history of manic or hypomanic episodes. These symptoms may indicate a diagnosis of bipolar affective disorder, either type 1 (with at least one manic episode) or type 2 (with at least one hypomanic episode).
    1. **When an SSRI is prescribed for clients diagnosed with bipolar affective disorder, it can cause alterations in neurotransmitters and trigger a hypomanic or manic episode.**
    2. This client is exhibiting signs of mania and is not ready for discharge.
    3. Although clients may attempt to mask their depression to be discharged, the symptoms noted in the question are signs of mania.
    4. When a client has decided not to take the medications and chooses not to share this decision with the team, the client may choose to "cheek," or hide medications in the mouth. This allows the client either to discard or hoard the medication for use at another time. If an individual takes SSRIs in an attempt to overdose, it would not cause a client to experience mania.

TEST-TAKING HINT: It is important for the test taker to understand the effects of psychotropic medications on neurotransmitters and how these may generate signs and symptoms of mania in clients with a diagnosis of bipolar affective disorder.

44. The nurse will administer *six tablets* in 1 day.

$$\frac{75 \text{ mg}}{x \text{ tab}} = \frac{37.5 \text{ mg}}{1 \text{ tab}} = 2 \text{ tabs}$$

$$\frac{150 \text{ mg}}{x \text{ tab}} = \frac{37.5 \text{ mg}}{1 \text{ tab}} = 4 \text{ tabs}$$

2 tabs + 4 tabs = 6 tabs/d

TEST-TAKING HINT: The test taker must note keywords in the questions, such as *daily*. The test taker first must calculate the number of tablets for each scheduled dose and then add these together to get the total daily number of tablets. Set up the ratio and proportion problem based on the number of milligrams contained in one tablet. The test taker can then solve this problem by cross multiplication and solving for *x* by division.

45. 1. Levomilnacipran is an SNRI used in the treatment of depression and anxiety. Levomilnacipran does not need to be taken with food for absorption but can be taken with food if a client experiences dyspepsia.
2. Lurasidone is an atypical antipsychotic medication used in the treatment of psychosis and mood instability. Lurasidone must be taken with at least 350 calories in order to be effectively absorbed.
3. Vilazodone is an SSRI used in the treatment of depression and anxiety. Vilazodone must be taken with at least 350 calories in order to be effectively absorbed.
4. Vortioxetine is an antidepressant used in the treatment of depression. This medication does not need to be taken with food but can be taken with food if a client experiences dyspepsia.
5. Risperidone is an atypical antipsychotic medication used in the treatment of psychosis. Risperidone does not need to be taken with food.

TEST-TAKING HINT: To answer this question correctly, the test taker must be familiar with specific administration requirements for different medications.

46. 1. Transcranial magnetic stimulation (TMS) is a procedure that does not require surgery or medications, is approved by the Food and Drug Administration (FDA), and has been shown to be safe and effective in the treatment of depression.
2. Cognitive-behavioral therapy (CBT) can help clients deal with symptoms associated with depression.
3. Light therapy can assist clients experiencing seasonal affective disorder (SAD) but is not effective with all subtypes of depression.
4. Vagus nerve stimulation (VNS) is a procedure in which a surgically implanted pacemaker-like device sends electrical pulses to stimulate the vagal nerve. This treatment has been FDA approved for clients experiencing treatment resistant depression.
5. Electroconvulsive therapy (ECT) is among the safest and most effective treatments available for depression. ECT causes a brief seizure in the brain and is one of the fastest ways to relieve symptoms in clients experiencing severe depression or suicidal ideation.

TEST-TAKING HINT: To answer this question correctly, the test taker must be familiar with nonpharmacological treatments for depressive symptoms.

47. 1. Although dextromethorphan/bupropion (Auvelity) has the active ingredient bupropion HCl, it is different than the generic because of the small addition of dextromethorphan HBr.
2. Although Auvelity is shown to work faster, it is because dextromethorphan impacts glutamate and not because of better absorption in the digestive track.
3. Auvelity is different because with the addition of dextromethorphan, the medication acts on the *N*-methyl-D-aspartate (NMDA) receptor affecting glutamate. Glutamate is the brain's primary "go" signal.
4. Auvelity affects norepinephrine and dopamine receptors; however, it does not affect serotonin, and therefore this is incorrect statement.

TEST-TAKING HINT: When reviewing medications for depression, the test-taker must also review all new medications approved by the Federal Drug Administration (FDA) and work on recognizing what makes them different from others already approved.

Bipolar and Related Disorders

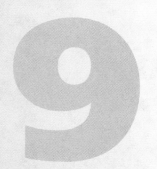

QUESTIONS

Theory

1. Which statement about the development of bipolar disorder is from a biochemical perspective?
    1. Family studies have shown that if one parent is diagnosed with bipolar disorder, the risk that a child will have the disorder is about 28%.
    2. In bipolar disorder, there may be possible alterations in normal electrolyte transfer across cell membranes, resulting in elevated levels of intracellular calcium and sodium.
    3. Magnetic resonance imaging reveals enlarged third ventricles, subcortical white matter, and periventricular hyperintensity in those diagnosed with bipolar disorder.
    4. Twin studies have indicated a concordance rate among monozygotic twins of 60% to 80%.

Nursing Process—Assessment

2. Which of the following nursing charting entries is documentation of a behavioral symptom of mania? **Select all that apply.**
    1. "Thoughts fragmented; flight of ideas noted."
    2. "Mood euphoric and expansive. Rates mood as 10/10."
    3. "Pacing halls throughout the day."
    4. "Easily distracted, unable to focus on goals."
    5. "Exhibits poor impulse control."

3. A nurse on an inpatient psychiatric unit receives report at 1500 hours. Which client would need to be assessed first?
   1. A client on one-to-one status because of active suicidal ideations.
   2. A client pacing the hall and experiencing irritability and flight of ideas.
   3. A client diagnosed with hypomania monopolizing time in the milieu.
   4. A client with a history of mania who is to be discharged in the morning.

Nursing Process—Diagnosis

4. A client diagnosed with cyclothymic disorder is newly admitted to an inpatient psychiatric unit. The client has a history of irritability and grandiosity, and is currently sleeping 2 hours a night. Which nursing diagnosis takes priority?
   1. Altered thought processes R/T biochemical alterations.
   2. Social isolation R/T grandiosity.
   3. Disturbed sleep patterns R/T agitation.
   4. Risk for violence: self-directed R/T depressive symptoms.

5. A newly admitted client diagnosed with bipolar I disorder is experiencing a manic episode. Which nursing diagnosis is a priority at this time?
   1. Risk for violence: other-directed R/T poor impulse control.
   2. Altered thought process R/T hallucinations.
   3. Social isolation R/T manic excitement.
   4. Low self-esteem R/T guilt about promiscuity.

Nursing Process—Planning

6. A client diagnosed with bipolar I disorder has a nursing diagnosis of disturbed thought process R/T biochemical alterations. Based on this diagnosis, which correctly written outcome would be appropriate?
   1. The client will not experience injury throughout the shift.
   2. The client will interact appropriately with others by day 3.
   3. The client will be compliant with prescribed medications.
   4. The client will distinguish reality from delusions by day 6.

7. The nurse is reviewing expected outcomes for a client diagnosed with bipolar I disorder. Number the outcomes presented in the order in which the nurse would address them.
   1. _____ The client exhibits no evidence of physical injury.
   2. _____ The client eats 70% of all finger foods offered.
   3. _____ The client is able to access available outpatient resources.
   4. _____ The client accepts responsibility for own behaviors.

8. A client diagnosed with bipolar II disorder has a nursing diagnosis of impaired social interactions R/T egocentrism. Which short-term, correctly written outcome is an appropriate expectation for this client problem?
   1. The client will have an appropriate one-on-one interaction with a peer by day 4.
   2. The client will exchange personal information with peers at lunchtime.
   3. The client will verbalize the desire to interact with peers by day 2.
   4. The client will initiate an appropriate social relationship with a peer.

Nursing Process—Implementation

9. A client seen in the emergency department (ED) is experiencing irritability, pressured speech, and increased levels of anxiety. Which would be the nurse's priority intervention?
   1. Place the client on a one-on-one observation to prevent injury.
   2. Ask the physician for a psychiatric consultation.
   3. Assess vital signs and complete a physical assessment.
   4. Reinforce relaxation techniques to decrease anxiety.

10. A client experiencing mania states, "Everything I do is great." Using a cognitive approach, which nursing response would be most appropriate?
    1. "Is there a time in your life when things didn't go as planned?"
    2. "Everything you do is great."
    3. "What are some other things you do well?"
    4. "Let's talk about the feelings you have about your childhood."

11. A newly admitted client is experiencing a manic episode. The client's nursing diagnosis is imbalanced nutrition, less than body requirements. Which of the following meals are most appropriate for this client? **Select all that apply.**
    1. Chicken fingers and French fries.
    2. Grilled chicken and a baked potato.
    3. Spaghetti and meatballs.
    4. Chili and crackers.
    5. Ham and cheese sandwich.

12. A provocatively dressed client diagnosed with bipolar I disorder is observed laughing loudly with peers in the milieu. Which nursing action is a priority in this situation?
    1. Join the milieu to assess the appropriateness of the laughter.
    2. Redirect clients in the milieu to structured social activities, such as cards.
    3. Privately discuss with the client the inappropriate provocative dress.
    4. Administer prn antianxiety medication to calm the client.

13. A client diagnosed with bipolar I disorder in the manic phase is yelling at another peer in the milieu. Which nursing intervention takes priority?
    1. Calmly redirect and remove the client from the milieu.
    2. Administer prescribed prn intramuscular injection for agitation.
    3. Ask the client to lower their voice while in the common area.
    4. Obtain an order for seclusion to help decrease external stimuli.

14. A client newly admitted with bipolar I disorder has a nursing diagnosis of risk for injury R/T extreme hyperactivity. Which nursing intervention is appropriate?
    1. Place the client in a room with another client experiencing similar symptoms.
    2. Use prn antipsychotic medications as ordered by the physician.
    3. Discuss consequences of the client's behaviors with the client daily.
    4. Reinforce previously learned coping skills to decrease agitation.

15. A client diagnosed with bipolar I disorder, most recent episode manic, is now ready for discharge. Which of the following resource services should be included in discharge teaching? **Select all that apply.**
    1. Financial and legal assistance.
    2. Crisis hotline.
    3. Individual psychotherapy.
    4. Support groups.
    5. Family education groups.

Nursing Process—Evaluation

16. A nursing instructor is teaching about the etiology of mood disorders. Which statement by a nursing student best indicates an understanding of the etiology of mood disorders?
    1. "When clients experience loss, they learn that it is inevitable and become hopeless and helpless."
    2. "There are alterations in the neurochemicals, such as serotonin, that cause the client's symptoms."
    3. "Evidence continues to support multiple causations related to an individual's susceptibility to mood symptoms."
    4. "Current research suggests that a genetic component affects the development of mood disorders."

17. A nursing instructor is teaching about the psychosocial theory related to the development of bipolar disorder. Which student statement indicates that learning has occurred?
    1. "The credibility of psychosocial theories in the etiology of bipolar disorder has strengthened in recent years."
    2. "Individuals are genetically predisposed to being diagnosed with bipolar disorder if a parent is mentally ill."
    3. "Following steroid, antidepressant, or amphetamine use, individuals can experience manic episodes."
    4. "The etiology of bipolar disorder is unclear, but it is possible that biological and psychosocial factors are influential."

18. A nurse working with a client diagnosed with bipolar I disorder attempts to recognize the motivation behind the client's use of grandiosity. Which is the rationale for this nurse's action?
    1. Understanding the reason behind a behavior would assist the nurse in accepting and relating to the client, not the behavior.
    2. Change in behavior cannot occur until the client can accept responsibility for their own actions.
    3. As self-esteem is increased, the client will meet individual needs without the use of manipulation.
    4. Positive reinforcement would enhance self-esteem and promote desirable behaviors.

19. A nursing instructor is teaching about the client's criteria for the diagnosis of bipolar II disorder. Which student statement indicates that learning has occurred?
    1. "Clients diagnosed with bipolar II disorder experience a full syndrome of mania and have a history of symptoms of depression."
    2. "Clients diagnosed with bipolar II disorder experience numerous episodes of hypomanic and dysthymic symptoms for at least 2 years."
    3. "Clients diagnosed with bipolar II disorder have mood disturbances that are directly associated with the physiological effects of a substance."
    4. "Clients diagnosed with bipolar II disorder experience recurrent bouts of depression with episodic occurrences of hypomanic symptoms."

Psychopharmacology

20. A client diagnosed with bipolar I disorder is experiencing auditory hallucinations and flight of ideas. Which medication combination would the nurse expect to be prescribed to treat these symptoms?
    1. Amitriptyline and divalproex sodium.
    2. Verapamil and topiramate.
    3. Lithium carbonate and clonazepam.
    4. Risperidone and lamotrigine.

21. A client prescribed lithium carbonate is experiencing an excessive output of dilute urine, tremors, and muscular irritability. These symptoms would lead the nurse to expect to assess which serum lithium level?
    1. 0.6 mEq/L.
    2. 1.5 mEq/L.
    3. 2.6 mEq/L.
    4. 3.5 mEq/L.

22. A client experiencing euphoria, racing thoughts, and irritability is brought into the emergency department when found nude in a residential area. Choose the numbered line of this illustration that graphically represents this client's mood disorder. Line number _____.

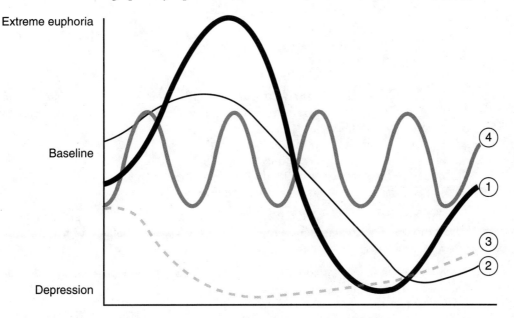

23. A client prescribed lithium carbonate 300 mg a.m. daily and 600 mg qhs presents in the emergency department with impaired consciousness, nystagmus, arrhythmias, and a history of recent seizure. Which serum lithium level would the nurse expect to assess?
  1. 3.7 mEq/L.
  2. 3.0 mEq/L.
  3. 2.5 mEq/L.
  4. 1.9 mEq/L.

24. A client is newly prescribed lithium carbonate. Which teaching point by the nurse takes priority?
  1. "Make sure your salt intake is consistent."
  2. "Limit your fluid intake to 2,000 mL/day."
  3. "Monitor your caloric intake because of potential weight gain."
  4. "Get yourself in a daily routine to assist in avoiding relapse."

25. Which list contains medications that the nurse may see prescribed to treat clients diagnosed with bipolar affective disorder (BPAD)?
  1. Lithium carbonate, loxapine, and carbamazepine.
  2. Gabapentin, thiothixene, and clonazepam.
  3. Divalproex sodium, asenapine, and olanzapine.
  4. Lamotrigine, risperidone, and benztropine.

26. The nurse is evaluating laboratory test results for a client prescribed lithium carbonate. The client's lithium level is 1.9 mEq/L. Which nursing intervention takes priority?
  1. Give next dose because the lithium level is normal for acute mania.
  2. Hold the next dose and continue the medication as prescribed the following day.
  3. Give the next dose after assessing for signs and symptoms of lithium toxicity.
  4. Immediately notify the physician and hold the dose until instructed further.

27. A client on an inpatient psychiatric unit is prescribed lamotrigine 50 mg daily. After client teaching, which client statement reflects understanding of important information related to lamotrigine?
  1. "I will call the doctor if I miss more than 5 days before restarting the medication."
  2. "I will schedule an appointment for my blood to be drawn at the laboratory next week."
  3. "I will call the doctor immediately if my temperature rises above 100°F."
  4. "I will stop my medication if I start having muscle rigidity of my face or neck."

28. A client diagnosed with bipolar affective disorder (BPAD) is prescribed divalproex sodium. Which of the following laboratory tests would the nurse need to monitor throughout drug therapy? **Select all that apply.**
    1. Platelet count.
    2. Aspartate aminotransferase (AST).
    3. Fasting blood sugar (FBS).
    4. Alanine aminotransferase (ALT).
    5. Serum divalproex sodium level.

29. A client diagnosed with bipolar affective disorder (BPAD) is prescribed carbamazepine. The client exhibits nausea, vomiting, and anorexia. Which is an appropriate nursing intervention at this time?
    1. Stop the medication and notify the physician.
    2. Hold the next dose until symptoms subside.
    3. Administer the next dose with food.
    4. Ask the physician for a stat carbamazepine level.

30. A client thought to be "cheeking" medications is prescribed lithium syrup 900 mg bid. The syrup contains 300 mg of lithium carbonate per 5 mL. At 0800, how many milliliters would the nurse administer? _____ mL.

31. A nurse is teaching a client about taking asenapine effectively. Which client statement indicates that learning has occurred?
    1. "I must take the medicine with a meal to help with absorption."
    2. "I must take the medicine in the morning to help with my depression."
    3. "I must monitor for signs and symptoms of serotonin syndrome."
    4. "I must place the medicine under my tongue."

32. The nurse reviews the medical record illustrated for a 40-year-old client hospitalized with an acute episode of bipolar depression.

Assessment Information	Lab and Dx Study Results	Medications Due Now
Irregular HR 100 BPM	Creatinine clearance: 100 mL/min	Lithium carbonate 1,800 mg oral daily
B/P 96/55	Serum lithium level: 3.7 mEq/L	Lorazepam 1 mg oral prn
30 mL urine output in last 3 hours	BUN: 90 mg/dL	Ondansetron 8 mg oral prn
Unaware of place and time	CIWA: <10	
Persistent nausea and vomiting		
Hand tremors		
C/O tinnitus		

Which action by the nurse takes priority?
1. Interview family related to client's substance abuse history.
2. Administer lorazepam 1 mg to decrease anxiety and notify health-care personnel (HCP).
3. Stay with the client and offer support.
4. Hold lithium carbonate and notify HCP.

The correct answer number and rationale for why it is the correct answer are given in **boldface blue type**. Rationales for why the other answer options are incorrect are given as well, but they are not in boldface type.

Theory

1. 1. Increased risk for the diagnosis of bipolar disorder based on family history is evidence of a genetic, not biochemical, perspective in the development of the disease.
   2. **Alterations in normal electrolyte transfer across cell membranes, resulting in elevated levels of intracellular calcium and sodium, is an example of a biochemical perspective in the development of bipolar disorder.**
   3. Enlarged third ventricles, subcortical white matter, and periventricular hyperintensity occur in individuals diagnosed with bipolar disorder. This theory is from a neuroanatomical, not biochemical, perspective in the development of the disease.
   4. Twin studies support evidence that heredity plays a major role in the etiology of bipolar disorder. This theory is from a genetic, not biochemical, perspective in the development of the disease.

TEST-TAKING HINT: The test taker needs to understand the various theories that are associated with the development of bipolar disorders to answer this question correctly. Only answer 2 is a theory from a biochemical perspective.

Nursing Process—Assessment

2. 1. When the nurse documents, "Thoughts fragmented, flight of ideas noted," the nurse is charting a cognitive, not behavioral, symptom of mania.
   2. When the nurse documents, "Mood euphoric and expansive. Rates mood as 10/10," the nurse is charting an affective, not behavioral, symptom of mania.
   3. **When the nurse documents, "Pacing halls throughout the day," the nurse is charting a behavioral symptom of mania. Psychomotor activities and uninhibited social and sexual behaviors are classified as behavioral symptoms.**

4. When the nurse documents, "Easily distracted, unable to focus on goals," the nurse is charting a cognitive, not behavioral, symptom of mania.
   5. **When the nurse documents "Exhibits poor impulse control," the nurse is charting a behavioral symptom of mania.**

TEST-TAKING HINT: The test taker must be able to differentiate the symptoms of mania as affective, cognitive, physiological, and behavioral to answer this question correctly.

3. 1. A client on one-to-one observation status is being monitored constantly by staff members and would not require immediate assessment.
   2. **A client's behavior of pacing the halls and experiencing irritability should be considered emergent and warrant immediate attention. Most assaultive behavior that occurs on an inpatient unit is preceded by a period of increasing hyperactivity. Because of these symptoms, this client would need to be assessed first.**
   3. Client behaviors that are experienced during hypomanic episodes are not as extreme as behaviors that may occur in manic episodes and would not require immediate assessment. The nurse may need to address the behavior of monopolizing time in the milieu, but this would be a less critical intervention.
   4. When clients meet discharge criteria, acute symptoms have been resolved. Assessment of client needs is important for discharge planning, but this client would not require immediate assessment.

TEST-TAKING HINT: When deciding priority assessments, the test taker must look for the client with the most critical problem who can pose a safety risk to self or others. In this question, answer 1 would meet safety criteria, but because this client already is being monitored by staff, this answer choice would take lower priority.

Nursing Process—Diagnosis

4. 1. Altered thought process is defined as a state in which an individual experiences an alteration in cognitive operations and activities. Nothing is presented in the question that would indicate this client is experiencing a disturbed thought process. Clients diagnosed

with bipolar I disorder, not cyclothymic disorder, may experience disturbed thought processes during manic episodes.

2. Social isolation is defined as aloneness experienced by the individual, perceived as imposed by others, and as a negative and threatened state. Nothing is presented in the question that would indicate this client is experiencing social isolation.

3. **Disturbed sleep pattern is defined as a time-limited disruption of sleep amount and quality. Because the client is sleeping only 2 hours a night, the client is meeting the defining characteristics of the nursing diagnosis of disturbed sleep patterns. This sleep problem is usually due to excessive hyperactivity and agitation.**

4. Risk for violence: self-directed is defined as behaviors in which an individual demonstrates that they can be physically, emotionally, or sexually harmful to self. Nothing is presented in the question that would indicate this client is experiencing risk for violence, self-directed.

TEST-TAKING HINT: To select the correct answer, the test taker must be able to correlate the client symptoms presented in the question with the nursing diagnosis that describes the client problem exhibited by these symptoms.

5. 1. **Risk for violence: other-directed is defined as behaviors in which an individual demonstrates that they can be physically, emotionally, or sexually harmful to others. Because of poor impulse control, irritability, and hyperactive psychomotor behaviors experienced during a manic episode, this client is at risk for violence directed toward others. Keeping everyone in the milieu safe is always a nursing priority.**

2. Altered thought process is defined as a state in which an individual experiences an alteration in cognitive operations and activities. Although a client at the peak of a manic episode may experience altered thought processes, of the diagnoses presented, this client problem would be less of a priority than maintaining safety.

3. Social isolation is defined as aloneness experienced by the individual and perceived as imposed by others and as a negative and threatened state. In a manic episode, the appropriate nursing diagnosis would be impaired social interaction, not social isolation, because of the presence of intrusive, not isolative, behaviors.

4. Low self-esteem is defined as a long-standing negative self-evaluation and feelings about

self or self-capabilities. During a manic episode, a client is more apt to experience grandiosity than to exhibit symptoms of low self-esteem.

TEST-TAKING HINT: The test taker must understand that during a manic episode, because of the client's experiencing poor impulse control, grandiosity, and irritability, the risk for violence toward others is increased and must be prioritized.

Nursing Process—Planning

6. 1. A client's being free of injury throughout a shift would be an appropriate outcome for the nursing diagnosis of risk for injury, not disturbed thought process.

2. A client's interacting appropriately by day 3 would be an appropriate outcome for the nursing diagnosis of impaired social interaction, not disturbed thought process.

3. A client adhering with prescribed medications would be an appropriate outcome for the nursing diagnosis of disturbed thought process R/T biochemical alterations. Medications address the biochemical alterations that cause disturbed thought in clients diagnosed with bipolar I disorder. The reason this outcome is an incorrect choice is because it does not contain a time frame and cannot be measured.

4. **Distinguishing reality from delusions by day 6 is an appropriate outcome for the nursing diagnosis of disturbed thought process R/T biochemical alterations. Altered thought processes have improved when the client can distinguish reality from delusions.**

TEST-TAKING HINT: To select the correct answer, the test taker must be able to pair the nursing diagnosis presented in the question with the correct client outcome. There always must be a correlation between the stated problem and the expectation for improvement. Also note that the correct outcome must be measurable and contain a time frame.

7. The outcomes should be numbered as follows: 1, 2, 4, 3.

1. **The nurse would first address the outcome that states, "The client exhibits no evidence of physical injury," because this outcome deals with client physical safety.**

2. **Next, the nurse would address the outcome that states, "The client eats 70% of all finger foods offered," because this**

outcome deals with the client's physical needs.

3. The nurse would next address the outcome that states, "The client accepts responsibility for own behaviors," because this outcome is realistic only later in treatment.

4. Finally, the nurse would address the outcome that states, "The client is able to access available outpatient resources," because this outcome would be appropriate only during the discharge process.

TEST-TAKING HINT: The test taker can use Maslow's hierarchy of needs to facilitate the ranking of client outcomes. In this question, answer 1 relates to safety, 2 relates to physical needs, and 4 relates to psychosocial needs. The time frame in which answer 3 would be accomplished (discharge) determines its ranking.

8. Egocentrism is defined as viewing everything in relation to self, or self-centeredness.

1. A client having an appropriate one-to-one interaction with a peer is a successful outcome for the nursing diagnosis of impaired social interactions. The test taker should note that this outcome is specific, client centered, positive, realistic, and measurable and includes a time frame.

2. Exchanging personal information with peers at lunchtime is an appropriate outcome for the nursing diagnosis of impaired social interactions R/T egocentrism. Exchanging information with other clients indicates interest in others, which shows a decrease in egocentrism. However, this outcome does not contain a time frame and so cannot be measured.

3. Although verbalizing a desire to interact with peers is an appropriate short-term outcome, this outcome addresses the nursing diagnosis of social isolation, not impaired social interactions.

4. Initiating an appropriate social relationship with a peer is an outcome related to the nursing diagnosis of impaired social interactions; however, because this outcome does not contain a time frame, it cannot be measured.

TEST-TAKING HINT: To answer this question correctly, the test taker needs to know the components of a correctly written outcome. Outcomes need to be specific, client centered, realistic, positive, and measurable and include a time frame.

Nursing Process—Implementation

9. 1. Before assuming the client's problem is psychological in nature and placing the client on a one-to-one observation, the nurse should rule out a physical cause for the symptoms presented.

2. Before assuming the client's problem is psychological in nature and requesting a psychiatric consultation, the nurse should rule out a physical cause for the symptoms presented.

3. The nurse first should assess vital signs and complete a physical assessment to rule out a physical cause for the symptoms presented. Many physical problems manifest in symptoms that seem to be caused by psychological problems.

4. By reinforcing relaxation techniques to decrease anxiety, the nurse has assumed, without sufficient assessment data, that the client's problems are caused by anxiety. Before making this assumption, the nurse should rule out a physical cause for the symptoms presented.

TEST-TAKING HINT: The test taker must recognize that many physical problems manifest themselves in symptoms that, on the surface, look psychological in nature. A nursing assessment should progress from initially gathering physiological data toward collecting psychological information.

10. 1. By asking, "Is there a time in your life when things didn't go as planned?" the nurse is using a cognitive approach to challenge the thought processes of the client.

2. By stating, "Everything you do is great," the nurse is using the therapeutic technique of restating. This is a general communication technique and is not considered a cognitive communication approach, which would challenge the client's thought processes.

3. By asking, "What are some other things you do well?" the nurse is using a cognitive approach by encouraging further discussion about strengths. However, the content of this communication is inappropriate because it reinforces the grandiosity being experienced by the client.

4. By stating, "Let's talk about the feelings you have about your childhood," the nurse is using an intrapersonal, not cognitive, approach by assessing the client's feelings rather than thoughts.

TEST-TAKING HINT: There are two aspects of this question of which the test taker must be aware. First, the test taker must choose a statement by the nurse that is cognitive in nature and then ensure the appropriateness of the statement.

11. Clients experiencing mania have excessive psychomotor activity that leads to an inability to sit still long enough to eat. Increased nutritional intake is necessary because of a high metabolic rate.
    1. **Chicken fingers and French fries are finger foods, which the client would be able to eat during increased psychomotor activity, such as pacing. Because these foods are high in caloric value, they also meet the client's increased nutritional needs.**
    2. Although grilled chicken and a baked potato would meet the client's increased nutritional needs, the baked potato is not a finger food and would be difficult for the client to eat during periods of hyperactivity.
    3. Although spaghetti and meatballs would meet the client's increased nutritional needs, this dinner would be difficult for the client to eat during periods of hyperactivity.
    4. Although chili and crackers would meet the client's increased nutritional needs, this dinner would be difficult for the client to eat during periods of hyperactivity.
    5. **A ham and cheese sandwich is finger food, which a client could easily eat during increased psychomotor activity, such as pacing.**

TEST-TAKING HINT: To answer this question correctly, the test taker must understand that the symptom of hyperactivity during a manic episode affects the client's ability to meet nutritional needs. The test taker should look for easily portable foods with high caloric value to determine the most appropriate meal for this client.

12. 1. Although it is important for the nurse to gather any significant data related to client behaviors in the milieu, this nurse already has made the determination that the client is provocatively dressed. Dressing provocatively can precipitate sexual overtures that can be dangerous to the client and must be addressed immediately.
    2. By redirecting clients to structured social activities, the nurse is not dealing with the assessed, critical problem of provocative dress.
    3. **Because dressing provocatively can precipitate sexual overtures that can be**

dangerous to the client, it is the priority of the nurse to discuss with the client the inappropriateness of this clothing choice.
    4. When the nurse administers antianxiety medications in an attempt to calm the client, the nurse is ignoring the assessed, critical problem of the client's provocative dress.

TEST-TAKING HINT: The test taker should note that answers 1, 2, and 4 all address the observed behavior of potentially insignificant laughter in the milieu. Only answer 3 addresses the actual critical problem of provocative dress.

13. 1. **When a client experiencing mania is yelling at other peers, it is the nurse's priority to address this situation immediately. Behaviors of this type can escalate into violence toward clients and staff members. By using a calm manner, the nurse avoids generating any further hostile behaviors, and by removing the client from the milieu, the nurse protects other clients on the unit.**
    2. Administering a prescribed prn intramuscular injection for agitation could be an appropriate intervention, but only after all less restrictive measures have been attempted.
    3. When the nurse asks an agitated client in a manic phase of bipolar I disorder to lower their voice in the common area, the nurse has lost sight of the fact that these behaviors are inherent in this client's diagnosis. The client who is yelling at another peer does not have the ability to alter behaviors in response to simple direction.
    4. Obtaining an order for seclusion to help decrease external stimuli could be an appropriate intervention, but only after all less restrictive measures have been attempted.

TEST-TAKING HINT: The test taker must remember that all less-restrictive measures must be attempted before imposing chemical or physical restraints. Understanding this would help the test taker to eliminate answers 2 and 4 immediately.

14. 1. Placing a hyperactive client diagnosed with bipolar I disorder with another hyperactive client would serve only to increase hyperactivity in both clients. When a client is in a manic phase of the disorder, the best intervention is to reduce environmental stimuli, assign a private room, and keep lighting and noise at a low level when possible.

2. A newly admitted client experiencing an extremely hyperactive episode as the result of bipolar I disorder would benefit from an antipsychotic medication to sedate the client quickly. A mood stabilizer may be given concurrently for maintenance therapy, and to prevent or diminish the intensity of subsequent manic episodes.

3. A client experiencing an extremely hyperactive episode as the result of bipolar I disorder would have difficulty comprehending the cause and effect of behaviors until medications begin to take effect.

4. Reinforcing previously learned coping skills with a client experiencing a hyperactive episode would increase, not decrease, agitation. This client is unable to focus on review of learned behaviors because of the distractibility inherent in mania.

TEST-TAKING HINT: To answer this question correctly, the test taker needs to understand that a client experiencing a manic episode must be de-escalated before any teaching, confronting, or enforcing can occur.

15. 1. During a manic episode, clients are likely to experience impulse control problems, which may lead to excessive spending. Having access to financial and legal assistance may help the client assess the situation and initiate plans to deal with financial problems.

2. Clients diagnosed with bipolar disorder can experience hyperactivity or depression, which may lead to ambivalence regarding their desire to live. Having access to a crisis hotline may help the client to de-escalate and make the difference between life and death decisions.

3. During a manic episode, a client most likely would have had difficulties in various aspects of interpersonal relationships, such as with family, friends, and coworkers. Individuals experiencing mania may be difficult candidates for psychotherapy because of their inability to focus. When the acute phase of the illness has passed, the client may decide to access an available resource to deal with interpersonal problems. Psychotherapy, in conjunction with medication maintenance treatment, and counseling may be useful in helping these individuals.

4. During a manic episode, a client would not be a willing candidate for any type of group therapy. However, when the acute phase of the illness has passed, this individual may want to access support groups to benefit therapeutically from peer support.

5. During a manic episode, a client may have jeopardized marriage or family functioning. Having access to a resource that would help this client restore adaptive family functioning may improve not only relationships but also noncompliance issues and dysfunctional behavioral patterns, and ultimately may reduce relapse rates. Family therapy is most effective with the combination of psychotherapeutic and pharmacotherapeutic treatment.

TEST-TAKING HINT: To answer this question correctly, the test taker must understand that during the manic phase of bipolar I disorder, clients engage in inappropriate behaviors that lead to future problems. It is important to provide outpatient resources to help clients avoid or minimize the consequences of their past behaviors.

Nursing Process—Evaluation

16. 1. Learning theorists believe that learned helplessness predisposes individuals to depression by imposing a feeling of lack of control over their life situations. They become depressed because they feel helpless; they have learned whatever they do is futile. However, this theory presents only one of the possible causes of mood disorders.

2. Neurobiological theorists believe that there are alterations in the neurochemicals, such as serotonin, that cause mood disorder symptoms. However, this theory presents only one of the possible causes of mood disorders.

3. When the student states that there is support for multiple causations related to an individual's susceptibility to mood symptoms, the student understands the content presented about the etiology of mood disorders.

4. Genetic theorists believe there is a strong genetic component affecting the development of mood disorders. However, this theory presents only one of the possible causes of mood disorders.

TEST-TAKING HINT: All answers presented include possible theories for the cause of mood disorders. To choose the correct answer, the test taker must understand that no one theory has been accepted as a definitive explanation of the etiology of mood disorders.

17. 1. The credibility of psychosocial theories that deal with the etiology of bipolar disorder has weakened, not strengthened, in recent years.
    2. The etiology of bipolar disorder is affected by genetic, biochemical, and physiological factors. If bipolar disorders were purely genetic, there would be a 100% concordance rate among monozygotic twins. Research shows the concordance rate among monozygotic twins is only 60% to 80%.
    3. Following steroid, antidepressant, or amphetamine use, individuals can experience manic episodes. The response to these medications, which cause these symptoms, is physiological, not psychosocial.
    4. **The etiology of bipolar disorder is unclear; however, research evidence shows that biological and psychosocial factors are influential in the development of the disorder.**

TEST-TAKING HINT: The test taker needs to understand the various theories that are associated with the development of bipolar disorders to answer this question correctly.

18. 1. **Grandiosity, which is defined as an exaggerated sense of self-importance, power, or status, is exhibited by clients diagnosed with bipolar affective disorder (BPAD). When the nurse understands the characteristics of this behavior, the nurse can better work with, and relate to, the client.**
    2. Because grandiosity is a symptom that can occur during a manic episode, it is unrealistic to think that a client diagnosed with bipolar I disorder has control over this behavior.
    3. Grandiosity exhibited by clients diagnosed with bipolar I disorder is a symptom that can occur during a manic episode and is not manipulative in nature.
    4. Grandiosity exhibited by clients diagnosed with bipolar I disorder is a symptom that can occur during a manic episode. The client's self-esteem is not tied to the symptom of grandiosity, so positive reinforcement would be ineffective.

TEST-TAKING HINT: The test taker first must note the nursing action being addressed in the question (attempting to recognize the motivation behind the client's use of grandiosity), and then look for a specific reason why the nurse implements this action (to accept and relate to the client, not the behavior).

19. 1. When a client experiences a full syndrome of mania with a history of symptoms of depression, the client meets the criteria for bipolar I, not bipolar II, disorder.
    2. When a client has experienced numerous episodes of hypomanic and dysthymic symptoms for the past 2 years, the client meets the criteria for cyclothymic disorder, not bipolar II disorder. Cyclothymic disorder is chronic in nature, and the symptoms experienced must be of insufficient severity or duration to meet the criteria for bipolar I or bipolar II disorder.
    3. When disturbances of mood can be associated directly with the physiological effects of a substance, the client is likely to be diagnosed with a substance-/medication-induced bipolar disorder, not bipolar II disorder.
    4. **Recurrent bouts of depression and episodic occurrences of hypomanic symptoms are diagnostic criteria for bipolar II disorder. Experiencing a full manic episode would indicate a diagnosis of bipolar I disorder and rule out a diagnosis of bipolar II disorder.**

TEST-TAKING HINT: The test taker must be able to distinguish among the criteria for various bipolar disorders to answer this question correctly.

Psychopharmacology

20. 1. Divalproex sodium is a mood stabilizer commonly prescribed to treat clients diagnosed with bipolar I disorder. Amitriptyline, a tricyclic antidepressant, would not address the symptoms described in the question and may precipitate a manic episode in clients diagnosed with bipolar I disorder.
    2. Both verapamil and topiramate are used as mood stabilizers in the treatment of bipolar I disorder, but neither medication would address the auditory hallucinations exhibited by the client in the question.
    3. Lithium carbonate is a mood stabilizer commonly prescribed to treat clients diagnosed with bipolar I disorder. Clonazepam, an antianxiety medication, may treat agitation and anxiety but would not address the auditory hallucinations experienced by the client.
    4. **Risperidone, an antipsychotic, directly addresses the auditory hallucinations experienced by the client. Lamotrigine,**

a mood stabilizer, would address the classic symptoms of bipolar I disorder.

TEST-TAKING HINT: The test taker first must recognize risperidone as an antipsychotic and lamotrigine as a mood stabilizer. Understanding the classification and action of these medications helps the test taker to link them to the symptoms experienced by the client.

21. 1. A client with a lithium serum level of 0.6 mEq/L would not experience any negative symptoms because this level indicates that the client's serum concentration is at the low end of normal.
    2. A client with a serum lithium level of 1.5 mEq/L may experience blurred vision, ataxia, tinnitus, persistent nausea and vomiting, and severe diarrhea. The client's symptoms described in the question do not support a serum lithium level of 1.5 mEq/L.
    3. **A client with a serum lithium level of 2.6 mEq/L may experience an excessive output of dilute urine, tremors, muscular irritability, psychomotor retardation, and mental confusion. The client's symptoms described in the question support a serum lithium level of 2.6 mEq/L.**
    4. A client with a serum lithium level of 3.5 mEq/L may experience impaired consciousness, nystagmus, seizures, coma, oliguria or anuria, arrhythmias, and myocardial infarction. The client's symptoms described in the question do not support a serum lithium level of 3.5 mEq/L.

TEST-TAKING HINT: To answer this question correctly, the test taker must be aware of the symptoms associated with various serum lithium levels.

22. Line 1 illustrates bipolar I disorder, which includes manic and depressive symptoms. The client in the question is exhibiting manic symptoms. Manic episodes are distinct periods of abnormal extreme euphoria, expansive mood, or irritable mood, lasting at least a week.

Line 2 illustrates bipolar II disorder, which is characterized by recurrent bouts of depressive symptoms with episodic occurrence of hypomanic symptoms. Hypomanic symptoms are a milder presentation of manic symptoms. The client in the question is exhibiting manic, not hypomanic symptoms.

Line 3 illustrates major depressive disorder, which is characterized by depressed mood and/or loss of interest and/or pleasure in usual activities. Client symptoms last at least 2 weeks with no history of manic behavior. The client in the question is exhibiting manic symptoms, so the diagnosis of major depressive disorder can be eliminated.

Line 4 illustrates cyclothymic disorder, which is characterized by chronic mood disturbance of at least 2 years' duration, involving numerous episodes of hypomanic and depressive symptoms of insufficient severity or duration to meet the criteria for bipolar I or bipolar II disorders.

TEST-TAKING HINT: To answer this question correctly, the test taker must be able to recognize the cyclic patterns of symptoms in the various mood disorders.

23. Lithium carbonate is a mood stabilizer that is used in clients diagnosed with bipolar affective disorder (BPAD). The margin between the therapeutic and toxic levels of lithium carbonate is very narrow. Serum lithium levels should be monitored once or twice a week after initial treatment until dosage and serum levels are stable. The maintenance level for lithium is 0.6 to 1.2 mEq/L.
    1. **Clients with a serum lithium level greater than 3.5 mEq/L may show signs such as impaired consciousness, nystagmus, seizures, coma, oliguria/anuria, arrhythmias, myocardial infarction, or cardiovascular collapse.**
    2. When the serum lithium level is 2.0 to 3.5 mEq/L, the client may exhibit signs such as excessive output of diluted urine, increased tremors, muscular irritability, psychomotor retardation, mental confusion, and giddiness.
    3. When the serum lithium level is 2.0 to 3.5 mEq/L, the client may exhibit signs such as excessive output of diluted urine, increased tremors, muscular irritability, psychomotor retardation, mental confusion, and giddiness.
    4. When the serum lithium level is 1.5 to 2.0 mEq/L, the client exhibits signs such as blurred vision, ataxia, tinnitus, persistent nausea, vomiting, and diarrhea.

TEST-TAKING HINT: The test taker must be able to pair the serum lithium level with the client's symptoms presented in the question. Lithium has a narrow therapeutic range, and levels outside this range place the client at high risk for injury.

24. Lithium carbonate is a mood stabilizer that is used in clients diagnosed with bipolar

affective disorder (BPAD). The margin between the therapeutic and toxic levels of lithium carbonate is very narrow.

1. **Lithium is similar in chemical structure to sodium, behaving in the body in much the same manner and competing with sodium at various sites in the body. If sodium intake is reduced, or the body is depleted of its normal sodium, lithium is reabsorbed by the kidneys, and this increases the potential for toxicity.**
2. When a client is prescribed lithium, it is important for the client to keep fluid intake around 2,500 to 3,000 mL/day.
3. Weight gain is a potential side effect of lithium therapy and would need to be monitored; however, risk for toxicity is a higher priority than weight gain.
4. It is important for clients to have some routine to assist them in remembering to take their medications regularly. This also helps clients maintain their sleep–wake cycle, which has been shown to be important to avoid relapse in clients diagnosed with BPAD. Although it is important to talk to the client about this, risk for toxicity is the highest priority because it is life threatening.

TEST-TAKING HINT: When a question is asking for the "priority," it is important for the test taker always to address safety concerns. In this question, the risk for toxicity related to salt intake could cause the client serious injury and possibly death. This intervention takes highest priority.

25. Many medications are used off-label for the treatment of bipolar affective disorder (BPAD). If a client is diagnosed with BPAD with psychotic features, an antipsychotic medication may be prescribed.
    1. Lithium carbonate is an antimanic medication, and carbamazepine is an anticonvulsant medication; both are used to assist with mood stabilization. Loxapine is an antipsychotic medication used for symptoms related to alterations in thought and is not approved by the Food and Drug Administration (FDA) to be used to stabilize mood.
    2. Gabapentin is an anticonvulsant medication used to assist with mood stabilization. Thiothixene is an antipsychotic medication used for symptoms related to alterations in thought and is not FDA approved to stabilize mood. Clonazepam is a benzodiazepine used for clients with anxiety. Benzodiazepines can

be used on a short-term basis to assist clients with agitation related to mania or depression; however, they are not used for long-term treatment to stabilize mood.
3. **Divalproex sodium, an anticonvulsant, is used in long-term treatment of BPAD. Asenapine and olanzapine, antipsychotic medications, have been approved by the FDA for the treatment of bipolar disorder.**
4. Lamotrigine is used as a mood stabilizer. Risperidone is an antipsychotic medication used for symptoms related to alterations in thought and is not FDA approved to stabilize mood. Benztropine is an antiparkinsonian agent and is used to assist clients with extrapyramidal symptoms from antipsychotic medications such as risperidone.

TEST-TAKING HINT: The test taker must understand that all parts of the answer must be correct for the answer to be correct. The test taker should review all medications used to stabilize mood. Many medications are used off-label to treat BPAD.

26. Lithium carbonate (lithium) is a mood stabilizer that is used in clients diagnosed with bipolar affective disorder (BPAD). The margin between the therapeutic and toxic levels of lithium carbonate is very narrow. The maintenance level for lithium is 0.6 to 1.2 mEq/L.
    1. The level necessary for managing acute mania is 1.0 to 1.5 mEq/L, and 1.9 mEq/L falls outside the therapeutic range. When the serum lithium level is 1.5 to 2.0 mEq/L, the client exhibits signs such as blurred vision, ataxia, tinnitus, persistent nausea, vomiting, and diarrhea.
    2. The nurse should hold, not continue, the next dose of lithium and discuss laboratory results with the physician prior to resuming the medication.
    3. Whether or not the client exhibits signs and symptoms of toxicity, based on the laboratory value noted in the question, the nurse would not give the next dose of lithium. If the serum level is not discussed with the physician, the client may be at risk for toxicity.
    4. **The nurse needs to notify the physician immediately of the serum lithium level, which is outside the therapeutic range, to avoid any risk for further toxicity.**

TEST-TAKING HINT: The test taker must understand the therapeutic laboratory value range for lithium. If one part of the answer is incorrect, the entire answer is incorrect. In answer 2, the

nurse's holding the medication but continuing the dose the next day would place the client at risk for injury and is an incorrect answer.

27. Lamotrigine is an anticonvulsant medication used as a mood stabilizer. This medication needs to be titrated slowly, or Stevens-Johnson syndrome, a potentially deadly rash, can result. Nurses need to be aware of this side effect and teach clients to follow dosing directions accurately.
    1. **When lamotrigine is titrated incorrectly, the risk for Stevens-Johnson syndrome increases. Clients need to be taught the importance of taking the medication as prescribed and accurately reporting adherence.**
    2. Lamotrigine does not require ongoing laboratory monitoring.
    3. Fever is a potential sign of neuroleptic malignant syndrome, a side effect of antipsychotic medications, not lamotrigine.
    4. Muscle rigidity of the face and neck is a potential side effect of all antipsychotic medications, not mood stabilizers such as lamotrigine.

TEST-TAKING HINT: To answer this question correctly, the test taker must understand the importance of titrating lamotrigine to avoid Stevens-Johnson syndrome.

28. Divalproex sodium is classified as an anticonvulsant and is used as a mood stabilizer in the treatment of clients diagnosed with bipolar affective disorder (BPAD). Side effects of this medication include prolonged bleeding times and liver toxicity.
    1. **Platelet counts need to be monitored before and during therapy with divalproex sodium because of the potential side effect of blood dyscrasias.**
    2. **Aspartate aminotransferase (AST) is a liver enzyme test that needs to be monitored before and during therapy with divalproex sodium because of the potential side effect of liver toxicity.**
    3. Fasting blood sugar measurements are not affected and are not indicated during treatment with divalproex sodium.
    4. **Alanine aminotransferase (ALT) is a liver enzyme test that needs to be monitored before and during therapy with divalproex sodium because of the potential side effect of liver toxicity.**
    5. **Divalproex sodium levels need to be monitored to determine therapeutic levels and assess potential toxicity.**

TEST-TAKING HINT: To answer this question correctly, the test taker first must understand that AST and ALT are liver function studies. Then the test taker must recognize that side effects of divalproex sodium therapy may include blood dyscrasias, liver toxicity, and the potential for divalproex sodium toxicity.

29. Carbamazepine is classified as an anticonvulsant and is used as a mood stabilizer in the treatment of clients diagnosed with bipolar affective disorder (BPAD). Nausea, vomiting, and anorexia all are acceptable side effects of carbamazepine.
    1. Because nausea, vomiting, and anorexia all are acceptable side effects, the nurse would not need to stop the medication and notify the physician.
    2. Because nausea, vomiting, and anorexia all are acceptable side effects, the nurse would not need to hold the next dose until symptoms subside.
    3. **When clients prescribed carbamazepine experience nausea, vomiting, and anorexia, it is important for the nurse to administer the medication with food to decrease these uncomfortable, but acceptable, side effects. If these side effects do not abate, other interventions may be necessary.**
    4. Although a carbamazepine level may need to be obtained, it is unnecessary for the nurse to request a stat carbamazepine level because these symptoms are acceptable.

TEST-TAKING HINT: To answer this question correctly, the test taker must recognize that nausea, vomiting, and anorexia are uncomfortable, but acceptable, side effects of carbamazepine therapy.

30. The nurse would administer **15 mL**.

$$\frac{900 \text{ mg}}{x \text{ mL}} = \frac{300 \text{ mg}}{5 \text{ mL}} = 15 \text{ mL}$$

TEST-TAKING HINT: The test taker must note that this question is asking for a single dosage that would be administered at 0800, not the total daily dosage. Set up the ratio and proportion problem based on the number of milligrams contained in 5 mL. The test taker can then solve this problem by cross multiplication and solving for x by division.

31. Asenapine is an atypical antipsychotic medication FDA approved for treatment of schizophrenia and bipolar disorder.
    1. Asenapine is administered sublingually and is absorbed through the mucous membrane, not in the stomach.

2. The client would take asenapine for mood stability or psychosis, not depression.

3. The client prescribed asenapine would need to monitor for tardive dyskinesia, extrapyramidal symptoms, and neuroleptic malignant syndrome, not serotonin syndrome. Antidepressant, not antipsychotic, medications may cause serotonin syndrome.

4. **The client prescribed asenapine would need to place the medication under the tongue to be absorbed through the mucous membrane. The nurse must teach the client to avoid eating or drinking for 10 minutes following administration.**

TEST-TAKING HINT: To answer this question correctly, the test taker must recognize asenapine as an antipsychotic medication and that it is administered sublingually.

32. The serum lithium carbonate level of 3.7 mEq/L should alert the nurse to assess for symptoms of lithium carbonate toxicity, which could be life threatening.

1. Interviewing the family related to the client's substance abuse history would provide important information related to this client's care, but this nursing intervention would not address the life-threatening problem of lithium carbonate toxicity and therefore is not the priority nursing action.

2. If anxiety was this client's presenting problem, administering lorazepam 1 mg would be an appropriate nursing intervention and there would be no need to notify the health-care personnel (HCP). However, this nursing intervention does not address the life-threatening problem of lithium carbonate toxicity and therefore is not the priority nursing action.

3. Staying with the client and offering support is always an appropriate nursing intervention. However, this nursing intervention does not address the life-threatening problem of lithium carbonate toxicity and therefore is not the priority nursing action.

4. **A serum lithium carbonate level of 3.7 mEq/L and the client symptoms as presented should alert the nurse to a possible life-threatening lithium carbonate toxicity. Administering another dose of lithium carbonate would exacerbate the client's critical condition. Holding lithium carbonate and notifying HCP is the priority nursing action.**

TEST-TAKING HINT: To answer this question correctly, the test taker must recognize that the maintenance level for lithium carbonate is 0.6 to 1.2 mEq/L. The margin between the therapeutic and toxic levels of lithium carbonate is very narrow. A lithium carbonate level of 3.7 mEq/L far exceeds the normal range and can result in a life-threatening situation.

Substance-Related and Addictive Disorders

KEYWORDS

The following words include English vocabulary, nursing/medical terminology, concepts, principles, or information relevant to content specifically addressed in this chapter or associated with topics presented in it. English dictionaries, your nursing textbooks, and medical dictionaries such as *Taber's Cyclopedic Medical Dictionary* are resources that can be used to expand your knowledge and understanding of these words and related information.

Acamprosate calcium

Al-Anon

Alcohol

Alcohol psychosis

Alcohol use disorder

Alcohol withdrawal

Alcoholic cardiomyopathy

Alcoholic myopathy

Alcoholics Anonymous (AA)

Amphetamines

Ascites

Bad trip

Barbiturates

Benzodiazepines

Binge

Blackouts

Blood alcohol level (BAL)

Buprenorphine-naloxone

Caffeine

CAGE questionnaire

Central nervous system (CNS) depressant

Central nervous system (CNS) stimulant

Chronic phase

Cirrhosis

Clinical Institute Withdrawal Assessment (CIWA)

Cocaine abuser

Cocaine intoxication

Codependency

Complicated withdrawal

Confabulation

Crack

Creatine phosphokinase (CPK)

Crucial phase

Denial

Detoxification (detox)

Disulfiram

Early alcoholic phase

Esophageal varices

Flunitrazepam

Gamma-glutamyl transferase

Gastroesophageal reflux disorder

Hereditary factor

Heroin abuse

Impairment

Intoxicated

Korsakoff's psychosis

Legal intoxication

Legal limit

Lorazepam

Lysergic acid diethylamide (LSD)

Methadone

Methamphetamines

Minimization

Naltrexone

Nicotine

Pancreatitis

Peripheral neuropathy

Phases of drinking progression

Phencyclidine (PCP)

Physical withdrawal

Physiological dependence

Prealcoholic phase

Projection

Rationalization

Snow

Sobriety

Sponsors

Standard of legal intoxication
Stimulant
Substance intoxication
Substance use disorder
Substance-impaired nurse
Thiamine deficiency

Tolerance
Toxicology screen
Tremors
Wernicke-Korsakoff syndrome
Wernicke's encephalopathy
Withdrawal

QUESTIONS

Theory

1. A nursing student is preparing a thesis on alcohol use disorder. Which facts should be included?
   1. The prevalence of alcohol use disorder varies within cultural groups.
   2. More females than males are diagnosed with alcohol use disorder.
   3. Drinking rates are highest among young adults and accelerate with increasing age.
   4. Nicotine dependence decreases with increasing levels of alcohol consumption.

2. The nurse is working with a 45-year-old client diagnosed with alcohol use disorder who has been drinking since age 20. Related to this client's stage of psychosocial development, what developmental data would the nurse expect to assess?
   1. The client may have trouble establishing intimate relationships.
   2. The client may have trouble trusting others.
   3. The client may review life, have serious regrets, and experience despair.
   4. The client may feel a sense of inferiority or inadequacy.

3. Using the principles of biological theory, what contributing factor puts a client at risk for the diagnosis of alcohol use disorder?
   1. The client is a child of a parent diagnosed with alcohol use disorder.
   2. The client is fixated in the oral stage of psychosocial development.
   3. The client is highly self-critical and has unconscious anxiety.
   4. The client is unable to relax or defer gratification.

4. Which of the following sociocultural factors increase a client's risk for the diagnosis of alcohol use disorder? **Select all that apply.**
   1. The client's twin sister has been diagnosed with alcohol use disorder.
   2. The client was raised in a home where alcohol use was the norm.
   3. The client is from a family that culturally accepts the use of alcohol.
   4. The client experiences pleasure when using alcohol and subsequently repeats the use.
   5. The client is influenced by morphine-like substances produced during alcohol use.

5. Which of the following nursing statements describe the personality factors that are implicated in the predisposition to a diagnosis of substance use disorder? **Select all that apply.**
   1. "Hereditary factors can predispose a client to the diagnosis of substance use disorders."
   2. "Alcohol produces morphine-like substances in the brain that are responsible for a predisposition to alcohol use disorder."
   3. "A punitive superego can predispose a client to substance use disorders."
   4. "A tendency toward addictive behaviors increases as low self-esteem, passivity, and an inability to relax or defer gratification increases."
   5. "Fixation at the oral stage of psychosexual development can predispose a client to the diagnosis of substance use disorders."

Defense Mechanisms

6. A client diagnosed with a substance use disorder states to the nurse, "My wife causes me to abuse methamphetamines. She uses and expects me to." This client is using which defense mechanism?
   1. Rationalization.
   2. Denial.
   3. Minimization.
   4. Projection.

7. A client admitted for chest pain related to cocaine use disorder states, "This is nothing but a little indigestion. What is all the fuss about?" This client is using which defense mechanism?
   1. Minimization.
   2. Denial.
   3. Rationalization.
   4. Projection.

8. A client who has recently relapsed from alcohol abstinence is seen in the outpatient mental health clinic. The client states, "I don't know what all the fuss is about. Can't I have a few drinks now and then?" Which nursing diagnosis applies to this client?
   1. Risk for injury.
   2. Risk for violence: self-directed.
   3. Ineffective denial.
   4. Powerlessness.

Nursing Process—Assessment

9. Which of the following assessment data should the nurse gather when confirming a diagnosis of alcohol use disorder? **Select all that apply.**
   1. Continued alcohol use despite recurrent interpersonal problems.
   2. Recurrent, alcohol-related legal problems.
   3. Recurrent alcohol use resulting in failure to fulfill major role obligations.
   4. A need for markedly decreased amounts of alcohol to achieve a desired effect.
   5. A disruption in physical and psychological functioning.

10. An intoxicated client is brought to the emergency department (ED) after spraining an ankle. The client states, "How did I get here? Who brought me to the hospital?" Which is the client most likely experiencing?
    1. A blackout.
    2. Denial.
    3. Minimization.
    4. Alcohol psychosis.

11. What situation places an individual at highest risk for mood and behavioral changes related to alcohol consumption?
    1. At a bar, a 180-lb college student drinks four beers in a 1-hour period.
    2. At a restaurant, a 160-lb woman drinks a glass of wine with a spaghetti dinner.
    3. At a football game, a 250-lb man drinks three beers with hot dogs.
    4. A 110-lb woman drinks a margarita with a Mexican combo platter.

12. Which of the following are parts of the CAGE questionnaire screening tool? **Select all that apply.**
    1. Have you ever felt you should cut down on your drinking?
    2. Have people annoyed you by criticizing your drinking?
    3. Have you ever felt guilty about your drinking?
    4. Have you ever had a drink in the morning to steady your nerves?
    5. Have you ever felt isolated, like you were in a cage?

13. A client with a long history of alcohol use disorder recently has been diagnosed with Wernicke-Korsakoff syndrome. Which of the following symptoms should the nurse expect to assess? **Select all that apply.**
    1. A sudden onset of muscle pain with elevations of creatine phosphokinase (CPK).
    2. Signs and symptoms of congestive heart failure.
    3. Loss of short-term and long-term memory and the use of confabulation.
    4. Inflammation of the stomach and gastroesophageal reflux disorder.
    5. Laboratory values that document severe thiamine deficiency.

14. A client with a history of alcohol use disorder complains of extreme muscle pain, swelling and weakness of extremities, and reddish-tinged urine. What laboratory value related to these symptoms would the nurse expect to assess?
    1. An elevated gamma-glutamyl transferase (GGT).
    2. An elevated enzyme-linked immunosorbent assay (ELISA).
    3. An elevated white blood cell count (WBC).
    4. An elevated creatine phosphokinase (CPK).

15. A client on an inpatient psychiatric unit is overheard stating, "I blew some snow yesterday while I was out on a pass with my family." What would the nurse expect to assess as a positive finding in this client's urine drug screen?
    1. Amphetamines.
    2. Cocaine.
    3. Barbiturates.
    4. Benzodiazepines.

16. The following clients are waiting to be seen in the ED. Which client should the nurse assess first?
    1. A client diagnosed with cocaine use disorder experiencing chest pain.
    2. An intoxicated client with a long history of alcohol use disorder.
    3. A client who recently experienced a "bad trip" from lysergic acid diethylamide (LSD).
    4. A woman who thinks she has been given flunitrazepam.

17. A client diagnosed with alcohol use disorder states that their spouse complains about their drinking but stocks the bar with gin. The nurse suspects codependency. Which of the following characteristics would the nurse expect the spouse to exhibit? **Select all that apply.**
    1. The spouse has a long history of egocentric tendencies.
    2. The spouse is a "people pleaser" and would do almost anything to gain approval.
    3. The spouse does not feel responsible for making the client happy.
    4. The spouse has an accurate understanding regarding their own identity.
    5. The spouse experiences a profound sense of powerlessness.

18. Which of the following are effective ways to identify a substance-impaired nurse? **Select all that apply.**
    1. A nurse who frequently administers medications to other nurses' clients.
    2. High absenteeism if the substance source is outside of the work area.
    3. Denial of substance abuse problems.
    4. A high incidence of incorrect narcotic counts.
    5. Poor concentration and difficulty in meeting deadlines.

19. When alcohol is consumed, what percentage is absorbed immediately into the bloodstream through which body organ?
    1. 20% is absorbed through the stomach wall.
    2. 30% is absorbed through the small intestine.
    3. 40% is absorbed through the large intestine.
    4. 50% is absorbed through the liver.

20. Which of the following statements are true regarding how the body processes alcohol? **Select all that apply.**
    1. Alcohol is absorbed slowly after processing through the liver.
    2. Similar to other foods, alcohol must be digested.
    3. Rapidity of absorption is influenced by various factors, such as a full stomach.
    4. Only moments after consumption, alcohol is excreted.
    5. The body burns alcohol at the rate of about 0.5 ounce per hour.

21. Which of the following behaviors are likely to be assessed in the prealcoholic phase of drinking progression? **Select all that apply.**
    1. Alcohol is used to relieve stressful situations.
    2. Alcohol is no longer a source of pleasure, but rather a drug that is required by the individual. Blackouts are experienced.
    3. Control is lost, and physiological dependence is evident.
    4. The individual is usually intoxicated more than sober, and emotional and physical disintegration occur.
    5. Tolerance to alcohol begins to develop.

22. The nurse is caring for a client on an inpatient substance use disorder unit. Because of the client's alcohol abuse, the client has lost family, job, and driver's license. What phase of drinking pattern progression is this client experiencing?
    1. Prealcoholic phase.
    2. Early alcoholic phase.
    3. Crucial phase.
    4. Chronic phase.

23. A nursing student is reviewing a client's chart. It is noted that the client is exhibiting signs of a drinking pattern in the early alcoholic phase. Which of the following behaviors would the student expect to note? **Select all that apply.**
    1. Use of alcohol as a stress reliever.
    2. Amnesia that occurs during or immediately after a period of drinking.
    3. Total loss of control over drinking behaviors.
    4. Continuous intoxication with few periods of sobriety.
    5. Secret drinking and preoccupation with drinking and maintaining alcohol supply.

24. Three days after surgery to correct a perforated bowel, a client begins to display signs and symptoms of tremors, increased blood pressure, and diaphoresis. What should the nurse suspect?
    1. Concealed hemorrhage.
    2. Alcohol or other central nervous system (CNS) depressants–induced withdrawal.
    3. Malignant hyperpyrexia.
    4. Neuroleptic malignant syndrome.

25. A newly admitted client with a long history of alcohol use disorder complains of burning and tingling sensations of the feet. The nurse would recognize these symptoms as indicative of which condition?
    1. Peripheral neuropathy.
    2. Alcoholic myopathy.
    3. Wernicke's encephalopathy.
    4. Korsakoff's psychosis.

26. A client with a long history of alcohol use disorder presents in the ED with a sudden onset of muscle pain, swelling, and weakness as well as reddish-tinged urine. What laboratory value would the nurse evaluate as evidence of this client's disorder?
    1. Increase in creatine phosphokinase (CPK).
    2. Increase in low-density lipoproteins (LDL).
    3. Decrease in fasting blood sugar (FBS).
    4. Decrease in aspartate aminotransferase (AST).

27. A client has been diagnosed with Wernicke-Korsakoff syndrome. Which describes this client's use of confabulation?
    1. The client has difficulty keeping thoughts focused and on topic.
    2. The client clearly discussed a field trip, when in reality no field trip occurred.
    3. The client jumps from one topic to another.
    4. The client lies about anxiety level rating to receive more anxiolytics.

28. A client with a long history of alcohol use disorder comes to the ED with frank hemoptysis. Which life-threatening complication of this disorder is the client experiencing, and what is the probable cause?
    1. Hepatic encephalopathy resulting from the inability of the liver to convert ammonia to urea for excretion.
    2. Thrombocytopenia resulting from the inability of the diseased liver to produce adequate amounts of prothrombin and fibrinogen.
    3. Hemorrhage of esophageal varices resulting from portal hypertension.
    4. Ascites resulting from impaired protein metabolism.

29. A client with a history of alcohol use disorder is seen in the ED 2 days after a binge of excessive alcohol consumption. The nurse suspects pancreatitis. Which symptoms would support the nurse's suspicion?
    1. Confusion, loss of recent memory, and confabulation.
    2. Elevated creatine phosphokinase (CPK) with congestive heart failure symptoms.
    3. Paralysis of the ocular muscles, diplopia, and ataxia.
    4. Constant, severe epigastric pain; nausea and vomiting; and abdominal distention.

30. What substance stimulates the CNS?
    1. Vodka.
    2. Crack.
    3. Lorazepam.
    4. Triazolam.

31. The nurse is educating a client about how to avoid sources of stimulation. What substance produces the least significant stimulation to the CNS?
    1. Brewed coffee.
    2. Excedrin Migraine.
    3. Tequila shooter.
    4. Filtered cigarettes.

32. All states had to conform to the _____ g/dL blood alcohol level (BAL) standard of legal intoxication by 2004 or risk loss of federal highway funding.

33. A client is admitted to the ED and is tested for BAL. The client has a BAL of 0.10 g/dL. What is an accurate interpretation of this laboratory value?
    1. The client is within the legal limits of BAL.
    2. The client is assessed as legally intoxicated.
    3. The client would be considered intoxicated depending on state laws.
    4. The client must perform other psychomotor tests to determine intoxication.

Nursing Process—Diagnosis

34. Which is the priority diagnosis for a client experiencing alcohol-induced withdrawal?
    1. Ineffective health maintenance.
    2. Ineffective coping.
    3. Risk for injury.
    4. Dysfunctional family processes: alcohol use disorder.

35. A client with a long history of alcohol use disorder has been recently diagnosed with alcoholic cardiomyopathy. Which correctly written nursing diagnosis would take priority?
    1. Altered perfusion R/T misuse of alcohol AEB decreased oxygen saturations.
    2. Altered coping R/T powerlessness AEB chronic alcohol abuse.
    3. Risk for injury R/T congestive heart failure.
    4. Activity intolerance R/T decreased perfusion.

36. Which is the priority diagnosis for a client experiencing cocaine-induced withdrawal?
    1. Powerlessness.
    2. Risk for injury.
    3. Ineffective health maintenance.
    4. Ineffective coping.

37. Which is the priority nursing diagnosis for a client experiencing alcohol-induced intoxication?
    1. Pain.
    2. Ineffective denial.
    3. Ineffective coping.
    4. Risk for aspiration.

Nursing Process—Planning

38. Which is true about the outcomes of nursing interventions for clients experiencing a substance use disorder?
    1. Outcomes are based on the *Diagnostic and Statistical Manual of Mental Disorders, Fifth Edition*.
    2. Outcomes are set by the North American Nursing Diagnosis Association (NANDA).
    3. Outcomes should be tailored to the individual's immediate needs and abilities.
    4. Outcomes should return the client to the highest level of wellness.

39. A client who is exhibiting symptoms of alcohol-induced withdrawal is admitted to the substance abuse unit for detoxification (detox). One of the nursing diagnoses for this client is ineffective health maintenance. Which is a correctly written long-term outcome for this nursing diagnosis?
    1. The client will agree to attend nutritional counseling sessions.
    2. The client will exhibit reduced medical complications related to alcohol use disorder within 6 months.
    3. The client will identify at least three effects of alcohol on the body by day 2 of hospitalization.
    4. The client will remain free from injury while withdrawing from alcohol.

40. When the nurse is planning relapse prevention strategies for clients diagnosed with substance use disorders, which should be the initial nursing approach?
    1. Address previously successful coping skills.
    2. Encourage rehearsing stressful situations that may lead to relapse.
    3. Present information simply, using easily understood terminology.
    4. Provide numerous choices of community resources.

Nursing Process—Implementation

41. A student nurse is assessing a newly admitted client who suffered a concussion after a driving under the influence (DUI) citation involving crack cocaine. The nursing instructor should recommend which strategy to obtain the most accurate data?
    1. "It is important to teach the effects of cocaine on the body."
    2. "After obtaining client permission, validate this information with family members."
    3. "Accurately record the client's statement related to the quantity of cocaine use."
    4. "Instruct the client regarding what will happen during the detox process."

42. Which nursing intervention is appropriate for a client who has a nursing diagnosis of risk for injury R/T alcohol-induced withdrawal?
    1. Monitor fluid intake and output.
    2. Provide the client with a quiet room free from environmental stimuli.
    3. Teach the client about the effects of alcohol on the body.
    4. Empathize with the client but confront denial.

43. Ineffective denial is the nursing diagnosis that is appropriate at this time for a client diagnosed with alcohol use disorder who has relapsed. What is the priority nursing intervention to address this problem?
    1. Help the client to analyze the effects of substance abuse on life situations.
    2. Set up an appointment for follow-up and provide community resources.
    3. Provide a stimulus-free environment.
    4. Monitor vital signs.

44. A client is admitted for benzodiazepine use disorder detox. This is the client's fourth detox, and the client's third detox was considered complicated. What would determine the nurse's priority intervention at this time?
    1. The nurse must use confrontation because the client will use defense mechanisms such as denial, projection, and displacement to protect ego strength.
    2. The nurse must provide empathetic support because the client will have little family support as a result of behaviors influenced by substance use disorder.
    3. The nurse must present the consequences of the client's actions because the client will have little motivation for change.
    4. The nurse should monitor the client closely and initiate seizure precautions because the client will be at high risk for seizures.

45. Which intervention takes priority when dealing with a client experiencing Wernicke-Korsakoff syndrome?
    1. Monitor parenteral vitamin B_1.
    2. Increase fluid intake.
    3. Provide prenatal vitamins.
    4. Encourage foods high in vitamin C.

46. A client diagnosed with alcohol use disorder is admitted to a substance disorder unit complaining of decreased exercise tolerance, lower extremity edema, arrhythmias, and dyspnea. Which nursing intervention would be appropriate for this client?
    1. Provide thiamine-rich foods.
    2. Administer ordered digoxin and furosemide.
    3. Reorient the client to person, place, and time.
    4. Encourage high-sodium foods.

47. A client on the substance use disorder unit states, "I used to be able to get a 'buzz on' with a few beers. Now it takes a six-pack." How should the nurse, in the role of teacher, address this remark?
    1. By assessing the client's readiness for learning and reviewing the criteria for alcohol-induced withdrawal.
    2. By explaining the effects of tolerance and telling the client that this is a sign of alcohol use disorder.
    3. By presenting the concept of minimization and how this affects a realistic view of the problems precipitated by alcohol use disorder.
    4. By confronting the client with the client's use of the defense mechanism of rationalization.

Nursing Process—Evaluation

48. The nurse has given a client information on alcohol use disorder recovery. Which client statement indicates that learning has occurred?
    1. "Once I have detoxed, my recovery is complete."
    2. "I understand that the goal of recovery is to decrease my drinking."
    3. "I realize that recovery is a lifelong process that comes about in steps."
    4. "Al-Anon can assist me in my recovery process."

49. Which of the following are considered therapeutic elements of 12-step programs such as Alcoholics Anonymous (AA)? **Select all that apply.**
    1. 12-step programs break down denial in an atmosphere of support.
    2. 12-step programs give clients a sense of community.
    3. 12-step programs help clients recognize the power they have over their addiction.
    4. 12-step programs provide clients with experts in the field of addiction.
    5. 12-step programs provide sponsors who acclimate clients back into social settings.

Psychopharmacology

50. What classification of drugs share a similar profile of symptoms with alcohol-induced intoxication and alcohol-induced withdrawal?
    1. Anxiolytics.
    2. Amphetamines.
    3. Cocaine.
    4. Phencyclidine (PCP).

51. A client with a long history of alcohol use disorder is showing signs of cognitive deficits. What drug would the nurse recognize as appropriate in assisting with this client's alcohol recovery?
    1. Disulfiram.
    2. Naltrexone.
    3. Lorazepam.
    4. Methadone.

52. Which drug would a nurse recognize as appropriate in assisting a client with recovery from long-standing heroin use disorder?
    1. Acamprosate calcium.
    2. Buprenorphine/naloxone.
    3. Disulfiram.
    4. Haloperidol.

53. A client receives lorazepam because of a high Clinical Institute Withdrawal Assessment (CIWA) score. What is the rationale for this pharmacological intervention?
    1. Lorazepam is a medication that decreases cravings in clients who are experiencing alcohol-induced withdrawal.
    2. Lorazepam is a deterrent therapy that helps to motivate clients to maintain alcohol abstinence.
    3. Lorazepam is a substitution therapy to decrease the intensity of withdrawal symptoms.
    4. Lorazepam is a CNS stimulant that decreases the CIWA score.

54. The nurse is planning a teaching session for a client who has recently been prescribed disulfiram as deterrent therapy for alcohol use disorder. What statement indicates that the client has accurate knowledge of this subject matter?
    1. "Over-the-counter cough and cold medication should not affect me while I am taking the disulfiram."
    2. "I'll have to stop using my alcohol-based aftershave while I am taking the disulfiram."
    3. "Disulfiram should decrease my cravings for alcohol and make my recovery process easier."
    4. "Disulfiram is used as a substitute for alcohol to help me avoid alcohol withdrawal symptoms."

55. A fasting blood glucose level value is to a *sliding scale insulin dosage* as a CIWA score is to:
1. An olanzapine dosage.
2. A lithium carbonate dosage.
3. A fluoxetine dosage.
4. A lorazepam dosage.

56. A client in treatment for alcohol use disorder enters the ED complaining of head and neck pain, dizziness, sweating, and confusion. BP 100/60 mm Hg, pulse 130, and respirations 26. Which question should the nurse ask to assess this situation further?
1. "Are you currently on any medications for the treatment of alcohol use disorder?"
2. "How long have you been abstinent from using alcohol?"
3. "Are you currently using any illegal street drugs?"
4. "Have you had any diarrhea or vomiting?"

57. A client currently hospitalized for the third alcohol detox in 1 year believes relapses are partially due to an inability to control cravings. Which prescribed medication would meet this client's need?
1. Buspirone.
2. Disulfiram.
3. Naltrexone.
4. Lorazepam.

58. A client experiencing alcohol-induced withdrawal is prescribed lorazepam 0.5 mg qid. The physician has ordered a CIWA to be completed every 4 hours. Additional prn lorazepam is based on the following scale:
CIWA score of 7 to 12: administer 0.5 mg of lorazepam. CIWA score of >12: administer 1 mg of lorazepam. The client's CIWA score at 0400 was 6, at 0800 was 14, at 1200 was 8, at 1600 was 10, at 2000 was 14, and at 2400 was 6. How many milligrams of lorazepam did the client receive in 1 day? _____ mg.

59. A nurse on an inpatient psychiatric unit assesses a client after visitation hours. The nurse documents the assessment data and reviews the client's medical record.

Assessment Information	Medications	Lab Results
Pupils contracted, small	Ativan 0.5 mg prn	UDS + opiates, alcohol
Confused, slurred speech	Naloxone 2 mg IM prn	
Pale, clammy	Tylenol 500 mg prn	
Sleepy, difficult to awake		
Disoriented		
BP: 80/50		
Resp: 12		
CIWA = 5		
Pulse: 46 beats/min, irregular		

Which nursing intervention is **most important?**
1. Contact the family to inquire about past and current drug use.
2. Administer lorazepam to assist the client with alcohol-induced withdrawal.
3. Recheck vitals and stay with the client to build rapport and trust.
4. Administer naloxone 2 mg IM due to apparent overdose of opiates.

The correct answer number and rationale for why it is the correct answer are given in **boldface blue type**. Rationales for why the other answer options are incorrect are given as well, but they are not in boldface type.

Theory

1. 1. **Evidence-based statistics indicate that the incidence of alcohol use disorder is higher among northern Europeans than among southern Europeans, high in Native Americans, and low in the Asian population.**
   2. Evidence-based statistics indicate that the prevalence of alcohol use disorder is higher for men than women.
   3. Evidence-based statistics indicate that drinking rates are highest among young adults and decline with increasing age.
   4. Evidence-based statistics indicate that nicotine dependence increases with increasing levels of alcohol dependence.

   TEST-TAKING HINT: The question requires that the test taker know that there are cultural differences in the prevalence of the diagnosis of alcohol use disorder. Research supports that these differences can be linked to a genetic predisposition. This evidence-based knowledge should motivate the nurse to explore a client's family history further.

2. 1. **Clients experiencing chronic alcohol use disorders often arrest in developmental progression at the age when the use began. In this situation, the client began abusing alcohol at age 20. According to Erikson's psychosocial theory, the client's developmental conflict at this age would have been intimacy versus isolation. The major developmental task at this age is to form an intense, lasting relationship or a commitment to another person, cause, institution, or creative effort. Because of developmental arrest, this client may have trouble establishing intimate relationships.**
   2. According to Erikson's psychosocial theory, trust is established in the infancy (birth to 1 year) stage of development. If this client's psychosocial development was arrested at age 20, the establishment of trust would not be affected directly by alcohol use disorder.
   3. According to Erikson's psychosocial theory, despair is the negative outcome of the old-age (65 years to death) stage of development. If this client's psychosocial development were arrested at age 20, despair would not as yet have been established because the client had not reached this age.
   4. According to Erikson's psychosocial theory, feeling a sense of inferiority or inadequacy is the negative outcome of the school-age (6 to 12 years) stage of development. If this client's psychosocial development was arrested at age 20, the establishment of identity would not be affected directly by the alcohol use disorder.

   TEST-TAKING HINT: To answer this question correctly, the test taker must understand and differentiate the developmental tasks at various stages of psychosocial development. Understanding that psychosocial development arrests because of substance use disorders allows the test taker to choose the correct stage based on the age at which the substance use disorder began.

3. Numerous factors have been implicated in the predisposition to substance use disorder. Currently, there is not a single theory that can adequately explain the etiology of this problem.
   1. **A hereditary factor is involved in the development of substance use disorders, especially when the substance is alcohol. Children of parents diagnosed with alcohol use disorder are three times more likely than other children to be diagnosed with this disorder. Genetic theory falls under the category of biological theory.**
   2. The psychodynamic, not biological, theory of etiology of substance use disorders focuses on a punitive superego and fixation at the oral stage of psychosexual development.
   3. Individuals with punitive superegos turn to alcohol to diminish unconscious anxiety. This is characteristic of psychoanalytic, not biological, theory.
   4. Theories have associated addictive behaviors with certain personality traits. Clients who have an inability to relax or to defer gratification are more likely to abuse substances. This is from a developmental, not biological, theory perspective.

   TEST-TAKING HINT: The question requires the test taker to distinguish among various

theories of etiology of substance use disorders. Understanding the principles of biological theory assists the test taker in choosing the correct answer.

4. 1. Monozygotic (identical) twins have a higher rate for concordance of alcohol use disorder than dizygotic (nonidentical) twins. This is an indication of the role hereditary factors play in the development of alcohol use disorder. This is a biological, not a sociocultural, factor that influences the risk for the development of this disorder.
   2. Adolescents are more likely to use substances if they have parents who provide a model for substance use. This modeling is a sociocultural factor that influences the risk for the development of alcohol use disorder.
   3. Factors within an individual's culture help to establish patterns of substance use by molding attitudes and influencing patterns of consumption based on cultural acceptance. Cultural and ethnic influences are sociocultural factors that influence the risk for the development of alcohol use disorder.
   4. Many substances create a pleasurable experience that encourages the user to repeat use. *Conditioning* describes how the intrinsically reinforcing properties of addictive drugs condition the individual to seek out and repeat the use of these drugs. Conditioning is a sociocultural factor that influences the risk for the development of alcohol use disorder.
   5. Alcohol use produces morphine-like substances in the brain that are linked to alcohol use disorder. This is an indication of a biochemical, not sociocultural, factor that influences the development of alcohol use disorder.

TEST-TAKING HINT: The question requires the test taker to distinguish among various factors that influence the risk for the development of alcohol use disorder.

5. Substance use disorder has also been associated with antisocial personality and depressive response personality styles.
   1. This statement is related to genetic, not personality, factors that predispose individuals to the diagnosis of substance use disorder.
   2. This statement is related to biochemical, not personality, factors that predispose individuals to the diagnosis of substance use disorder.
   3. This statement is related to developmental, not personality, factors that predispose

individuals to the diagnosis of substance use disorder.
   4. This true statement is related to the personality factors that predispose individuals to the diagnosis of substance use disorder.
   5. This true statement is related to the personality factors that predispose individuals to the diagnosis of substance use disorder.

TEST-TAKING HINT: To help differentiate among the various factors that predispose individuals to substance use disorder, the test taker should try noting the category of factors next to the answer choices.

Defense Mechanisms

6. 1. Rationalization is an attempt to make excuses or formulate logical reasons to justify unacceptable feelings or behaviors. This defense is often used by clients diagnosed with substance use disorder; however, the situation described is not reflective of this defense mechanism.
   2. Denial is used when a client refuses to acknowledge the existence of a real situation or the feelings associated with it. This defense is often used by clients diagnosed with substance use disorder; however, the situation described is not reflective of this defense mechanism.
   3. Clients diagnosed with substance use disorder often minimize problems caused by their addiction; however, the situation described is not reflective of this defense mechanism.
   4. When a client attributes feelings or impulses unacceptable to the client to another person, the client is using the defense mechanism of projection. In the question, the client is projecting the responsibility for decisions about his use of methamphetamines to his wife.

TEST-TAKING HINT: Rationalization and projection are often confused. The test taker should look for an element of blame or transference of the client's feelings or thoughts to another when a client uses projection. The test taker should look for "excuse making" when rationalization is used.

7. 1. Clients diagnosed with substance use disorder often minimize problems caused by their addiction. The client in the question is not admitting that a cardiac problem exists. The client does not just minimize the problem but denies the problem by interpreting it as indigestion.

2. Denial is used when a client refuses to acknowledge the existence of a real situation or the feelings associated with it. When this client states that chest pain is a "little indigestion," the client is using denial to avoid facing a serious complication of cocaine abuse.

3. Rationalization is an attempt to make excuses or formulate logical reasons to justify unacceptable feelings or behaviors. This defense is often used by clients diagnosed with substance use disorder, but the situation presented is not reflective of this defense mechanism.

4. When a client attributes feelings or impulses unacceptable to the client to another person, the client is using the defense mechanism of projection. This defense is often used by clients diagnosed with substance use disorder, but the situation described is not reflective of this defense mechanism.

TEST-TAKING HINT: Minimization and denial are used by clients diagnosed with substance use disorder to avoid looking at problems caused by addiction. To answer this question correctly, the test taker must distinguish the difference. When using denial, the client refuses to recognize the problem. Using minimization, the client recognizes the problem but discounts its effect.

8. 1. A client is at risk for injury as a result of internal or external environmental conditions interacting with the individual's adaptive and defensive resources. Nothing is presented in the question to indicate that this client is at risk for injury. If the client were exhibiting signs and symptoms of alcohol-induced withdrawal, the diagnosis of risk for injury would apply.

2. Risk for violence: self-directed is identified when a client is at risk for behaviors in which an individual demonstrates that they can be physically, emotionally, or sexually harmful to self. Nothing is presented in the question to indicate that this client is at risk for self-directed violence.

3. **Ineffective denial is defined as the conscious or unconscious attempt to disavow knowledge or meaning of an event to reduce anxiety or fear, leading to the detriment of health. The client in the question is denying the need to continue abstinence from alcohol.**

4. Powerlessness is defined as the perception that one's own action would not significantly affect an outcome—a perceived lack of control over a current situation or immediate happening. Nothing is

presented in the question to indicate that this client is experiencing powerlessness.

TEST-TAKING HINT: The test taker must understand the behaviors that indicate the use of the defense mechanism of denial to answer this question correctly. The test taker must use only the information presented in the question to determine the nursing diagnosis for the client. Other nursing diagnoses may apply to clients with specific medical conditions, but the answer must be based on the symptoms presented in the question.

Nursing Process—Assessment

9. Alcohol use disorder is described as a maladaptive pattern of alcohol use leading to clinically significant impairment or distress.

1. Continued alcohol use despite recurrent interpersonal problems is a symptom of alcohol use disorder.

2. Recurrent, alcohol-related legal problems are symptoms of alcohol use disorder.

3. Recurrent alcohol use resulting in failure to fulfill major role obligations is a symptom of alcohol use disorder.

4. A need for markedly increased, not decreased, amounts of alcohol to achieve the desired effect is evidence of tolerance. Tolerance is a symptom of alcohol use disorder.

5. Use of alcohol causes problems with interpersonal relationships, and the individual may become socially isolated. This is a symptom of alcohol use disorder.

TEST-TAKING HINT: The question requires that the test taker be able to recognize the signs and symptoms of alcohol use disorder.

10. 1. **Blackouts are brief periods of amnesia that occur during or immediately after a period of drinking. Because this client cannot remember recent events and was intoxicated on admission, the client is likely experiencing a blackout.**

2. Denial is the refusal to acknowledge the existence of a real situation or the feelings associated with it or both. Denial is a common defense mechanism used by clients diagnosed with alcohol use disorder to enable them to ignore the consequences of their behaviors. The use of denial is not described in the question.

3. Minimization is used when the client discounts the amount of alcohol consumed and the effect drinking has had on their life. This defensive behavior usually occurs in the early alcoholic phase of drinking

pattern progression. Minimization defenses are not described in the question.

4. Alcohol psychosis is a loss of contact with reality that results from acute or chronic alcohol use. This psychosis can be experienced during alcohol-induced withdrawal. The symptoms of alcohol psychosis are not described in the question.

TEST-TAKING HINT: To answer this question correctly, the test taker should look for client symptoms in the question that indicate what the client is experiencing and evaluate only the symptoms presented.

11. 1. **The body burns alcohol at about 0.5 ounce per hour, so behavioral changes would not be expected in an individual who slowly consumes only one average-size drink per hour. By consuming four drinks in a 1-hour period, however, this individual is likely to experience behavioral and mood changes.**
2. Because it usually takes at least 1 hour to eat out at a restaurant, the individual would be able to metabolize the wine at a pace that avoids behavioral and mood changes. Because the wine is consumed with food, the effect of the alcohol would be diminished further.
3. The individual's body size and the presence of food in the stomach would contribute to a diminished alcohol effect on the body and not put this individual at risk for behavioral and mood changes.
4. The intake of food, consumed with the margarita, would diminish the effect of alcohol on the body and not put this individual at risk for behavioral and mood changes.

TEST-TAKING HINT: To answer this question correctly, it is important for the test taker to consider an individual's size, whether there is food in the stomach, and how fast the individual consumes alcohol. These are all factors that influence the effects of alcohol on behavior and mood.

12. The CAGE questionnaire screening tool is an assessment tool used to determine if an individual abuses alcohol.
1. **Feeling the need to "Cut down" on drinking is the "C" of the CAGE assessment tool.**
2. **Feeling "Annoyed" when criticized about drinking is the "A" of the CAGE assessment tool.**
3. **Feeling "Guilty" about drinking is the "G" of the CAGE assessment tool.**
4. **"Eye opener," or having a drink in the morning to steady nerves, is the "E" of the CAGE assessment tool.**

5. Although clients experiencing alcohol use disorder tend to isolate themselves from others, this is not a question contained in the CAGE assessment tool.

TEST-TAKING HINT: To answer this question correctly, the test taker must know that CAGE is a mnemonic in which each letter represents a question in the CAGE assessment tool. This mnemonic assists the practitioner in remembering the categories of assessment addressed by this tool.

13. Wernicke-Korsakoff syndrome is the most serious form of thiamine deficiency in clients diagnosed with alcohol use disorder. If thiamine replacement therapy is not undertaken quickly, death will ensue.
1. A sudden onset of muscle pain with elevations of creatine phosphokinase (CPK) is an indication of alcoholic myopathy, not Wernicke-Korsakoff syndrome.
2. Signs and symptoms of congestive heart failure are indications of alcoholic cardiomyopathy, not Wernicke-Korsakoff syndrome.
3. **Loss of short-term and long-term memory and the use of confabulation are symptoms of Wernicke-Korsakoff syndrome. The treatment of this syndrome is alcohol abstinence and thiamine replacement.**
4. The effects of alcohol on the stomach include inflammation of the stomach lining characterized by epigastric distress, nausea, vomiting, and distention. These are not symptoms of Wernicke-Korsakoff syndrome.
5. **Wernicke-Korsakoff syndrome is caused by severe thiamine deficiency. The nurse would expect to see this reflected in thiamine laboratory value levels.**

TEST-TAKING HINT: To answer this question correctly, the test taker should study the various effects alcohol has on the body and match these effects with any symptoms presented.

14. Creatine phosphokinase (CPK) is elevated with alcoholic myopathy. The symptoms of alcoholic myopathy include extreme muscle pain, swelling and weakness of extremities, and reddish-tinged urine.
1. An elevated gamma-glutamyl transferase is an indication of chronic alcohol use disorder but is not indicative of the alcohol myopathy that is described in the question.
2. Enzyme-linked immunosorbent assay tests for the presence of antibodies to HIV, the virus that causes AIDS. This serological test would not be performed to substantiate the symptom of alcoholic myopathy.

3. An elevation in white blood cell count would indicate the presence of an infectious process. A white blood cell count would not be performed to substantiate the symptom of alcoholic myopathy.
4. **An elevated CPK is an indication of alcoholic myopathy. The described client's symptoms are indicative of this complication of alcohol use disorder.**

TEST-TAKING HINT: To answer this question correctly, the test taker must recognize that alcohol myopathy would cause an elevation in CPK.

15. 1. Street names for amphetamines include meth, speed, crystal, ice, Adam, ecstasy, Eve, and XTC.
2. **Street names for cocaine include snow, coke, blow, toot, lady, flake, and crack.**
3. Street names for barbiturates include yellow jackets, yellow birds, red devils, blue angels, jellybeans, rainbows, and double trouble.
4. Street names for benzodiazepines include Vs, roaches, dolls, and dollies.

TEST-TAKING HINT: The test taker must be able to recognize common names for street drugs to answer this question correctly.

16. 1. **Cocaine-induced intoxication typically produces an increase in myocardial demand for oxygen and an increase in heart rate. Severe vasoconstriction may occur and can result in myocardial infarction, ventricular fibrillation, and sudden death. Because the client in the question is presenting with chest pain and has a history of cocaine use disorder, the nurse should prioritize the assessment of this client.**
2. A client would need immediate assessment if experiencing alcohol-induced withdrawal, not intoxication. This client would be at risk only if the intoxication was severe with extreme central nervous system (CNS) depression. Because alcohol-induced withdrawal begins within 4 to 12 hours of cessation or reduction in heavy and prolonged alcohol use, the nurse has time to assess this client for alcohol-induced withdrawal. Compared with the clients described, this client would not take priority.
3. There is no physical withdrawal from hallucinogens such as lysergic acid diethylamide (LSD). A client experiencing a bad trip should be monitored closely to prevent self-injury as a result of extreme hyperactivity, hallucinations, and psychosis.

Overdose symptoms also can include seizures. Because the client described is not experiencing LSD overdose symptoms, this client would not take priority.
4. Flunitrazepam is commonly used to treat insomnia, and is referred to as a date rape drug. The effects of this drug include hypotension, confusion, visual disturbances, urinary retention, and aggressive behavior. It is important to assess for these symptoms and any signs of sexual assault. Psychological support also is necessary. None of the effects of flunitrazepam are life threatening, so compared with the clients described, this client would not take priority.

TEST-TAKING HINT: It is difficult to choose a priority assessment when presented with clients in the emergency department (ED). The test taker should look for signs and symptoms of conditions that can cause severe harm or death and for the time frame of the presenting problem to determine whether it is current and emerging, or whether the nurse has some time to defer assessment.

17. 1. A codependent individual would have a long history of focusing thoughts and behaviors on other people rather than self.
2. **A codependent individual tends to be a "people pleaser" and would do almost anything to gain approval from others.**
3. For a codependent individual to feel good, the partner must be happy and behave in appropriate ways. If the partner is not happy, the codependent person feels responsible for making them happy.
4. A codependent individual is confused about their own identity. In a relationship, a codependent person derives self-worth from the partner, whose feelings and behaviors determine how the codependent individual should feel and behave.
5. **A codependent individual has unmet autonomy needs and a profound sense of powerlessness.**

TEST-TAKING HINT: To answer this question correctly, the test taker needs to recognize the characteristics of an unhealthy dependence on another person.

18. Substance use disorder becomes a more serious problem when the impaired individual is responsible for the lives of others on a daily basis. All of the following are characteristic of an impaired nurse.
1. **An impaired nurse may look for the opportunity to administer medications to other nurses' clients, and there may**

be client complaints of inadequate pain control.

2. An impaired nurse has high absentee-ism if the substance source is outside the work area. Conversely, the nurse may rarely miss work if the substance source is within the work area.

3. It is easy to overlook a problem when dealing with impaired nurses. Denial on the part of the impaired nurse and nurse colleagues is the refusal to acknowledge the existence of the situation or the feelings associated with it.

4. There may be an increase in "wasting" of drugs, higher incidences of incorrect narcotic counts, and a higher record of signing out drugs for other nurses.

5. Poor concentration, difficulty in meeting deadlines, inappropriate responses, and poor memory and recall are usually apparent late in the disease process.

TEST-TAKING HINT: To answer this question correctly, it is important for the test taker to recognize and identify the characteristics of impairment that may occur in the workplace.

19. In contrast to foods, alcohol does not need to be digested.

1. **20% of a single dose of alcohol is absorbed directly and immediately into the bloodstream through the stomach wall.**

2. 80%, not 30%, is processed only slightly more slowly through the upper intestinal tract and into the bloodstream.

3. 0%, not 40%, of alcohol is absorbed through the large intestine.

4. 0%, not 50%, of alcohol is absorbed through the liver. The liver filters alcohol from the bloodstream.

TEST-TAKING HINT: The keyword *immediately* determines the correct answer to this question. Immediate absorption of alcohol occurs only in the stomach.

20. 1. Alcohol is absorbed into the bloodstream rapidly, not slowly, through the stomach wall before being processed through the liver.

2. In contrast to foods, alcohol does not need to be digested.

3. Rapidity of absorption is influenced by various factors. Absorption is delayed when the drink is sipped, rather than gulped; when the stomach contains food, rather than being empty; and when the drink is wine or beer, rather than distilled alcohol.

4. Only moments after alcohol is consumed, it can be found in all tissues, organs, and secretions of the body. It is not immediately excreted. Alcohol still can be found in the urine 12 hours after ingestion.

5. The body burns alcohol at the rate of about 0.5 ounce per hour. Because of this, behavioral changes would not be expected to occur in an individual who slowly consumed only one average-sized drink per hour.

TEST-TAKING HINT: To answer this question correctly, the test taker should review the characteristics of how the body processes alcohol.

21. There are four phases through which an individual's pattern of drinking progresses: the prealcoholic phase, early alcoholic phase, crucial phase, and chronic phase.

1. In the prealcoholic phase, alcohol is used to relieve the everyday stress and tensions of life.

2. The early alcoholic phase begins with blackouts. Alcohol has become required rather than a source of pleasure or relief for the individual.

3. Control is lost, and physiological dependence is evident in the crucial, not prealcoholic, phase of drinking progression.

4. In the chronic, not prealcoholic, phase, the individual is usually intoxicated more often than sober, and emotional and physical disintegration occur.

5. Tolerance begins to develop in the prealcoholic phase of drinking progression.

TEST-TAKING HINT: The test taker must understand the phases of an individual's drinking pattern progression to recognize characteristics of each phase.

22. 1. Tolerance to alcohol develops in the prealcoholic phase, but significant losses have not yet occurred.

2. Common behaviors that occur in the early alcoholic phase are sneaking drinks or secret drinking and preoccupation with drinking and maintaining the supply of alcohol. The individual experiences guilt and becomes defensive about drinking, but significant losses have not yet occurred.

3. In the crucial phase, the client's focus is totally on alcohol. The client is willing to lose everything that was once important in an effort to maintain the addiction. The losses presented in the question are evidence of this crucial phase.

4. Emotional disintegration is evidenced by profound helplessness and self-pity in the chronic phase. Impairment in reality testing may result in psychosis. Clients experience alcohol-related physical problems in almost every system of the body. The client described in this question does not exhibit the extremes of these symptoms.

TEST-TAKING HINT: The test taker needs to understand that in the crucial phase of drinking it is common for the individual to have experienced the loss of job, marriage, family, friends, and, especially, self-respect.

23. 1. In the prealcoholic, not early alcoholic, phase, alcohol is used to relieve the everyday stress and tensions of life.
    2. **When an individual experiences blackouts, they have entered the early alcoholic phase. Blackouts are brief periods of amnesia that occur during or immediately after a period of drinking.**
    3. Control is lost, and physiological dependence is evident in the crucial, not early alcoholic, phase of alcohol use disorder.
    4. An individual is usually intoxicated more often than sober, and emotional and physical disintegration occur in the chronic, not early alcoholic, phase of alcohol use disorder.
    5. **When an individual is experiencing secret drinking, preoccupation with drinking, and maintaining alcohol supply, they have entered the early alcoholic phase.**

TEST-TAKING HINT: The test taker must distinguish between blacking out and passing out. When a client passes out, they are unconscious. This is due to CNS depression resulting from the consumption of high amounts of alcohol, a CNS depressant. When a blackout is experienced, the individual seems to be functioning but later remembers nothing of the situation.

24. 1. Concealed hemorrhage occurs internally from a blood vessel that is no longer sutured or cauterized. The early symptoms include restlessness (not tremors), anxiety, and thirst. Pulse increases and blood pressure decreases, not increases.
    2. **Tremors, increased blood pressure, and diaphoresis all are signs of CNS rebound that occurs on withdrawal from any CNS depressant. The 3-day time frame presented in the question is the typical period in which a withdrawal syndrome might occur.**

3. Malignant hyperpyrexia is a severe form of pyrexia that occurs because of the use of muscle relaxants and general inhalation anesthesia. This condition is rare and occurs during or immediately after surgery. In the question, there is no mention of the client's having an elevated temperature.
4. Neuroleptic malignant syndrome is a rare, but potentially fatal, complication of neuroleptic drug treatment. In the question, there is no mention that the client has received any antipsychotic medications.

TEST-TAKING HINT: This question requires that the test taker recognize the importance of always reviewing a client's history. Any history of CNS depressant use disorder should be noted to alert the nurse for the potential problem of substance-induced withdrawal. The client's history should be validated with significant others and family because the defense mechanism of denial may be used by the client to minimize substance use.

25. 1. **Peripheral neuropathy, characterized by peripheral nerve damage, results in pain, burning, tingling, or prickly sensations of the extremities. Researchers believe it is the direct result of deficiencies in the B vitamins, particularly thiamine.**
    2. Clients with acute alcoholic myopathy present with a sudden onset of muscle pain, swelling, and weakness; a reddish tinge in the urine caused by myoglobin, a breakdown product of muscle that is excreted in the urine; and a rapid increase in muscle enzymes in the blood. The symptoms described in the question do not reflect acute alcoholic myopathy.
    3. Wernicke's encephalopathy is the most serious form of thiamine deficiency. Symptoms include paralysis of the ocular muscles, diplopia, ataxia, somnolence, and stupor. The symptoms described in the question do not reflect Wernicke's encephalopathy.
    4. Korsakoff's psychosis is identified by symptoms of confusion, loss of recent memory, and confabulation. It also is believed to be caused by a thiamine deficiency. The symptoms described in the question do not reflect Korsakoff's psychosis.

TEST-TAKING HINT: To answer this question correctly, the test taker needs to match the symptoms described with the disorders presented.

26. 1. An increase in CPK, a muscle enzyme that is released when muscle tissue

is damaged, occurs with alcoholic myopathy. Clients with acute alcoholic myopathy present with a sudden onset of muscle pain, swelling, and weakness. Reddish-tinged urine is caused by myoglobin, a breakdown product of muscle, excreted in the urine.

2. Low-density lipoproteins (LDL) are not increased when a client is experiencing alcoholic myopathy. The enzyme lactate dehydrogenase (LDH) does increase.

3. There is no decrease in fasting blood sugar (FBS) when a client is experiencing alcoholic myopathy.

4. There is no decrease in aspartate aminotransferase (AST) when a client is experiencing alcoholic myopathy. Because AST is a liver function test, it may be elevated if liver damage has occurred because of a long history of alcohol use disorder.

TEST-TAKING HINT: To answer this question correctly, the test taker must know the signs and symptoms of alcoholic myopathy and understand what laboratory values reflect this diagnosis.

27. 1. A client diagnosed with Wernicke-Korsakoff syndrome may have difficulty keeping thoughts focused, but this is not an example of confabulation.

2. **Confabulation is the filling in of a memory gap with detailed fantasy believed by the teller. The purpose is to maintain self-esteem. Clients diagnosed with Wernicke-Korsakoff syndrome use confabulation to fill in missing recent memories.**

3. When a client jumps from one topic to another in rapid succession, the client is experiencing the thought process alteration of flight of ideas. This is not a description of confabulation.

4. A client who confabulates actually believes the story presented. Confabulation is an unconscious defense mechanism used to protect the client's self-esteem. This is different from a client who consciously lies to manipulate for self-gratification.

TEST-TAKING HINT: The test taker must understand the concept of unconscious confabulation and differentiate it from tangential thinking (answer 1), flight of ideas (answer 3), and conscious lying (answer 4).

28. 1. Hepatic encephalopathy is a complication of cirrhosis of the liver resulting from chronic alcohol use disorder. It is caused by the inability of the liver to convert ammonia to

urea for excretion. The continued increase in serum ammonia results in progressively impaired mental functioning, apathy, euphoria or depression, sleep disturbance, increasing confusion, and progression to coma and eventual death. Hemorrhage is not a symptom of this complication.

2. Thrombocytopenia is a complication of cirrhosis of the liver resulting from chronic alcohol use disorder. It is caused by the inability of the diseased liver to produce adequate amounts of prothrombin and fibrinogen. This places the client at risk for hemorrhage, but this client is experiencing the actual problem of frank hemoptysis.

3. **Esophageal varices are veins in the esophagus that become distended because of excessive pressure from defective blood flow through the cirrhotic liver, causing portal hypertension. When pressure increases, these varicosities can rupture, resulting in hemorrhage. The frank hemoptysis experienced by the client indicates ruptured esophageal varices.**

4. Ascites occurs in response to portal hypertension caused by cirrhosis of the liver resulting from chronic alcohol use disorder. Increased pressure results in the seepage of fluid from the surface of the liver into the abdominal cavity, causing an enlarged, protuberant abdomen. Impaired protein metabolism contributes to this complication of cirrhosis. The client's presenting symptoms do not reflect the complication of ascites.

TEST-TAKING HINT: The test taker must examine the client symptoms described in the question. If the test taker understands the pathophysiology of the physical effects of alcohol use disorder, the correct complication and symptom can easily be matched.

29. 1. Confusion, loss of recent memory, and confabulation are symptoms of Korsakoff's psychosis, not pancreatitis.

2. Elevated CPK and signs and symptoms of congestive heart failure are symptoms of alcoholic cardiomyopathy, not pancreatitis.

3. Paralysis of the ocular muscles, diplopia, and ataxia are symptoms of Wernicke's encephalopathy, not pancreatitis.

4. **Constant, severe epigastric pain; nausea and vomiting; and abdominal distention are signs of acute pancreatitis, which can occur one or two days after a binge of excessive alcohol consumption.**

TEST-TAKING HINT: To answer this question correctly, the test taker must be able to differentiate among the signs and symptoms of various complications of alcohol use disorder.

30. Crack is a cocaine alkaloid that is extracted from its powdered hydrochloride salt by mixing it with sodium bicarbonate and allowing it to dry into small "rocks."
    1. Vodka is a distilled alcohol. Alcohol is a CNS depressant, not stimulant.
    2. **Crack cocaine is classified as a stimulant. It is the most potent stimulant derived from natural origin. Cocaine is extracted from the leaves of the coca plant.**
    3. Lorazepam is a benzodiazepine. This classification of drug depresses, rather than stimulates, the CNS and is often used to treat anxiety disorders.
    4. Triazolam is a nonbarbiturate hypnotic, not a stimulant, that is used to treat sleep disorders by depressing the CNS.

TEST-TAKING HINT: The test taker must understand the term *crack* to answer this question correctly. Crack is a cocaine alkaloid and is classified as a stimulant.

31. Caffeine is a CNS stimulant. The two most widely used stimulants are caffeine and nicotine.
    1. A 5- to 6-ounce cup of brewed coffee contains 90 to 125 mg of caffeine.
    2. Excedrin Migraine is a combination of aspirin and acetaminophen and contains 65 mg of caffeine.
    3. **Tequila is distilled liquor. Alcohol is a CNS depressant, not a stimulant.**
    4. Any cigarettes, including those with filters, contain nicotine, a CNS stimulant.

TEST-TAKING HINT: To answer this question correctly, the test taker must be able to identify products containing nicotine and caffeine, and recognize that these products stimulate the CNS. Nicotine is contained in all tobacco products. Caffeine is readily available in every supermarket and grocery store as a common ingredient in over-the-counter medications, coffee, tea, colas, and chocolate.

32. The standard of intoxication varies from state to state but the federally imposed standard of alcohol intoxication is a blood alcohol level (BAL) of **0.08 g/dL**. This is mandated in all 50 states.

TEST-TAKING HINT: To answer this question correctly, the test taker needs to know the BAL that indicates intoxication. This is often referred to as the *legal limit*.

33. The federally imposed standard of intoxication is a BAL of 0.08 g/dL or greater.
    1. Because the client's BAL is 0.10 g/dL, which is greater than the 0.08 g/dL legal limit, the client is assessed as legally intoxicated.
    2. **With a BAL of 0.10, which is greater than the 0.08 g/dL legal limit, the client is considered legally intoxicated.**
    3. All states must conform to the federally imposed BAL limit of 0.08 g/dL for intoxication. Individual state law would not be a consideration.
    4. Intoxication is determined by a BAL of 0.08 g/dL or greater. No other psychomotor tests are necessary.

TEST-TAKING HINT: To answer this question correctly, the test taker must know that the legal BAL for intoxication is 0.08 g/dL and that this level is federally mandated.

Nursing Process—Diagnosis

34. 1. Ineffective health maintenance is the inability to identify, manage, or seek out help to maintain health. This is an appropriate nursing diagnosis for many clients diagnosed with substance use disorder, not alcohol-induced withdrawal. With substance use disorder, all activities of life are focused on obtaining and using the substance of abuse, rather than maintaining health. Risk for injury is a higher priority for clients experiencing alcohol-induced withdrawal because of risk for CNS overstimulation rebound.
    2. Ineffective coping is the inability to form a valid appraisal of stressors, inadequate choices of practiced responses, or inability to use available resources. This is an appropriate nursing diagnosis for many clients diagnosed with substance use disorder, not substance-induced withdrawal. These clients use substances to cope, rather than adaptive behaviors or problem-solving. Risk for injury is a higher priority for clients experiencing alcohol-induced withdrawal because of the risk for CNS overstimulation rebound.
    3. **Risk for injury is the result of either internal or external environmental conditions interacting with the individual's adaptive and defensive resources. It is the priority diagnosis for a client experiencing alcohol-induced withdrawal. Withdrawal of CNS depressants (alcohol) causes a rebound stimulation of the CNS, leading to alcohol-induced withdrawal**

and puts the client at risk for injury. This alcohol-induced withdrawal may include symptoms of elevated blood pressure, tachycardia, hallucinations, and seizures.

4. Dysfunctional family processes are the chronic disorganization of psychosocial, spiritual, and physiological functions of the family unit that leads to conflict, denial of problems, resistance to change, ineffective problem-solving, and a series of self-perpetuating crises. This is an appropriate nursing diagnosis for many clients diagnosed with substance use disorder, not substance-induced withdrawal. Risk for injury is a higher priority for clients experiencing alcohol-induced withdrawal because of the risk for CNS overstimulation rebound.

TEST-TAKING HINT: When prioritizing nursing diagnoses, the test taker always must give priority to client safety. This question asks for a priority diagnosis for alcohol-induced withdrawal. The other diagnoses are appropriate for alcohol use disorder, not withdrawal.

35. 1. Alcoholic cardiomyopathy results from the effects of alcohol on the heart by the accumulation of lipids causing the heart to enlarge and weaken, leading to congestive heart failure. Symptoms include decreased exercise tolerance, tachycardia, dyspnea, edema, palpitations, and nonproductive cough. Altered perfusion related to palpitations as evidenced by decreased oxygen saturations would address and prioritize these client problems.

2. Although most clients experiencing alcohol use disorder use alcohol to cope with stressors and can feel powerless, this nursing diagnosis does not address the client's problem of alcoholic cardiomyopathy.

3. This nursing diagnosis is incorrectly written. You cannot include a medical diagnosis within a nursing diagnosis. Nursing diagnoses address client problems that are within the nurse's scope of practice. Also, the risk for injury does not address the alcoholic cardiomyopathy presented in the question.

4. Activity intolerance is a symptom of alcoholic cardiomyopathy. Altered perfusion is prioritized because, if this can be resolved, the activity intolerance also would be corrected.

TEST-TAKING HINT: When prioritizing nursing diagnoses, the test taker first must make sure the diagnosis is correctly written, and then make sure the diagnosis addresses the client problem presented in the question. After safety is prioritized, the test taker must choose the diagnosis that, if resolved, would solve other client problems.

36. 1. When a client withdraws from cocaine, the withdrawal symptoms are more psychological than physical. The intensely pleasurable effects of the drug create the potential for extraordinary psychological dependency, leading to powerlessness over the addiction. Powerlessness is the perception that one's own action would not significantly affect an outcome. This client's priority diagnosis is powerlessness.

2. Cocaine is a CNS stimulant, not a depressant, so there is no rebound of the nervous system during withdrawal and less chance of physical injury.

3. Ineffective health maintenance is the inability to identify, manage, or seek out help to maintain health. This is an appropriate nursing diagnosis for many clients diagnosed with substance use disorder, not substance-induced withdrawal. With these clients, all activities of life are focused on obtaining and using the substance of abuse rather than on maintaining health.

4. Ineffective coping is the inability to form a valid appraisal of stressors, inadequate choices of practiced responses, or inability to use available resources. This is an appropriate nursing diagnosis for many clients diagnosed with substance use disorder, not substance-induced withdrawal. These clients use substances rather than adaptive behaviors or problem-solving to cope.

TEST-TAKING HINT: To answer this question correctly, the test taker must recognize the effects of cocaine-induced withdrawal. This knowledge helps eliminate answer 2. Answers 3 and 4 can be eliminated because they relate to cocaine use disorder rather than cocaine-induced withdrawal.

37. 1. The symptoms of alcohol-induced intoxication include lack of inhibition related to sexual or aggressive impulses, mood lability, impaired judgment, impaired social or occupational functioning, slurred speech, unsteady gait, nystagmus, and flushed face, not pain. Because alcohol is a CNS depressant, intoxication would decrease, rather than increase, pain.

2. Ineffective denial is the conscious or unconscious attempt to disavow knowledge or meaning of an event to reduce anxiety

or fear, leading to the detriment of health. This may be an appropriate diagnosis for a client experiencing alcohol-induced intoxication, but of the diagnoses presented, it is not the priority.

3. Ineffective coping is the inability to form a valid appraisal of stressors, inadequate choices of practiced responses, or inability to use available resources. This may be an appropriate diagnosis for a client experiencing alcohol-induced intoxication, but of the diagnoses presented, it is not the priority.

4. **Alcohol depresses the CNS and, with significant intake, can render an individual unconscious. The effects of alcohol on the stomach include inflammation of the stomach lining characterized by epigastric distress, nausea, vomiting, and distention. These effects of alcohol could lead to aspiration, making this the most life-threatening, priority client problem.**

TEST-TAKING HINT: To answer this question correctly, the test taker must know the effects of alcohol on the body. When asked for a priority nursing diagnosis, it is important to choose the answer that addresses client safety, in this case aspiration.

Nursing Process—Planning

38. 1. The *Diagnostic and Statistical Manual of Mental Disorders*, Fifth Edition, Text Revision (*DSM-5-TR*) classifies mental illness and presents guidelines and diagnostic criteria for various mental disorders. The *DSM-5-TR* does not set outcomes for nursing interventions for clients experiencing substance use disorders.

2. The North American Nursing Diagnosis Association (NANDA) has formulated an approved list of client problems stated in nursing diagnosis terminology. The NANDA does not set outcomes for nursing interventions for clients experiencing substance use disorders.

3. An outcome is a specific client expectation related to nursing interventions based on an established nursing diagnosis. Nursing outcomes provide direction for selection of appropriate nursing interventions and evaluation of client progress. Because clients with substance use disorder problems have different strengths, backgrounds, and supports, outcomes of treatment should be tailored to the individual's immediate needs and abilities. This is an individualized process that should not be standardized.

4. Nursing outcomes provide direction for selection of appropriate nursing interventions and evaluation of client progress. These nursing interventions, not outcomes, help a client to return to the highest level of wellness. Outcomes alone, without appropriate interventions, would set expectations only, not assist the client in reaching those expectations.

TEST-TAKING HINT: To answer this question correctly, the test taker should look for a true statement about client outcomes. Understanding the use of the *DSM-5-TR* and the NANDA classification of client problems eliminates answers 1 and 2 immediately.

39. 1. That the client will agree to attend nutritional counseling sessions is a short-term outcome for the nursing diagnosis of ineffective health maintenance. Also, this outcome is written incorrectly because it does not contain a measurable time frame.

2. **A long-term outcome for the nursing diagnosis of ineffective health maintenance for the client described is that the client will exhibit reduced medical complications related to substance use disorder within 6 months. This outcome is directly related to health maintenance and is long term in nature.**

3. That the client will identify three effects of alcohol on the body by day 2 of hospitalization is a short-term, not long-term, outcome for the nursing diagnosis of ineffective health maintenance.

4. That the client will remain free from injury while withdrawing from alcohol is not an outcome that relates to the nursing diagnosis of ineffective health maintenance. This outcome would relate to the nursing diagnosis of potential for injury related to alcohol-induced withdrawal.

TEST-TAKING HINT: The test taker should focus on two key concepts in this question—first, the nursing diagnosis being addressed and then the long-term nature of the outcome. Because answer 2 has no time frame incorporated in the outcome and cannot be measured, it can be eliminated immediately.

40. 1. Addressing previously successful coping skills is a good nursing intervention for planning relapse prevention strategies, but it must be in the context of a simple approach.

2. Encouraging rehearsing stressful situations that may lead to relapse is a good nursing intervention for planning relapse prevention strategies, but it must be in the context of a simple approach.

3. Because 40% to 50% of clients who abuse substances have mild to moderate cognitive problems while actively using, relapse prevention strategies initially should be approached simply. All interventions should be in the context of simple planning to be fully comprehended by the client.

4. Providing numerous choices of community resources such as Alcoholics Anonymous (AA) is a good nursing intervention for planning relapse prevention strategies, but it must be in the context of a simple approach.

TEST-TAKING HINT: The keyword *initially* helps the test taker determine the correct answer. All of the interventions are correct for planning relapse prevention strategies, but without a simple approach none of them may be understood effectively by the client.

Nursing Process—Implementation

41. 1. It is inappropriate to begin any teaching with a client who has recently experienced a head injury. In this situation, attention and concentration could be limited, making learning difficult.

2. After obtaining client permission, the student should validate any information received from this client with family members because clients diagnosed with substance use disorder tend to minimize or deny substance use.

3. The student should not necessarily accept the client's statement about cocaine use as factual because clients diagnosed with substance use disorder tend to minimize or deny substance use.

4. Because there is no physical dependency related to cocaine use disorder, there would be no need to instruct this client about the detoxification (detox) process.

TEST-TAKING HINT: To choose the correct answer to this question, the test taker must focus on the client's current situation. This recognition would eliminate answer 1. Understanding that cocaine has no physical withdrawal symptoms eliminates answer 4.

42. 1. Monitoring fluid intake and output is a nursing intervention that does not directly relate to the nursing diagnosis of risk for injury R/T alcohol withdrawal.

2. Providing clients who are experiencing alcohol-induced withdrawal with a quiet room free from environmental stimuli is a nursing intervention that directly relates to the nursing diagnosis of risk for injury R/T alcohol-induced withdrawal. Alcohol-induced withdrawal is a pattern of physiological responses to the discontinuation of alcohol use. It is life threatening, with a mortality rate of 25% caused by a rebound reaction to CNS depression leading to increased neurological excitement potentially causing seizures and death. Increased environmental stimuli would exacerbate this problem. Decreasing stimuli would help to avoid injury resulting from alcohol-induced withdrawal.

3. When clients withdraw from alcohol, they are in a health crisis, a life-threatening situation. Teaching would be ineffective because of increased anxiety generated by this life-threatening situation.

4. When clients withdraw from alcohol, they are in a health crisis, a life-threatening situation. It would be ineffective to confront denial at this time.

TEST-TAKING HINT: The test taker must understand the critical nature of alcohol-induced withdrawal to be able to determine the nursing intervention that directly relates to this client's problem. During crisis situations, various nursing interventions, such as teaching the client, can be eliminated immediately because the nurse's focus should be on maintaining client safety and reducing injury.

43. 1. The first step in decreasing the use of denial is for clients to see the relationship between substance use and personal problems. The nurse can assist with this by helping the client analyze the effects of substance abuse on life situations.

2. Setting up follow-up appointments and providing community resources are effective nursing interventions to help prevent relapse, but they do not directly address the nursing diagnosis of ineffective denial.

3. Providing a stimulus-free environment is a nursing intervention related to prevention of injury during alcohol-induced withdrawal. This intervention does not directly address the nursing diagnosis of ineffective denial.

4. It is critical to monitor vital signs when a client is experiencing alcohol-induced

withdrawal because of the life-threatening nature of withdrawal symptoms. However, monitoring vital signs does not address the client problem of ineffective denial.

TEST-TAKING HINT: The test taker must note the nursing diagnosis assigned to the client in the question to determine the appropriate nursing intervention. Other nursing interventions may apply to clients with specific medical conditions, but the correct answer choice must be based on the nursing diagnosis presented in the question.

44. A benzodiazepine is a CNS depressant. During CNS depressant-induced withdrawal, the CNS rebounds, potentially causing life-threatening complications such as seizures. Repeated episodes of withdrawal seem to kindle even more serious withdrawal episodes, including the production of withdrawal seizures that can result in brain damage. A complicated withdrawal is a withdrawal in which complications such as seizures have occurred.
    1. The nurse's priority intervention is not the use of confrontation to deal with the defense mechanisms of denial, projection, and displacement. Because of this client's high risk for complicated withdrawal, client safety takes priority.
    2. The nurse's priority intervention is not providing empathetic support. Because of this client's high risk for complicated withdrawal, client safety takes priority.
    3. The nurse's priority intervention is not presenting the consequences of the client's actions. Because of this client's high risk for complicated withdrawal, client safety takes priority.
    4. **Because of this client's high risk for complicated withdrawal, the nurse should monitor the client closely and initiate seizure precautions. Client safety takes priority.**

TEST-TAKING HINT: The test taker first must recognize the situation presented in the question that puts the client at high risk for complications from benzodiazepine-induced withdrawal. After this risk is determined, safety interventions must be prioritized.

45. Wernicke's encephalopathy and Korsakoff's psychosis are two disorders that occur as a direct result of chronic alcohol use disorder and are considered together in the United States as Wernicke-Korsakoff syndrome.
    1. Intravenous thiamine, vitamin B_1, is the treatment of choice and a priority when a client is experiencing the life-threatening complication of Wernicke-Korsakoff syndrome. This syndrome is caused by a thiamine deficiency resulting from poor intake of vitamin B_1 and poor absorption of this vitamin.
    2. Increasing fluid intake would not be an intervention indicated or prioritized for a client diagnosed with Wernicke-Korsakoff syndrome.
    3. A client diagnosed with chronic alcohol use disorder is probably experiencing nutritional deficits. These deficits occur because caloric intake is supplied by alcohol rather than nutritious foods. Prenatal vitamins do contain the B complex, including B_1, but not in sufficient amounts to counteract the effects of Wernicke-Korsakoff syndrome.
    4. Encouraging foods high in vitamin C would not be an intervention indicated or prioritized for a client diagnosed with Wernicke-Korsakoff syndrome.

TEST-TAKING HINT: To answer this question correctly, the test taker must know the cause of Wernicke-Korsakoff syndrome and not confuse overall nutritional deficits with the specific thiamine deficiency that leads to Wernicke-Korsakoff syndrome in clients diagnosed with alcohol use disorder.

46. 1. The symptoms presented in the question are not symptoms that reflect a thiamine deficiency. Peripheral neuropathy, alcoholic myopathy, and Wernicke-Korsakoff syndrome all are caused by thiamine deficiencies. The symptoms presented are not indicative of these disorders.
    2. **The effect of alcohol on the heart is an accumulation of lipids in the myocardial cells, resulting in enlargement and weakened cardiac function. The clinical findings of alcoholic cardiomyopathy present as symptoms of congestive heart failure. Besides total abstinence from alcohol, treatment includes digitalis, sodium restriction, and diuretics.**
    3. No cognitive alterations are presented in the question. Reorienting the client to person, place, and time would not address the physical problems presented.
    4. The symptoms presented indicate that the client is experiencing alcoholic cardiomyopathy. Treatment should include sodium restriction, not an increase in sodium intake.

TEST-TAKING HINT: To answer this question correctly, the test taker must relate the client's history of alcohol use disorder to the physical symptoms presented. When the client's cardiomyopathy has been identified, the choice of intervention should be clear.

47. 1. It is important always to assess a client's readiness for learning before any teaching. Because this client is experiencing tolerance, which is a symptom of substance use disorder, reviewing the criteria for alcohol-induced withdrawal is misdirected.

2. **Tolerance is the need for markedly increased amounts of a substance to achieve intoxication or desired effects. Tolerance is a characteristic of alcohol use disorder. Because the client is experiencing tolerance, the nurse in the role of teacher should present this information.**

3. Minimization is a type of thinking in which the significance of an event is minimized or undervalued. There is nothing in the question that indicates that the client is using minimization.

4. Rationalization is a defense mechanism by which an individual attempts to make excuses or formulate logical reasons to justify unacceptable feelings or behaviors. Nothing in the question indicates that the client is using rationalization.

TEST-TAKING HINT: To answer this question correctly, the test taker first needs to recognize and understand the characteristics of tolerance. The test taker then can choose the appropriate teaching priority for the client described in the question.

Nursing Process—Evaluation

48. 1. Detox from alcohol is the first and easiest step in the recovery process. After detox, the day-to-day recovery process begins.

2. The goal of recovery is abstinence from alcohol, not to decrease the amount of alcohol consumed.

3. **Recovery is a lifelong process and comes about in steps. AA is a self-help group that can assist with recovery. Its slogan is "One day at a time."**

4. Al-Anon is a support group for spouses and friends of alcoholics. AA is a support group specifically for clients diagnosed with alcohol use disorder.

TEST-TAKING HINT: This is essentially a true/false question. Only one answer choice can be true. The test taker should either look for the true statement or eliminate the false statements. The

test taker also must know the focus of Al-Anon to understand that it is not a support group for clients diagnosed with alcohol use disorder.

49. A 12-step program is designed to help an individual refrain from addictive behaviors and foster individual growth and change.

1. **A 12-step program helps break down denial in an atmosphere of support, understanding, and acceptance. Clients work with sponsors within the support group to accomplish this goal.**

2. **A 12-step program helps clients establish a relationship between a person's feelings of belonging and treatment outcomes. When clients feel socially involved with others in the support group, they have a higher rate of continuation of treatment and lower relapse rates.**

3. The first step of the "12 Steps" of Alcoholics Anonymous is to admit powerlessness, not power, over alcohol.

4. A 12-step program is a self-help organization. Individuals are helped to maintain sobriety by the assistance of peers with similar problems, not experts in the field.

5. Sponsors who are provided by a 12-step program assist fellow clients diagnosed with alcohol use disorder with individual growth and change. Change must be the responsibility of the client and not imposed by the sponsor. Social settings, friends, and lifestyles need to be modified to achieve sobriety and avoid relapse.

TEST-TAKING HINT: The test taker must understand the principles of 12-step programs such as AA and Narcotics Anonymous (NA) to choose appropriate reasons for the success of these programs.

Psychopharmacology

50. 1. **Alcohol is a CNS depressant. Alcohol-induced intoxication symptoms are related to this depression, and withdrawal symptoms are related to a rebound of the CNS. Because anxiolytics (antianxiety medications such as barbiturates) also depress the CNS, they share similar features of alcohol-induced intoxication and withdrawal.**

2. Amphetamines are CNS stimulants. They stimulate the CNS while alcohol depresses it. There are few physical withdrawal effects from the cessation of

amphetamines. Amphetamine-induced withdrawal is psychological, not physical, in nature, including depression, anxiety, fatigue, and cravings.

3. Cocaine is a CNS stimulant. It stimulates the CNS while alcohol depresses it. There are few physical withdrawal effects from the cessation of cocaine. Cocaine-induced withdrawal is psychological, not physical, in nature, including depression, anxiety, fatigue, cravings, and paranoid thinking.

4. Phencyclidine (PCP) is a hallucinogen. The effects produced by hallucinogens are highly unpredictable, in contrast to the effects of alcohol. There is no withdrawal from PCP.

TEST-TAKING HINT: To determine the correct answer, the test taker must be able to distinguish between the similarities of the signs and symptoms of alcohol-induced intoxication and withdrawal, and the signs and symptoms of anxiolytic-induced intoxication and withdrawal.

51. 1. Disulfiram is a drug that can be administered to individuals diagnosed with alcohol use disorder as a deterrent to drinking. Ingestion of alcohol when disulfiram is in the body results in a syndrome of symptoms that can produce discomfort. Clients must be able to understand the need to avoid all alcohol and any food or over-the-counter medication that contains alcohol. Clients with cognitive deficits would not be candidates for disulfiram therapy.

2. **Naltrexone is an opiate antagonist that can decrease some of the reinforcing effects of alcohol and decrease cravings. This would be an appropriate drug to assist this client with alcohol recovery.**

3. Lorazepam is a CNS depressant used as substitution therapy during alcohol-induced withdrawal to decrease the excitation of the CNS and prevent complications. There is no indication in the question that this client is experiencing alcohol-induced withdrawal.

4. Methadone is used as substitution therapy for opioid-, not alcohol-, induced withdrawal.

TEST-TAKING HINT: The test taker must be familiar with the psychopharmacology used for intoxication and withdrawal of various substances to answer this question correctly. Recognizing that this client has cognitive deficits would eliminate answer 1 immediately. Because the assistance is needed for recovery, not withdrawal, answer 3 can be eliminated.

52. 1. Acamprosate calcium is an amino acid derivative that is helpful in the maintenance of abstinence in alcohol, not heroin, use disorder.

2. **Buprenorphine/naloxone is approved by the Food and Drug Administration for assistance with recovery from opioid addiction.**

3. Disulfiram is a drug that can be used as a deterrent to drinking for individuals who abuse alcohol, not heroin.

4. Haloperidol is an antipsychotic medication that is not used for heroin recovery.

TEST-TAKING HINT: To answer this question correctly, the test taker needs to understand the use of psychopharmacology in the treatment of substance use disorder and substance-induced withdrawal.

53. Lorazepam is a CNS depressant used in alcohol detox.

1. Lorazepam does not decrease cravings associated with alcohol use disorder.

2. Disulfiram, not lorazepam, is a deterrent therapy to motivate clients to avoid alcohol.

3. **Lorazepam is substitution therapy to decrease the intensity of withdrawal symptoms. The dosage depends on the severity of symptoms experienced during alcohol-induced withdrawal, and this is objectively measured by the use of the Clinical Institute Withdrawal Assessment (CIWA) score.**

4. Lorazepam is a CNS depressant, not stimulant, that works to decrease the client's withdrawal symptoms and lower the CIWA score.

TEST-TAKING HINT: The test taker must understand the action of the drug lorazepam to recognize its use in substitution therapy.

54. Disulfiram is a drug that can be administered to individuals diagnosed with alcohol use disorder as a deterrent to drinking. Ingestion of alcohol when disulfiram is in the body results in a syndrome of symptoms that can produce discomfort. Clients must be able to understand the need to avoid all alcohol and any food or over-the-counter medication that contains alcohol.

1. Over-the-counter cough and cold medications often contain alcohol. This alcohol would negatively affect a client who is taking disulfiram.

2. Alcohol can be absorbed through the skin. Alcohol-based aftershaves should be avoided when taking disulfiram. This

client's statement indicates that the client has accurate knowledge related to this important information.

3. Disulfiram is used as deterrent therapy and does not decrease alcohol cravings. Acamprosate calcium is a drug that is used for maintenance of alcohol abstinence by decreasing cravings.

4. Disulfiram is used as deterrent therapy, not substitution therapy. Benzodiazepines are the most frequently prescribed group of drugs used for substitution therapy during alcohol-induced withdrawal.

TEST-TAKING HINT: The test taker must understand the purpose of the use of disulfiram and its potential side effects to recognize the client's statement that contains correct information regarding this medication.

55. Insulin is prescribed based on a sliding scale of fasting blood glucose levels. A CIWA tool assesses symptoms of alcohol-induced withdrawal. Medications that immediately calm the central nervous system (CNS) are prescribed based on this CIWA score.

1. Olanzapine is an antipsychotic and would not be used to treat alcohol-induced withdrawal.

2. Lithium carbonate is a mood stabilizer and does not have an immediate, calming effect on the CNS. This drug is not used for alcohol-induced withdrawal.

3. Fluoxetine is an antidepressant and does not have an immediate, calming effect on the CNS. This drug is not used for alcohol-induced withdrawal.

4. A CIWA score is an evaluation of symptoms experienced by a client undergoing alcohol-induced withdrawal. As the score increases, the client's potential for serious complications increases, and CNS depressant medications must be administered. These types of medications calm the CNS, decrease elevated blood pressure, and prevent seizures. Lorazepam is a benzodiazepine, which is an antianxiety medication that provides an immediate, calming effect on the CNS. Other benzodiazepines, such as chlordiazepoxide and diazepam, also can be used for the symptoms of alcohol-induced withdrawal.

TEST-TAKING HINT: To answer this question correctly, the test taker must be familiar with several terms, such as *CIWA* and *sliding scale*. The test taker also needs to understand the effects of alcohol-induced withdrawal on the CNS, necessitating the administration of CNS depressants.

56. A client with a history of alcohol use disorder can be prescribed disulfiram to deter the drinking of alcohol. If the client drinks alcohol while taking disulfiram, the client may experience symptoms such as flushed skin, throbbing head and neck, respiratory difficulty, dizziness, nausea and vomiting, sweating, hyperventilation, tachycardia, hypotension, weakness, blurred vision, and confusion.

1. In asking about medications for the treatment of alcohol use disorder, the nurse understands that the symptoms assessed are similar to the symptoms of a client who consumes alcohol while taking disulfiram.

2. Asking about abstinence does not address the symptoms assessed.

3. Asking about any illegal street drugs may be important; however, this does not address the symptoms assessed.

4. Although some of the symptoms, such as low blood pressure and tachycardia, can be signs of dehydration, the other symptoms assessed are not. It is important for the nurse to think critically about all the symptoms presented.

TEST-TAKING HINT: To answer this question correctly, the test taker must recognize signs and symptoms that indicate that alcohol has been consumed while taking disulfiram. Also, the test taker should note that this client is currently in treatment for alcohol use disorder. This information would lead the test taker to consider the possibility of disulfiram use.

57. 1. Buspirone, an antianxiety agent, would not assist this client in decreasing cravings.

2. Disulfiram is a medication prescribed to assist individuals in avoiding alcohol consumption. The client described in the question is complaining of cravings; disulfiram does not decrease an individual's cravings but instead deters alcohol use because of the potential uncomfortable symptoms that occur with use of alcohol. An individual taking disulfiram and consuming alcohol experiences symptoms such as flushed skin, throbbing head and neck, respiratory difficulty, dizziness, nausea and vomiting, sweating, hyperventilation, tachycardia, hypotension, weakness, blurred vision, and confusion.

3. Naltrexone, a narcotic antagonist, can be used in the treatment of alcohol use disorder. It works on the same

receptors in the brain that produce the feelings of pleasure when heroin or other opiates bind to them, but it does not produce the "narcotic high" and is not habit forming. Naltrexone would help the client abstain from alcohol by decreasing cravings.

4. Lorazepam is a benzodiazepine that is used to assist clients going through alcohol-induced withdrawal, but it would not assist in decreasing cravings.

TEST-TAKING HINT: To answer this question correctly, the test taker must distinguish among medications used to decrease cravings, to deter alcohol consumption, and to assist with alcohol-induced withdrawal.

58. The client received **5 mg** in 1 day.

CIWA score at 0400 = 6   0 mg
CIWA score at 0800 = 14   1 mg
CIWA score at 1200 = 8   0.5 mg
CIWA score at 1600 = 10   0.5 mg
CIWA score at 2000 = 14   1 mg
CIWA score at 2400 = 6 + <u>0 mg</u>
                          3 mg (prn)
0.5 mg × 4 = 2 mg (standing dose)
3 mg + 2 mg = 5 mg/day

TEST-TAKING HINT: The test taker must recognize that to arrive at the correct daily dosage, the prn and standing dosages must be added together.

59. The assessed client data indicate a potential for opiate overdose.
1. Although the nurse may want to call the family to inquire about drug use, based on the assessed information and vital signs, the most important intervention by the nurse would be first treat symptoms of opiate overdose.

2. Based on the assessment data and vitals, the client is not experiencing alcohol-induced withdrawal. The client's CIWA is under 10. Mild alcohol withdrawal is less than or equal to 10. A moderate alcohol withdrawal scores 11–15, and severe withdrawal is any score equal to or greater than 16. Administering lorazepam at this time would further decrease respiratory rate, decrease CNS functioning and cause worsening symptoms.

3. Although the nurse may want to recheck the vital signs, the reason for this intervention would not be to build rapport and trust. The client's symptoms indicate opiate overdose. If this situation is not addressed by appropriate interventions, the client may experience worsening symptoms that may lead to death.

4. **The nurse must recognize the client's assessed symptoms as an opiate overdose. Symptoms of opiate overdose include cold, clammy skin; bluish skin around the lips and under the fingernails; breathing problems, including slowed or irregular breathing, leading to respiratory arrest; extreme sleepiness; inability to wake up; intermittent loss of consciousness; pinpoint pupils; vomiting; marked confusion; delirium; or acting drunk. Administering naloxone 2 mg IM will address and reverse the opiate overdose.**

TEST-TAKING HINT: The test-taker must recognize the possible danger of family or friends bringing drugs to the client during visitation. With this risk in mind, the nurse would then need to identify the symptoms the client is experiencing as opiate overdose and respond appropriately.

Schizophrenia Spectrum and Other Psychotic Disorders

KEYWORDS

The following words include English vocabulary, nursing/medical terminology, concepts, principles, or information relevant to content specifically addressed in this chapter or associated with topics presented in it. English dictionaries, your nursing textbooks, and medical dictionaries such as *Taber's Cyclopedic Medical Dictionary* are resources that can be used to expand your knowledge and understanding of these words and related information.

Akathisia

Akinesia

Altered thought processes

Anhedonia

Anticholinergic side effects

Antipsychotic medications

Associative looseness

Auditory hallucinations

Bizarre delusions

Blunted affect

Brief psychotic disorder

Catatonia

Clang association

Concrete thinking

Delusion of influence

Delusional disorder

Delusional thinking

Delusions

Delusions of grandeur

Delusions of persecution

Depersonalization

Disorganized thinking

Distortions of reality

Disturbed sensory perception

Disturbed thought process

Dopamine hypothesis

Dystonia

Echolalia

Echopraxia

Ego boundaries

Erotomanic delusion

Extrapyramidal symptoms

Flat affect

Grandiose delusion

Hallucinations

Hyperpyrexia

Illusion

Magical thinking

Muscle rigidity

Negative symptoms

Neologism

Neuroleptic malignant syndrome (NMS)

Nihilistic delusion

Paranoia

Persecutory delusion

Pharmacotherapy

Positive symptoms

Primitive behavior

Prodromal phase

Pseudoparkinsonism

Psychosocial therapies

Psychotherapy

Religiosity

Residual phase

Schizoaffective disorder

Schizoid personality disorder

Schizophrenia

Schizophrenia spectrum disorders

Schizophreniform disorder

Social isolation

Somatic delusion

Unconscious identification

Waxy flexibility

Word salad

QUESTIONS

Theory

1. Although symptoms of schizophrenia occur at various times in the life span, what client would more likely be diagnosed?
   1. A 10-year-old girl.
   2. A 20-year-old man.
   3. A 50-year-old woman.
   4. A 65-year-old man.

2. A nursing instructor is teaching about the etiology of schizophrenia. What statement by the nursing student indicates an understanding of the content presented?
   1. "Schizophrenia is a disorder of the brain that can be cured with the correct treatment."
   2. "A person inherits schizophrenia from a parent."
   3. "Problems in the structure of the brain cause schizophrenia."
   4. "There are many potential causes for this disease, and its etiology is controversial."

3. What is required for effective treatment of schizophrenia?
   1. Concentration on pharmacotherapy alone to alter imbalances in affected neurotransmitters.
   2. Comprehensive efforts, which include pharmacotherapy and psychosocial care.
   3. Emphasis on social and living skills training to help the client fit into society.
   4. Group and family therapy to increase socialization skills.

4. When one fraternal twin has been diagnosed with schizophrenia, the other twin has approximately a _____ % chance of developing the disease.

5. When one identical twin has been diagnosed with schizophrenia, the other twin has approximately a _____ % chance of developing the disease.

6. From a biochemical influence perspective, which accurately describes the etiology of schizophrenia?
   1. Adopted children with non-schizophrenic parents, raised by parents diagnosed with schizophrenia, have a higher incidence of this disease.
   2. An excess of dopamine-dependent neuronal activity occurs in the brain.
   3. A higher incidence of schizophrenia occurs after there is prenatal exposure of the mother to influenza.
   4. Poor parent–child interaction and dysfunctional family systems occur.

Nursing Process—Assessment

7. A nurse is working with a client diagnosed with schizoid personality disorder. What symptom of this diagnosis should the nurse expect to assess, and at what risk is this client for acquiring schizophrenia?
   1. Delusions and hallucinations—high risk.
   2. Limited range of emotional experience and expression—high risk.
   3. Indifferent to social relationships—low risk.
   4. Loner who appears cold and aloof—low risk.

8. A nurse is assessing a client with a long history of being a loner and having few social relationships. This client's parent has been diagnosed with schizophrenia. The nurse would suspect that this client is in what phase of the development of schizophrenia?
   1. Phase I—premorbid phase.
   2. Phase II—prodromal phase.
   3. Phase III—schizophrenia.
   4. Phase IV—residual phase.

9. A client diagnosed with schizophrenia is experiencing social withdrawal, flat affect, and impaired role functioning. To distinguish whether this client is in the prodromal or residual phase of schizophrenia, what question would the nurse ask the family?
   1. "Have these symptoms followed an active period of schizophrenic behaviors?"
   2. "How long have these symptoms been occurring?"
   3. "Has the client had a change in mood?"
   4. "Has the client been diagnosed with any developmental disorders?"

10. The nurse is assessing a client diagnosed with schizophrenia with catatonic features. Which of the following symptoms should the nurse expect the client to exhibit? **Select all that apply.**
    1. Catalepsy.
    2. Waxy flexibility.
    3. Pressured speech.
    4. Posturing.
    5. Stereotypy.

11. Schizophrenia is identified in the *Diagnostic and Statistical Manual of Mental Disorders, Fifth Edition, Text Revision* (*DSM-5-TR*), as a spectrum disorder based on the severity of symptoms. Which of the following accurately describes this diagnostic category? **Select all that apply.**
    1. Degree of severity of the schizophrenia spectrum is determined by the number of psychotic symptoms.
    2. Schizotypal personality disorder initiates the schizophrenia spectrum.
    3. Symptoms within the schizophrenia spectrum are directly attributable to toxins.
    4. Degree of severity of the schizophrenia spectrum is determined by the duration of psychotic symptoms.
    5. Schizophrenia spectrum disorders can carry the additional specification of *with catatonic features*.

12. A student nurse is assessing a 20-year-old client who is experiencing auditory hallucinations. The student states, "I believe the client has schizophrenia." Which of the following instructor responses is the most appropriate? **Select all that apply.**
    1. "How long has the client experienced these symptoms?"
    2. "Has the client taken any drug or medication that could cause these symptoms?"
    3. "It is not within your scope of practice to assess for a medical diagnosis."
    4. "Does this client have any mood problems?"
    5. "What kind of relationships has this client established?"

13. A 21-year-old client, being treated for asthma with a steroid medication, has been experiencing delusions of persecution and disorganized thinking for the past 6 months. Which factor may rule out a diagnosis of schizophrenia?
    1. The client has experienced signs and symptoms for only 6 months.
    2. The client must hear voices to be diagnosed with schizophrenia.
    3. The client's age is not typical for this diagnosis.
    4. The client is receiving medication that could lead to thought disturbances.

14. A client is brought to the emergency department after being found wandering the streets and talking to unseen others. Which situation is further evidence of a diagnosis of schizophrenia for this client?
    1. The client exhibits a developmental disorder, such as autism spectrum disorder.
    2. The client has a medical condition that could contribute to the symptoms.
    3. The client experiences manic or depressive signs and symptoms.
    4. The client's signs and symptoms last for 6 months.

15. A client on an inpatient psychiatric unit refuses to take medications because "the pill has a special code written on it that will make it poisonous." What kind of delusion is this client experiencing?
    1. An erotomanic delusion.
    2. A grandiose delusion.
    3. A persecutory delusion.
    4. A somatic delusion.

16. The nurse is performing an admission assessment on a client diagnosed with schizophrenia who is experiencing paranoid thinking. To receive the most accurate assessment information, which should the nurse consider?
    1. This client will be able to make a significant contribution to history data collection.
    2. Data will need to be gained by reviewing old records and, with permission, talking with family.
    3. This client's assessment will be easy because of the consistent nature of the symptoms.
    4. The nurse should use a very friendly approach to show empathy and to put the client at ease.

17. The nurse is interviewing a client who states, "The dentist put a filling in my tooth; I now receive transmissions that control what I think and do." The nurse accurately documents this symptom with which charting entry?
    1. "Client is experiencing a delusion of persecution."
    2. "Client is experiencing a delusion of grandeur."
    3. "Client is experiencing a somatic delusion."
    4. "Client is experiencing a delusion of influence."

18. The children's saying "Step on a crack and you break your mother's back" is an example of which type of thinking?
    1. Concrete thinking.
    2. Thinking using neologisms.
    3. Magical thinking.
    4. Thinking using clang associations.

19. The nurse is assessing a client diagnosed with schizophrenia. The client states, "We wanted to take the bus, but the airport took all the traffic." Which charting entry accurately documents this symptom?
    1. "The client is experiencing associative looseness."
    2. "The client is attempting to communicate by the use of word salad."
    3. "The client is experiencing delusional thinking."
    4. "The client is experiencing an illusion involving planes."

20. The nurse reports that a client diagnosed with schizophrenia is experiencing religiosity. Which client statement would confirm this finding?
    1. "I see Jesus in my bathroom."
    2. "I read the Bible every hour so that I will know what to do next."
    3. "I have no heart. I'm dead and in heaven today."
    4. "I can't read my Bible because the CIA has poisoned the pages."

21. The nurse states, "It's time for lunch." A client diagnosed with schizophrenia responds, "It's time for lunch, lunch, lunch." Which type of communication process is the client using, and what is the underlying reason for its use?
    1. Echopraxia, which is an attempt to identify with the person speaking.
    2. Echolalia, which is an attempt to acquire a sense of self and identity.
    3. Unconscious identification to reinforce weak ego boundaries.
    4. Depersonalization to stabilize self-identity.

22. Clients diagnosed with schizophrenia may have difficulty knowing where their ego boundaries end and others' begin. Which client behavior reflects this deficit?
    1. The client eats only prepackaged food.
    2. The client believes that family members are adding poison to food.
    3. The client looks for actual animals when others state, "It's raining cats and dogs."
    4. The client imitates other people's physical movements.

23. The nurse documents that a client diagnosed with schizophrenia is expressing a flat affect. What is an example of this symptom?
    1. The client laughs when told of the death of their parent.
    2. The client sits alone and does not interact with others.
    3. The client exhibits no emotional expression.
    4. The client experiences no emotional feelings.

24. Which client is most likely to benefit from group therapy?
    1. A client diagnosed with schizophrenia being followed up in an outpatient clinic.
    2. A client diagnosed with schizophrenia newly admitted to an inpatient unit for stabilization.
    3. A client experiencing an exacerbation of the signs and symptoms of schizophrenia.
    4. A client diagnosed with schizophrenia who is not adherent with antipsychotic medications.

25. In the United States, which diagnosis has the lowest percentage of occurrence?
    1. Major depressive disorder.
    2. Generalized anxiety disorder.
    3. Obsessive-compulsive disorder.
    4. Schizophrenia.

Nursing Process—Diagnosis

26. A client who is hearing and seeing things others do not is brought to the emergency department. Laboratory values indicate a sodium level of 160 mEq/L. Which nursing diagnosis would take priority?
    1. Altered thought processes R/T low blood sodium levels.
    2. Altered communication processes R/T altered thought processes.
    3. Risk for impaired tissue integrity R/T dry oral mucous membranes.
    4. Imbalanced fluid volume R/T increased serum sodium levels.

27. A client diagnosed with schizophrenia is experiencing anhedonia. Which nursing diagnosis addresses the client's problem that this symptom may generate?
    1. Disturbed thought processes.
    2. Disturbed sensory perception.
    3. Risk for suicide.
    4. Impaired verbal communication.

28. A client diagnosed with a thought disorder is experiencing clang associations. Which nursing diagnosis reflects this client's problem?
    1. Impaired verbal communication.
    2. Risk for violence.
    3. Ineffective health maintenance.
    4. Disturbed sensory perception.

29. A disheveled client diagnosed with schizophrenia has body odor and halitosis. Which nursing diagnosis reflects this client's current problem?
    1. Social isolation.
    2. Impaired home maintenance.
    3. Interrupted family processes.
    4. Self-care deficit.

30. A client's family is having a difficult time accepting the client's diagnosis of schizophrenia, and this has led to family conflict. Which nursing diagnosis reflects this problem?
    1. Impaired home maintenance.
    2. Interrupted family processes.
    3. Social isolation.
    4. Disturbed thought processes.

31. A client diagnosed with schizophrenia who is experiencing paranoid thinking tells the nurse about three previous suicide attempts. Which nursing diagnosis would take priority and reflect this client's problem?
    1. Disturbed thought processes.
    2. Risk for suicide.
    3. Violence: directed toward others.
    4. Risk for altered sensory perception.

32. A client has the nursing diagnosis of impaired home maintenance R/T regression. Which behavior confirms this diagnosis?
    1. The client fails to take antipsychotic medications.
    2. The client states, "I haven't bathed in a week."
    3. The client lives in an unsafe and unclean environment.
    4. The client states, "You can't draw my blood without crayons."

Nursing Process—Planning

33. Which outcome should the nurse expect from a client with a nursing diagnosis of social isolation?
    1. The client will recognize distortions of reality by day 4.
    2. The client will use appropriate verbal communication when interacting by day 3.
    3. The client will actively participate in unit activities by discharge.
    4. The client will rate anxiety as 5/10 by discharge.

34. Which outcome should the nurse expect from a client diagnosed with schizophrenia who is hearing and seeing things others do not hear and see?
    1. The client will recognize distortions of reality by discharge.
    2. The client will demonstrate the ability to trust by day 2.
    3. The client will recognize delusional thinking by day 3.
    4. The client will experience no auditory hallucinations by discharge.

35. A client admitted to an inpatient setting has not been adherent with antipsychotic medications prescribed for schizophrenia. Which outcome related to this client's problem should the nurse expect the client to achieve?
    1. The client will maintain anxiety at a reasonable level by day 2.
    2. The client will take antipsychotic medications by discharge.
    3. The client will communicate to staff any paranoid thoughts by day 3.
    4. The client will take responsibility for self-care by day 4.

36. A client taking olanzapine has a nursing diagnosis of altered sensory perception R/T command hallucinations. Which outcome would be appropriate for this client's problem?
    1. The client will verbalize feelings related to depression and suicidal ideations.
    2. The client will limit caloric intake because of the side effect of weight gain.
    3. The client will notify staff members of bothersome hallucinations.
    4. The client will tell staff members if experiencing thoughts of self-harm.

Nursing Process—Implementation

37. An unhoused client, diagnosed with schizophrenia, is seen in the mental health clinic complaining of insects infesting arms and legs. Which intervention should the nurse implement first?
    1. Check the client for body lice.
    2. Present reality regarding somatic delusions.
    3. Explain the origin of persecutory delusions.
    4. Refer for inpatient hospitalization because of substance-induced psychosis.

38. A client states to the nurse, "I see headless people walking down the hall at night." Which nursing response is appropriate?
   1. "What makes you think there are headless people here?"
   2. "Let's think about this. A headless person would not be able to walk down the hall."
   3. "It must be frightening. I realize this is real to you, but I see no headless people."
   4. "I don't see those people you are talking about."

39. A client with a nursing diagnosis of disturbed thought processes has an expected outcome of recognizing delusional thinking. Which intervention would the nurse first implement to address this problem?
   1. Reinforce and focus on reality.
   2. Appreciate that the client has experienced disturbing delusional thinking.
   3. Indicate that the nurse does not share the belief.
   4. Present logical information to refute the delusional thinking.

40. A client is in the active phase of schizophrenia and is experiencing paranoid thinking. Which nursing intervention would aid in facilitating other interventions?
   1. Assign consistent staff members.
   2. Convey acceptance of the client's delusional belief.
   3. Help the client understand that anxiety causes paranoid thinking.
   4. Encourage participation in group activities.

41. A client newly admitted to an inpatient psychiatric unit is scanning the environment continuously. Which nursing intervention is most appropriate to address this client's behavior?
   1. Offer self to build a therapeutic relationship with the client.
   2. Assist the client in formulating a plan of action for discharge.
   3. Involve the family in discussions about dealing with the client's behaviors.
   4. Reinforce the need for medication adherence on discharge.

42. Which interaction is most reflective of an appropriate psychotherapeutic approach when interacting with a client diagnosed with schizophrenia?
   1. The nurse should exhibit exaggerated warmth to counteract client loneliness.
   2. The nurse should profess friendship to decrease social isolation.
   3. The nurse should attempt closeness with the client to decrease suspiciousness.
   4. The nurse should establish a relationship by respecting the client's dignity.

43. The nurse is educating the family members of a client diagnosed with schizophrenia about the effects of psychotherapy. Which statement should be included in the teaching plan?
   1. "Psychotherapy is a short-term intervention that is usually successful."
   2. "Much patience is required during psychotherapy because clients often relapse."
   3. "Major changes in client symptoms can be attributed to immediate psychotherapy."
   4. "Independent functioning can be gained by immediate psychotherapy."

44. A client diagnosed with schizoid personality disorder asks the nurse in the mental health clinic, "Does this mean I will get schizophrenia?" What nursing response would be most appropriate?
   1. "Does that possibility upset you?"
   2. "Not all clients diagnosed with schizoid personality disorders progress to schizophrenia."
   3. "Few clients diagnosed with schizophrenia show evidence of early personality changes."
   4. "What do you know about schizophrenia?"

45. Which intervention used for clients diagnosed with schizophrenia is a behavioral therapy approach?
   1. Offer opportunities for learning about psychotropic medications.
   2. Attach consequences to adaptive and maladaptive behaviors.
   3. Establish trust within a relationship.
   4. Encourage discussions of feelings related to delusions.

46. Which intervention used for clients diagnosed with schizophrenia is a milieu therapy approach?
    1. Assist family in dealing with life stressors caused by interactions with the client.
    2. Engage in one-to-one interactions to discuss family dynamics.
    3. Role-play to enhance motor and interpersonal skills.
    4. Emphasize the rules and expectations of social interactions mediated by peer pressure.

Nursing Process—Evaluation

47. Which of the following clients have the greatest chances of positive prognoses after being diagnosed with schizophrenia? **Select all that apply.**
    1. A client diagnosed at age 35.
    2. A male client experiencing a gradual onset of signs and symptoms.
    3. A female client whose signs and symptoms began after a rape.
    4. A client who has a family history of schizophrenia.
    5. A client who has a family history of a mood disorder diagnosis.

48. The nurse is teaching a client diagnosed with schizophreniform disorder about what may affect a good prognosis. Which of the following features should the nurse include? **Select all that apply.**
    1. Confusion and perplexity at the height of the psychotic episode.
    2. Good premorbid social and occupational functioning.
    3. Absence of blunted or flat affect.
    4. Predominance of negative symptoms.
    5. Onset of psychotic symptoms within 4 weeks of noticeable behavioral change.

49. Which symptom experienced by a client diagnosed with schizophrenia would predict a less positive prognosis?
    1. Hearing hostile voices.
    2. Thinking the TV is controlling their behavior.
    3. Continuously repeating what has been said.
    4. Having little or no interest in work or social activities.

50. The nurse is educating the family of a client diagnosed with schizophrenia about the importance of medication adherence. Which statement indicates that learning has occurred?
    1. "After stabilization, the relapse rate is high, even if antipsychotic medications are taken regularly."
    2. "My brother will have only about a 30% chance of relapse if he takes his medications consistently."
    3. "Because the disease is multifaceted, taking antipsychotic medications has little effect on relapse rates."
    4. "Because schizophrenia is a chronic disease, taking antipsychotic medications has little effect on relapse rates."

Psychopharmacology

51. The nurse documents that a client diagnosed with schizophrenia is experiencing anticholinergic side effects from long-term use of thioridazine. Which symptoms has the nurse noted?
    1. Akinesia, dystonia, and pseudoparkinsonism.
    2. Muscle rigidity, hyperpyrexia, and tachycardia.
    3. Hyperglycemia and diabetes.
    4. Dry mouth, constipation, and urinary retention.

52. A client has a history of schizophrenia, controlled by haloperidol. During an assessment, the nurse notes continuous restlessness. Which medication would the nurse expect the physician to prescribe for this client?
    1. Haloperidol.
    2. Fluphenazine decanoate.
    3. Clozapine.
    4. Benztropine mesylate.

53. A client diagnosed with schizrenia takes clozapine 200 mg daily. Laboratory results reveal RBC 4.7 million/mcL, ANC 800/mcL, and TSH 1.3 mIU/L. Which of the following would the nurse expect the physician to order?
    1. Levothyroxine sodium 150 mcg daily.
    2. Ferrous sulfate 100 mg tid.
    3. Discontinue clozapine.
    4. Discontinue clozapine and start levothyroxine sodium 150 mcg daily.

54. The nurse is discussing the side effects experienced by a female client taking antipsychotic medications. The client states, "I haven't had a period in 4 months." Which client teaching should the nurse include in the plan of care?
    1. Antipsychotic medications can cause a decreased libido.
    2. Antipsychotic medications can interfere with the effectiveness of birth control.
    3. Antipsychotic medications can cause amenorrhea, but ovulation still occurs.
    4. Antipsychotic medications can decrease red blood cells, leading to amenorrhea.

55. For the past year, a client has received haloperidol. The nurse administering the client's next dose notes a twitch on the right side of the client's face and tongue movements. Which nursing intervention takes priority?
    1. Give haloperidol and benztropine 1 mg IM prn per order.
    2. Assess for other signs of hyperglycemia resulting from the use of the haloperidol.
    3. Check the client's temperature and assess mental status.
    4. Hold the haloperidol and call the physician.

56. A client has been prescribed ziprasidone 40 mg bid. Which of the following interventions are important related to this medication? **Select all that apply**.
    1. Obtain a baseline electrocardiogram (EKG) initially and periodically throughout treatment.
    2. Teach the client to take the medication with meals.
    3. Monitor the client's pulse because of the possibility of palpitations.
    4. Institute seizure precautions and monitor closely.
    5. Watch for signs and symptoms of a manic episode.

57. A client prescribed quetiapine 50 mg bid has a nursing diagnosis of risk for injury R/T sedation. Which nursing intervention appropriately addresses this client's problem?
    1. Assess for homicidal and suicidal ideations.
    2. Remove clutter from the environment to prevent injury.
    3. Monitor orthostatic changes in pulse or blood pressure.
    4. Evaluate for auditory and visual hallucinations.

58. A client is newly prescribed hydroxyzine 50 mg qhs and clozapine 25 mg bid. Which is an appropriate nursing diagnosis for this client?
    1. Risk for injury R/T serotonin syndrome.
    2. Risk for injury R/T possible seizure.
    3. Risk for injury R/T clozapine toxicity.
    4. Risk for injury R/T depressed mood.

59. Which atypical antipsychotic medication has the highest potential for a client to experience serious side effects?
    1. Haloperidol.
    2. Chlorpromazine.
    3. Risperidone.
    4. Clozapine.

60. A woman is prescribed risperidone 1 mg bid. At her 3-month follow-up, the client states, "I knew it was a possible side effect, but I can't believe I am not getting my period anymore." Which is a priority teaching need?
    1. "Sometimes amenorrhea is a temporary side effect of medications and should resolve itself."
    2. "I am sure this was very scary for you. How long has it been since your last menstrual cycle?"
    3. "Although your menstrual cycles have stopped, there is still a potential for you to become pregnant."
    4. "Maybe the amenorrhea is not due to your medication. Have your menstrual cycles been regular in the past?"

61. A client is exhibiting sedation, auditory hallucinations, dystonia, and grandiosity. The client is prescribed haloperidol 5 mg tid and trihexyphenidyl 4 mg bid. Which statement about these medications is accurate?
    1. Trihexyphenidyl would assist the client with sedation.
    2. Trihexyphenidyl would assist the client with auditory hallucinations.
    3. Haloperidol would assist the client in decreasing grandiosity.
    4. Haloperidol would assist the client with dystonia.

62. A client is prescribed aripiprazole 10 mg a.m. daily. The client complains of sedation and dizziness. Vital signs reveal B/P 100/60 mm Hg, pulse 80, respiration rate 20, and temperature 97.4°F. Which nursing diagnosis takes priority?
    1. Risk for nonadherence R/T irritating side effects.
    2. Knowledge deficit R/T new medication prescribed.
    3. Risk for injury R/T orthostatic hypotension.
    4. Activity intolerance R/T dizziness and drowsiness.

63. A client recently prescribed fluphenazine complains to the nurse of severe muscle spasms. On examination, heart rate is 110, blood pressure is 160/92 mm Hg, and temperature is 101.5°F. Which nursing intervention takes priority?
    1. Check the chart for a prn order of benztropine mesylate because of increased extrapyramidal symptoms.
    2. Hold the next dose of fluphenazine and call the physician immediately to report the findings.
    3. Schedule an examination with the client's physician to evaluate cardiovascular function.
    4. Ask the client about any recreational drug use and ask the physician to order a drug screen.

64. Lithium carbonate is to mania as clozapine is to:
    1. Anxiety.
    2. Depression.
    3. Psychosis.
    4. Akathisia.

65. A client is prescribed risperidone 4 mg bid. After the client is caught "cheeking" medications, liquid medication is prescribed. The label reads 0.5 mg/mL. How many milliliters would be administered daily? _____ mL.

66. A client has an order for "ziprasidone 20 mg IM q4h prn for agitation with a maximum daily dose of 40 mg/day." Administration times are documented in the medication record. Which times indicate safe medication administration?
    1. 0800 and 1100.
    2. 1200, 1700, and 2100.
    3. 0900, 1200, and 2100.
    4. 1300 and 1700.

67. A client is prescribed clozapine 12.5 mg am daily and 50 mg qhs. Clozapine is available in 25-mg tablets. How many tablets would be administered daily? _____ tablets.

68. An instructor is teaching students about psychiatric medications. Which of the following antipsychotic medications need to be given with food? **Select all that apply.**
    1. Ziprasidone.
    2. Vilazodone.
    3. Lurasidone.
    4. Aripiprazole.
    5. Asenapine.

69. Which of the following medications would be given to a client, in an outpatient setting, diagnosed with schizophrenia experiencing nonadherence? **Select all that apply.**
    1. Olanzapine IM (Zyprexa Relprevv).
    2. Ziprasidone IM (Geodon IM).
    3. Haloperidol Lactate (Haldol Lactate).
    4. Aripiprazole IM (Abilify Maintena).
    5. Paliperidone IM (Invega Trinza).

70. Which of the following oral antipsychotic medications could be administered on an inpatient psychiatric unit to prevent a client from "cheeking," or hiding medication in the mouth? **Select all that apply.**
    1. Mirtazapine.
    2. Olanzapin.
    3. Paliperidone.
    4. Aripiprazole.
    5. Asenapine.

71. A client is prescribed olanzapine. Which of the following client statements indicate that teaching regarding this medication has been effective? Select all that apply.
    1. "I must stay in the facility and be monitored for 3 hours after receiving the injection."
    2. "I cannot drive for the remainder of the day."
    3. "I must register paperwork with the drug company."
    4. "I need to notify staff if I get overly tired or confused."
    5. "After my first three injections, the risk of adverse reaction decreases."

72. After taking antipsychotic medications for several months, a client begins to experience uncontrolled facial and body movements. Which of the following medications, approved by the Food and Drug Administration (FDA), would the nurse anticipate the physician to prescribe? **Select all that apply.**
    1. Benztropine.
    2. Diphenhydramine.
    3. Trihexyphenidyl.
    4. Valbenazine.
    5. Deutetrabenazine.

73. Which of the following client statements is true as it relates to treatment of tardive dyskinesia (TD)? **Select all that apply.**
    1. "My psychiatrist ordered both physical and occupational therapy to help lessen the symptoms of TD."
    2. "Unless the antipsychotic medication is discontinued, the muscle movements will continue."
    3. "The doctor ordered deutetrabenazine with my current antipsychotic to help with the twitching."
    4. "I am going to start taking valbenazine daily to stop the muscle movements of my face and tongue."
    5. "There are no psychotropic medications used to treat muscle movements associated with TD."

The correct answer number and rationale for why it is the correct answer are given in **boldface blue type**. Rationales for why the other answer options are incorrect are given as well, but they are not in boldface type.

Theory

1. 1. Children are not typically diagnosed with schizophrenia spectrum disorder. Thought processes must be fully developed before alterations in thought can be diagnosed.
   2. **Symptoms of schizophrenia generally appear in late adolescence or early adulthood. Some studies have indicated that symptoms occur earlier in men than in women.**
   3. Although symptoms of schizophrenia can occur during middle or late adulthood, this is not typical.
   4. Although symptoms of schizophrenia can occur during middle or late adulthood, this is not typical.

   TEST-TAKING HINT: Thought processes such as magical and concrete thinking, which occur normally in childhood thought development, are not symptoms of schizophrenia. This knowledge assists the test taker in eliminating answer 1.

2. The definitive cause of schizophrenia is still uncertain. Most likely, no single factor can be implicated in the etiology; rather, the disease probably results from a combination of influences, including biological, psychological, and environmental factors.
   1. Schizophrenia is a disorder of the brain for which many physical factors of possible etiological significance have been identified. At this time, there is no cure for schizophrenia.
   2. Offspring of a parent diagnosed with schizophrenia have a 5% to 10% or higher risk of acquiring the disease. How schizophrenia is inherited is uncertain. No reliable biological marker has yet been found.
   3. With the use of neuroimaging technologies, structural brain abnormalities have been observed in individuals diagnosed with schizophrenia. Ventricular enlargement is the most consistent finding; however, sulci enlargement and cerebellar atrophy also are reported. These changes may be a

result rather than a cause of schizophrenia. The definitive cause of schizophrenia is still uncertain.
   4. **The etiology of schizophrenia remains unclear. No single theory or hypothesis has been postulated that substantiates a clear-cut etiology for this disease. The more research that is conducted, the more evidence is compiled to support the concept of multiple causes in the development of schizophrenia. The most current theory seems to be that schizophrenia is a biologically based disease with a genetic component. The onset of the disease also is influenced by factors in the internal and external environment.**

   TEST-TAKING HINT: All answers presented are possible theories for the cause of schizophrenia. To choose the correct answer, the test taker must understand that no one theory has been accepted as a definitive cause of the disease of schizophrenia.

3. 1. There is not now, and probably never will be, a single treatment that cures schizophrenia. Antipsychotic drugs, also called neuroleptics, are effective in the treatment of acute and chronic manifestations of schizophrenia and in maintenance therapy to prevent exacerbation of symptoms. The efficacy of antipsychotic drugs is enhanced by adjunct psychosocial therapy.
   2. **Effective treatment of schizophrenia requires a comprehensive, multidisciplinary effort, including pharmacotherapy and various forms of psychosocial care. Psychosocial care includes social and living skills training, rehabilitation, and family therapy.**
   3. Social and living skills training is only one aspect of the treatment for schizophrenia. Psychotic manifestations of the illness may subside with the use of antipsychotic drugs. Antipsychotic drugs assist clients in being more cooperative with the psychosocial therapies that help the client fit into society.
   4. Group and family therapy is only one aspect of the treatment for schizophrenia. Psychotic manifestations of the illness may subside with the use of antipsychotic drugs. Antipsychotic drugs assist clients in being more cooperative with the psychosocial therapies that increase socialization skills.

TEST-TAKING HINT: All answers presented are possible interventions that support various theories for the causation of schizophrenia. To choose the correct answer, the test taker must understand that no one intervention has been accepted as a definitive treatment for the disease of schizophrenia. Pharmacotherapy coupled with psychosocial therapies has been recognized as the most effective approach to controlling the symptoms of schizophrenia.

4. When one fraternal (dizygotic) twin has been diagnosed with schizophrenia, the other twin has approximately a **15%** chance of developing the disease.

TEST-TAKING HINT: To answer this question correctly, the test taker must review the statistics of twin studies related to the development of schizophrenia. The keyword *fraternal* determines the correct percentage.

5. When one identical (monozygotic) twin has been diagnosed with schizophrenia, the other twin has approximately a **50%** chance of developing the disease.

TEST-TAKING HINT: To answer this question correctly, the test taker must review the statistics of twin studies related to the development of schizophrenia. The keyword *identical* determines the correct percentage.

6. 1. Research indicates that children born of parents without schizophrenia and raised by parents diagnosed with schizophrenia do not seem to suffer more often from the disease than the general population.
   2. **The dopamine hypothesis suggests that schizophrenia may be caused by an excess of dopamine-dependent neuronal activity in the brain. This excess activity may be related to increased production, or release, of the substance at nerve terminals; increased receptor sensitivity; too many dopamine receptors; or a combination of these mechanisms. This etiological theory is from a biochemical influence perspective.**
   3. Research has shown a higher incidence of schizophrenia after prenatal exposure to influenza. This theory of the etiology of schizophrenia is from a physiological, not biochemical influence, perspective.
   4. Poor parent-child interaction and dysfunctional family systems do not cause schizophrenia. Stress in a family system may precipitate symptoms in an individual who possesses a genetic vulnerability to schizophrenia.

TEST-TAKING HINT: The test taker must note the keyword *biochemical*. There are numerous etiological theories for schizophrenia, but the question is asking for a biochemical perspective. A neurochemical perspective would relate to a neurochemical imbalance, such as an increased level of dopamine. A physiological perspective would include functional and structural abnormalities.

Nursing Process—Assessment

7. 1. Clients diagnosed with schizoid personality disorder do not typically experience delusions and hallucinations. Not all individuals who demonstrate the characteristics of schizoid personality disorder progress to schizophrenia, but most individuals diagnosed with schizophrenia show evidence of the characteristics of schizoid personality disorder premorbidly.
   2. **Individuals diagnosed with schizoid personality disorder are indifferent to social relationships and have a very limited range of emotional experience and expression. They do not enjoy close relationships and prefer to be loners. They appear cold and aloof. Not all individuals who demonstrate the characteristics of schizoid personality disorder progress to schizophrenia, but most individuals diagnosed with schizophrenia show evidence of the characteristics of schizoid personality disorder premorbidly, putting them at high risk for schizophrenia.**
   3. Individuals diagnosed with schizoid personality disorder are typically indifferent to social relationships, but this diagnosis puts them at high, not low, risk for a later diagnosis of schizophrenia.
   4. Individuals diagnosed with schizoid personality disorder are typically loners who appear cold and aloof, but this diagnosis puts them at high, not low, risk for a later diagnosis of schizophrenia.

TEST-TAKING HINT: To answer this question correctly, the test taker must realize that if one part of an answer is incorrect, the entire answer is incorrect. In answer 1, the first part of the answer is incorrect, eliminating this as a correct choice. In answers 3 and 4, the second part of the answer is incorrect, eliminating these choices.

8. 1. Personality in the premorbid development phase of schizophrenia often exhibits social maladjustment, social

withdrawal, irritability, and antagonist thoughts and behaviors. **Behavioral measurements that have been noted include being very shy and withdrawn, having poor peer relationships, and doing poorly in school.**

2. Characteristics of the prodromal phase include social withdrawal; impairment in role functioning; eccentric behaviors; neglect of personal hygiene and grooming; blunted or inappropriate affect; disturbances in communication; bizarre ideas; unusual perceptual experiences; and lack of initiative, interests, or energy. The length of this phase varies; it may last for many years before progressing to schizophrenia. The symptoms presented in the question are not reflective of the prodromal phase of the development of schizophrenia.

3. In the active phase of schizophrenia, psychotic symptoms are prominent. Two or more of the following symptoms must be present for a significant portion of time during a 1-month period: delusions, hallucinations, disorganized speech, grossly disorganized or catatonic behavior, and negative symptoms (affective flattening, alogia, or avolition). The client in the question does not present with these symptoms.

4. Schizophrenia is characterized by periods of remission and exacerbation. A residual phase usually follows an active phase of the illness. Symptoms during the residual phase are similar to those of the prodromal phase, with flat affect and impairment in role function being prominent. There is no indication in the question that the client has recently experienced an active phase of schizophrenia.

TEST-TAKING HINT: Understanding the relationship of inherited risk for the development of schizophrenia and the phases of its development will assist the test taker in choosing the correct answer to this question.

9. 1. It is important for the nurse to know if this client has recently experienced an active phase of schizophrenia to distinguish the symptoms presented as indications of the prodromal or residual phase of schizophrenia. Schizophrenia is characterized by periods of remission and exacerbation. A residual phase usually follows an active phase of the illness. Symptoms during the residual phase are similar to those of the prodromal phase, with flat affect and impairment in role function being prominent.

2. Duration of symptoms is a criterion for the diagnosis of schizophrenia, but this knowledge does not help the nurse determine whether this client is in the prodromal or residual phase of schizophrenia.

3. It is important to rule out schizoaffective and mood disorders when determining the diagnosis of schizophrenia, but this knowledge does not help the nurse determine whether this client is in the prodromal or residual phase of schizophrenia.

4. If there is a history of an autism spectrum disorder or another pervasive developmental disorder, the additional diagnosis of schizophrenia is made only if prominent delusions or hallucinations also are present for at least 1 month. This determination must be made before diagnosing the client with schizophrenia, but this knowledge does not help the nurse determine whether this client is in the prodromal or residual phase of schizophrenia.

TEST-TAKING HINT: This question is asking for the test taker to determine whether the client is in the prodromal or residual phase. Only answer 1 deals with this distinction. All other answers are important information related to the client's meeting the criteria for a diagnosis of schizophrenia, but these answers do not deal with phase distinction.

10. 1. Catalepsy is the passive induction of a posture held against gravity. It is a diagnostic criterion for a catatonia specifier to the diagnosis of schizophrenia.

2. **Waxy flexibility is a condition by which the individual diagnosed with schizophrenia passively yields all movable parts of the body to any efforts made at placing them in certain positions. It is a diagnostic criterion for a catatonia specifier to the diagnosis of schizophrenia.**

3. Pressured speech is a tendency to speak rapidly and frenziedly, as if motivated by an urgency not apparent to the listener. Mutism (no, or very little, verbal responses), not pressured speech, is a diagnostic criterion for a catatonia specifier to the diagnosis of schizophrenia.

4. **Posturing is the spontaneous and active maintenance of a posture against gravity. It is a diagnostic criterion for a catatonia specifier to the diagnosis of schizophrenia.**

5. **Stereotypy is repetitive, abnormally frequent, non-goal-directed movements. It is a diagnostic criterion for a catatonia specifier to the diagnosis of schizophrenia.**

TEST-TAKING HINT: The test taker must review the diagnostic criteria for a catatonia specifier in order to answer this question correctly.

11. 1. It is accurate that the degree of severity of the schizophrenia spectrum is determined by the number of psychotic symptoms.
    2. It is accurate that schizotypal personality disorder initiates the schizophrenia spectrum.
    3. Symptoms within the schizophrenia spectrum should not be directly attributable to toxins.
    4. It is accurate that the degree of severity of the schizophrenia spectrum is determined by the duration of psychotic symptoms.
    5. It is accurate that schizophrenia spectrum disorders can carry the additional specification of *with catatonic features*.

TEST-TAKING HINT: The test taker must recognize that schizophrenia is a spectrum of disorders that is organized to reflect a gradient of psychopathology from least to most severe.

12. 1. The duration of symptoms is an important assessment finding to determine the diagnosis of schizophrenia. One diagnostic criterion for this diagnosis is that symptoms need to be present for a significant amount of time during a 1-month period and last for 6 months.
    2. The use of a substance may rule out the diagnosis of schizophrenia. One diagnostic criterion for this diagnosis is that the presenting symptoms are not due to the direct physiological effects of the use or abuse of a substance or medication.
    3. Even though nurses do not diagnose medical conditions such as schizophrenia, nurses must assess the signs and symptoms that meet the criteria for this diagnosis. This assists the nurse in the implementation of appropriate nursing interventions based on client problems.
    4. The presence of mood disorders is an important finding to assess to determine the diagnosis of schizophrenia. Schizoaffective disorder, depressive disorder with psychotic features, and bipolar disorder with psychotic features must be ruled out for the client to meet the criteria for this diagnosis. No major depressive, manic, or mixed episodes should have occurred concurrently with the active-phase symptoms.

If mood episodes have occurred during the active-phase symptoms, their total duration should have been brief, relative to the duration of the active and residual periods.

   5. The ability to form relationships is an important finding to assess to determine the diagnosis of schizophrenia. One diagnostic criterion for this diagnosis is a disturbance in one or more major areas of functioning, such as work, interpersonal relationships, or self-care. When the onset is in adolescence, there should be a failure to achieve expected levels of interpersonal or academic functioning.

TEST-TAKING HINT: To answer this question correctly, the test taker must be familiar with the diagnostic criteria for the diagnosis of schizophrenia.

13. 1. The client in the question has experienced two symptoms for a 6-month period; therefore, the diagnosis of schizophrenia cannot be ruled out. The diagnostic criteria for the diagnosis of schizophrenia state that two or more symptoms of the disease must be present for a significant amount of time during a 1-month period and last for 6 months.
    2. This client is not experiencing auditory hallucinations, but this in itself does not rule out the diagnosis of schizophrenia. Although auditory hallucinations are classic symptoms of schizophrenia, other symptoms also may lead to the diagnosis. Delusions, disorganized speech, grossly disorganized or catatonic behavior, affective flattening, alogia, and avolition are other symptoms that can occur.
    3. Symptoms of schizophrenia generally appear in late adolescence or early adulthood. The client described falls within this age range; therefore, schizophrenia cannot be ruled out.
    4. Steroid medications could precipitate the thought disorders experienced by the client and potentially rule out the diagnosis of schizophrenia. According to the diagnostic criteria for this diagnosis, the thought disturbance cannot be due to the direct physiological effects of a substance.

TEST-TAKING HINT: To answer this question correctly, the test taker must be familiar with the diagnostic criteria for the diagnosis of schizophrenia. This question asks what would potentially eliminate the diagnosis of schizophrenia; the test taker should look for incorrect or inappropriate criteria.

14. 1. A history of a developmental disorder would not be further evidence for a diagnosis of schizophrenia. If there is a history of an autism spectrum disorder or another pervasive developmental disorder, the additional diagnosis of schizophrenia is made only if prominent delusions or hallucinations also are present for at least 1 month. This determination must be made before making the diagnosis of schizophrenia.

2. The presence of a medical condition that contributes to the client's signs and symptoms of schizophrenia is not further evidence of this diagnosis. To meet the criteria for a diagnosis of schizophrenia, the client's symptoms must not be due to the direct physiological effects of a general medical condition.

3. Experiencing manic or depressive signs and symptoms is not further evidence for the diagnosis of schizophrenia. Schizoaffective, depressive, and bipolar disorders must be excluded for the client to meet the criteria for this diagnosis.

4. **The client's signs and symptoms lasting for 6 months is further evidence for the diagnosis of schizophrenia. Two or more characteristic symptoms must be present for a significant amount of time during a 1-month period and must last for 6 months to meet the criteria for the diagnosis of schizophrenia.**

TEST-TAKING HINT: To answer this question correctly, the test taker must be familiar with the diagnostic criteria for the diagnosis of schizophrenia. This question asks what would contribute to the diagnosis of schizophrenia; the test taker should look for correct and appropriate criteria.

15. 1. An erotomanic delusion is a type of delusion in which the individual believes that someone, usually of higher status, is in love with them. The situation described in the question does not reflect this type of delusion.

2. A grandiose delusion is a type of delusion in which the individual has an irrational idea regarding self-worth, talent, knowledge, or power. The situation described in the question does not reflect this type of delusion.

3. **A persecutory delusion is a type of delusion in which the individual believes they are being malevolently treated in some way. Frequent themes include being conspired against, cheated, spied**
on, followed, poisoned or drugged, maliciously maligned, harassed, or obstructed in the pursuit of long-term goals. The situation described in the question reflects this type of delusion.

4. A somatic delusion is a type of delusion in which individuals believe they have some sort of physical defect, disorder, or disease. The situation described in the question does not reflect this type of delusion.

TEST-TAKING HINT: The root word of *persecutory* is *persecute*, which means "to afflict or harass constantly so as to injure or distress." Knowing the definition of persecute should assist the test taker in choosing the correct answer.

16. 1. Clients experiencing paranoid thinking are seldom able to make a significant contribution to their history because of thought disorders, altered perceptions, and communication problems.

2. **Background assessment information must be gathered from numerous sources, including old records and, with permission, family members. A client in an acute episode who is experiencing paranoid thinking would be unable to provide accurate and insightful assessment information because of deficits in communication and thought.**

3. Assessment of a client diagnosed with schizophrenia is a complex, not simple, process. The nurse must gather as much information as possible to gain a total symptomatic clinical picture of the client. This is difficult because of the client's thought and communication deficits.

4. A client experiencing paranoid thinking has problems with trust. An overly friendly approach is often misinterpreted as an attempt at manipulation.

TEST-TAKING HINT: The test taker must understand client limitations when active signs and symptoms of schizophrenia are present. This knowledge helps the test taker to recognize the need to use other sources to obtain assessment information.

17. 1. A delusion of persecution occurs when a client feels threatened and believes that others intend harm or persecution. The statement of the client is not reflective of a delusion of persecution.

2. A delusion of grandeur occurs when a client has an exaggerated feeling of importance, power, knowledge, or identity. The statement of the client is not reflective of a delusion of grandeur.

3. A somatic delusion occurs when a client has a false idea about the functioning of their body. The statement of the client is not reflective of a somatic delusion.

4. **A delusion of influence or control occurs when a client believes certain objects or persons have control over their behavior. The statement of the client is reflective of a delusion of influence.**

TEST-TAKING HINT: To answer this question correctly, the test taker must understand the definition of the various types of delusions and be able to recognize these delusions in the statements and behaviors of clients.

18. 1. Concrete thinking is a literal interpretation of the environment. It is normal during the cognitive development of childhood. When experienced by clients diagnosed with schizophrenia, it is a regression to an earlier level of cognitive development. The statement presented is not reflective of concrete thinking.

2. A neologism is the invention of new words that are meaningless to others but have symbolic meaning to the individual experiencing psychosis. The statement presented is not reflective of a neologism.

3. **Magical thinking occurs when the individual believes that their thoughts or behaviors have control over specific situations or people. It is commonly seen during cognitive development in childhood. The statement presented is an example of magical thinking.**

4. A clang association is a choice of words that is governed by sounds. Clang associations often take the form of rhyming. An example of a clang association is "Bang, rang, sang. My cat has a fang." The statement presented is not reflective of a clang association.

TEST-TAKING HINT: There are many terms related to the symptoms experienced by clients diagnosed with schizophrenia. To answer this type of question, the test taker must understand the meaning of these terms and recognize examples of these symptoms.

19. 1. **Associative looseness is thinking characterized by speech in which ideas shift from one unrelated subject to another. The client is unaware that the topics are not connected. The client statement is an example of associative looseness.**

2. Word salad is a group of words that are strung together in a random fashion without any logical connection. The client

statement presented is not an example of word salad.

3. Delusions are false personal beliefs that are inconsistent with the client's cultural background. The client statement presented is not an example of a delusion.

4. Illusions are misperceptions or misinterpretations of real external stimuli. The client statement presented is not an example of an illusion.

TEST-TAKING HINT: The concepts of *loose associations* and *word salad* can be confused because there is disconnection of meaning in both. The test taker needs to understand that when looseness of association is present, phrases may be understood, but their meaning is not linked. In word salad, words are isolated, and no meaning is communicated.

20. 1. The statement "I see Jesus in my bathroom" is an example of a visual hallucination. A visual hallucination is a false visual perception not associated with real external stimuli. This is not an example of religiosity.

2. **The statement "I read the Bible every hour so that I will know what to do next" is evidence of the symptom of religiosity. Religiosity is an excessive demonstration of, or obsession with, religious ideas and behavior. The client may use religious ideas in an attempt to provide rational meaning and structure to behavior.**

3. The statement "I have no heart. I'm dead and in heaven today" is evidence of a nihilistic delusion. A nihilistic delusion is a false idea that the self, a part of the self, others, or the world is nonexistent.

4. The statement "I can't read my Bible because the CIA has poisoned the pages" is evidence of a paranoid delusion. Individuals experiencing paranoia have extreme suspiciousness of others, of their actions, or of their perceived intentions.

TEST-TAKING HINT: The test taker should not confuse the theme of a visual hallucination, which is a false perception, with the delusion or false belief of religiosity. Even though the client in the question sees a religious figure, the client is experiencing a visual hallucination, not religiosity.

21. 1. When clients purposely imitate movements made by others, they are exhibiting echopraxia. The behaviors presented in the question are not reflective of echopraxia.

2. **When clients diagnosed with schizophrenia repeat words that they hear,**

they are exhibiting echolalia. This is an indication of alterations in the client's sense of self. Weak ego boundaries cause these clients to lack feelings of uniqueness. Echolalia is an attempt to identify with the person speaking.

3. Unconscious identification is an ego defense mechanism used by clients diagnosed with schizophrenia in an attempt to strengthen ego boundaries. The need to imitate the actions or physical characteristics of others is a result of their confusion with self-identity. The behaviors presented in the question are not reflective of unconscious identification. When a psychiatrist grows a beard and smokes a cigar in an attempt to emulate Sigmund Freud, the psychiatrist is exhibiting unconscious identification.

4. When clients diagnosed with schizophrenia experience feelings of unreality, they are exhibiting depersonalization. The client may have a sense of observing themself from a distance or thinking that parts of their body may have changed in size. The behaviors presented in the question are not reflective of depersonalization.

TEST-TAKING HINT: The test taker needs to understand that all parts of an answer must be correct. In this question, all answer choices include correct reasons for the use of various defenses. Only answer 2, however, correctly identifies the echolalia presented in the question.

22. 1. A client's eating only prepackaged foods is a behavior that reflects paranoid thinking. Individuals experiencing this type of thinking have extreme suspiciousness of others and of their actions or intentions. Paranoid thinking is not indicative of problems with ego boundaries.

2. Believing that their family members are adding poison to food is an example of delusions of persecution. Experiencing delusions of persecution does not reflect that the client has difficulty knowing where their ego boundaries end and others' begin.

3. When clients look for actual animals when others state, "It's raining cats and dogs," they are experiencing concrete thinking. Concreteness, or literal interpretations of the environment, represents a regression to an earlier level of cognitive development. Concrete thinking does not indicate that the client has difficulty knowing where their ego boundaries end and others' begin.

4. When clients imitate other people's physical movements, they are experiencing echopraxia. The behavior of echopraxia is an indication of alterations in the client's sense of self. These clients have difficulty knowing where their ego boundaries end and others' begin. Weak ego boundaries cause these clients to lack feelings of uniqueness. Echopraxia is an attempt to identify with others.

TEST-TAKING HINT: It is important to recognize the various defenses used by clients diagnosed with schizophrenia to deal with the symptoms of their disease. Alterations in thought such as paranoia and delusions of persecution can also be experienced. The correct answer choice in this question is the symptom that reflects the client's difficulty knowing where their ego boundaries end and others' begin.

23. 1. When a client laughs when told of the death of their parent, the client is experiencing inappropriate affect. The client's emotional tone is incongruent with the circumstances. This behavior is not reflective of flat affect.

2. When clients do not interact with others, they are experiencing social isolation. This behavior is not reflective of flat affect.

3. Flat affect is described as affect devoid of emotional tone. Having no emotional expression is an indication of flat affect.

4. Even with a flat affect, the client continues to experience feelings; however, these emotions are not represented in facial expressions.

TEST-TAKING HINT: The test taker must distinguish a flat affect from the inability to feel emotions to answer this question correctly.

24. 1. Group therapy for clients diagnosed with schizophrenia has been shown to be effective, particularly in an outpatient setting and when combined with medication management.

2. Inpatient treatment usually occurs when symptoms and social disorganization are at their most intense. Because these clients experience lower functioning levels, they are not appropriate candidates for group therapy.

3. A less stimulating environment is most beneficial for clients experiencing an exacerbation of the signs and symptoms of schizophrenia. Because group therapy can be an intensive and highly stimulating environment, it may be counterproductive early in treatment.

4. Group therapy for clients diagnosed with schizophrenia has been shown to be effective when combined with medication management. Because the psychotic manifestations of the illness subside with use of antipsychotic drugs, clients are generally more cooperative with psychosocial therapies such as group therapy. Without the effects of psychotropic drugs, group therapy may not be as beneficial.

TEST-TAKING HINT: To answer this question correctly, the test taker must understand the common signs and symptoms of schizophrenia that may hinder clients from benefiting from group therapy. It also is important to realize the effect that antipsychotic medications have on the ability of these clients to participate in therapeutic groups.

25. 1. In the United States, the prevalence of major depressive disorder is approximately 17%.
    2. In the United States, the prevalence of generalized anxiety disorder is approximately 5%.
    3. In the United States, the prevalence of obsessive-compulsive disorder is approximately 3%.
    4. **In the United States, the prevalence of schizophrenia is approximately 1%. It is recorded that 1.7 million American adults are diagnosed with the brain disorder of schizophrenia.**

TEST-TAKING HINT: The test taker must differentiate among the prevalence rates of schizophrenia and other mental health disorders to answer this question correctly.

Nursing Process—Diagnosis

26. 1. The client presented in the question is experiencing altered thought processes as a result of hypernatremia, not hyponatremia. The appropriate physical condition must be corrected for the psychotic symptoms to improve.
    2. **As a result of experiencing psychotic symptoms secondary to electrolyte imbalance, this client may have impaired communication. Altered thought processes lead to an inability to communicate effectively. Correcting the physical problem, which is the priority, would improve the client's ability to communicate.**
    3. Because the client is experiencing hypernatremia, the client is at risk for impaired tissue integrity related to dry oral mucous membranes. Correcting the physical problem, which is the priority, would reduce the client's risk for impaired tissue integrity.
    4. All physiological problems must be corrected before evaluating a client experiencing symptoms of schizophrenia. In this situation, the psychotic symptoms may be related to the critically high sodium level. If the cause is physiological in nature, the nurse's priority is to assist in correcting the physiological problem. If the client's fluid volume imbalance is corrected, the psychotic symptoms, which are due to the medical condition of hypernatremia, would be eliminated, resulting in an improvement in sensory perceptual symptoms. This would improve the client's ability to communicate effectively and decrease the risk of dry mucous membranes.

TEST-TAKING HINT: To answer this question correctly, the test taker first must recognize a critically high sodium level and note the word *priority*. When choosing a priority nursing diagnosis, the test taker always must focus on the NANDA-I stem, which is the statement of the client problem, and choose the diagnosis that, if resolved, also would solve other client problems.

27. 1. Disturbed thought processes is defined as a disruption in cognitive operations and activities. An example of a disturbed thought process is a delusion. The nursing diagnosis of disturbed thought processes does not address the symptom of anhedonia.
    2. Disturbed sensory perception is defined as a change in the amount or patterning of incoming stimuli (either internally or externally initiated), accompanied by a diminished, exaggerated, distorted, or impaired response to such stimuli. An example of a disturbed sensory perception is a hallucination. The nursing diagnosis of disturbed sensory perception does not address the symptom of anhedonia.
    3. **Risk for suicide is defined as a risk for self-inflicted, life-threatening injury. The negative symptom of anhedonia is defined as the inability to experience pleasure. This is a particularly distressing symptom that generates hopelessness and compels some clients to attempt suicide.**
    4. Impaired verbal communication is defined as the decreased, delayed, or absent ability to receive, process, transmit, and use a

system of symbols. The nursing diagnosis of impaired verbal communication does not address the symptom of anhedonia.

TEST-TAKING HINT: To answer this question correctly, the test taker first must understand the definition of *anhedonia*. When this symptom of schizophrenia is understood, the test taker can discern the client problem that this distressful symptom may generate.

28. 1. Impaired verbal communication is defined as the decreased, delayed, or absent ability to receive, process, transmit, and use a system of symbols. Clang associations are choices of words that are governed by sound. Words often take the form of rhyming. An example of a clang association is "It is cold. I am bold. The gold has been sold." This type of language is an impairment to verbal communication.
   2. Risk for violence is defined as a risk for behaviors in which an individual demonstrates that they can be physically, emotionally, or sexually harmful either to self or to others. The symptom described in the question does not reflect the nursing diagnosis of risk for violence.
   3. Ineffective health maintenance is defined as the inability to identify, manage, or seek out help to maintain health. Nonadherence with antipsychotic medications is one form of ineffective health maintenance that is common in clients diagnosed with thought disorders, but there is no indication that the client described in the question has this problem.
   4. Disturbed sensory perception is defined as a change in the amount or patterning of incoming stimuli (either internally or externally initiated), accompanied by a diminished, exaggerated, distorted, or impaired response to such stimuli. An example of a disturbed sensory perception is a visual hallucination. The symptom presented in the question does not reflect the nursing diagnosis of disturbed sensory perception.

TEST-TAKING HINT: To answer this question correctly, the test taker must first understand the definition of clang associations. When this symptom of schizophrenia is understood, the test taker can discern the client problem that this symptom may generate.

29. 1. Social isolation is defined as aloneness experienced by the individual and perceived as imposed by others and as a negative or threatened state. Even though poor hygiene may cause others to avoid this client, the statement in the question does not indicate that social isolation is a current client problem.
   2. Impaired home maintenance can be related to regression, withdrawal, lack of knowledge or resources, or impaired physical or cognitive functioning in clients experiencing thought disturbances. This is evidenced by an unsafe, unclean, disorderly home environment. No information is presented in the question that indicates impaired home maintenance is a client problem.
   3. The nursing diagnosis of interrupted family processes is defined as a change in family relationships or functioning or both. The situation described does not reflect this nursing diagnosis.
   4. Self-care deficit is defined as the impaired ability to perform or complete activities of daily living. The client's symptoms of body odor, halitosis, and a disheveled appearance are directly related to a self-care deficit problem.

TEST-TAKING HINT: The test taker must determine the nursing diagnosis that relates directly to the client's presented symptoms. In this question, although others may avoid the client because of poor personal hygiene, there is no evidence of current social isolation in the question.

30. 1. Impaired home maintenance can be related to regression, withdrawal, lack of knowledge or resources, or impaired physical or cognitive functioning in clients experiencing these symptoms of schizophrenia. This is evidenced by an unsafe, unclean, disorderly home environment. There is no information in the question that indicates impaired home maintenance is the problem.
   2. The nursing diagnosis of interrupted family processes is defined as a change in family relationships or functioning or both. This nursing diagnosis is reflected in the family's conflict related to an inability to accept the family member's diagnosis of schizophrenia.
   3. Social isolation is defined as aloneness experienced by the individual and perceived as imposed by others and as a negative or threatened state. No evidence is presented in the question that would indicate social isolation is the problem.
   4. The nursing diagnosis of disturbed thought processes is defined as the disruption in cognitive operations and activities. An example of a disturbed thought process is a delusion. No evidence is presented in

the question that would indicate disturbed thought processes are present.

TEST-TAKING HINT: The only nursing diagnosis that relates to a problem with family dynamics is interrupted family processes. All of the other nursing diagnoses relate to individual client problems and can be eliminated.

31. 1. The nursing diagnosis of disturbed thought processes is defined as the disruption in cognitive operations and activities. An example of a disturbed thought process is a delusion. Thinking about suicide is not a disturbed thought process. The content, not process, of thought that the client is experiencing reflects the client's risk for suicide. No evidence is presented in the question that would indicate disturbed thought processes are present.

2. **Risk for suicide is defined as the risk for self-inflicted, life-threatening injury. A past history of suicide attempts greatly increases the risk for suicide and makes this an appropriate diagnosis for this client. Because client safety is always the main consideration, this diagnosis should be prioritized.**

3. Violence: directed toward others is defined as behaviors in which an individual demonstrates that they can be physically, emotionally, or sexually harmful to others. Although clients experiencing paranoid thinking can lash out defensively when a threat is perceived, there is no evidence in the question that would indicate that this is a problem.

4. Risk for disturbed sensory perception is defined as being at risk for a change in the amount or patterning of incoming stimuli (either internally or externally initiated), accompanied by a diminished, exaggerated, distorted, or impaired response to such stimuli. An example is an auditory hallucination. Although clients with a diagnosis of paranoid schizophrenia are at risk for disturbed sensory perception because of the nature of their disease, there is no evidence in the question that would indicate the client is at risk for this problem.

TEST-TAKING HINT: It is important for the test taker to choose a nursing diagnosis that reflects the client symptom or situation described in the question. Paranoid thinking puts a client at risk for various problems, including violence toward others and disturbed sensory perception. This client's history of suicide attempts determines the appropriate

choice and prioritization of the nursing diagnosis of risk for suicide.

32. 1. When a client fails to take antipsychotic medications, the client is experiencing the problem of ineffective health maintenance R/T nonadherence, not impaired home maintenance.

2. When the client states, "I haven't bathed in a week," the client is presenting evidence of self-care deficit, not impaired home maintenance.

3. **Impaired home maintenance can be related to regression, withdrawal, lack of knowledge or resources, or impaired physical or cognitive functioning in clients experiencing the symptoms of schizophrenia. This is evidenced by an unsafe, unclean, disorderly home environment.**

4. When the client states, "You can't draw my blood without crayons," the client is experiencing concrete thinking, or a literal interpretation of the environment. It represents a regression to an earlier level of cognitive development; however, this is reflective of an altered thought process nursing diagnosis, not a symptom of the nursing diagnosis of impaired home maintenance.

TEST-TAKING HINT: To answer this question correctly, the test taker should note that answers 3 and 4 are symptoms of regressive behaviors but only 3 is related to a home maintenance problem.

Nursing Process—Planning

33. 1. Recognizing distortions of reality by day 4 is an outcome for the nursing diagnosis of disturbed thought processes, not social isolation.

2. Using appropriate verbal communication when interacting with others by day 3 is an outcome for the nursing diagnosis of impaired verbal communication, not social isolation. Impaired communication can lead to social isolation, but it is not directly related.

3. **Actively participating in unit activities by discharge is an outcome for the nursing diagnosis of social isolation. Participation in unit activities indicates interaction with others on the unit, which leads to decreased social isolation.**

4. Rating anxiety as 5/10 by discharge is an outcome for the nursing diagnosis of anxiety, not social isolation. If anxiety is

decreased, the client is more apt to interact with others, but the stated outcome is not directly related to social isolation.

TEST-TAKING HINT: The test taker needs to look for a direct connection between the nursing diagnosis presented and the outcome choices.

34. 1. When a client is hearing and seeing things others do not, the client is experiencing a hallucination, which is an altered sensory perception. A hallucination is defined as a false sensory perception not associated with real external stimuli. Hallucinations may involve any of the five senses. Because schizophrenia is a chronic disease, some individuals, even when compliant with antipsychotic medications, continue to experience hallucinations. Recognizing distortions of reality by discharge is an appropriate outcome for the nursing diagnosis of altered sensory perception.
2. Demonstrating the ability to trust by day 2 is not an outcome directly related to the client problem of hearing and seeing things others do not. Also, trust takes time to develop, and expecting trust by day 2 is unrealistic.
3. Recognizing delusional thinking by day 3 is an inappropriate outcome for the client who is hearing and seeing things others do not. This client is experiencing hallucinations, not delusions. A delusion is a false personal belief not consistent with a person's intelligence or cultural background. The individual continues to have the belief despite obvious proof that it is false or irrational.
4. Experiencing no auditory hallucinations by discharge is an unrealistic outcome for the client problem of hearing and seeing things others do not. Schizophrenia is a chronic disease. Medication and therapy can decrease the signs and symptoms of the disease, but to expect the signs and symptoms to disappear completely by discharge is unrealistic.

TEST-TAKING HINT: To answer this question correctly, the test taker must recognize schizophrenia as a chronic and incurable disease. Expecting distortions of reality to disappear by discharge is unrealistic, whereas simply being aware of the distortions of reality is a realistic outcome.

35. 1. Anxiety is not addressed in this question as this client's problem. If the client is non-adherent with antipsychotic medications because of paranoid thinking, anxiety may be present. An outcome of decreased anxiety is not directly related to the client's described nonadherent behaviors. Also, a "reasonable" level of anxiety is not specific or measurable.
2. Taking antipsychotic medications by discharge is an appropriate outcome for this client's problem of nonadherence. The outcome is realistic, client centered, and measurable.
3. Communicating to staff any paranoid thoughts by day 3 is not an outcome that is directly related to the client's nonadherence issue. No information is presented to indicate that the reason for the client's nonadherence is paranoid thinking. If paranoid thinking is the cause of the nonadherence, this outcome may be appropriate.
4. Taking responsibility for self-care by day 4 is an inappropriate outcome for the client problem of nonadherence with antipsychotic medications. This outcome would be appropriate for a self-care deficit problem.

TEST-TAKING HINT: To answer this question correctly, the test taker must choose the outcome that is directly related to the client's medication nonadherence. It is important not to read anything into the question. Overthinking questions usually results in incorrect answers.

36. 1. Expecting the client to verbalize feelings related to depression and any suicidal ideations is appropriate for a nursing diagnosis of risk for suicide, not altered sensory perception R/T command hallucinations.
2. Weight gain is a side effect of many antipsychotic drugs, including olanzapine. The outcome of limiting caloric intake because of the side effect of weight gain does not relate to the nursing diagnosis of altered sensory perception R/T command hallucinations.
3. When the client has the insight to recognize hallucinations and report them to staff members, the client is in better touch with reality and moving toward remission. This is an outcome that relates to the client's problem of altered sensory perception. Reporting to staff members also can assist in preventing the client from following through with the commands given by auditory hallucinations.
4. Expecting the client to tell staff members if the client is experiencing thoughts of self-harm is an outcome that is appropriate for a nursing diagnosis of risk for violence: self-directed, not altered sensory perception.

TEST-TAKING HINT: To answer this question correctly, the test taker needs to determine the

problem being addressed in the question. The answers may address side effects of olanzapine, but the question asks for the client problem outcome based on the nursing diagnosis of altered sensory perception R/T command hallucinations.

Nursing Process—Implementation

37. 1. Before assuming that the client is experiencing a somatic delusion, the nurse first must rule out a physical cause for the client's symptoms, such as body lice. A somatic delusion occurs when an individual has an unsubstantiated belief that they are experiencing a physical defect, disorder, or disease.
    2. After ruling out a physical cause for symptoms, the nurse would then present reality.
    3. If this client is experiencing a delusion, it would be somatic, not persecutory. Also, using logic to counteract a delusion is not effective.
    4. Substance-induced psychosis is the presence of prominent hallucinations and delusions that are judged to be directly attributable to the physiological effect of a substance. No information is presented in the question that would indicate this client is experiencing substance-induced psychosis.

TEST-TAKING HINT: When asked to choose the first nursing intervention to be implemented, the test taker must look for an intervention that rules out physical causes before determining that symptoms are psychological in nature.

38. 1. Challenging an altered sensory perception does not assist the client with reality orientation and can generate hostile, defensive behaviors.
    2. Presenting logical reasons and challenging altered sensory perceptions serves no useful purpose. Hallucinations are not eliminated and may be aggravated by this approach.
    3. Empathizing with the client about the altered perception encourages trust and promotes further client communication about hallucinations. The nurse must follow this by presenting the reality of the situation. Clients must be assisted in accepting that the perception is unreal to maintain reality orientation.
    4. By using terms such as "those people," the nurse has unwittingly implied validation of the altered perception. Hallucinations should not be reinforced.

TEST-TAKING HINT: The test taker first must recognize the client problem as an alteration in sensory perception (hallucination). When a client is out of touch with reality, the nurse first must communicate empathy and understanding followed by the presentation of reality. The test taker should eliminate answers that belittle the client or logically argue against the hallucination.

39. 1. It is important to reinforce and focus on reality when a client is experiencing disturbed thought processes; however, this is not the first intervention that the nurse should implement.
    2. When the nurse conveys understanding that the client is experiencing delusional thinking, the nurse is showing empathy for the client's situation and building trust. This should be the first step to address the problem of disturbed thought processes. All further interventions would be based on the relationship's being established by generating trust.
    3. It is important to indicate that the nurse does not share the client's delusional thought; however, this is not the initial intervention that the nurse should implement.
    4. Presenting logical information to refute delusional thinking serves no useful purpose because fixed delusional ideas are not eliminated by this approach. This also may impede the establishment of a trusting relationship.

TEST-TAKING HINT: The keyword in this question is *first*. Other answer choices may be appropriate, but the correct choice is the intervention that should be implemented first. All interventions would be better accepted if they are implemented in a trusting environment.

40. 1. Individuals experiencing paranoid thinking have extreme suspiciousness of others and their actions. It is difficult to establish trust with clients experiencing paranoia. All interventions would be suspect. Only by assigning consistent staff members would there be hope to establish a trusting nurse–client relationship and increase the effectiveness of further nursing interventions.
    2. The nurse should convey acceptance of the client and the client's need for the false belief, not the client's false belief itself. The nurse should present, focus on, and reinforce reality.

3. Paranoid thinking can generate anxiety, but anxiety does not cause paranoid thinking. The cause of this alteration in thinking is the chemical imbalance in the brain due to schizophrenia.

4. Individuals experiencing paranoid thinking have extreme suspiciousness of others and their actions. When the client is in the active phase of this disease, group activities can be misinterpreted. This would not be an appropriate nursing intervention at this time.

TEST-TAKING HINT: To answer this question correctly, the test taker must understand the need first to establish trust with a client experiencing paranoia. Assigning consistent staff members is one way to foster trust. Other interventions would be more effective after trust is established.

41. 1. The client described in the question is exhibiting signs of paranoia. Clients with this symptom have trouble trusting others. The nurse should use the therapeutic technique of offering self to assist in building a trusting therapeutic relationship with this client.

2. Because this client is newly admitted and requires stabilization, the client is not ready to formulate a plan of action for discharge. Also, because of paranoid thinking, the client would not be able to trust and work with the nurse to formulate a discharge plan.

3. The nurse needs to work with the client first to build a trusting relationship. The nurse then needs to assess the client's acceptance of family involvement before including family members in discussions about dealing with the client's behaviors.

4. The nurse should reinforce the need for medication adherence; however, a therapeutic relationship should be established prior to client education for the client to trust the nurse and value the information presented.

TEST-TAKING HINT: When reading a question, the test taker must note the client's admission status (newly admitted or ready for discharge). Is the client in an inpatient or outpatient setting? This information would affect the answer choice. It is important always to think about timewise interventions. If this client were stabilized and ready for discharge, the other three answers could be considered.

42. 1. Exaggerated warmth and professions of friendship are likely to be met with confusion and suspicion when dealing with clients diagnosed with schizophrenia.

2. The client diagnosed with schizophrenia is desperately lonely yet defends against kindness, compassion, and trust. The nurse needs to maintain a professional relationship, and professing friendship is inappropriate.

3. The client diagnosed with schizophrenia is likely to respond to attempts at closeness with suspiciousness, anxiety, aggression, or regression. It is important for the nurse to maintain professional boundaries.

4. **Successful interventions may best be achieved with honesty, simple directness, and a manner that respects the client's privacy and human dignity.**

TEST-TAKING HINT: To answer this question correctly, the test taker must understand that establishing a relationship with a client diagnosed with schizophrenia is often particularly difficult and should not be forced.

43. 1. Psychotherapy for clients diagnosed with schizophrenia is a long-term, not short-term, endeavor. The therapist must accept the fact that a great deal of client behavioral change may not occur.

2. **The psychotherapist requires much patience when treating clients diagnosed with schizophrenia. Depending on the severity of the illness, psychotherapeutic treatment may continue for many years before clients regain some degree of independent functioning.**

3. Psychotherapeutic treatment may continue for many years before clients regain some degree of independent functioning. Even with immediate psychotherapy, behavioral changes may not occur.

4. There is no guarantee that clients diagnosed with schizophrenia who receive immediate psychotherapy will gain independent functioning.

TEST-TAKING HINT: The test taker must understand that psychotherapy may have limited effects because of the chronic nature of schizophrenia. Noting the word *immediate* in answers 3 and 4 will lead the test taker to eliminate these choices.

44. 1. This response from the nurse does not address the client's concern and does not offer the information that the client has requested.

2. Not all individuals who demonstrate the characteristics of schizoid personality disorder progress to schizophrenia. However, most individuals diagnosed

with schizophrenia show evidence of having schizoid personality characteristics in the premorbid state.

3. Most, not few, clients diagnosed with schizophrenia show evidence of having schizoid personality characteristics in the premorbid state.

4. Although it is important to assess a client's previous knowledge before beginning any teaching, this response from the nurse does not address the client's concern and does not offer the information that the client has requested.

TEST-TAKING HINT: When asked to choose the correct response of the nurse, the test taker must make sure that the response addresses the client question or concern. Only answer 2 addresses this client's concern.

45. 1. Offering opportunities to learn about psychotropic medications is a cognitive, not behavioral, therapy approach.
2. **When the nurse attaches consequences to adaptive or maladaptive behaviors, the nurse is using a behavioral therapy approach. Behavior therapy can be a powerful treatment tool for helping clients change undesirable behaviors.**
3. When the nurse establishes trust within a relationship, the nurse is using an interpersonal, not behavioral, therapy approach.
4. When the nurse encourages discussions of feelings related to delusions, the nurse is using an intrapersonal, not behavioral, therapy approach.

TEST-TAKING HINT: The test taker must distinguish between the various treatment modalities for clients diagnosed with schizophrenia. The use of consequences for behaviors is the hallmark of behavioral therapy and should be recognized as such.

46. 1. When the nurse assists the family to deal with life stressors caused by interactions with the client, the nurse is using a family therapy, not milieu therapy, approach. Even when families seem to cope well, there is a notable impact on the mental health status of relatives when a family member is diagnosed with schizophrenia.
2. When the nurse offers one-to-one interactions to discuss family dynamics, the nurse is using an interpersonal, not milieu, therapy approach.
3. When the nurse uses role-play to enhance motor and interpersonal skills, the nurse is using a social skills training, not milieu,

therapy approach. The educational procedure in social skills training focuses on role-play. Social skills training is a type of behavioral therapy in which the nurse can serve as a role model for acceptable behaviors.

4. **When the nurse emphasizes the rules and expectations of social interactions mediated by peer pressure, the nurse is using a milieu therapy approach. Milieu therapy emphasizes group and social interaction. Rules and expectations are mediated by peer pressure for normalization of adaptation.**

TEST-TAKING HINT: The test taker must distinguish among the various treatment modalities for clients diagnosed with schizophrenia. Rules and realistic client expectations are the hallmarks of milieu therapy and should be recognized as such.

Nursing Process—Evaluation

47. 1. Symptoms of schizophrenia generally appear in late adolescence or early adulthood. Onset at a later age is associated with a more positive prognosis.
2. Gradual, insidious onset of symptoms is associated with a poorer prognosis than abrupt onset of symptoms precipitated by a stressful event. Being male also is associated with a poor prognosis.
3. **Abrupt onset of symptoms precipitated by a stressful event, such as rape, is associated with a more positive prognosis. Being female also is associated with a more positive prognosis.**
4. A family history of schizophrenia is associated with a poor prognosis.
5. **A family history of mood disorder is associated with a more positive prognosis.**

TEST-TAKING HINT: To answer this question correctly, the test taker must be able to differentiate the factors associated with a good prognosis and a poor prognosis for the diagnosis of schizophrenia.

48. 1. **Confusion and perplexity at the height of the psychotic episode is a feature of schizophreniform disorder that is thought to lead to a good prognosis. When the client is exhibiting perplexity, there is an element of insight that is absent in the more severe cases of cognitive impairment. This insight may lead to a future positive prognosis.**

2. Good premorbid social and occupational functioning is a feature of schizophreniform disorder that is thought to lead to a good prognosis.

3. Absence of blunted or flat affect is a feature of schizophreniform disorder that is thought to lead to a good prognosis.

4. If negative symptoms are predominant, a good prognosis for schizophreniform disorder is unlikely.

5. When the onset of prominent psychotic symptoms is within 4 weeks of the first noticeable change in usual behavior or functioning, a good prognosis is likely.

TEST-TAKING HINT: Because answers 3 and 4 are opposites, the test taker can eliminate one of these choices. Because clients who experience negative symptoms of schizophrenia generally have a poor prognosis, answer 4 is a good choice to eliminate.

49. Positive symptoms of schizophrenia tend to reflect an excess or distortion of normal function, whereas negative symptoms reflect a diminution or loss of normal function. Individuals who exhibit mostly negative symptoms often show structural brain abnormalities on computed tomography (CT) scan and respond poorly to treatment, leading to a poor prognosis. Clients exhibiting a predominance of positive symptoms have a better prognosis. Individuals who exhibit mostly positive symptoms show normal brain structure on CT scan and relatively good responses to treatment.

1. Hearing hostile voices, or auditory hallucinations, is a positive symptom of schizophrenia. Because this client is exhibiting a positive symptom, the client has the potential for a better prognosis.

2. When the client thinks the TV is controlling their behavior, the client is experiencing the positive symptom of a delusion of control or influence. Because this client is exhibiting a positive symptom, the client has the potential for a better prognosis.

3. When a client continuously repeats what has been said, the client is exhibiting the positive symptom of echolalia. Because this client is exhibiting a positive symptom, the client has the potential for a better prognosis.

4. When a client has little or no interest in work or social activities, the client is exhibiting the negative symptom of apathy. Apathy is indifference to, or disinterest in, the environment. Flat affect is a manifestation of emotional apathy.

Because this client is exhibiting a negative symptom, the client has the potential for a poorer prognosis.

TEST-TAKING HINT: To answer this question correctly, the test taker must distinguish between positive and negative symptoms and understand that experiencing negative symptoms adversely affects the prognosis of schizophrenia.

50. 1. Without drug treatment, the relapse rate of a client diagnosed with schizophrenia can be approximately 70% to 80%. With continuous antipsychotic drug treatment, this rate can be reduced to approximately 30%.

2. Research shows that with continuous antipsychotic drug treatment, the relapse rate of clients diagnosed with schizophrenia can be reduced to approximately 30%.

3. Schizophrenia is a multifaceted disease; however, antipsychotic medications are very effective in treating the symptoms of schizophrenia and can reduce the relapse rate if taken consistently.

4. Schizophrenia is a chronic disease; however, research has shown that if antipsychotic medications are taken consistently, relapse rates decrease.

TEST-TAKING HINT: Even if the test taker does not know the percentage of relapse rates, the correct answer can be chosen if it is known that antipsychotic medications are effective in reducing the symptoms of schizophrenia.

Psychopharmacology

51. 1. Akinesia, dystonia, and pseudoparkinsonism are extrapyramidal, not anticholinergic, side effects caused by the use of antipsychotic drugs such as thioridazine.

2. Muscle rigidity, hyperpyrexia, and tachycardia are symptoms that indicate the client is experiencing neuroleptic malignant syndrome (NMS), not anticholinergic side effects of thioridazine. NMS is a rare but potentially fatal complication of treatment with neuroleptic drugs.

3. Research has shown that clients receiving atypical antipsychotic medications are at increased risk for developing hyperglycemia and diabetes. Thioridazine is classified as a typical antipsychotic. Hyperglycemia and diabetes are not anticholinergic side effects.

4. Dry mouth, constipation, and urinary retention are anticholinergic side effects of antipsychotic medications

such as thioridazine. Anticholinergic side effects are caused by agents that block parasympathetic nerve impulses. Thioridazine has a high incidence of anticholinergic side effects.

TEST-TAKING HINT: The test taker must distinguish among the various categories of side effects and the symptoms that may occur with antipsychotic therapy to answer this question correctly.

52. Akathisia, which is uncontrollable restlessness, is an extrapyramidal side effect of antipsychotic medications.
    1. Continuous restlessness and fidgeting (akathisia) are the extrapyramidal side effects caused by the use of antipsychotic drugs such as haloperidol. If an increased dose of haloperidol is prescribed, the symptom of akathisia would increase, not decrease.
    2. Continuous restlessness and fidgeting (akathisia) are the extrapyramidal side effects caused by the use of antipsychotic drugs such as fluphenazine decanoate. If fluphenazine decanoate is prescribed, the symptom of akathisia would increase, not decrease.
    3. Continuous restlessness and fidgeting (akathisia) are the extrapyramidal side effects caused by the use of antipsychotic drugs such as clozapine. If clozapine is prescribed, the symptom of akathisia would increase, not decrease.
    4. Benztropine mesylate is an anticholinergic medication used for the treatment of extrapyramidal symptoms such as akathisia. The nurse would expect the physician to prescribe this drug for the client's symptoms of restlessness.

TEST-TAKING HINT: To answer this question correctly, the test taker must recognize the symptom presented in the question as an extrapyramidal side effect of haloperidol and then be able to distinguish between an antipsychotic and an anticholinergic medication.

53. 1. Levothyroxine sodium is used as replacement or substitution therapy in diminished or absent thyroid function. TSH is thyroid-stimulating hormone. An increased TSH indicates low thyroid functioning. The normal range of TSH is 0.4 to 4.0 mIU/L. This client's TSH level is within the normal range, so this medication should not be indicated.
    2. This client's red blood cell (RBC) count is 4.7 million/mcL, which is within the

normal range for males (4.6 to 6) and females (4 to 5). Because these values do not indicate anemia, the nurse would not expect replacement iron (ferrous sulfate) to be ordered.
    3. A normal adult value of absolute neutrophil count (ANC) is >1,500/mcL. This client's ANC is 800/mcL, indicating moderate neutropenia, which is a potentially fatal blood disorder. There is a significant risk for neutropenia with clozapine therapy. The nurse would expect the physician to discontinue clozapine.
    4. The first part of this choice is correct, but the second part is incorrect. This client's TSH level is normal, so levothyroxine sodium would not be indicated.

TEST-TAKING HINT: The test taker first must recognize the ANC count as critically low and the TSH value as normal. Recognizing a low ANC as moderate neutropenia would lead the test taker to expect the physician to discontinue clozapine. The test taker also must remember that all parts of the answer must be correct or the entire answer is considered incorrect. This would eliminate answer 4 because levothyroxine sodium would not be indicated.

54. 1. Antipsychotic medications can cause a decreased libido, but the client's symptom does not warrant this teaching.
    2. There is no evidence that antipsychotic medications can interfere with the effectiveness of birth control.
    3. Antipsychotic medications can cause amenorrhea, but ovulation still occurs. If this client does not understand this, there is a potential for pregnancy. This is vital client teaching information that must be included in the plan of care.
    4. There is no evidence that antipsychotic medications can decrease red blood cells, leading to amenorrhea.

TEST-TAKING HINT: The test taker must recognize the side effects of antipsychotic medications to answer this question correctly. The test taker also must understand terminology such as *amenorrhea* to determine what is being asked in the question.

55. Haloperidol is a typical antipsychotic used in the treatment of schizophrenia. A side effect of antipsychotic medications is tardive dyskinesia, a syndrome characterized by bizarre facial and tongue movements, a stiff neck, and difficulty swallowing. All clients receiving long-term treatment with antipsychotic

medications are at risk, and the symptoms are potentially irreversible.

1. Although benztropine may be given to assist with the signs of tardive dyskinesia, because tardive dyskinesia is potentially irreversible, it is important that the nurse hold the medication and talk with the physician before giving the next dose of haloperidol.

2. Antipsychotic medications, such as haloperidol, can cause metabolic changes, and the client would need to be monitored. However, the symptoms in the question do not reflect hyperglycemia.

3. Another side effect of antipsychotic medications is neuroleptic malignant syndrome (NMS). The signs and symptoms of NMS are muscle rigidity, hyperpyrexia (107°F), tachycardia, tachypnea, fluctuations in blood pressure, diaphoresis, and rapid deterioration of mental status to stupor or coma. The symptoms in the question do not reflect NMS.

4. **The symptoms noted in the question reflect tardive dyskinesia, a potentially irreversible side effect of antipsychotic medications, and the nurse must hold the haloperidol to avoid permanent damage, and call the physician.**

TEST-TAKING HINT: The test taker should review and understand different side effects of antipsychotic medications and appropriate nursing interventions to deal with the symptoms of these side effects. Also, remember that if a portion of a choice is incorrect, the entire choice is incorrect, as in answer 1.

56. Ziprasidone is an atypical antipsychotic used to treat symptoms related to altered thought processes.

    1. **Ziprasidone has the potential, in rare cases, to elongate the QT interval; a baseline and periodic electrocardiogram (EKG) would be necessary.**

    2. **Ziprasidone needs to be taken with meals for it to be absorbed effectively. It is important for the nurse to teach the client the need to take ziprasidone with meals.**

    3. **Palpitations can be a side effect of ziprasidone and would need to be monitored.**

    4. Seizure precautions are needed with bupropion and clozapine, not ziprasidone.

    5. A manic episode is not a side effect of ziprasidone.

TEST-TAKING HINT: To choose the appropriate interventions, the test taker must be aware of potential risks and special needs of clients who are prescribed ziprasidone.

57. Quetiapine is an atypical antipsychotic used in the treatment of schizophrenia. A significant side effect of quetiapine is sedation.

    1. Although the nurse would want to monitor for homicidal and suicidal ideations, this answer does not relate to the nursing diagnosis noted in the question.

    2. **Removing clutter from the client's environment would assist the client to avoid injury due to tripping and falling. It is important for the nurse to ensure the environment is clutter free, especially when the client may be experiencing sedation.**

    3. There is a potential for orthostatic changes when a client is prescribed quetiapine. However, orthostatic changes are not related to the "sedation" noted in the nursing diagnosis.

    4. Although it is important for the nurse to evaluate for auditory and visual hallucinations while a client is taking quetiapine, such evaluation does not relate to the stated nursing diagnosis.

TEST-TAKING HINT: When a nursing diagnosis is presented in the question, the test taker should make sure the intervention chosen relates to all aspects of the stated nursing diagnosis: the NANDA-I stem, the *related to* statement, and the *as evidenced by* data.

58. Hydroxyzine is an antihistamine medication used to treat anxiety, and clozapine is an atypical antipsychotic with many side effects.

    1. Although hydroxyzine affects serotonin, clozapine does not have much impact on serotonin, and the risk for serotonin syndrome is low.

    2. **A side effect of clozapine is that it lowers the seizure threshold. The nurse would need to place the client taking clozapine on seizure precautions.**

    3. There is no test for clozapine blood levels. Signs that too much clozapine has been taken include, but are not limited to, excessive sedation or hypersalivation.

    4. Hydroxyzine and clozapine are not used for treating depression, and this answer is incorrect.

TEST-TAKING HINT: To answer this question correctly, the test taker must understand that a potential side effect of clozapine is seizure activity and that this can place the client at risk for injury.

59. 1. Although haloperidol can have the listed side effects, haloperidol is a "typical" antipsychotic. The question is asking for an "atypical" antipsychotic medication.

2. Although chlorpromazine can have the listed side effects, chlorpromazine is a "typical" antipsychotic. The question is asking for an "atypical" antipsychotic medication.

3. Risperidone and clozapine are both atypical antipsychotics; however, based on studies, clozapine, not risperidone, has the highest potential for serious side effects.

4. **Clozapine, an "atypical" antipsychotic, has side effects including sedation, weight gain, and hypersalivation. Because of these side effects and the life-threatening side effect of neutropenia, clozapine usually is used as a last resort after other failed medication trials. Diagnostic laboratory tests need to be performed weekly for 6 months, every other week for the next 6 months, and then monthly as long as the clozapine is prescribed.**

TEST-TAKING HINT: The test taker must note important words in the question. When the word *atypical* is noted, answers 1 and 2 can be eliminated immediately because they are typical antipsychotics.

60. 1. Amenorrhea is a side effect of antipsychotic medications, such as risperidone, and when it occurs it resolves only if the client is taken off the medication.

2. Empathy related to the concern is appropriate, but asking the client further questions, such as how long they have been without their period, is an assessment. The question is asking for further teaching needs, and assessing further does not answer the question.

3. **It is important for nurses to teach clients taking antipsychotic medications about the potential for amenorrhea and that, even though they are not regularly having their menstrual cycle, ovulation still may occur.**

4. Asking the client for more information regarding her amenorrhea would be appropriate, but it does not answer the question. The question is asking for further teaching needs, and asking about regularity of past periods is an assessment.

TEST-TAKING HINT: The test taker must note important words in the question, such as *teaching*. In this question, answers 2 and 4 can be eliminated immediately because they are assessment interventions and not teaching interventions.

61. 1. Trihexyphenidyl, an anticholinergic medication, is prescribed to counteract extrapyramidal symptoms, which are side effects of all antipsychotic medications.

Dystonia—involuntary muscular movements (or spasms) of the face, arms, legs, and neck—is an extrapyramidal symptom. Sedation is a side effect of haloperidol, not an extrapyramidal symptom, and is not affected by trihexyphenidyl.

2. Haloperidol, an antipsychotic, not trihexyphenidyl, is used to treat auditory hallucinations.

3. **Haloperidol, an antipsychotic, would decrease an individual's grandiosity, which is one of many symptoms of schizophrenia.**

4. Haloperidol, similar to all antipsychotic medications, causes dystonia. Medications such as trihexyphenidyl are used to counteract extrapyramidal symptoms, such as dystonia.

TEST-TAKING HINT: This is essentially a true/false question. The test taker should check the accuracy of the information presented in the answer choices. The test taker also must understand the meaning of the terms *dystonia* and *grandiosity* to answer this question correctly.

62. Aripiprazole is an atypical antipsychotic medication. It is prescribed for individuals diagnosed with schizophrenia.

1. Nonadherence is a concern; however, it is not a priority nursing diagnosis.

2. Knowledge deficit is a concern; however, it is not a priority nursing diagnosis.

3. **Risk for injury R/T orthostatic hypotension, which is a side effect of the aripiprazole, is a priority diagnosis. It is important for nurses to recognize when a client is at increased risk for injury because of side effects such as orthostatic hypotension.**

4. Activity intolerance is a concern; however, it is not a priority nursing diagnosis.

TEST-TAKING HINT: When a question calls for prioritization, the test taker must consider the problem that would place the client in immediate danger.

63. Severe muscle spasms, increased heart rate, hypertension, and hyperpyrexia all are symptoms of neuroleptic malignant syndrome (NMS). NMS is a rare but potentially fatal complication of treatment with neuroleptic drugs.

1. The symptoms are not indicative of extrapyramidal symptoms, which include, but are not limited to, tremors, dystonia, akinesia, and akathisia.

2. **Because NMS is related to the use of neuroleptic medications, such as fluphenazine, the next dose should be held, and the client's physician should**

be notified immediately because this is a life-threatening situation.

3. Elevated blood pressure and pulse rate in this situation are not due to cardiac problems but are due to NMS from the use of neuroleptic medications.

4. Drug use can cause the listed symptoms, but when the nurse understands the relationship between neuroleptics and NMS, the nurse understands the client is at risk for this life-threatening condition.

TEST-TAKING HINT: The test taker should review the side effects of neuroleptic medications, such as NMS, extrapyramidal symptoms, and tardive dyskinesia, to prioritize nursing interventions.

64. Lithium carbonate is a mood stabilizing medication that is used to treat symptoms of bipolar affective disorder (BPAD). Symptoms of BPAD include, but are not limited to, mania, labile mood, and depressive symptoms.

1. Benzodiazepines and selective serotonin reuptake inhibitors (SSRIs) are medications to assist clients with anxiety. Nurses need to remember that SSRIs begin to show an effect in 2 to 3 weeks and reach full effect around 6 to 8 weeks of regular use.

2. Medications that assist clients with depression are monoamine oxidase inhibitors, tricyclic antidepressants, and SSRIs.

3. **Clozapine, an atypical antipsychotic, is used to treat symptoms of schizophrenia, such as, but not limited to, psychoses.**

4. Akathisia is an extrapyramidal symptom that occurs as a result of the use of antipsychotic medications. Medications to treat extrapyramidal symptoms such as akathisia are anticholinergic or antihistamine drugs.

TEST-TAKING HINT: When answering an analogy, the test taker must recognize the relationships between the subject matter within the question.

65. The nurse will administer **16 mL** daily.

$$\frac{0.5 \text{ mg}}{1 \text{ mL}} = \frac{4 \text{ mg}}{\times \text{ mL}} = 8 \text{ mL}$$

8 mL × 2 doses (bid) = 16 mL

TEST-TAKING HINT: The test taker must note keywords in the question, such as *daily*. The individual dose for this medication calculates as 8 mL, but the daily dose is 16 mL. Set up the ratio and proportion problem based on the number of milligrams contained in 1 mL. The test taker can solve this problem by cross multiplication and solving for *x* by division.

66. 1. The medication is ordered q4h. Because there are only 3 hours between 0800 and 1100, the medication was administered incorrectly.

2. Although there are 4 hours between administration times in this answer, the client would have received 60 mg/day of ziprasidone, exceeding the maximum daily dose.

3. This documentation of administration has only 3 hours between 0900 and 1200, not q4h per order; if given three times in 1 day (= 60 mg), it would exceed the maximum daily dose of 40 mg/day.

4. **The medication administration record documenting that ziprasidone was administered at 1300 and 1700 is 4 hours apart (q4h) and equals the maximum daily dose of 40 mg/day. This would be appropriate documentation of the order "ziprasidone 20 mg IM q4h for agitation with a maximum daily dose of 40 mg/day."**

TEST-TAKING HINT: To answer this question correctly, the test taker first must note how often the prn medication can be administered and then be able to understand how the maximum daily dose would affect the number of times the medication can be administered.

67. The nurse will administer **2.5 tablets** daily.

$$\frac{12.5 \text{ mg}}{\times \text{ tab}} = \frac{25 \text{ mg}}{1 \text{ tab}} = 0.5 \text{ tab}$$

$$\frac{50 \text{ mg}}{\times \text{ tab}} = \frac{25 \text{ mg}}{1 \text{ tab}} = 2 \text{ tab}$$

0.5 tab + 2 tabs = 2.5 tabs/d

TEST-TAKING HINT: The test taker must note keywords in the question, such as *daily*. The test taker first must calculate the number of tablets for each scheduled dose and then add these together to get the total daily number of tablets. Set up the ratio and proportion problem based on the number of milligrams contained in 1 tablet. The test taker can then solve this problem by cross multiplication and solving for *x* by division.

68. 1. Ziprasidone is an antipsychotic medication that needs to be given with at least 350 calories to facilitate absorption.

2. Although vilazodone needs to be taken with food for absorption, vilazodone is an antidepressant, not antipsychotic medication.

3. **Lurasidone is an antipsychotic medication that needs to be given with at least 350 calories to facilitate absorption.**

4. Aripiprazole is an antipsychotic medication; however, it does not need to be taken with food to be absorbed.

5. Asenapine is an antipsychotic medication; however, asenapine must dissolve under

the tongue for absorption. The nurse must teach the client to avoid all food and liquid for at least 10 minutes following administration.

TEST-TAKING HINT: To answer this question correctly, the test taker must recognize important words in the question. This question is asking for an antipsychotic medication, which immediately eliminates answer 2.

69. 1. Olanzapine IM is a long-acting antipsychotic injection that can be given every 4 weeks to assist with medication adherence for a client diagnosed with schizophrenia.
    2. Ziprasidone IM is a short-acting antipsychotic injection used in acute care, not outpatient settings, for clients experiencing extreme agitation or acute psychosis.
    3. Haloperidol Lactate is a short-acting antipsychotic injection used in acute care, not outpatient settings, for clients experiencing extreme agitation or acute psychosis. Haloperidol decanoate is a long-acting injection given every 3 to 4 weeks in an outpatient setting to assist clients with medication adherence.
    4. Aripiprazole IM is a long-acting antipsychotic injection given every 4 weeks in an outpatient setting to assist clients with medication adherence.
    5. Paliperidone IM is a long-acting antipsychotic injection given every 3 months in an outpatient setting to assist clients with medication adherence. Normally, a client will be stabilized on paliperidone IM every 4 weeks for 6 months, 1 year before changing to the every 3-month Invega Trinza injection.

TEST-TAKING HINT: To answer this question correctly, the test taker must recognize keywords in the stem of the question. This question is asking for medications to help with medication adherence in an outpatient setting, and therefore numbers 2 and 3 can be eliminated.

70. 1. Mirtazapine is an antidepressant, not an antipsychotic medication. Mirtazapine will dissolve rapidly in saliva and would ensure medication adherence for those depressed clients suspected of "cheeking" medications.
    2. Olanzapine is an atypical antipsychotic medication that will dissolve rapidly in saliva and would ensure medication adherence for those suspected of cheeking medications.
    3. Paliperidone is an atypical antipsychotic long-acting injection, not an oral medication.
    4. Aripiprazole is an atypical antipsychotic medication that will dissolve rapidly in saliva and would ensure medication adherence for those suspected of cheeking medications.
    5. Asenapine is an atypical antipsychotic medication that will dissolve rapidly in saliva when administered sublingually and would ensure medication adherence for those suspected of cheeking medications.

TEST-TAKING HINT: To answer this question correctly, the test taker must recognize keywords in the question. The words *oral medication* and *antipsychotic* would assist the test taker in immediately eliminating answer 1, which is an antidepressant, and answer 3, which is an injection.

71. Olanzapine is a long-acting antipsychotic medication given IM every 4 weeks to assist with medication adherence. Post-injection delirium/sedation syndrome is an adverse reaction which can occur after receiving olanzapine. Signs and symptoms include sedation (coma) and delirium (agitation, anxiety, confusion, and disorientation). These symptoms are associated with a rapid rise in serum levels.
    1. The client stating that they need to stay in the facility for 3 hours shows understanding of the need to be monitored during that time for any signs and symptoms of post-injection delirium/sedation syndrome. Highest risk occurs during the first hour after the injection but can occur 3 hours after.
    2. The client stating that they will be unable to drive for the remainder of the day shows understanding of the need for the client to avoid activities that can cause danger to self or others if post-injection delirium/sedation syndrome occurs.
    3. The client stating they need to complete registration with the drug company shows understanding of the process to obtain Zyprexa Relprevv. Because of the risk of post-injection delirium/sedation syndrome, the facility, the nurse giving the injection, and the client must all be registered with Eli Lilly's Zyprexa Relprevv program.

4. The client stating they need to notify staff immediately if sedation or confusion occur shows understanding of the recognition of early signs of post-injection delirium/sedation syndrome.

5. There is a cumulative risk for post-injection delirium/sedation syndrome with each injection, and therefore the client is incorrect in stating the risk decreases after the first three injections.

TEST-TAKING HINT: To answer this question correctly, the test taker must recognize the increased risk of post-injection delirium/sedation syndrome and familiarize themself with the added educational needs of clients prescribed Zyprexa Relprevv.

72. The uncontrollable movements of the head, neck, tongue and/or other parts of the body are a side effect of antipsychotic medications. These symptoms are called tardive dyskinesia (TD).
   1. Benztropine is an antiparkinson medication used to treat movement disorders due to antipsychotic medications called dystonia and parkinsonism, not TD.
   2. Diphenhydramine is an allergy medication at times used to treat movement disorders due to antipsychotic medications, such as dystonia and parkinsonism, not TD.
   3. Trihexyphenidyl is an antiparkinson medication used to treat movement disorders due to antipsychotic medications, such as dystonia and parkinsonism, not TD.
   4. Valbenazine is a medication used to treat TD.
   5. Deutetrabenazine is a medication used to treat TD.

TEST-TAKING HINT: To answer this question the test taker must recognize the presenting symptoms as tardive dyskinesia and then be aware

of which medications are approved by the Food and Drug Administration (FDA) to treat this disorder.

73. Tardive dyskinesia (TD) is a rare side effect of antipsychotic medications. Symptoms include uncontrollable stiff, jerky movements of the face and body. Examples are eye blinking, tongue protrusion, or arm/leg or trunk movements. If not addressed, symptoms can become permanent.
   1. To help treat TD, the psychiatric prescriber could order both physical and occupational therapy to help manage the symptoms.
   2. In the past the only treatment was to discontinue the antipsychotic medication. Today there have been two medications developed to be administered alone or with the offending agent to help reduce symptoms of TD.
   3. **The medication deutetrabenazine is one of two medications that can be prescribed to help treat the symptoms of TD and can be taken in conjunction with the offending antipsychotic.**
   4. **The medication valbenazine is one of two medications that can be prescribed to help treat the symptoms of TD.**
   5. In the past the only treatment was to discontinue the antipsychotic medication. Today there have been two medications developed to be administered alone or with the offending agent to help reduce symptoms of TD such as muscle movements.

TEST-TAKING HINT: To answer this question correctly, the test-taker must review newest medications and treatments for clients experiencing side effects from psychotropic medications, such as TD.

Personality Disorders

KEYWORDS

The following words include English vocabulary, nursing/medical terminology, concepts, principles, or information relevant to content specifically addressed in this chapter or associated with topics presented in it. English dictionaries, your nursing textbooks, and medical dictionaries such as *Taber's Cyclopedic Medical Dictionary* are resources that can be used to expand your knowledge and understanding of these words and related information.

CLUSTER A
Paranoid personality disorder
Schizoid personality disorder
Schizotypal personality disorder
CLUSTER B
Antisocial personality disorder
Borderline personality disorder
Histrionic personality disorder
Narcissistic personality disorder
CLUSTER C
Avoidant personality disorder
Dependent personality disorder

Denial
Extrapyramidal symptoms (EPS)
Grandiose
Impulse control disorders
Limit setting
Magical thinking
Mahler's theory of object relations
Obsessive-compulsive personality disorder
Passive-aggressive traits
Self-injurious behaviors
Self-mutilation
Splitting

QUESTIONS

Theory

1. Which predisposing factor would be implicated in the etiology of paranoid personality disorder?
   1. The individual may have been subjected to parental demands, criticism, and perfectionistic expectations.
   2. The individual may have been subjected to parental indifference, impassivity, or formality.
   3. The individual may have been subjected to parental bleak and unfeeling coldness.
   4. The individual may have been subjected to parental antagonism and harassment.

2. The nurse is assessing a client diagnosed with borderline personality disorder. According to Mahler's theory of object relations, which describes the client's unmet developmental need?
   1. The need for survival and comfort.
   2. The need for awareness of an external source for fulfillment.
   3. The need for awareness of separateness of self.
   4. The need for internalization of a sustained image of a love object/person.

3. Using interpersonal theory, which statement is true regarding development of paranoid personality disorder?
   1. Studies have revealed a higher incidence of paranoid personality disorder among relatives of clients with schizophrenia.
   2. Clients diagnosed with paranoid personality disorder frequently have been family scapegoats and subjected to parental antagonism and harassment.
   3. There is an alteration in the ego development so that the ego is unable to balance the id and superego.
   4. During the anal stage of development, the client diagnosed with paranoid personality disorder has problems with control within their environment.

Defense Mechanisms

4. When confronted, a client diagnosed with narcissistic personality disorder states, "Contrary to what everyone believes, I do not think that the whole world owes me a living." This client is using what defense mechanism?
   1. Minimization.
   2. Denial.
   3. Rationalization.
   4. Projection.

5. A client diagnosed with borderline personality disorder coyly requests diazepam. When the physician refuses, the client becomes angry and demands to see another physician. What defense mechanism is the client using?
   1. Undoing.
   2. Splitting.
   3. Altruism.
   4. Reaction formation.

Nursing Process—Assessment

6. A client with diabetes is admitted to a medical floor for medication stabilization and has a history of antisocial personality disorder. Which documented behaviors would support this diagnosis? **Select all that apply.**
   1. "Labile mood and affect, and old scars noted on wrists bilaterally."
   2. "Appears younger than stated age with flamboyant hair and makeup."
   3. "Began cursing when confronted with drug-seeking behaviors."
   4. "Demands foods prepared by personal chef to be delivered to room."
   5. "Attempted to use insincere flattery to obtain extra snacks."

7. Irresponsible, guiltless behavior is to a client diagnosed with cluster B personality disorder as avoidant, dependent behavior is to a client diagnosed with a:
   1. Cluster A personality disorder.
   2. Cluster B personality disorder.
   3. Cluster C personality disorder.
   4. Cluster D personality disorder.

8. A client tells the nurse, "When I was a waiter, I used to spit in the dinners of annoying customers." This statement would be associated with which personality trait?
   1. Paranoid personality trait.
   2. Schizoid personality trait.
   3. Passive-aggressive personality trait.
   4. Antisocial personality trait.

9. A client diagnosed with a personality disorder insists that a grandmother, through reincarnation, has come back to life as a pet kitten. The thought process described is reflective of which personality disorder?
   1. Obsessive-compulsive personality disorder.
   2. Schizotypal personality disorder.
   3. Borderline personality disorder.
   4. Schizoid personality disorder.

10. A client diagnosed with a personality disorder states, "You are the very best nurse on the unit and not at all like that mean nurse who never lets us stay up later than 9 p.m." This statement would be associated with which personality disorder?
    1. Borderline personality disorder.
    2. Schizoid personality disorder.
    3. Dependent personality disorder.
    4. Paranoid personality disorder.

11. A male client diagnosed with a personality disorder boasts to the nurse that he has to fight off female attention and is the highest paid in his company. These statements are reflective of which personality disorder?
    1. Obsessive-compulsive personality disorder.
    2. Avoidant personality disorder.
    3. Schizotypal personality disorder.
    4. Narcissistic personality disorder.

12. A nurse encourages an angry client to attend group therapy. Knowing that the client has been diagnosed with a cluster B personality disorder, which client response might the nurse expect?
    1. Sarcastically states, "That group is only for crazy people with problems."
    2. Scornfully states, "No, can't you see that I'm having a séance with my mom?"
    3. Suspiciously states, "No, that room has been bugged."
    4. Hesitantly states, "OK, but only if I can sit next to you."

13. A client has been diagnosed with a cluster A personality disorder. Which of the following client statements would reflect cluster A characteristics? **Select all that apply.**
    1. "I'm the best chef on the East Coast."
    2. "My dinner has been poisoned."
    3. "I have to wash my hands 10 times before eating."
    4. "I just can't eat when I'm alone."
    5. "When my mom died, her spirit entered my cat."

14. Personality disorders are grouped in clusters according to their behavioral characteristics. In which cluster are the disorders correctly matched with their behavioral characteristics?
    1. Cluster C: antisocial, borderline, histrionic, narcissistic disorders; anxious or fearful characteristic behaviors.
    2. Cluster A: avoidant, dependent, obsessive-compulsive disorders; odd or eccentric characteristic behaviors.
    3. Cluster A: antisocial, borderline, histrionic, narcissistic disorders; dramatic, emotional, or erratic characteristic behaviors.
    4. Cluster C: avoidant, dependent, obsessive-compulsive disorders; anxious or fearful characteristic behaviors.

15. Which behavior would the nurse expect to observe if a client is diagnosed with paranoid personality disorder?
    1. The client sits alone at lunch and states, "Everyone wants to hurt me."
    2. The client is irresponsible and exploits other peers in the milieu for cigarettes.
    3. The client is shy and refuses to talk to others because of poor self-esteem.
    4. The client sits with peers and allows others to make decisions for the entire group.

16. Which diagnostic criterion describes a characteristic of schizotypal personality disorder?
    1. Neither desires nor enjoys close relationships, including being part of a family.
    2. Is preoccupied with unjustified doubts about the loyalty of friends and associates.
    3. Considers relationships to be more intimate than they actually are.
    4. Exhibits behavior or appearance that is odd, eccentric, or peculiar.

17. Which of the following diagnostic criteria describe the characteristics of borderline personality disorder? **Select all that apply.**
    1. Arrogant, haughty behaviors or attitudes.
    2. Frantic efforts to avoid real or imagined abandonment.
    3. Recurrent suicidal and self-mutilating behaviors.
    4. Unrealistic preoccupation with fears of being left to take care of self.
    5. Chronic feelings of emptiness.

18. Which of the following diagnostic criteria describe the characteristics of avoidant personality disorder? **Select all that apply.**
    1. Fears shame and/or ridicule; does not form intimate relationships.
    2. Has difficulty making everyday decisions without reassurance from others.
    3. Is unwilling to be involved with people unless certain of being liked.
    4. Shows perfectionism that interferes with task completion.
    5. Views self as socially inept, unappealing, and inferior.

19. When assessing a client diagnosed with histrionic personality disorder, the nurse might identify which characteristic behavior?
    1. Odd beliefs and magical thinking.
    2. Grandiose sense of self-importance.
    3. Preoccupation with orderliness and perfection.
    4. Attention-seeking flamboyance.

20. When assessing a client exhibiting passive-aggressive personality traits, which characteristic behavior might the nurse identify?
    1. The client exhibits behaviors that attempt to split the staff.
    2. The client shows reckless disregard for the safety of self or others.
    3. The client has unjustified doubts about the trustworthiness of friends.
    4. The client seeks subtle retribution when feeling others have wronged them.

21. Although there are differences among the three personality disorder clusters, there also are some traits common to all individuals diagnosed with personality disorders. Which of the following are common traits? **Select all that apply.**
    1. Failure to accept the consequences of their own behavior.
    2. Self-injurious behaviors.
    3. Reluctant to take personal risks.
    4. Copes by altering environment instead of self.
    5. Lack of insight.

Nursing Process—Diagnosis

22. A client diagnosed with antisocial personality disorder states, "My kids are so busy at home and school, they don't miss me or even know I'm gone." Which nursing diagnosis applies to this client?
    1. Risk for injury.
    2. Risk for violence: self-directed.
    3. Ineffective denial.
    4. Powerlessness.

23. A client diagnosed with borderline personality disorder superficially cut both wrists, is disruptive in group, and is splitting staff. Which nursing diagnosis would take priority?
    1. Risk for self-mutilation R/T need for attention.
    2. Ineffective coping R/T inability to deal directly with feelings.
    3. Anxiety R/T fear of abandonment AEB splitting staff.
    4. Risk for suicide R/T past suicide attempt.

24. A client diagnosed with schizoid personality disorder chooses solitary activities, lacks close friends, and appears indifferent to criticism. Which nursing diagnosis would be appropriate for this client's problem?
    1. Anxiety R/T poor self-esteem AEB lack of close friends.
    2. Ineffective coping R/T inability to communicate AEB indifference to criticism.
    3. Altered sensory perception R/T threat to self-concept AEB magical thinking.
    4. Social isolation R/T discomfort with human interaction AEB avoiding others.

25. A client exhibiting passive-aggressive personality traits continuously complains to the marriage counselor about a nagging spouse who criticizes their indecisiveness. Which nursing diagnosis reflects this client's problem?
    1. Social isolation R/T decreased self-esteem.
    2. Impaired social interaction R/T inability to express feelings openly.
    3. Powerlessness R/T spousal abuse.
    4. Self-esteem disturbance R/T unrealistic expectations of spouse.

Nursing Process—Planning

26. A nurse is discharging a client diagnosed with narcissistic personality disorder. Which employment opportunity is most likely to be recommended by the treatment team?
    1. Home builder.
    2. Air traffic controller.
    3. Night security guard at the zoo.
    4. Prison warden.

27. Which client situation requires the nurse to prioritize the implementation of limit setting?
    1. A client making sexual advances toward a staff member.
    2. A client telling staff that another staff member allows food in the bedrooms.
    3. A client verbally provoking another client who is paranoid.
    4. A client refusing medications to receive secondary gains.

28. A client newly admitted to an inpatient psychiatric unit is diagnosed with schizotypal personality disorder. The client states, "I envision my future death by fire." Which is the most appropriate nursing response?
    1. "I don't know what you mean by envisioning your future death."
    2. "Your future death? Can you please tell me more about that?"
    3. "I was wondering if you want to come to group to talk about that."
    4. "I can see your thoughts are bothersome. How can I help?"

29. A client experiencing suicidal ideations is diagnosed with borderline personality disorder. Which correctly written short-term outcome is most beneficial for the client?
    1. The client will be free from self-injurious behavior.
    2. The client will express feelings without inflicting self-injury by discharge.
    3. The client will socialize with peers in the milieu by day 3.
    4. The client will acknowledge their role in altered interpersonal relationships.

30. A client diagnosed with an avoidant personality disorder has the nursing diagnosis of social isolation R/T severe malformation of the spine AEB "I can't be around people, looking like this." Which correctly written, short-term outcome is appropriate for this client's problem?
   1. The client will see self as straight and tall by the time of discharge.
   2. The client will see self as valuable after attending assertiveness training courses.
   3. The client will be able to participate in one therapy group by end of shift.
   4. The client will join in a charade game to decrease social isolation.

31. A client diagnosed with an obsessive-compulsive personality disorder has a nursing diagnosis of anxiety R/T interference with hand washing AEB "I'll go crazy if you don't let me do that." Which correctly written short-term outcome is appropriate for this client?
   1. During a 3-hour period after admission to the unit, the client will refrain from hand washing.
   2. The client will wash hands only at appropriate bathroom and meal intervals.
   3. The client will refrain from hand washing throughout the night.
   4. Within 72 hours of admission, the client will notify staff when signs and symptoms of anxiety escalate.

Nursing Process—Implementation

32. A client diagnosed with antisocial personality disorder demands, at midnight, to speak to the ethics committee about the involuntary commitment process. Which nursing statement is appropriate?
   1. "I realize you're upset; however, this is not the appropriate time to explore your concerns."
   2. "Let me give you a sleeping pill to help put your mind at ease."
   3. "It's midnight, and you are disturbing the other clients."
   4. "I will document your concerns in your chart for the morning shift to discuss with the ethics committee."

33. A client diagnosed with antisocial personality disorder is caught smuggling cigarettes into the nonsmoking clinical area. Which initial nursing intervention is appropriate?
   1. Confront the client about the behavior.
   2. Tell the client's primary nurse about the situation.
   3. Remind all clients of the no smoking policy in the community meeting.
   4. Teach alternative coping mechanisms to assist with anxiety.

34. After being treated in the emergency department (ED) for self-inflicted lacerations to wrists and arms, a client with a diagnosis of borderline personality disorder is admitted to the psychiatric unit. Which nursing intervention takes priority?
   1. Administer tranquilizing drugs.
   2. Observe client frequently.
   3. Encourage client to verbalize hostile feelings.
   4. Explore alternative ways of handling frustration.

35. A 15-year-old client living in a residential facility has a nursing diagnosis of ineffective coping R/T abuse AEB defiant responses to adult rules. Which of the following interventions would address this nursing diagnosis appropriately? **Select all that apply.**
   1. Set limits on manipulative behavior.
   2. Refuse to engage in controversial and argumentative encounters.
   3. Obtain an order for tranquilizing medications.
   4. Encourage the discussion of angry feelings.
   5. Remove all dangerous objects from the client's environment.

36. A client diagnosed with a borderline personality disorder is given a nursing diagnosis of disturbed personal identity R/T unmet dependency needs AEB the inability to be alone. Which nursing intervention would be appropriate?
    1. Ask the client directly, "Have you thought about killing yourself?"
    2. Maintain a low level of stimuli in the client's environment.
    3. Frequently orient the client to reality and surroundings.
    4. Help the client identify values and beliefs.

37. A client diagnosed with a dependent personality disorder has a nursing diagnosis of social isolation R/T parental abandonment AEB fear of involvement with individuals not in the immediate family. Which nursing intervention would be appropriate?
    1. Address inappropriate interactions during group therapy.
    2. Recognize when client is playing one staff member against another.
    3. Role-model positive relationships.
    4. Encourage client to discuss conflicts evident within the family system.

38. A client diagnosed with paranoid personality disorder needs information regarding medications. Which nursing intervention would best assist this client in understanding prescribed medications?
    1. Ask the client to join the medication education group.
    2. Provide one-to-one teaching in the client's room.
    3. During rounds, have the physician ask if the client has any questions.
    4. Let the client read the medication information handout.

Nursing Process—Evaluation

39. A nursing student is studying the historical aspects of personality disorder. Which entry on the examination indicates that learning has occurred?
    1. Zeus, in the 3rd century BCE, identified, described, and applied the theory of object relations.
    2. Hippocrates, in the 4th century BCE, identified four fundamental personality styles.
    3. Narcissus, in 923 CE, introduced the word *personality* from the Greek term "persona."
    4. Achilles, in 866 CE, described the pathology of personality as a complex behavioral phenomenon.

40. A nursing student is learning about narcissistic personality disorder. Which of the following student statements indicate that learning has occurred? **Select all that apply.**
    1. "These clients have peculiarities of ideation."
    2. "These clients require constant approval and affirmation."
    3. "These clients are impulsive and self-destructive."
    4. "These clients express a grandiose sense of self-importance."
    5. "These clients have a deep need for admiration."

41. A nursing instructor is teaching about personality disorder characteristics. Which student statement indicates that learning has occurred?
    1. "Clients diagnosed with personality disorders need frequent hospitalizations."
    2. "Clients perceive their behaviors as uncomfortable and disorganized."
    3. "Personality disorders cannot be cured or controlled successfully with medication."
    4. "Practitioners have a good understanding about the etiology of personality disorders."

Psychopharmacology

42. A client diagnosed with dependent personality disorder has a nursing diagnosis of altered sleep pattern R/T impending divorce. The client is prescribed oxazepam prn. Which is an appropriate, correctly written outcome for this nursing diagnosis?
    1. The client verbalizes a decrease in tension and racing thoughts.
    2. The client expresses understanding about the medication side effects by day 2.
    3. The client sleeps 4 to 6 hours a night by day 3.
    4. The client notifies the nurse when the medication is needed.

43. A client diagnosed with paranoid personality disorder is prescribed risperidone. The client is noted to have restlessness and weakness in the lower extremities and is drooling. Which nursing intervention would be most important?
    1. Hold the next dose of risperidone and document the findings.
    2. Monitor vital signs and encourage the client to rest in their room.
    3. Give the ordered prn dose of trihexyphenidyl.
    4. Get a fasting blood sugar measurement because of potential hyperglycemia.

44. A client diagnosed with obsessive-compulsive personality disorder is admitted to a psychiatric unit in a highly agitated state. The physician prescribes a benzodiazepine. Which of the following medications should the nurse expect to administer? **Select all that apply.**
    1. Clonazepam.
    2. Lithium carbonate.
    3. Clozapine.
    4. Olanzapine.
    5. Chlordiazepoxide.

The correct answer number and rationale for why it is the correct answer are given in **boldface blue type**. Rationales for why the other answer options are incorrect are given as well, but they are not in boldface type.

Theory

1. 1. Individuals diagnosed with narcissistic, not paranoid, personality disorder most likely would be subjected to parental demands, criticism, and perfectionistic expectations.
   2. Individuals diagnosed with schizotypal, not paranoid, personality disorder most likely would be subjected to parental indifference, impassivity, or formality.
   3. Individuals diagnosed with schizoid, not paranoid, personality disorder most likely would be subjected to parental bleak and unfeeling coldness.
   4. **Individuals diagnosed with paranoid personality disorder most likely would be subjected to parental antagonism and harassment. These individuals likely served as scapegoats for displaced parental aggression and gradually relinquished all hope of affection and approval. They learned to perceive the world as harsh and unkind, a place calling for protective vigilance and mistrust.**

   TEST-TAKING HINT: To answer this question correctly, the test taker must study and understand the predisposing factors involved in personality disorders. The test taker also needs to understand that although personality disorders are diagnosed in adulthood, they usually begin in childhood and adolescence and often are rooted in parental behaviors and attitudes.

2. According to Mahler's theory of object relations, the infant passes through six phases from birth to 36 months. If the infant is successful, a sense of separateness from the parenting figure is established.
   1. Phase 1 (birth to 1 month) is the normal autism phase of Mahler's development theory. The main task of this phase is survival and comfort. According to Mahler's theory, fixation in this phase may predispose the child to autistic spectrum disorders.
   2. Phase 2 (1 to 5 months) is the symbiosis phase. The main task of this phase is the development of the awareness of an external source of need fulfillment. According to Mahler's theory, fixation in this phase may predispose the child to adolescent or adult-onset psychotic disorders.
   3. **Phase 3 (5 to 36 months) is the separation-individuation phase. The main task of this phase is the primary recognition of separateness from the mother figure. According to Mahler's theory, fixation in this phase may predispose the child to borderline personality disorder.**
   4. Consolidation is the third subcategory of the separation-individuation phase. With the achievement of consolidation, the child is able to internalize a sustained image of the mothering figure as enduring and loving. The child also is able to maintain the perception of the mother as a separate person in the outside world, leading to successful personality development.

   TEST-TAKING HINT: The test taker first must understand Mahler's theory of object relations and then recognize that clients diagnosed with borderline personality disorder have deficits during the separation-individuation phase.

3. 1. Biological, not interpersonal, theory attributes a higher incidence of paranoid personality disorder to relatives of clients with schizophrenia.
   2. **An example of an interpersonal theory of development might involve a client whose background reflects parental emotional abuse to the extent that paranoid personality disorder eventually will be diagnosed.**
   3. Intrapersonal, not interpersonal, theory would discuss the alteration in the ego development and the inability to balance the id and superego.
   4. Intrapersonal, not interpersonal, theory would discuss alterations in the anal stage of development.

   TEST-TAKING HINT: *Intrapersonal* theory and *interpersonal* theory are sometimes confused. To answer this question correctly, the test taker can best differentiate these terms by thinking of the comparison between *interpersonal* and *interstate* (an interstate is a road between states, and interpersonal is between two persons). *Intrapersonal* means existing or occurring within one person's mind or self.

Defense Mechanisms

4. 1. Clients diagnosed with a narcissistic personality disorder may attempt to minimize problems brought about by their effect on others, but the situation described is not reflective of the defense mechanism of minimization.
   2. **Denial is used when a client refuses to acknowledge the existence of a real situation or associated feelings. When the client states, "I don't think the whole world owes me a living," denial is being used to avoid facing others' perceptions.**
   3. Rationalization is an attempt to make excuses or formulate logical reasons to justify unacceptable feelings or behaviors. Clients diagnosed with narcissistic personality disorder often use this defense, but the situation described is not reflective of the defense mechanism of rationalization.
   4. When a client attributes unacceptable feelings or impulses to another person, the client is using the defense mechanism of projection. Clients diagnosed with narcissistic personality disorder often use this defense, but the situation described is not reflective of the defense mechanism of projection.

   TEST-TAKING HINT: To answer this question correctly, the test taker needs to understand that although narcissistic individuals may use any defense mechanism, the client in this question is refusing to recognize others' perceptions. The test taker needs to study and recognize examples of the defense mechanism of denial.

5. Ego defenses are either adaptive or pathological. They can be grouped into four categories: mature defenses, neurotic defenses, immature defenses, and psychotic defenses.
   1. The defense mechanism of undoing is the symbolic negation or cancellation of thoughts or experiences that one finds intolerable. The only thing that the manipulative client in the question finds intolerable is the physician who refuses to give the requested drug.
   2. **The client in the question is using the defense mechanism of splitting. An individual diagnosed with borderline personality disorder sees things as either all good or all bad. In the question, when the client's manipulative charm does not work in obtaining the drug from the "good" physician, the client determines that the physician is now "bad" and seeks another physician to meet their needs.**

3. The defense mechanism of altruism is considered a mature defense and is used when emotional conflicts and stressors are dealt with by meeting the needs of others. The client in the question is meeting no one else's needs but their own.
4. The defense mechanism of reaction formation prevents unacceptable or undesirable thoughts or behaviors from being expressed by exaggerating the opposite thoughts or types of behaviors. The client in the question does not perceive their thoughts or behaviors as either unacceptable or problematic and is not exaggerating the opposite behavior.

TEST-TAKING HINT: To answer this question correctly, the test taker must recognize the behavior in the question as pathological. In understanding this, the test taker can eliminate answer 3 immediately.

Nursing Process—Assessment

6. 1. Borderline personality disorder, not antisocial personality disorder, is characterized by a marked instability in interpersonal relationships, mood, and self-image. These clients also exhibit self-destructive behaviors, such as cutting.
   2. Histrionic personality disorder, not antisocial personality disorder, is characterized by a pervasive pattern of excessive emotionality and attention-seeking behavior. In their attempt to be the center of attention, these clients also exhibit inappropriate sexual, seductive, or provocative behavior.
   3. **Antisocial personality disorder is characterized by a pattern of socially irresponsible, exploitive, and guiltless behavior. These clients disregard the rights of others and frequently fail to conform to social norms with respect to lawful behaviors. They are also deceitful, impulsive, irritable, and aggressive.**
   4. Narcissistic personality disorder, not antisocial personality disorder, is characterized by a constant need for attention; a grandiose sense of self-importance; and preoccupations with fantasies of success, power, brilliance, and beauty. These clients have a sense of entitlement and unreasonable expectations of special treatment.
   5. Antisocial personality disorder is characterized by a pattern of socially irresponsible, exploitive, and guiltless behavior. These clients disregard rules,

authority, and social norms. They will frequently use insincere flattery and manipulation for their own gain.

TEST-TAKING HINT: To answer this question correctly, the test taker must recognize characteristic behaviors that reflect various personality disorders.

7. Irresponsible and guiltless behavior is a characteristic of an individual diagnosed with an antisocial personality disorder, which is grouped in the cluster B classification.
    1. Cluster A categorizes behaviors that are odd or eccentric, and it comprises the following disorders: (1) paranoid personality disorder, which is characterized by a pervasive and unwarranted suspiciousness and mistrust of people; (2) schizoid personality disorder, which is characterized by an inability to form close, personal relationships; and (3) schizotypal personality disorder, which is characterized by peculiarities of ideation, appearance, behavior, and deficits in interpersonal relatedness that are not severe enough to meet the criteria for schizophrenia.
    2. Cluster B categorizes behaviors that are dramatic, emotional, or erratic, and it comprises the following disorders: (1) antisocial personality disorder, which is characterized by a pattern of socially irresponsible, exploitive, and guiltless behavior; (2) borderline personality disorder, which is characterized by a marked instability in interpersonal relationships, mood, and self-image; (3) histrionic personality disorder, which is characterized by a pervasive pattern of excessive emotionality and attention-seeking behavior; and (4) narcissistic personality disorder, which is characterized by a constant need for attention; a grandiose sense of self-importance; and preoccupations with fantasies of success, power, brilliance, and beauty.
    3. Cluster C categorizes behaviors that are anxious or fearful, and it comprises the following disorders: (1) avoidant personality disorder, which is characterized by social withdrawal brought about by extreme sensitivity to rejection; (2) dependent personality disorder, which is characterized by allowing others to assume responsibility for major areas of life because of one's inability to function independently; and (3) obsessive-compulsive personality disorder, which is characterized by a pervasive pattern of perfectionism and inflexibility.

4. There is no *Diagnostic and Statistical Manual of Mental Disorders*, Fifth Edition, Text Revision (*DSM-5-TR*) cluster D classification.

TEST-TAKING HINT: To answer this question correctly, the test taker must understand that there are three clusters of personality disorders, A, B, and C. This eliminates answer 4 immediately.

8. A personality trait is an enduring pattern of perceiving, relating to, and thinking about the environment and oneself that is exhibited in a wide range of social and personal contexts. Personality disorders occur when these traits become inflexible and maladaptive, and cause either significant functional impairment or subjective distress.
    1. Clients exhibiting paranoid personality traits are characterized by a pervasive and unwarranted suspiciousness and mistrust of people. These characteristics are not reflected in the question.
    2. Clients exhibiting schizoid personality traits are characterized by an inability to form close, personal relationships. These characteristics are not reflected in the question.
    3. **Clients exhibiting passive-aggressive personality traits are characterized by a passive resistance to demands for adequate performance in occupational and social functioning. The client in the question is demonstrating passive-aggressive traits toward customers whom they find annoying.**
    4. Clients exhibiting antisocial personality traits are characterized by a pattern of socially irresponsible, exploitive, and guiltless behaviors. These characteristics are not reflected in the question.

TEST-TAKING HINT: To answer this question correctly, the test taker must be able to link the behaviors noted in the question with the correct personality trait.

9. 1. Cluster C includes dependent, avoidant, and obsessive-compulsive personality disorders. Clients diagnosed with obsessive-compulsive personality disorder are characterized by difficulty in expressing emotions, along with a pervasive pattern of perfectionism and inflexibility. The characteristics of this disorder are not reflected in the question.
    2. Cluster A includes paranoid, schizoid, and schizotypal personality disorders. Clients diagnosed with schizotypal personality disorder are characterized by peculiarities of ideation, appearance, and behavior; magical thinking; and deficits

in interpersonal relatedness that are not severe enough to meet the criteria for schizophrenia. In the question, this client's statement reflects ideations of magical thinking.

3. Cluster B includes antisocial, borderline, histrionic, and narcissistic personality disorders. Clients diagnosed with borderline personality disorder are characterized by a marked instability in interpersonal relationships, mood, and self-image. These behaviors are not described in the question.

4. Cluster A includes paranoid, schizoid, and schizotypal personality disorders. Clients diagnosed with schizoid personality disorder are characterized by an inability to form close, personal relationships. In contrast to schizotypal behavior, a client with this disorder would be incapable of establishing any type of personal alliance the way the client presented in the question has established with their grandmother.

TEST-TAKING HINT: To answer this question correctly, the test taker needs to understand the differences between schizoid and schizotypal personality disorders.

10. 1. **Cluster B includes antisocial, borderline, histrionic, and narcissistic personality disorders. Clients diagnosed with borderline personality disorder are characterized by a marked instability in interpersonal relationships, mood, and self-image. Clients with this disorder attempt to pit one individual against another. This is known as *splitting* and is related to an inability to integrate and accept positive and negative feelings. Splitting is a primitive ego defense mechanism that is common in individuals with borderline personality disorder. In the question, the client's statement typifies splitting behavior.**

2. Cluster A includes paranoid, schizoid, and schizotypal personality disorders. Clients diagnosed with schizoid personality disorder are characterized by an inability to form close, personal relationships. The behaviors exhibited by the client described are not associated with this personality disorder.

3. Cluster C includes dependent, avoidant, and obsessive-compulsive personality disorders. Clients diagnosed with obsessive-compulsive disorder are characterized by difficulty in expressing emotions, along with a pervasive pattern of perfectionism

and inflexibility. This client is not displaying any features of a cluster C disorder.

4. Cluster A includes paranoid, schizoid, and schizotypal personality disorders. Clients diagnosed with paranoid personality disorder are characterized by a pervasive and unwarranted suspiciousness and mistrust of people. The behaviors exhibited by the client described are not associated with this personality disorder.

TEST-TAKING HINT: To answer this question correctly, the test taker first must recognize the behaviors in the question as splitting behaviors. Next, the test taker must understand that splitting behaviors are commonly seen in clients diagnosed with borderline personality disorder.

11. The concept of narcissism has its roots in Greek mythology, where Narcissus drowns himself after falling in love with his watery reflection. It is estimated that this disorder occurs in 2% to 16% of the clinical population and less than 1% of the general population. It is diagnosed more often in men than in women.

1. Cluster C includes dependent, avoidant, and obsessive-compulsive personality disorders. Clients diagnosed with obsessive-compulsive personality disorder are characterized by difficulty in expressing emotions, along with a pervasive pattern of perfectionism and inflexibility. Nowhere in the stem does it mention that the client is perfectionistic or inflexible.

2. Cluster C includes dependent, avoidant, and obsessive-compulsive personality disorders. Clients diagnosed with avoidant personality disorder are characterized by a pervasive pattern of social inhibition, feelings of inadequacy, and hypersensitivity to negative evaluation.

3. Cluster A includes paranoid, schizoid, and schizotypal personality disorders. Clients diagnosed with schizotypal personality disorder are characterized by peculiarities of ideation, appearance, and behavior and deficits in interpersonal relatedness that are not severe enough to meet the criteria for schizophrenia. Nowhere in the question does this client demonstrate schizotypal behaviors.

4. **Cluster B includes antisocial, borderline, histrionic, and narcissistic personality disorders. Clients diagnosed with narcissistic personality disorder are characterized by a constant need for attention, a grandiose sense of self-importance, and**

preoccupations with fantasies of success, power, brilliance, and beauty, all of which this client is displaying.

TEST-TAKING HINT: To answer this question correctly, the test taker must be able to link the behaviors noted in the question to the appropriate personality disorder.

12. Clients diagnosed with a cluster B personality disorder do not believe that they have any problems and frequently blame others for their behaviors.
    1. In the question, the client's statement would represent a typical response from someone who was diagnosed with an antisocial personality disorder. These clients also display patterns of socially irresponsible, exploitive, and guiltless behaviors that reflect a disregard for the rights of others. Cluster B includes antisocial, borderline, histrionic, and narcissistic personality disorders. Clients diagnosed with cluster B personality disorders exhibit behaviors that are dramatic, emotional, or erratic.
    2. This client statement would represent a typical response from a client diagnosed with schizotypal personality disorder. These clients also are characterized by peculiarities of ideation with odd and eccentric behaviors. Cluster A includes paranoid, schizoid, and schizotypal personality disorders.
    3. This client statement would represent a typical response from a client diagnosed with paranoid personality disorder. These clients are characterized by a pervasive and unwarranted suspiciousness and mistrust of people, as portrayed in the question. Cluster A includes paranoid, schizoid, and schizotypal personality disorders.
    4. This client statement would represent a typical response from a client diagnosed with dependent personality disorder. These clients are characterized by the inability to function independently and by allowing others to assume responsibility for major areas of life. Cluster C includes dependent, avoidant, and obsessive-compulsive personality disorders.

TEST-TAKING HINT: To answer this question correctly, the test taker must be able to link the behaviors noted in the question with the appropriate personality disorder. If the test taker understands that clients diagnosed with a cluster A disorder may exhibit suspiciousness, answer 3 can be eliminated immediately.

13. 1. This statement might be voiced by a client diagnosed with narcissistic personality disorder. Cluster B includes antisocial, borderline, histrionic, and narcissistic personality disorders. This cluster's characteristic behaviors are dramatic, emotional, or erratic.
    2. This statement might be voiced by a client diagnosed with paranoid personality disorder. Cluster A includes paranoid, schizoid, and schizotypal personality disorders. This cluster's characteristic behaviors are odd or eccentric and include patterns of suspiciousness and mistrust.
    3. This statement might be voiced by a client diagnosed with obsessive-compulsive personality disorder. Cluster C includes dependent, avoidant, and obsessive-compulsive personality disorders. This cluster's characteristic behaviors are anxious and fearful.
    4. This statement might be voiced by a client diagnosed with dependent personality disorder. Cluster C includes dependent, avoidant, and obsessive-compulsive personality disorders. This cluster's characteristic behaviors are anxious and fearful.
    5. This statement might be voiced by a client diagnosed with schizotypal personality disorder. This cluster's characteristic behaviors are odd or eccentric and include patterns of suspiciousness and mistrust.

TEST-TAKING HINT: To answer this question correctly, the test taker must be able to link the cluster noted in the question with the appropriate client statement.

14. 1. Cluster B, not cluster C, consists of antisocial, borderline, histrionic, and narcissistic personality disorders. Being anxious or fearful is the correct description for clients diagnosed with a cluster C personality disorder.
    2. Cluster C, not cluster A, includes avoidant, dependent, and obsessive-compulsive personality disorders. Cluster A consists of paranoid, schizoid, and schizotypal personality disorders, with characteristic behaviors described as odd or eccentric.
    3. Cluster B, not cluster A, consists of antisocial, borderline, histrionic, and narcissistic personality disorders. These disorders are correctly described as dramatic, emotional, or erratic.
    4. Cluster C includes avoidant, dependent, and obsessive-compulsive personality

disorders. Anxious or fearful is the correct description for clients diagnosed with a cluster C personality disorder.

TEST-TAKING HINT: To answer this question correctly, the test taker must review which personality disorders make up clusters A, B, and C and then the characteristic behaviors of clients diagnosed with these disorders. The test taker also must understand that when one part of the answer choice is incorrect, the whole answer choice is incorrect.

15. 1. Individuals with paranoid personality disorder would be isolative and believe that others were out to get them. The behavior presented reflects a client diagnosed with this disorder.
2. Individuals with antisocial personality disorder, not paranoid personality disorder, would be irresponsible and try to exploit others in the milieu.
3. Individuals with avoidant, not paranoid, personality disorder would be shy and refuse to talk with others because of poor self-esteem.
4. Individuals with dependent, not paranoid, personality disorder would sit with peers and allow others to make decisions for the entire group.

TEST-TAKING HINT: To answer this question correctly, the test taker needs to review the signs and symptoms of the different personality disorders and be able to recognize them in various presented behaviors.

16. 1. Having no close relationship with either friends or family is described as a characteristic of schizoid, not schizotypal, personality disorder.
2. Preoccupation with unjustified doubts and suspicions is often a principal aberration associated with paranoid, not schizotypal, personality disorder. Individuals with paranoid personality disorder are extremely oversensitive and tend to misinterpret even minute cues within the environment, magnifying and distorting them into thoughts of trickery and deception. Paranoid behaviors are not commonly associated with individuals diagnosed with schizotypal personality disorders.
3. Individuals diagnosed with histrionic, not schizotypal, personality disorder have a tendency to be self-dramatizing, attention seeking, overly gregarious, and seductive. Because they have difficulty maintaining long-lasting relationships, they tend to exaggerate the intimacy of a relationship. In contrast,

individuals diagnosed with schizotypal personality disorders are aloof and isolated and behave in a bland and apathetic manner.
4. Magical thinking and odd beliefs that influence behavior and are inconsistent with subcultural norms are defined as criteria for schizotypal personality disorder, which is often described as *latent schizophrenia*. Clients with this diagnosis are odd and eccentric but do not decompensate to the level of schizophrenia.

TEST-TAKING HINT: To differentiate between schizotypal and schizoid personality disorders, the test taker should remember that clients diagnosed with *schizotypal* personality disorder *typically* are odd and eccentric, and clients diagnosed with *schizoid* personality disorder are *void* of close relationships.

17. 1. This criterion describes narcissistic, not borderline, personality disorder, which is characterized by a pervasive pattern of grandiosity (in fantasy or behavior), a need for admiration, and a lack of empathy for others.
2. This criterion describes borderline personality disorder, which is characterized by a pervasive pattern of instability of interpersonal relationships. Having real or imagined feelings of abandonment is the first criterion of this disorder.
3. Recurrent suicidal and self-mutilating behavior is a diagnostic criterion that describes borderline personality disorder.
4. This criterion describes dependent, not borderline, personality disorder, which is characterized by a pervasive and excessive need to be cared for, leading to submissive and clinging behavior.
5. Having chronic feelings of emptiness is a diagnostic criterion that describes borderline personality disorder.

TEST-TAKING HINT: To answer this question correctly, the test taker must understand that all four disorders in cluster B may have many characteristics that overlap; however, each cluster has at least one defining characteristic. In the case of borderline personality, feelings of abandonment, self-mutilating behavior, and feelings of emptiness are the key components of this disorder.

18. 1. Clients diagnosed with avoidant personality disorder show a pervasive pattern of social inhibitions, feelings of inadequacies, and hypersensitivity to negative evaluation, and find it difficult to form intimate relationships.

2. Clients diagnosed with dependent, not avoidant, personality disorder are unable to assume the responsibility for making decisions. They have problems with doing things on their own and have difficulties initiating projects.
3. Clients diagnosed with avoidant personality disorder are extremely sensitive to rejection and need strong guarantees of uncritical acceptance.
4. Clients diagnosed with obsessive-compulsive, not avoidant, personality disorder display a pervasive pattern of preoccupation with orderliness and perfectionism. The tendency to be rigid and unbending about rules and procedures often makes task completion a problem.
5. Although there may be a strong desire for companionship, a client with avoidant personality disorder has such a pervasive pattern of inadequacy, social inhibition, and withdrawal from life that the desire for companionship is negated.

TEST-TAKING HINT: To answer this question correctly, the test taker should note that an individual diagnosed with an avoidant personality disorder is generally unwilling to get involved with another person unless certain of being liked.

19. 1. Clients diagnosed with schizotypal, not histrionic, personality disorder exhibit odd beliefs and magical thinking that influence behavior and are inconsistent with subcultural norms (e.g., belief in clairvoyance, telepathy, or sixth sense). These clients present with a pervasive pattern of social and interpersonal deficits marked by acute discomfort with close relationships.
2. Clients diagnosed with narcissistic, not histrionic, personality disorder are preoccupied with fantasies of unlimited success, brilliance, beauty, or ideal love. Through a grandiose sense of self, this individual expects to be recognized as superior without commensurate achievements.
3. Clients diagnosed with obsessive-compulsive, not histrionic, personality disorder have a pervasive pattern of preoccupation with orderliness, perfection, and mental and interpersonal control at the expense of flexibility, openness, and efficiency.
4. Clients diagnosed with histrionic personality disorder have a pervasive pattern of excessive emotionality and attention-seeking behaviors. These individuals are uncomfortable in situations in which

they are not the center of attention and have a style of speech that is excessively impressionistic and lacking in detail.

TEST-TAKING HINT: To answer this question correctly, the test taker must pair characteristic behaviors with various personality disorders. For clients diagnosed with histrionic personality disorder, it may help the test taker to remember, "Life is a stage, and they are the director."

20. 1. Clients diagnosed with borderline personality disorder, not passive-aggressive traits, have a pattern of unstable and intense interpersonal relationships characterized by alternating between extremes of idealization and devaluation. This client behavior manifests itself in a major defense mechanism referred to as splitting.
2. Clients diagnosed with antisocial personality disorder, not passive-aggressive traits, have a sense of entitlement and a lack of remorse, believing they have the right to hurt others. These individuals have little regard for the safety of self or others and are repeatedly involved in altercations.
3. Clients diagnosed with paranoid personality disorder, not passive-aggressive traits, suspect that others will exploit, harm, or deceive them. These individuals have recurrent suspicions, without justification, regarding friends and relatives.
4. Clients exhibiting passive-aggressive traits believe another individual has wronged them, and they may go to great lengths to seek retribution or to get even. This is done in a subtle and passive manner rather than by discussing their feelings with the offending individual.

TEST-TAKING HINT: To answer this question correctly, the test taker must recognize the characteristics associated with passive-aggressive personality traits.

21. 1. A common trait among individuals diagnosed with a personality disorder is the failure to accept the consequences of their own behavior. Although these individuals can identify correct and appropriate behavior, they repeatedly avoid change and cling to patterns that meet their unhealthy needs.
2. Self-injurious behaviors, such as self-mutilation or cutting, are characteristics specific to borderline personality disorder. This trait is not commonly associated with other disorders.

3. Reluctance in taking personal risks or engaging in any new activities for fear of embarrassment is a particular trait seen in avoidant personality disorders. This trait is not commonly associated with other disorders.

4. **A common trait among individuals diagnosed with a personality disorder is their response to stress. When feeling threatened, these individuals cope by attempting to change the environment instead of changing themselves.**

5. **A common trait among individuals diagnosed with a personality disorder is the lack of insight. These individuals lack understanding of the impact of their behaviors on others.**

TEST-TAKING HINT: To answer this question correctly, the test taker must note that the essential characteristics of personality disorders are pervasive, maladaptive, and chronic.

Nursing Process—Diagnosis

22. 1. Risk for injury is defined as when a client is at risk for injury as a result of internal or external environmental conditions interacting with the individual's adaptive and defensive resources. Nothing presented in the question would indicate that this client is at risk for injury.

2. Risk for violence: self-directed is defined as when a client is at risk for behaviors in which an individual demonstrates that they can be physically, emotionally, or sexually harmful to self. Nothing presented in the question would indicate that this client is at risk for violence: self-directed.

3. **Ineffective denial is defined as the conscious or unconscious attempt to disavow knowledge or meaning of an event to reduce anxiety or fear. The client presented in the question is denying their children's need for parental support by turning the situation around and making themself sound like the victim who is not needed.**

4. Powerlessness is defined as the perception that one's own action would not significantly affect an outcome, a perceived lack of control over a current situation or immediate happening. Although the client in the question would like to be perceived as powerless over the situation, nothing presented in the question would indicate that this client is experiencing powerlessness.

TEST-TAKING HINT: To answer this question correctly, the test taker needs to use the information presented in the question to determine the nursing diagnosis for this client.

23. 1. **Repetitive, self-mutilating behaviors are classic manifestations of borderline personality disorder. These individuals seek attention by self-mutilating until pain is felt in an effort to counteract feelings of emptiness. Some clients reported that "to feel pain is better than to feel nothing." Because these clients often inflict injury on themselves, this diagnosis must be prioritized to ensure client safety.**

2. This client is expressing ineffective coping by self-mutilating, exhibiting disruptive behaviors, and splitting staff. However, because the client is self-mutilating, client safety must be prioritized.

3. Although clients diagnosed with borderline personality disorder may exhibit anxiety, because the client is self-mutilating, client safety must be prioritized.

4. Although self-mutilation acts can be fatal, most commonly they are manipulative gestures designed to elicit a rescue response from significant others. Nothing in the question indicates the client has a history of a suicide attempt, so the "related to" statement of this diagnosis is incorrect.

TEST-TAKING HINT: To answer this question correctly, the test taker needs to link the behaviors presented in the question with the nursing diagnosis that describes this client's problem. Client safety should always be prioritized.

24. 1. Anxiety is defined as a vague, uneasy feeling of discomfort or dread accompanied by an autonomic response. The client in the question is experiencing feelings of indifference, not anxiety.

2. This client is expressing ineffective coping by choosing solitary activities, avoiding socialization, and exhibiting indifference to criticism, but there is nothing in the question that indicates the client is unable to communicate. The "related to" statement of this diagnosis is incorrect.

3. The nursing diagnosis of altered sensory perception generally is reserved for clients experiencing hallucinations or delusions or both. Nothing in the question indicates that this client is experiencing hallucinations, delusions, or magical thinking.

4. Clients diagnosed with schizoid personality disorder are unsociable and prefer to work in isolation. These individuals are characterized primarily by a profound defect in the ability to form personal relationships or to respond to others in any meaningful or emotional way. They display a lifelong pattern of social withdrawal, and their discomfort with human interaction is very apparent. This client is choosing solitary activities and lacks friends. The nursing diagnosis of social isolation is appropriate in addressing this client's problem.

TEST-TAKING HINT: To answer this question correctly, the test taker needs to link the behaviors described in the question with the nursing diagnosis that reflects the client's problem.

25. 1. Social isolation is defined as aloneness experienced by the individual and perceived as imposed by others and as a negative or threatening state. There is nothing in the question indicating that this client is experiencing social isolation.
2. Impaired social interaction is defined as the insufficient or excessive quantity or ineffective quality of social exchange. When the client in the question complains about a nagging spouse who criticizes their indecisiveness, they are passively expressing covert aggression. This negative expression impedes the client's ability to interact appropriately and to express feelings openly, which leads to the correct nursing diagnosis, impaired social interaction.
3. Powerlessness is defined as a perceived lack of control over a current situation or immediate happening. As a tactic of interpersonal behavior, passive-aggressive individuals commonly switch among the roles of the martyr, the affronted, the aggrieved, the misunderstood, the contrite, the guilt ridden, the sickly, and the overworked. These roles empower, not render powerless, the passive-aggressive individual. Also, nothing in the question suggests that the client's spouse is abusive.
4. Self-esteem disturbance is defined as a negative self-evaluation and feelings about self or self-capabilities. Nothing in the question indicates the client is experiencing low self-esteem. The spouse wanting the client to make decisions is not an unrealistic expectation. By stating that their spouse's expectations are unrealistic, the

client is attempting to make this situation the spouse's fault, not their own.

TEST-TAKING HINT: To answer this question correctly, the test taker needs to link the behaviors described in the question with the nursing diagnosis that reflects the client's problem.

Nursing Process—Planning

26. 1. The flexibility and mobility of construction work, which uses physical versus interpersonal skills, may be best suited for a client diagnosed with antisocial personality disorder. These clients tend to exploit and manipulate others, and construction work would provide less opportunity for the client to exhibit these behaviors. A client diagnosed with narcissistic personality disorder would not be suited for this job.
2. Individuals with obsessive-compulsive personality disorder are inflexible and lack spontaneity. They are meticulous and work diligently and patiently at tasks that require accuracy and discipline. They are especially concerned with matters of organization and efficiency and tend to be rigid and unbending about rules and procedures, making them, and not the client described in the question, good candidates for the job of air traffic controller.
3. Clients diagnosed with schizoid personality disorder are unable to form close, personal relationships. These clients are comfortable with animal companionship, making a night security job at the zoo an ideal occupation. A client diagnosed with narcissistic personality disorder would not be suited for this job.
4. Individuals diagnosed with narcissistic personality disorder have an exaggerated sense of self-worth and believe they have an inalienable right to receive special consideration. They tend to exploit others to fulfill their own desires. Because they view themselves as superior beings, they believe they are entitled to special rights and privileges. Because of the need to control others inherent in the job of prison warden, this would be an appropriate job choice for a client diagnosed with narcissistic personality disorder.

TEST-TAKING HINT: To answer this question correctly, the test taker must be familiar with the characteristics of the various personality disorders and how these traits would affect employment situations.

27. 1. Although limit setting is needed, this situation does not pose a threat, and immediate limiting setting would not be indicated.
    2. The client in this situation is attempting to split the staff. Although the nurse needs to set limits on the client's manipulative behavior, there is no potential physical threat, so limit setting in this situation does not take priority.
    3. **A paranoid client has the potential to strike out defensively if provoked. Because safety is the nurse's first concern, and this situation poses a physical threat, this situation takes priority and needs immediate intervention by the nurse.**
    4. Attention-seeking by refusing medications is a secondary gain that the nurse may want to address with the client. This situation presents no physical threat, however, and is not the nurse's immediate concern.

TEST-TAKING HINT: When the word *prioritize* is used in a question, the test taker must pay attention to which situation the nurse would need to address first. Safety is always the priority.

28. 1. Although the nurse may want to further assess the client's perception of future death, the nurse would not ask a question that supports this altered thought process. It is important for the nurse to make it clear that the visions of future death are not real before assessing further.
    2. Asking the client to elaborate about the visions allows the client to continue with altered thoughts. The nurse would want to ask specific questions and then move on to assisting the client in dealing with the uncomfortable feelings.
    3. Asking the client to come to group to talk further about the visions does not support the client's feelings and encourages the client to continue to focus on the altered thoughts.
    4. **Acknowledging the client's feelings about the altered thoughts is an important response. The nurse supports the client's feelings but not the altered thoughts. At the same time, the nurse explores ways to help the client feel comfortable.**

TEST-TAKING HINT: To answer this question correctly, the test taker must remember that when a client is experiencing altered thoughts, it is important for the nurse to be empathetic about the feelings that occur. The nurse never wants to make statements that reinforce altered thoughts, however real they may be to the client.

29. 1. Although it is important for the client to be safe and free from self-injurious behaviors, this outcome does not have a time frame and is incorrectly written.
    2. **The client's being able to express feelings without inflicting self-injury by discharge is an outcome that reinforces the priority for client safety, is measurable, and has a time frame.**
    3. Although it is important for the client to be able to socialize with peers in the milieu, it is not the priority outcome.
    4. The ultimate outcome for a client diagnosed with borderline personality disorder is to understand better how specific personal behaviors affect interpersonal skills. Because this outcome does not have a time frame and does not reinforce the priority of safety, it is incorrect.

TEST-TAKING HINT: To answer this question correctly, the test taker needs to review the criteria for outcomes, making sure that all answers are measurable, specific, client-centered, and positive and have a time frame. Answers 1 and 4 can be eliminated immediately because they do not have a time frame.

30. The hallmark of a client diagnosed with avoidant personality disorder is social isolation. The cause of social isolation in these clients is the fear of criticism and rejection.
    1. This is an idealistic, but unrealistic, outcome. The client has a deformity that needs to be dealt with realistically. There is nothing deformed about the client's mind, character, principles, or value system. It is up to the nurse to explore the client's strengths and develop, through a plan of care, the client's positive, rather than negative, attributes.
    2. Seeing self as valuable is a positive step in increasing self-esteem and self-worth; however, it does not relate to the nursing diagnosis of social isolation. Also, the completion of the course most likely would extend beyond discharge, and positive results would be considered a long-term, not short-term, outcome.
    3. **This short-term outcome is stated in observable and measurable terms. This outcome sets a specific time for achievement (by end of shift). It is short and specific (one therapy group), and it is written in positive terms, all of which**

should contribute to the final goal of the client having increased social interaction.

4. This is not a measurable outcome because it does not include a time frame and therefore can be eliminated.

TEST-TAKING HINT: To answer this question correctly, the test taker must look for an outcome that has a time frame and is positive, realistic, measurable, and client centered.

31. 1. Expecting the client to abstain from ritualistic hand washing on admission is an unrealistic outcome. To do this would heighten, rather than lower, the client's anxiety level. There is no mention of a time frame, so this outcome cannot be measured.

2. This outcome has no specific measurable time frame. Although this might be a reasonable client outcome if started after treatment has begun, it might be an unreasonable expectation if implemented too soon after admission. Only after the client has learned new coping skills can ritualistic behaviors be decreased without increasing anxiety levels.

3. Although this may eventually be a reasonable client expectation, there is no mention of a time frame, so this outcome cannot be measured.

4. **This short-term outcome is stated in observable and measurable terms. This outcome sets a specific time for achievement (within 72 hours). It is specific (signs and symptoms), and it is written in positive terms. When the client can identify signs and symptoms of increased anxiety, the next step of problem-solving can begin.**

TEST-TAKING HINT: To answer this question correctly, the test taker must note that outcomes need to be realistic for clients diagnosed with personality disorders to achieve success. An outcome that may be inappropriate on admission may be attainable and appropriate by discharge.

Nursing Process—Implementation

32. 1. **In this situation, the nurse empathizes with the client's concerns and then sets limits on inappropriate behaviors in a matter-of-fact manner.**

2. Offering a sleeping pill in this situation avoids the client's frustrations and the need to set limits on inappropriate behaviors.

3. "It's midnight, and you are disturbing the other clients" is a judgmental response and does not deal with the client's concerns or the inappropriate behavior.

4. Documenting the client's concerns in the chart placates the client and avoids addressing the client's concerns directly. Here, the nurse is transferring responsibility to other staff members versus dealing with the immediate situation. This interaction allows the client to split staff.

TEST-TAKING HINT: To answer this question correctly, the test taker must remember that when setting limits on manipulative behaviors, the nurse always should give reasons for the limits and deal with the situation in a timely manner.

33. 1. **It is important to address an individual's behavior in a timely manner to set appropriate limits. Limit setting is to be done in a calm but firm manner. A client diagnosed with antisocial personality disorder may have no regard for rules or regulations, which necessitates limit setting by the nurse.**

2. Limit setting needs to be applied immediately, by all staff members, to avoid client manipulation and encourage responsible and appropriate behaviors.

3. Although the nurse may want to remind all clients about unit rules, the word *initial* makes this answer incorrect. Initially, the nurse needs to confront the behavior.

4. The word *initial* makes this answer incorrect. Addressing inappropriate or testing behaviors must be a priority to bring into the client's awareness the consequences of inappropriate actions. The nurse should follow up limit setting at a later time with constructive discussions regarding the cause and effects of inappropriate behaviors.

TEST-TAKING HINT: The test taker must note important keywords in the question, such as *initial*, *priority*, or *most important*. These words assist the test taker in determining the correct answer.

34. 1. Giving the client tranquilizing medications, such as anxiolytics or antipsychotics, may have a calming effect and reduce aggressive behavior, but it does not address the client's priority safety issue. Tranquilizing medications are considered a chemical restraint and would be used only when all other, less-restrictive measures have been attempted.

2. **The priority nursing intervention is to observe the client's behavior frequently.**

The nurse should do this through routine activities and interactions to avoid appearing watchful and suspicious. Close observation is required so that immediate interventions can be implemented as needed.

3. Encouraging the client to verbalize hostile feelings may help the client to come to terms with unresolved issues, but it does not address the client's priority safety need.
4. It is important to explore alternative ways of handling frustration, such as physical activities. Although this may relieve pent-up frustration, it does not address the client's priority safety need.

TEST-TAKING HINT: To answer this question correctly, the test taker must note important words in the question, such as *priority*. Physical safety is a major concern, and client safety must be considered a priority whenever the nurse formulates a nursing plan of care.

35. The nursing diagnosis of ineffective coping is defined as the inability to form a valid appraisal of stressors, inadequate choices of practiced responses, or inability to use available resources.
    1. **Setting limits on manipulative behaviors is an appropriate intervention to discourage dysfunctional coping, such as oppositional and defiant behaviors. It is important to convey to the client that inappropriate behaviors are not tolerated.**
    2. **By refusing to engage in debate, argument, rationalization, or bargaining with a client, the nurse has intervened effectively to decrease manipulative behaviors and has decreased the opportunity for oppositional and defiant behaviors.**
    3. Tranquilizing medications may have a calming effect; however, nothing in the question indicates the client is agitated or anxious. Tranquilizing medications are considered a chemical restraint and would be used only when all other, less-restrictive measures have been attempted.
    4. **Dealing with feelings honestly and directly discourages ineffective coping. The client may cope with anger inappropriately by displacing this anger onto others.**
    5. When a client is a danger to self or others, ensuring safety in the environment is a priority. However, nothing in the question indicates any need for this intervention.

TEST-TAKING HINT: To answer this question correctly, the test taker must recognize interventions that directly affect defiant behaviors.

36. The definition of the nursing diagnosis of disturbed personal identity is the inability to distinguish between self and others.
    1. This intervention addresses suicidal behavior, but nothing in the question suggests that this client has suicidal ideations.
    2. This intervention decreases agitation and aggressive behavior, but nothing in the question suggests that this client needs this type of intervention.
    3. Presenting reality is a necessary intervention when a client is experiencing a thought process problem, but nothing in the question suggests that this client needs this type of intervention.
    4. **This client has been diagnosed with borderline personality disorder resulting from fixation in an earlier developmental level. This disruption during the establishment of the client's value system has led to disturbed personal identity. When the nurse helps the client to identify internalized values, beliefs, and attitudes, the client begins to distinguish personal identity.**

TEST-TAKING HINT: To answer this question correctly, the test taker must be able to link the appropriate nursing intervention with the stated nursing diagnosis.

37. 1. Inappropriate interactions are associated with the nursing diagnosis of impaired social interaction, not social isolation. Also, nothing in the question indicates the client is exhibiting inappropriate interactions.
    2. A client playing one staff member against another is known as splitting. Nothing in the question indicates that the client is attempting to split staff.
    3. **Role-modeling positive relationships would provide a motivation to initiate interactions with others outside the client's family. This is an appropriate intervention for the nursing diagnosis of social isolation.**
    4. There is no mention of conflict within the family. The conflict that is being addressed is the client's inability to reach beyond the family system because of unresolved abandonment issues.

TEST-TAKING HINT: To answer this question correctly, the test taker must find the nursing interaction that addresses the problem of

social isolation. Role-modeling positive interactions is an appropriate nursing intervention for this problem. Understanding the difference between social isolation and impaired social interaction assists the test taker in eliminating answer 1 immediately.

38. 1. When a client is diagnosed with paranoid personality disorder, the client may have difficulty participating in a group activity and may miss important information regarding medications.
2. **When a client is diagnosed with paranoid personality disorder, one-to-one teaching in a client's room would decrease the client's paranoia, support a trusting relationship, and allow the client to ask questions. The nurse also would be able to evaluate the effectiveness of medication teaching.**
3. When a client is diagnosed with paranoid personality disorder, the client may feel uncomfortable asking questions during rounds, and the client may miss important information about the prescribed medications.
4. Although it may be a good idea to give a client diagnosed with paranoid personality disorder written material to refer to, if the nurse does not encourage a trusting relationship by one-to-one teaching, the client may not feel comfortable asking questions. The client may miss important information, and the nurse would have no way of noting whether the teaching was effective.

TEST-TAKING HINT: The test taker must review important information regarding dealing with clients exhibiting paranoia and understand the interventions that the nurse may use to assist in building a successful and therapeutic nurse–client relationship.

Nursing Process—Evaluation

39. 1. Zeus did not play a part in the historical aspects of personality disorders. He was a figure of Greek mythology, the chief deity, and son of Cronus and Rhea. In 1975, Mahler, Pine, and Berman developed the theory of object relations, which deals with infants passing through six phases from birth to 36 months, when a sense of separateness from the parenting figure is finally established.
2. In the 4th century BC, Hippocrates, also known as the father of medicine,

identified four fundamental personality styles that he concluded stemmed from excesses in the four humors: the irritable and hostile choleric (yellow bile), the pessimistic melancholic (black bile), the overly optimistic and extroverted sanguine (blood), and the apathetic phlegmatic (phlegm).
3. Although the word *personality* is from the Greek term *persona*, Narcissus cannot be credited with this introduction. Narcissus, according to Greek mythology, was a beautiful youth who, after Echo's death, was made to pine away for the love of his own reflection while gazing into spring water. The roots for narcissistic personality disorder can be traced back to this well-known Greek myth.
4. Achilles did not play a part in the historical aspects of personality disorders. He was a mythical Greek warrior and leader in the Trojan War.

TEST-TAKING HINT: To answer this question correctly, the test taker must study the historical aspects of personality disorders and understand how Hippocrates described the concept of personality.

40. 1. Schizotypal, not narcissistic, personality disorder is characterized by peculiarities of ideation, appearance, and behavior; magical thinking; and deficits in interpersonal relatedness that are not severe enough to meet the criteria for schizophrenia.
2. Histrionic, not narcissistic, personality disorder is characterized by a pervasive pattern of excessive emotionality, attention-seeking behavior, and the seeking of constant affirmation of approval and acceptance from others.
3. Borderline, not narcissistic, personality disorder is characterized by a marked instability in interpersonal relationships, mood, and self-image. These clients are impulsive and self-destructive. They lack a clear sense of identity and have fluctuating attitudes toward others.
4. **Narcissistic personality disorder is characterized by a grandiose sense of self-importance and preoccupations with fantasies of success, power, brilliance, and beauty. These clients sometimes may exploit others for self-gratification.**
5. **Clients diagnosed with narcissistic personality disorder have a deep need for admiration and exhibit a lack of empathy for others.**

TEST-TAKING HINT: To answer this question correctly, the test taker must be able to distinguish among behaviors exhibited by clients diagnosed with various personality disorders.

41. 1. Most personality-disordered individuals, although functioning inconsistently in subcultural norms, maintain themselves in the community. Therefore, individuals with a diagnosis of a personality disorder might never be hospitalized.
    2. In contrast to a client diagnosed with anxiety disorders, depressive disorders, schizophrenia spectrum disorders, or other mental disorders, clients with personality disorders experience no feelings of discomfort or disorganization with their inappropriate behaviors.
    3. It is important for nurses to understand that for individuals diagnosed with personality disorders, no prescribed medications are available to cure or control these disorders. Clients' inappropriate behaviors and skewed perceptions often lead to anxiety or depression or both; therefore, anxiolytics, antidepressants, and antipsychotics sometimes are prescribed.
    4. Although there are many different theories related to the development of personality disorders, it is unclear why some individuals develop personality disorders and others do not.

TEST-TAKING HINT: To answer this question correctly, the test taker needs to review theories regarding the etiology of personality development and treatment modalities for individuals diagnosed with a personality disorder.

Psychopharmacology

42. Oxazepam is a benzodiazepine used in the treatment of anxiety disorders.
    1. There is no time frame on this outcome; therefore, it is incorrectly written.
    2. This outcome would be appropriate for the nursing diagnosis of knowledge deficit, not altered sleep pattern.
    3. This outcome relates directly to the stated nursing diagnosis (altered sleep pattern), is measurable (sleeps 4 to

6 hours a night) and has a time frame (by day 3).
    4. There is no time frame included in this outcome; therefore, it is not measurable.

TEST-TAKING HINT: To answer this question correctly, the test taker must recognize the appropriate outcome as it relates to the stated nursing diagnosis and must also note that outcomes must be client specific, attainable, positive, and measurable and must include a time frame.

43. Risperidone is an atypical antipsychotic medication used in the treatment of paranoia. Restlessness, weakness in lower extremities, and drooling are extrapyramidal symptoms (EPS) caused by antipsychotic medications.
    1. It is unnecessary to hold the next dose of risperidone because the symptoms noted are not life threatening and can be corrected using an anticholinergic medication, such as trihexyphenidyl.
    2. The client in the question is experiencing EPS. Having EPS would not alter the client's vital signs.
    3. The symptoms noted are EPS caused by antipsychotic medications. These can be corrected by using anticholinergic medications, such as trihexyphenidyl, benztropine, or diphenhydramine.
    4. Although antipsychotic medications can cause hyperglycemia, the symptoms noted in the question are not related to hyperglycemia.

TEST-TAKING HINT: To answer this question correctly, the test taker must review the various side effects of antipsychotic medications and the interventions that address these side effects.

44. 1. Clonazepam is a benzodiazepine medication.
    2. Lithium carbonate is a mood stabilizer, or antimanic, not a benzodiazepine.
    3. Clozapine is an atypical antipsychotic, not a benzodiazepine.
    4. Olanzapine is an antipsychotic, not a benzodiazepine.
    5. Chlordiazepoxide is a benzodiazepine medication.

TEST-TAKING HINT: To answer this question correctly, the test taker must be able to recognize various classifications of psychotropic medications.

Somatic Symptom and Dissociative Disorders

The following words include English vocabulary, nursing/medical terminology, concepts, principles, or information relevant to content specifically addressed in this chapter or associated with topics presented in it. English dictionaries, your nursing textbooks, and medical dictionaries such as *Taber's Cyclopedic Medical Dictionary* are resources that can be used to expand your knowledge and understanding of these words and related information.

Body dysmorphic disorder

Conversion disorder (functional neurological symptom disorder)

Depersonalization/derealization disorder

Dissociative amnesia

Dissociative amnesia with dissociative fugue

Dissociative identity disorder (DID)

Factitious disorder

Illness anxiety disorder

Somatic symptom disorder

Specified somatic symptom disorder

QUESTIONS

Theory

1. Which statement describes the etiology of illness anxiety disorder from a psychodynamic theory perspective?
   1. The client expresses physical complaints, which are less threatening than facing underlying feelings of poor self-esteem.
   2. Emotions associated with traumatic events are viewed as morally or ethically unacceptable and are transferred into physical symptoms.
   3. The client's family has difficulty expressing emotions openly and resolving conflicts verbally; this is dealt with by focusing on the ill family member.
   4. The deficiency of endorphins seems to correlate with an increase in incoming sensory stimuli.

2. Which statement describes the etiology of somatic symptom disorder from a biochemical theory perspective?
   1. Unexpressed emotions are translated into symptoms of pain.
   2. A deficiency of endorphins affects incoming sensory stimuli.
   3. There is an increased incidence of this disorder in first-degree relatives.
   4. Harmony around the illness replaces discord within the family.

3. Which statement describes the etiology of somatic symptom disorder from a learning theory perspective?
   1. Studies have shown that there is an increase in the predisposition of somatic symptom disorder in first-degree relatives.
   2. Positive reinforcement of somatic symptoms encourages behaviors to continue.
   3. A client views self as bad and considers physical suffering as deserved and required for atonement.
   4. The use of physical symptoms is a response to repressed severe anxiety.

4. Which statement supports a psychodynamic theory in the etiology of dissociative disorders?
   1. Dysfunction in the hippocampus affects memory.
   2. Dissociate reactions may be precipitated by excessive cortical arousal.
   3. Coping capacity is overwhelmed by a set of traumatic experiences.
   4. Repression is used as a way to protect the client from emotional pain.

5. A frightened client diagnosed with dissociative amnesia tells the nurse, "I don't know who I am. What is wrong with me?" Which nursing response reflects a neurobiological perspective?
   1. "You appear to have repressed disturbing and distressing feelings from your conscious awareness."
   2. "Sometimes these symptoms are found in individuals with temporal lobe epilepsy or severe migraine headaches."
   3. "When individuals have experienced some sort of trauma, the primary self needs to escape from reality."
   4. "It has been found that these symptoms are seen more often when first-degree relatives have similar symptoms."

Nursing Process—Assessment

6. A client is suspected to be experiencing a conversion disorder. Which of the following would the nurse expect to assess? **Select all that apply.**
   1. Deep tendon reflexes intact.
   2. Muscle wasting.
   3. The client is unaware of the link between anxiety and physical symptoms.
   4. Physical symptoms are explained by a physiological cause.
   5. A lack of concern toward the alteration in function.

7. A client is diagnosed with illness anxiety disorder. Which of the following assessment data validate this diagnosis? **Select all that apply.**
   1. Preoccupation with disease processes and organ function.
   2. Long history of doctor shopping.
   3. Physical symptoms are managed by using the defense mechanism of denial.
   4. Depression and obsessive-compulsive traits are common.
   5. Social and occupational functioning may be impaired.

8. A client diagnosed with a specified somatic symptom disorder states, "I want to thank the staff for being so understanding when I am in pain." This is an example of a _____ gain.

9. A client admitted with dissociative amnesia with dissociative fugue is being evaluated. Which of the following assessment information would indicate that the client is ready for discharge? **Select all that apply.**
   1. The client is able to maintain reality during stressful situations.
   2. The client is able to verbalize why alternate personalities exist.
   3. The client is able to discuss feelings such as depersonalization.
   4. The client is able to integrate subpersonalities into a whole personality.
   5. The client is observed using relaxation techniques when visibly upset.

10. Which client situation supports a potential diagnosis of a dissociative amnesia with dissociative fugue?
    1. A Canadian client enters the emergency department (ED) in New York City without understanding who they are or how they got there.
    2. A client known as being shy and passive comes into the ED angry and demanding their address or phone number.
    3. A client known as being shy and passive comes into the ED and is unable to recall their address and phone number.
    4. A client seen in the ED complains of feeling detached from the current situation.

11. Which of the following chronic or transient medical conditions can be associated with amnestic disorders? **Select all that apply.**
    1. Cerebral anoxia.
    2. Cardiac arrhythmias.
    3. Migraine.
    4. Psoriasis.
    5. Cerebrovascular disease.

12. An amnestic disorder can result from the use of which of the following substances? **Select all that apply.**
    1. Toxins.
    2. Medications.
    3. Aspartame.
    4. Sedatives.
    5. Alcohol.

Nursing Process—Diagnosis

13. A client, who is fearful of an upcoming deployment to Iraq, experiences paralysis and is diagnosed with a conversion disorder. Which nursing diagnosis takes priority?
    1. Impaired skin integrity R/T muscle wasting.
    2. Body image disturbance R/T immobility.
    3. Anxiety R/T fears about a combat injury.
    4. Activity intolerance R/T paralysis.

14. A client diagnosed with illness anxiety disorder states, "I have so many symptoms, and yet no one can find out what is wrong with me. I can't do this anymore." Which nursing diagnosis would take priority?
    1. Altered role performance R/T multiple hospitalizations.
    2. Knowledge deficit R/T the link between anxiety and expressed symptoms.
    3. Risk for suicide R/T client statement, "I can't do this anymore."
    4. Self-care deficit R/T client statement, "I can't do this anymore."

15. A client diagnosed with somatic symptom disorder visits multiple physicians because of various, vague symptoms involving many body systems. Which nursing diagnosis takes priority?
    1. Risk for injury R/T treatment from multiple physicians.
    2. Anxiety R/T unexplained multiple somatic symptoms.
    3. Ineffective coping R/T psychosocial distress.
    4. Fear R/T multiple physiological complaints.

16. A client diagnosed with depersonalization/derealization disorder has a short-term outcome that states, "The client will verbalize an alternate way of dealing with stress by day 4." Which nursing diagnosis reflects the problem that this outcome addresses?
    1. Disturbed sensory perception R/T severe psychological stress.
    2. Ineffective coping R/T overwhelming anxiety.
    3. Self-esteem disturbance R/T dissociative events.
    4. Anxiety R/T repressed traumatic events.

Nursing Process—Planning

17. A client diagnosed with conversion disorder has a nursing diagnosis of disturbed sensory perception R/T anxiety AEB paralysis. Which short-term outcome would be appropriate for this client?
    1. The client will demonstrate recovery of lost function by discharge.
    2. The client will use one effective coping mechanism to decrease anxiety by day 3.
    3. The client will express feelings of fear about paralysis by day 1.
    4. The client will acknowledge underlying anxiety by day 4.

18. A client diagnosed with a specified somatic symptom disorder is experiencing pain. The client has been assigned a nursing diagnosis of ineffective coping R/T repressed anxiety. Which is an appropriate correctly written outcome for this client?
    1. The client will verbalize a pain rating of 0/10 by the end of the day.
    2. The client will substitute one effective coping strategy for one physical complaint by discharge.
    3. The client will express a realistic perception of their distorted self-image by discharge.
    4. The client will rate anxiety as less than 3/10.

19. It is documented in the client's chart "R/O somatic symptom disorder." The client complains of diarrhea, stomach cramping, and "feeling warm." Number the following nursing actions in the priority order in which the nurse would complete them.
    1. _____ Monitor vital signs.
    2. _____ Assess level of understanding about the effects of anxiety on the body.
    3. _____ Assess the level of anxiety, using an anxiety scale of 1 to 10.
    4. _____ Encourage the client to write down their feelings.
    5. _____ Teach and encourage relaxation techniques and note effectiveness.

20. A client diagnosed with dissociative identity disorder (DID) has been hospitalized for 7 days. The client has a nursing diagnosis of ineffective coping R/T repressed severe anxiety. Which correctly written outcome would be appropriate?
    1. The client will recover deficits in memory by day 14.
    2. The client will be aware of alternate personalities by day 14.
    3. The client will demonstrate the ability to perceive stimuli accurately.
    4. The client will demonstrate one adaptive way to deal with stress by day 14.

Nursing Process—Implementation

21. A client diagnosed with illness anxiety disorder complains to the nurse about others doubting the seriousness of the client's disease. The client is angry, frustrated, and anxious. Which nursing intervention takes priority?
    1. Remind the client that laboratory tests showed no evidence of physiological problems.
    2. Document the client's unwillingness to accept anxiety as the source of the illness.
    3. Discuss with the client's family ways to avoid secondary gains associated with physical complaints.
    4. Acknowledge the client's frustration without fostering continued focus on physical illness.

22. During group therapy, a client diagnosed with a specified somatic symptom disorder monopolizes the group by discussing back pain. Which nursing statement is an appropriate response in this situation?
    1. "I can tell this is bothering you. Let's briefly discuss this further after group."
    2. "Let's see if anyone in the group has ideas on how to deal with pain."
    3. "We need to get back to the topic of dealing with anxiety."
    4. "Let's check in and see how others in the group are feeling."

23. A client who currently complains of vague weakness and multisystem symptoms has been diagnosed with a somatic symptom disorder. Which nursing intervention takes priority?
    1. Discuss the client's symptoms to provide secondary gains.
    2. Discuss the stressor that the client is experiencing.
    3. Evaluate signs and symptoms, vital signs, and laboratory tests.
    4. Teach the client appropriate coping mechanisms to deal with stress.

24. A newly admitted client is diagnosed with dissociative identity disorder (DID). Which nursing intervention is a priority?
    1. Establish an atmosphere of safety and security.
    2. Identify relationships among subpersonalities and work with each equally.
    3. Teach new coping skills to replace dissociative behaviors.
    4. Process events associated with the origins of the disorder.

25. A newly admitted client diagnosed with depersonalization/derealization disorder has a nursing diagnosis of anxiety R/T family stressors. Which nursing intervention would be most helpful in building a trusting nurse–client relationship?
    1. Identify stressors that increase anxiety levels.
    2. Encourage use of adaptive coping mechanisms to decrease stress.
    3. Discuss events surrounding episodes of depersonalization.
    4. Reassure the client of safety and security during periods of anxiety.

Nursing Process—Evaluation

26. The nurse is teaching a client diagnosed with somatic symptom disorder ways to assist in recognizing links between anxiety and somatic symptoms. Which client statement would indicate that the intervention was effective?
    1. "My anxiety is currently 2 out of 10."
    2. "I would like you to talk with my family about my problem."
    3. "I would like assertiveness training to communicate more effectively."
    4. "Journaling has helped me to understand how stress affects me physically."

27. A client diagnosed with illness anxiety disorder has a nursing diagnosis of ineffective coping R/T repressed anxiety AEB physical illness concerns. The client states, "Exercising will prepare me for my returning illness." Which accurately evaluates this client's statement?
    1. The client is experiencing a positive outcome because the client is using exercise to cope effectively with the expressed physical symptoms.
    2. The client is experiencing a positive outcome exhibited by understanding the link between anxiety and the illness.
    3. The client is experiencing a negative outcome because exercise is irrelevant in avoiding future illnesses.
    4. The client is experiencing a negative outcome based on the continuous focus on physical illness, rather than the underlying cause of physical symptoms.

28. The nursing student is learning about depersonalization/derealization disorder. Which of the following student statements indicate that learning has occurred? **Select all that apply.**
    1. "Clients experiencing depersonalization/derealization disorder have an alteration in the perception of the external environment."
    2. "The symptoms of depersonalization/derealization disorder are rare, and few adults experience transient episodes."
    3. "Depersonalization/derealization disorder is characterized by a temporary change in the quality of self-awareness."
    4. "The alterations in perceptions are experienced as relaxing and are rarely accompanied by other symptoms."
    5. "Clients experiencing the symptoms of depersonalization/derealization disorder have a distorted sense of time."

29. After childhood sexual abuse, a client diagnosed with dissociative identity disorder (DID) has an outcome that states, "The client will verbalize causative factors for the development of multiple personalities." Which charting entry documents a successful outcome?
    1. "Able to state the particular function of each of the different personalities."
    2. "Discussed history of childhood sexual abuse."
    3. "Was able to be redirected to topic at hand during group therapy."
    4. "Verbalizes understanding that treatment may be lengthy."

Psychopharmacology

30. In which situation is lorazepam used appropriately?
    1. Long-term treatment of clients diagnosed with conversion disorder caused by anxiety.
    2. Long-term treatment of clients diagnosed with illness anxiety disorder.
    3. Short-term treatment of clients diagnosed with hypertension caused by atherosclerosis.
    4. Short-term treatment of clients diagnosed with conversion disorder.

31. In which of the following situations is buspirone used appropriately? **Select all that apply.**
    1. Long-term treatment of clients diagnosed with illness anxiety disorder.
    2. Long-term treatment of clients diagnosed with neurocognitive disorder.
    3. Short-term treatment of clients diagnosed with conversion disorder.
    4. Short-term treatment of clients diagnosed with a somatic symptom disorder.
    5. Long-term treatment of clients diagnosed with dissociative identity disorder.

32. A client diagnosed with illness anxiety disorder is prescribed clonazepam for underlying anxiety. Which of the following teachings should be included in this client's plan of care? **Select all that apply.**
    1. Monitor blood pressure and pulse.
    2. Administer the medication to the client at night to avoid daytime sedation.
    3. Encourage the client to avoid drinking alcohol while taking the medication.
    4. Remind the client to wear sunscreen to address photosensitivity.
    5. Advise the client to avoid abruptly stopping the medication.

The correct answer number and rationale for why it is the correct answer are given in **boldface blue type**. Rationales for why the other answer options are incorrect are given as well, but they are not in boldface type.

Theory

1. 1. **Because clients diagnosed with illness anxiety disorder are less threatened by physical complaints than poor self-esteem, they tend to use somatic symptoms as ego defenses. This describes the etiology of illness anxiety disorder from a psychodynamic theory perspective.**
   2. When clients view emotions associated with traumatic events as morally or ethically unacceptable, the transference of these emotions into physical symptoms describes the etiology of a conversion disorder, not illness anxiety disorder.
   3. Shifting focus to the ill family member when family conflicts cannot be resolved is a family dynamic, not psychodynamic, description of the etiology of illness anxiety disorder.
   4. Deficiencies of endorphins have been linked to the etiology of pain experienced by clients diagnosed with specified somatic symptom disorder, not illness anxiety disorder.

   TEST-TAKING HINT: To answer this question correctly, the test taker needs to distinguish the various theory perspectives related to the development of illness anxiety disorder. Only answer 1 describes the etiology of this disorder from a psychodynamic theory perspective.

2. 1. Unexpressed emotions translating into symptoms of pain explains the etiology of specified somatic symptom disorder from a psychodynamic, not biochemical, theory perspective.
   2. **Decreased levels of serotonin and endorphins may play a role in the etiology of somatic symptom disorders. This explains the etiology of these disorders from a biochemical theory perspective.**
   3. An increased incidence of this disorder in first-degree relatives explains the etiology of somatic symptom disorders from a genetic, not biochemical, theory perspective.
   4. Harmony around the illness, which replaces discord in the family, explains the etiology of somatic symptom disorders from a family dynamic, not biochemical, theory perspective.

   TEST-TAKING HINT: To answer this question correctly, the test taker needs to distinguish among the various theory perspectives related to the development of somatic symptom disorders. All answers describe the etiology of these disorders; however, only answer 2 is from a biochemical theory perspective.

3. 1. An increase in the predisposition of somatic symptom disorders in first-degree relatives explains the etiology of this disorder from a genetic, not a learning, theory perspective.
   2. **Positive reinforcement of somatic complaints virtually guarantees the repetition of these learned behaviors. This describes the etiology of somatic symptom disorder from a learning theory perspective.**
   3. A client's viewing self as bad and then believing physical symptoms are ways to punish self explains the etiology of somatic symptom disorder from a psychodynamic, not a learning, theory perspective.
   4. The use of physical symptoms as a response to repressed severe anxiety explains the etiology of somatic symptom disorder from a psychodynamic, not a learning, theory perspective.

   TEST-TAKING HINT: To answer this question correctly, the test taker should be familiar with the different theories associated with the development of somatic symptom disorder. All answers describe the etiology of somatic symptom disorder, but only answer 2 is from a learning theory perspective.

4. 1. Dysfunction in the hippocampus supports a neurobiological, not psychodynamic, theory in the etiology of dissociative disorders. There may be dysfunction in areas of the brain that affect memory, not only in the hippocampus but also in the mammillary bodies, the dorsomedial thalamus, and the inferior temporal cortices.
   2. Dissociate reactions precipitating excessive cortical arousal, which triggers reactive inhibition of signals at synapses in sensorimotor pathways, supports a neurobiological, not psychodynamic, theory.
   3. Evidence points to the etiology of dissociative disorders as a set of traumatic experiences that overwhelms the individual's capacity to cope. However, this supports the psychological

trauma, not psychodynamic, theory in the etiology of dissociative disorders.

4. Dissociative behaviors occur when individuals repress distressing mental contents from conscious awareness. The repression of mental contents is perceived as a coping mechanism for protecting the client from emotional pain that has arisen from disturbing external circumstances or anxiety-provoking internal urges and feelings. This supports a psychodynamic theory in the etiology of dissociative disorders.

TEST-TAKING HINT: The test taker must be able to differentiate among the various theories for the etiology of the diagnosis of dissociative disorders to answer this question correctly.

5. The characteristic feature of dissociative amnesia is the inability to recall important personal information, usually of a traumatic or stressful nature, that is too extensive to be explained by ordinary forgetfulness, and is not due to substance use or other medical conditions.
1. This nursing response, related to repressed feelings, is from an intrapersonal, not neurobiological, perspective. Intrapersonal theories include Freud's psychodynamic theory. He believed that disassociate behaviors occurred when individuals repressed distressing mental contents from conscious awareness.
2. Some clinicians have suggested a possible correlation between neurological alterations and dissociative disorders. This nurse's response correlates the relationship between temporal lobe epilepsy or severe migraine headaches or both to the diagnosis of dissociative amnesia and is from a neurobiological perspective.
3. A psychological trauma theorist would propose that a set of traumatic experiences would overwhelm an individual's capacity to cope by any means other than dissociation. This nurse's response, which deals with escape from reality to avoid traumatic events, reflects a psychological trauma perspective, not a neurobiological perspective.
4. This nurse's response is related to a genetic predisposition. Research suggests that dissociative identity disorder (DID) is more common in first-degree relatives of individuals with the disorder than in the general population. This nursing response is from a genetic, not neurobiological, perspective and addresses DID, not dissociative amnesia.

TEST-TAKING HINT: The test taker needs to distinguish among the various etiological theories associated with the diagnosis of dissociative

amnesia. It is important to look for biological structure and function of body systems when asked for neurobiological theory.

Nursing Process—Assessment

6. Conversion disorder is a loss of, or change in, body function resulting from a psychological conflict, the physical symptoms of which cannot be explained by any known medical disorder or pathological mechanism.
1. Individuals diagnosed with a conversion disorder would have intact deep tendon reflexes, whereas an individual with an actual impairment would not have intact deep tendon reflexes.
2. Individuals diagnosed with conversion disorders would have no muscle wasting.
3. Individuals diagnosed with conversion disorders are unaware of the link between anxiety and physical symptoms.
4. Individuals diagnosed with a conversion disorder complain of physical symptoms that have no basis in organic pathology.
5. Individuals diagnosed with conversion disorders exhibit lack of concern for functional alterations. This condition is referred to as *la belle indifference*. Clients with an actual impairment would exhibit considerable concern regarding any alteration in function.

TEST-TAKING HINT: To answer this question correctly, the test taker needs to recognize the signs and symptoms of conversion disorders.

7. 1. Preoccupation with disease processes and organ function is common when a client is diagnosed with illness anxiety disorder. The nurse can differentiate illness anxiety disorder from somatic symptom disorder because in somatic symptom disorder the complaints are general in nature and cannot be connected to specific disease processes or body systems.
2. A long history of doctor shopping is common when a client is diagnosed with illness anxiety disorder. Doctor shopping occurs because the client with illness anxiety disorder is convinced that there is a physiological problem and continues to seek assistance for this problem even after confirmation that no actual physiological illness exists.
3. The client diagnosed with illness anxiety disorder exaggerates, rather than denies, physical symptoms.

4. Anxiety and depression are common, and obsessive-compulsive traits frequently are associated with illness anxiety disorder.

5. Clients diagnosed with illness anxiety disorder are convinced, and will insist, that their symptoms are related to organic pathology or loss of function. This impairs social and occupational functioning.

TEST-TAKING HINT: To answer this question correctly, the test taker needs to recognize the potential symptoms experienced by clients diagnosed with illness anxiety disorder.

8. This is an example of a **secondary** gain. Secondary gains occur when clients obtain attention or support that they might not otherwise receive. This client's statement indicates that the client has received attention from staff members as a result of complaints of pain.

TEST-TAKING HINT: To answer this question correctly, the test taker must be able to recognize situations in which clients receive secondary gain in the form of attention or support or both.

9. Dissociative fugue is a subtype of dissociative amnesia. It is characterized by a sudden unexpected travel away from customary places of daily activities or by bewildered wandering, with inability to recall some or all of one's past. This is usually precipitated by severe, psychosocial stress.
   1. Because stress is the underlying cause of dissociative amnesia with dissociative fugue, the client's ability to maintain reality during stressful situations would indicate that the client meets discharge criteria.
   2. The client's ability to verbalize why alternate personalities exist would be a discharge criterion for a diagnosis of dissociative identity disorder (DID), not dissociative amnesia with dissociative fugue.
   3. The client's ability to discuss feelings such as depersonalization is an important step in understanding the diagnosis of DID, not dissociative amnesia with dissociative fugue. Because DID is not this client's diagnosis, this ability would not be a criterion for discharge.
   4. The client's ability to integrate subpersonalities into a whole personality is an important step in the resolution of DID, not dissociative amnesia with dissociative fugue. Because DID is not this client's diagnosis, this ability would not be a criterion for discharge.
   5. Because stress is the underlying cause of dissociative amnesia with dissociative fugue, the client's ability to use relaxation

techniques when visibly upset would indicate that the client meets discharge criteria.

TEST-TAKING HINT: The test taker must distinguish between DID and dissociative amnesia with dissociative fugue diagnostic criteria to answer this question correctly.

10. 1. The characteristic feature of dissociative amnesia with dissociative fugue is a sudden, unexpected travel away from home with inability to recall some or all of one's past. This is usually precipitated by severe, psychosocial stress. A situation in which a client has no idea who they are or how they arrived in a foreign city is an example of symptoms experienced during dissociative amnesia with dissociative fugue.
    2. Dissociative identity disorder (DID) is characterized by the existence of two or more personalities in a single individual. Although further assessments must be performed, the change in known personality characteristics presented may be evidence of DID, not dissociative amnesia with dissociative fugue.
    3. Dissociative amnesia is an inability to recall important personal information, usually of a traumatic or stressful nature, that is too extensive to be explained by ordinary forgetfulness and is not related to the direct effects of substance use or a neurological or other general medical condition. Dissociative amnesia with the specifier of dissociative fugue is the apparent purposeful travel or bewildered wandering that is associated with amnesia for identity or other important autobiographical information. Further assessments must be done to rule out the effects of substances or other general medical conditions. This client would not meet the criteria for a diagnosis of dissociative amnesia with dissociative fugue.
    4. Depersonalization disorder is characterized by a temporary change in the quality of self-awareness that often takes the form of feelings of unreality, changes in body image, feelings of detachment from the environment, or a sense of observing oneself from outside the body. Although further assessments must be done, this client's complaints of feeling detached may be evidence of depersonalization disorder, not dissociative amnesia with dissociative fugue.

TEST-TAKING HINT: The test taker must be able to recognize the symptoms of various

dissociative disorders to distinguish dissociative amnesia with dissociative fugue.

11. Amnestic disorders are characterized by an inability to learn new information and an inability to recall previously learned information. These disorders differ from neurocognitive disorders in that there is no impairment in abstract thinking or judgment and no personality change.
    1. Cerebral anoxia is an oxygen-depriving condition that can result in an amnestic disorder.
    2. Cardiac arrhythmias can cause cerebral anoxia, which can result in an amnestic disorder.
    3. Migraine headaches may result in symptoms including, but not limited to, mood changes, depression, fatigue, and occasionally amnesia.
    4. Psoriasis is a common chronic disease of the skin whose symptoms do not include any form of amnesia.
    5. Cerebrovascular disease can cause cerebral anoxia, which may result in an amnestic disorder.

TEST-TAKING HINT: The test taker must understand which medical conditions are associated with amnestic disorders to answer this question correctly.

12. 1. Toxins, such as lead, mercury, carbon monoxide, organophosphates, and industrial solvents, are associated with, and contribute to, substance-induced persisting amnestic disorder.
    2. Medications, such as anticonvulsants and methotrexate, are associated with, and contribute to, substance-induced persisting amnestic disorder.
    3. Aspartame is an artificial, low-calorie sweetener. It is not associated with substance-induced persisting amnestic disorder.
    4. Sedatives, such as hypnotics and anxiolytics, are associated with, and contribute to, substance-induced persisting amnestic disorder.
    5. Alcohol, including whiskey, wine, beer, or other fermented or distilled liquors, is associated with, and contributes to, substance-induced persisting amnestic disorder.

TEST-TAKING HINT: To answer this question correctly, the test taker must understand the effects various substances may have on a client's cognition.

Nursing Process—Diagnosis

13. 1. Because there is no true tissue damage, a client experiencing paralysis related to a conversion disorder would not have muscle wasting leading to impaired skin integrity.
    2. There is no body image disturbance when a client is experiencing a conversion disorder. Clients diagnosed with this disorder tend to be indifferent to physical symptoms and impaired functioning. This indifference is called *la belle indifference*.
    3. The underlying cause of a conversion disorder is anxiety. In this case, the paralytic condition is caused by anxiety related to the risk of possible combat injury. Anxiety must be prioritized over all other nursing diagnoses.
    4. The nursing diagnosis of activity intolerance R/T paralysis may be an appropriate nursing diagnosis because mobility is affected in conversion disorders. However, because anxiety is the root of this client's problem, it must be prioritized.

TEST-TAKING HINT: To answer this question correctly, the test taker needs to understand that physical symptoms of a conversion disorder are unconscious expressions of underlying anxiety.

14. 1. Because of preoccupation with illness and continued absenteeism, altered role performance may be an appropriate nursing diagnosis for a client diagnosed with illness anxiety disorder. Because of the client statement "I can't do this anymore," this nursing diagnosis does not take priority at this time.
    2. A client diagnosed with illness anxiety disorder does not understand the link between anxiety and the expressed symptoms. This makes the nursing diagnosis of knowledge deficit appropriate; however, because the client has expressed feelings of hopelessness, this nursing diagnosis does not take priority at this time.
    3. Because depression is common in individuals diagnosed with illness anxiety disorder, the client statement "I can't do this anymore" alerts the nurse to the possibility of suicidal ideations. This nursing diagnosis would take priority.
    4. The client statement "I can't do this anymore" is not related to the client's inability to perform activities of daily living but is an expression of hopelessness. There is no evidence presented that would indicate a self-care deficit.

TEST-TAKING HINT: When looking for a priority nursing diagnosis, the test taker should look for any information in the question that indicates that the client is a safety risk. Safety is the nurse's first priority. When a depressed client verbalizes being "tired" or states, "I can't do this anymore," the nurse needs to assess the client for suicidal ideations.

15. 1. Risk for injury is increased when multiple physicians treat clients without fully understanding other physician treatment plans. It is common for a client diagnosed with somatic symptom disorder to have the potential for dangerous combinations of medications or treatments, or both.
    2. This client may be experiencing anxiety related to various, vague symptoms. This nursing diagnosis does not address the risk for injury caused by the potential for dangerous combinations of medications or treatments when multiple physicians treat the client. This diagnosis is not currently prioritized.
    3. This client may be experiencing ineffective coping as evidenced by visiting multiple physicians in an attempt to meet psychological needs. This nursing diagnosis does not address the risk for injury caused by the potential for dangerous combinations of medications or treatments when multiple physicians treat the client. This diagnosis is not currently prioritized.
    4. This client may be experiencing fear related to the threatening nature of the various, vague symptoms. This nursing diagnosis does not address the risk for injury caused by the potential for dangerous combinations of medications or treatments when multiple physicians treat the client. This diagnosis is not currently prioritized.

TEST-TAKING HINT: When the test taker is asked to choose a priority nursing diagnosis, it is important to discern the diagnosis pertinent to the situation presented and then to prioritize according to Maslow's hierarchy of needs, which prioritizes physical over psychological needs.

16. 1. The outcome of verbalizing alternate ways of dealing with stress would apply to the nursing diagnosis of ineffective coping, not disturbed sensory perception. An outcome that would support the nursing diagnosis of disturbed sensory perception would be, "The client will maintain a sense of reality during stressful situations."
    2. The outcome of verbalizing alternate ways of dealing with stress would apply to the nursing diagnosis of ineffective coping R/T overwhelming anxiety.
    3. The outcome of verbalizing alternate ways of dealing with stress would apply to the nursing diagnosis of ineffective coping, not self-esteem disturbance. An outcome that would support a nursing diagnosis of self-esteem disturbance would be, "The client will verbalize one positive aspect about self."
    4. The outcome of verbalizing alternate ways of dealing with stress would apply to the nursing diagnosis of ineffective coping, not anxiety. An outcome that would support a nursing diagnosis of anxiety would be, "The client will verbalize an anxiety level at or below 4/10."

TEST-TAKING HINT: The test taker first must understand what problem the expected client outcome addresses, then look for a nursing diagnosis that documents this problem.

Nursing Process—Planning

17. 1. The client demonstrating recovery of lost function by discharge is an appropriate short-term outcome for the stated nursing diagnosis of disturbed sensory perception. The outcome is client specific, realistic, related to the stated nursing diagnosis, and measurable and has a time frame. When the nurse is dealing with a client diagnosed with a conversion disorder, the problem resolves itself as the client's anxiety decreases. It is realistic to expect this client to experience a significant decrease in anxiety by discharge and subsequent recovery of lost function.
    2. Using effective coping mechanisms would be an outcome for the nursing diagnosis of ineffective coping, not disturbed sensory perception.
    3. The client experiencing paralysis that accompanies a conversion disorder would not experience fear. This indifference to an otherwise disturbing symptom is referred to as *la belle indifference*.
    4. Acknowledging underlying anxiety would be related to the nursing diagnosis of anxiety, not disturbed sensory perception.

TEST-TAKING HINT: To answer this question correctly, the test taker must pair the nursing diagnosis presented in the question with the appropriate short-term client outcome expectation.

18. 1. Although pain is a major symptom experienced by clients diagnosed with specified somatic symptom disorder, the outcome of pain reduction is not an expectation for the nursing diagnosis of ineffective coping related to repressed anxiety.
2. **If the client is able to use coping strategies instead of resorting to physical complaints, the client has learned to cope effectively with anxiety. This is a positive outcome related to the nursing diagnosis of ineffective coping R/T repressed anxiety.**
3. Expressing realistic perceptions of distorted self-image by discharge is an outcome related to clients diagnosed with body dysmorphic disorder, not specified somatic symptom disorder.
4. Rating anxiety as less than 3/10 may be desirable for clients diagnosed with specified somatic symptom disorder; however, this outcome does not address an altered coping problem, and it does not contain a measurable time frame.

TEST-TAKING HINT: The test taker needs to understand that all outcomes must be client centered, specific, realistic, positive, and measurable and must include a time frame. If any one of these components is missing, the outcome is incorrectly written. Because a measurable time frame is not included, answer 4 can be eliminated immediately.

19. The order of priority is 1, 3, 2, 4, 5.
1. **The nurse first must assess the situation and monitor vital signs to see if there are any alterations and to detect an actual physical problem.**
2. Next, the nurse must attempt to determine whether anxiety is the cause of the somatic complaints by objectively assessing anxiety levels with an anxiety scale.
3. The nurse then assesses the client's understanding of the link between anxiety and the expressed somatic complaints to plan effective teaching.
4. The nurse encourages journaling to assist the client in beginning to link feelings to the expression of physical symptoms.
5. Finally, the nurse teaches the client relaxation techniques, encourages their use, and notes their effectiveness. This teaching gives the client a tool to reduce anxiety levels.

TEST-TAKING HINT: The nursing process is a helpful tool when deciding the priority of interventions. Also, the ranking of interventions can be based on Maslow's hierarchy of needs.

20. 1. Recovery of deficits in memory is an appropriate outcome for the nursing diagnosis of disturbed thought processes, not ineffective coping.
2. Verbalizing awareness of multiple personalities is an appropriate outcome for the nursing diagnosis of disturbed personal identity, not ineffective coping.
3. The ability to perceive stimuli accurately is an appropriate outcome for the nursing diagnosis of disturbed sensory perception, not ineffective coping. Also, this outcome is written incorrectly because it does not contain a time frame.
4. **A client diagnosed with dissociative identity disorder (DID) is coping with stress by self-dissociation into multiple personalities. The client's being able to demonstrate adaptive coping mechanisms in dealing with stress reflects a positive outcome for the nursing diagnosis of ineffective coping.**

TEST-TAKING HINT: To answer this question correctly, the test taker must pair the stated nursing diagnosis presented in the question with the appropriate client outcome.

Nursing Process—Implementation

21. 1. Because clients are so convinced that their symptoms are related to organic pathology, they adamantly reject negative test results. This confrontation only increases client frustration.
2. It is not a conscious choice for the client to be unwilling to accept anxiety as the source of the physical illness. The client is truly unaware that anxiety is the root of the problem.
3. Families may need assistance in developing ways to avoid providing clients secondary gains, which foster continued focus on physical complaints. Because this intervention does not address the frustration and anger this client is experiencing, however, it does not take priority.
4. **Clients diagnosed with illness anxiety disorder are convinced that their symptoms are related to organic pathology and are often angry and frustrated by anyone doubting their illness. Empathizing with the client about anger and frustration assists in building a therapeutic relationship. The nurse–client**

relationship is the foundation for all other interventions and takes priority at this time.

TEST-TAKING HINT: The test taker must recognize that any anger and frustration exhibited by clients diagnosed with illness anxiety disorder must be addressed empathetically and in a timely manner to avoid the escalation of this unhealthy behavior.

22. 1. It is important to empathize with individuals diagnosed with specified somatic symptom disorder; however, it is equally important to limit discussion of symptoms to avoid reinforcement and secondary gain. By telling the client that the nurse and client can discuss the client's complaints briefly at a future time, the nurse empathizes with the client and limits the client's monopolization of the group.
    2. When the nurse seeks from the group solutions for dealing with pain, the nurse has unwittingly provided the client with the secondary gain of group attention. This also validates the client's somatic symptom.
    3. By ignoring the client's need for attention, the nurse fails to express empathy and does not acknowledge what the client is experiencing. This may impede the establishment of a nurse–client relationship.
    4. When the nurse redirects attention to others in the group, the nurse has avoided acknowledging the client's feelings. The client may feel ignored, rejected, and belittled. This response by the nurse may impede any further client contributions to the group.

TEST-TAKING HINT: To answer this question correctly, the test taker must be aware of appropriate nursing responses that would discourage secondary gains and symptom reinforcement for clients diagnosed with specified somatic symptom disorder who are experiencing pain.

23. 1. There are psychological implications to the diagnosis of somatic symptom disorders. One is a primary gain, which enables the client to avoid anxiety-producing activities. Another is a secondary gain, which provides emotional support or attention that the client might not otherwise receive without the somatic symptoms. Discussions about symptoms may reinforce secondary gains and should be avoided by the nurse.
    2. It is important for the nurse to begin discussions about the underlying cause of a somatic symptom disorder; however, this intervention does not take priority.

It is necessary first to assess physiological alterations to rule out an actual medical condition.
    3. The nurse must first rule out signs and symptoms of an actual physical condition before assuming that the disorder is somatic in nature. Monitoring signs and symptoms, vital signs, and laboratory tests can rule out a physiological problem.
    4. The nurse may want to teach the client diagnosed with a somatic symptom disorder the link between anxiety and somatic symptoms. The client must first be medically cleared, however, for this to be an appropriate intervention.

TEST-TAKING HINT: To answer this question correctly, the test taker needs to recognize the importance of ruling out actual physical problems before assuming that a client's symptoms are somatic in nature.

24. 1. A growing body of evidence points to the etiology of dissociative identity disorder (DID) as a set of traumatic experiences that overwhelms the individual's capacity to cope by any means other than dissociation. It is a priority for the nurse to establish an atmosphere of safety and security in which trust can be established. Trust must be established before a client would feel comfortable to discuss highly charged, past traumatic events.
    2. Although it is important for the nurse to identify relationships among subpersonalities and work with each equally, this intervention would be ineffective if the client did not feel safe or secure.
    3. Although it is important for the nurse to teach new coping skills to deal with dissociative behaviors, this intervention would be ineffective if the client did not feel safe or secure.
    4. Although it is important for the nurse to process events associated with the origins of the disorder, this intervention would be ineffective if the client did not feel safe or secure.

TEST-TAKING HINT: The test taker must understand that at the root of DID is a traumatic event, and for the client to discuss concerns, a trusting therapeutic nurse–client relationship must take priority.

25. 1. Although it is important to identify stressors early in treatment, this nursing intervention does not directly address the establishment of a trusting nurse–client relationship.

2. Although it is important to encourage the use of adaptive coping mechanisms to decrease stress, this nursing intervention does not directly address the establishment of a trusting nurse–client relationship.

3. It is important for the nurse to discuss events surrounding episodes of depersonalization to gain further assessment data. Compared with the other interventions presented, however, this intervention would not be the most helpful in building a trusting nurse–client relationship.

4. For the nurse to build a trusting nurse–client relationship, the nurse must assure the client of safety and security during periods of anxiety. When safety has been established, other interventions may be implemented.

TEST-TAKING HINT: To answer this question correctly, the test taker must understand that the question asks for an intervention that would be most helpful in building a trusting nurse–client relationship. Clients need to feel safe and secure before any relationship can be established and any further interventions can be implemented effectively.

Nursing Process—Evaluation

26. 1. When the client communicates levels of anxiety, the client is providing assessment information, rather than information that indicates a recognition of the link between anxiety and somatic symptoms.

2. When the client requests information for family members, the client is indicating a possible knowledge deficit related to somatic symptom disorder. This request does not indicate that the client has an understanding regarding the link between anxiety and somatic symptoms.

3. A request for assertiveness training is not related to the nurse's teaching regarding the link between anxiety and somatic symptoms.

4. When the client states that awareness of feelings has been accomplished through journaling, the client is communicating recognition of the link between anxiety and somatic symptoms. This recognition is evidence that teaching in this area has been successful.

TEST-TAKING HINT: To answer this question correctly, the test taker must link the client's evaluative statement to the teaching presented in the question. Only answer 4 shows that the

client is aware of the link between anxiety and somatic symptoms.

27. 1. Although exercise relieves stress and is a positive coping strategy, expecting a recurrence of physical illness would indicate that the client continues to cope ineffectively by not recognizing anxiety as the underlying cause of the physical illness.

2. Expecting a recurrence of physical illness would indicate ineffective coping. Not recognizing anxiety as the underlying cause of the physical illness contributes to this negative outcome.

3. Because exercise relieves stress, it can be a positive coping strategy. However, expecting a recurrence of physical illness indicates that the client continues to cope ineffectively. Not recognizing anxiety as the underlying cause of the physical illness contributes to this negative outcome.

4. Expecting a recurrence of physical illness would indicate a negative outcome for the nursing diagnosis of ineffective coping. Continuing to focus on coping with illness shows that the client has not developed the understanding that anxiety is the underlying cause of the physical illness.

TEST-TAKING HINT: At first glance, the client's statement about exercise appears to be a positive outcome for the nursing diagnosis of ineffective coping R/T repressed anxiety. The test taker must understand that the underlying problem that this client is facing is not the illness itself but the anxiety that underlies the illness. Because client exercise is an attempt to deal with the illness, and not the anxiety, a negative outcome remains for the diagnosis of ineffective coping.

28. 1. Derealization is an alteration in the perception of the external environment. If a client is diagnosed with depersonalization/derealization disorder, objects in the environment are perceived as altered in size or shape. Other people in the environment may seem automated or mechanical.

2. The symptoms associated with depersonalization are common, but depersonalization/derealization disorder is diagnosed only if the symptoms cause significant distress or impairment in functioning. It is estimated that approximately half of all adults experience transient episodic symptoms of depersonalization.

3. Clients diagnosed with depersonalization/derealization disorder experience temporary changes in the quality of self-awareness. These changes may include feelings of unreality, changes in body image, feelings of detachment from the environment, or a sense of observing oneself from outside the body.

4. The alterations in perceptions are experienced as bothersome, not relaxing, and are commonly accompanied by anxiety, depression, fear of going insane, obsessive thoughts, somatic complaints, and disturbances in the subjective sense of time.

5. Clients diagnosed with depersonalization/derealization disorder experience perceptual alterations including a distorted sense of time.

TEST-TAKING HINT: The test taker must understand the difference between the symptoms of depersonalization and depersonalization/derealization disorder to answer this question correctly.

29. 1. In the diagnosis of dissociative identity disorder (DID), multiple personalities are unique and composed of a complex set of memories, behavior patterns, and social relationships. The client, being able to state the particular function of each of the different personalities, focuses on distinguishing among the various personalities, not on the reasons for their existence.

2. Research has shown that the etiology of DID is usually based on a long history of childhood physical or sexual abuse, or both. Discussing a past history of sexual abuse would connect these traumatic events to the reason why the client's multiple personalities exist and would support a successful outcome.

3. The ability of the client to be redirected does not address the outcome of increasing the awareness of causative factors for the development of the client's multiple personalities.

4. The ability of the client to verbalize an understanding of the long-term treatment needed to address the diagnosis of DID does not address the outcome of increasing the awareness of causative factors for the development of the client's multiple personalities.

TEST-TAKING HINT: The test taker must understand that the charting entries presented may be accurate evaluations of a client diagnosed with DID; however, only answer 2 evaluates the client's understanding of causative factors.

Psychopharmacology

30. Lorazepam is a benzodiazepine used for short-term treatment of anxiety disorders and for alcohol withdrawal.

1. Lorazepam is used for the short-term, not long-term, treatment of clients diagnosed with a conversion disorder.

2. Lorazepam is used for the short-term, not long-term, treatment of clients diagnosed with illness anxiety disorder.

3. Lorazepam may be used for short-term treatment of hypertension secondary to anxiety, not atherosclerosis.

4. Because anxiety is the underlying cause of conversion disorder, lorazepam may be used for short-term treatment of clients diagnosed with this disorder.

TEST-TAKING HINT: To answer this question correctly, the test taker needs to understand that benzodiazepines are used for short-term, not long-term, treatment of anxiety and anxiety-related disorders.

31. Buspirone is an antianxiety medication that takes 3 to 4 weeks to be effective. Often, clients are prescribed a short-acting benzodiazepine along with buspirone to treat acute anxiety or anxiety-related disorders.

1. Buspirone may be used in the long-term treatment of clients diagnosed with illness anxiety disorder.

2. It is inappropriate to use buspirone for clients diagnosed with neurocognitive disorders because anxiety is not the underlying cause of this diagnosis.

3. Buspirone can be used for the long-term, not short-term, treatment of clients diagnosed with a conversion disorder.

4. Buspirone can be used for the long-term, not short-term, treatment of clients diagnosed with a somatic symptom disorder.

5. Buspirone may be used in the long-term treatment of clients diagnosed with dissociative identity disorder.

TEST-TAKING HINT: To answer this question correctly, the test taker should understand the uses of buspirone in the treatment of anxiety and anxiety-related disorders.

32. 1. Orthostatic hypotension is a side effect of clonazepam, a benzodiazepine; however, monitoring blood pressure and pulse is an assessment intervention, not a teaching need.

2. Sedation is a side effect of clonazepam, a benzodiazepine; however, administering

this medication to the client at night is an intervention, not a teaching need.

3. It is important to teach the client to avoid drinking alcohol while taking clonazepam. Clonazepam and alcohol are central nervous system depressants and taken together produce an additive central nervous system depressant effect, placing the client at risk for injury. Because of the risk for injury, this intervention is prioritized.

4. Reminding the client to wear sunscreen is a teaching intervention; however, photosensitivity is a side effect of tricyclic antidepressants and antipsychotic medications, not benzodiazepines such as clonazepam.

5. Due to the potential for substance-induced withdrawal, it is important for the nurse to advise clients to avoid abruptly stopping clonazepam, a benzodiazepine. Symptoms of withdrawal from benzodiazepines include irritability, increased tension, hand tremor, sweating, confusion, palpitations, hallucinations, and seizures.

TEST-TAKING HINT: The test taker must note important words in the question, such as *teaching*. The test taker can eliminate answers 1 and 2 immediately because these are interventions that do not relate to teaching.

14

Neurocognitive Disorders

KEYWORDS

The following words include English vocabulary, nursing/medical terminology, concepts, principles, or information relevant to content specifically addressed in this chapter or associated with topics presented in it. English dictionaries, your nursing textbooks, and medical dictionaries such as *Taber's Cyclopedic Medical Dictionary* are resources that can be used to expand your knowledge and understanding of these words and related information.

Agnosia

Alzheimer's disease

Amnestic disorders

Amygdala

Aphasia

Apraxia

Cerebral anoxia

Confabulation

Creutzfeldt-Jakob disease

Delirium

Disturbance of consciousness

Frontal lobe

Hippocampus

Huntington's disease

Hypervigilance

Impaired orientation

Mini-mental state examination (MMSE)

Neurocognitive disorder (NCD)

Parietal lobe

Parkinson's disease

Perseveration

Pick's disease

Primary prevention

Prion

Pseudodementia

Secondary prevention

Slow virus

Substance-induced intoxication

Substance-induced withdrawal

Tertiary prevention

QUESTIONS

Theory

1. The physician tells family members that their parent, who is experiencing confusion and memory loss, has a reversible form of a neurocognitive disorder (NCD). Which is the likely cause of this disorder?
   1. Multiple sclerosis.
   2. Multiple small brain infarcts.
   3. Electrolyte imbalance.
   4. Human immunodeficiency virus disease.

2. A client diagnosed with a neurocognitive disorder (NCD) due to Alzheimer's disease is displaying signs and symptoms of anxiety, fear, and paranoia. An alteration in which area of the brain is responsible for these signs and symptoms?
   1. Frontal lobe.
   2. Parietal lobe.
   3. Hippocampus.
   4. Amygdala.

3. Which statement best explains the pathophysiology associated with a neurocognitive disorder (NCD) due to Parkinson's disease?
   1. The disease results from atrophy in the frontal and temporal lobes.
   2. A transmissible agent known as a slow virus, or prion, is associated with this disease.
   3. A loss of nerve cells located in the substantia nigra is associated with this disease.
   4. The disease results from damage in the basal ganglia and the cerebral cortex.

Nursing Process—Assessment

4. Number the symptoms of a neurocognitive disorder (NCD) due to Alzheimer's disease as they progress through stages of the disease process.
   1. _____ Client is bedfast and aphasic.
   2. _____ Client has no apparent memory decline.
   3. _____ Client begins to lose things and forget names.
   4. _____ Client is unable to recall the day, season, or year.
   5. _____ Client needs some assistance with hygiene.
   6. _____ Client forgets major events in personal history.
   7. _____ Client gets lost when driving a car.

5. On a 24-hour assessment, the nurse documents that a client diagnosed with a neurocognitive disorder (NCD) due to Alzheimer's disease presents with aphasia. Which client behavior supports this finding?
   1. The client is sad and has no ability to experience pleasure.
   2. The client is extremely emaciated and appears to be wasting away.
   3. The client is having difficulty forming words.
   4. The client is no longer able to speak.

6. A client diagnosed with a neurocognitive disorder (NCD) due to Alzheimer's disease was admitted 72 hours ago. The client states, "Last night I went on a wonderful dinner cruise." This is which type of communication, and what is the underlying reason for its use?
   1. The client is using confabulation to achieve secondary gains.
   2. The client is using confabulation to protect the ego.
   3. The client is using perseveration to divert attention.
   4. The client is using perseveration to maintain self-esteem.

7. After a neurocognitive disorder (NCD) has been ruled out, a client is diagnosed with pseudodementia (depression). Which of the following client symptoms would support this diagnosis? **Select all that apply.**
   1. Slow progression of symptoms.
   2. Impaired attention and concentration.
   3. Diminished appetite.
   4. Symptoms diminish as the day progresses.
   5. Oriented to time and place with no wandering.

8. A client presents in the emergency department with an acute decline in cognitive ability. The nurse's assessment should include which of the following? **Select all that apply.**
   1. Family history and a mini-mental state examination (MMSE).
   2. Laboratory tests and vital signs.
   3. Toxicology screen for illegal substances.
   4. Open-ended questions to obtain information.
   5. Familiarizing the client with the milieu.

9. The nurse suspects a client is experiencing delirium. Which specific assessment information would support this suspicion?
   1. A decreased level of consciousness with intermittent hypervigilance.
   2. Slow onset of confusion and agitation.
   3. Onset is insidious and relentless.
   4. The symptoms last for 1 month or longer.

10. Studies have indicated that drastically reduced levels of acetylcholine are noted in the brains of individuals diagnosed with a neurocognitive disorder (NCD) due to Alzheimer's disease. Which cognitive deficit is primarily associated with this reduction?
   1. Loss of memory.
   2. Loss of purposeful movement.
   3. Loss of sensory ability to recognize objects.
   4. Loss of language ability.

11. A neurocognitive disorder (NCD) is classified in the *Diagnostic and Statistical Manual of Mental Disorders*, Fifth Edition, Text Revision (*DSM-5-TR*), as either mild or major. Which of the following diagnostic criteria are correctly matched with these classifications? **Select all that apply.**
   1. Client who is concerned about a significant decline in cognitive function: Mild NCD.
   2. Cognitive deficits that interfere with independence in everyday activities: Major NCD.
   3. Cognitive deficits that do not occur exclusively in the context of delirium: Major NCD.
   4. Cognitive deficits that are not better explained by another medical condition: Mild NCD.
   5. Neuropsychological testing that shows substantial impairment in cognitive performance: Major NCD.

Nursing Process—Diagnosis

12. A client newly diagnosed with vascular neurocognitive disorder (NCD) isolates self because of consistently poor role performance and increased loss of independent functioning. Which correctly written nursing diagnosis reflects this client's problem?
   1. Disturbed thought processes R/T decreased cerebral circulation AEB disorientation.
   2. Risk for injury R/T poor role performance AEB decreased functioning.
   3. Disturbed body image R/T loss of independent functioning AEB tearful, sad affect.
   4. Low self-esteem R/T loss of independent functioning AEB social isolation.

13. An 80-year-old client admitted to the emergency department is experiencing fever, dysuria, and urinary frequency. The client is combative and seeing things others do not see. Which nursing diagnosis reflects this client's problem?
   1. Disturbed sensory perceptions R/T infection AEB visual hallucinations.
   2. Risk for violence: self-directed R/T disorientation.
   3. Self-care deficit R/T decreased perceived need AEB disheveled appearance.
   4. Social isolation R/T decreased self-esteem.

Nursing Process—Planning

14. A client diagnosed with a neurocognitive disorder (NCD) has a nursing diagnosis of risk for injury R/T extreme psychomotor agitation. Which would be an appropriate, correctly written short-term outcome related to this problem?
   1. The client will remain free from physiological harm during this shift.
   2. The client will ask the nurse for assistance when becoming agitated.
   3. The client will verbalize staff appreciation by day three.
   4. The client will demonstrate performance of activities of daily living (ADLs) on discharge.

15. A nursing diagnosis of self-care deficit R/T memory loss AEB inability to fulfill ADLs is assigned to a client diagnosed with a neurocognitive disorder (NCD) due to Alzheimer's disease. Which is an appropriate, correctly written, short-term outcome?
    1. The client participates in ADLs with assistance by discharge.
    2. The client accomplishes ADLs without assistance after discharge.
    3. By time of discharge, the client will exhibit feelings of self-worth.
    4. The client will not experience physical injury.

Nursing Process—Implementation

16. A client who is delirious yells out to the nurse, "You are an idiot. Get me your supervisor!" Which is the best nursing response in this situation?
    1. "You need to calm down and listen to what I'm saying."
    2. "You're very upset. I'll call my supervisor."
    3. "You're going through a difficult time. I'll stay with you."
    4. "Why do you feel that my calling the supervisor will solve anything?"

17. A client diagnosed with a neurocognitive disorder (NCD) states, "I can't believe it's the Fourth of July and it's snowing outside." Which is the nurse's most appropriate response?
    1. "What makes you think it's the Fourth of July?"
    2. "How can it be July in winter?"
    3. "Today is Tuesday, March 12. Look, your lunch is ready."
    4. "I'll check to see if it's time for your prn haloperidol (Haldol)."

18. In writing a plan of care for a client diagnosed with a neurocognitive disorder (NCD), the nurse considers which of the following secondary prevention interventions? **Select all that apply.**
    1. Reinforce speech with nonverbal techniques by pointing to and touching items.
    2. Keep surroundings simple by reducing clutter.
    3. Offer family ethics consultation or hospice assistance if appropriate.
    4. Place a large, visible clock and calendar in client's room.
    5. Talk to family members about genetic predisposition regarding NCD.

19. In working with a client with a late-stage neurocognitive disorder (NCD) due to Alzheimer's disease, which is a priority nursing intervention?
    1. Assist the client in consuming fluids and food to prevent electrolyte imbalance.
    2. Reorient the client to place and time frequently to reduce confusion and fear.
    3. Encourage the client to participate in ADLs promoting self-worth.
    4. Assist with ambulation to avoid injury from falls.

20. A client diagnosed with a neurocognitive disorder (NCD) has a nursing diagnosis of altered thought process R/T disorientation and confusion. Which nursing intervention should be implemented first?
    1. Use tranquilizing medications and soft restraints.
    2. Continuously orient client to reality and surroundings.
    3. Assess client's level of disorientation and confusion.
    4. Remove potentially harmful objects from client's room.

Nursing Process—Evaluation

21. A nursing student is studying delirium. Which of the following student statements indicates that learning has occurred? **Select all that apply.**
    1. "The symptoms of delirium develop over a short time."
    2. "Delirium permanently affects the ability to learn new information."
    3. "Symptoms of delirium include the development of aphasia, apraxia, and agnosia."
    4. "Delirium is a disturbance of consciousness."
    5. "Delirium is always secondary to another condition."

22. A family member of a client who is being treated for symptoms of a modest decline in cognitive function asks the nurse, "Is my parent's problem reversible?" Which is the most appropriate nursing response?
    1. "Treatment sometimes can reverse a mild NCD."
    2. "Unfortunately, major NCD is not reversible."
    3. "Unfortunately, mild NCD is not reversible."
    4. "Treatment sometimes can reverse major NCD."

Psychopharmacology

23. On discharge, a client diagnosed with a neurocognitive disorder (NCD) is prescribed donepezil hydrochloride. Which would the nurse include in a teaching plan for the client's family?
    1. "Donepezil is a sedative/hypnotic used for short-term treatment of insomnia."
    2. "Donepezil is an Alzheimer's treatment used for mild to moderate NCD."
    3. "Donepezil is an antipsychotic used for clients diagnosed with NCD."
    4. "Donepezil is an antianxiety agent used for clients diagnosed with NCD."

24. An emaciated client diagnosed with delirium is experiencing sleeplessness, auditory hallucinations, and vertigo. Meclizine has been prescribed. Which client response supports the effectiveness of this medication?
    1. The client no longer hears voices.
    2. The client sleeps through the night.
    3. The client maintains balance during ambulation.
    4. The client has an improved appetite.

25. A client is prescribed quetiapine 50 mg qhs for aggression associated with dementia. The target dose is 200 mg/d. The quetiapine is to be increased by 50 mg/d. On what day of treatment would the client reach the target dose?
    1. Day _____.

The correct answer number and rationale for why it is the correct answer are given in **boldface blue type**. Rationales for why the other answer options are incorrect are given as well, but they are not in boldface type.

Theory

1. 1. Multiple sclerosis is a chronic, not reversible, autoimmune inflammatory disease of the central nervous system. Because this underlying condition is irreversible, the accompanying neurocognitive disorder (NCD) likewise would be irreversible.
   2. Multiple small brain infarcts result from a failure of blood supply to the cerebral area. Multiple small brain infarcts cause permanent and irreversible necrosis, leading to vascular NCD.
   3. **Imbalance in electrolytes can have catastrophic effects on the body, including confusion, memory loss, and disorientation. The NCD of delirium is reversible with the restoration of the electrolyte balance.**
   4. NCD due to HIV infection is a neuropathological syndrome, possibly caused by chronic HIV encephalitis and myelitis. This syndrome is manifested by cognitive and behavioral symptoms, particularly confusion. Because this underlying condition is irreversible, the accompanying NCD likewise is irreversible.

   TEST-TAKING HINT: To answer this question correctly, the test taker should recognize that NCDs can be reversible or irreversible. Chronic disorders produce neurocognitive deficits that are more apt to be permanent. Recognizing the chronic nature of answers 1, 2, and 4 can eliminate these choices.

2. 1. When there is an alteration in the frontal lobe, the nurse should expect to see impaired reasoning ability. Because of this, clients are unable to solve problems and perform familiar tasks. Symptoms of anxiety, fear, and paranoia are not associated with this alteration.
   2. When there is an alteration in the parietal lobe, the nurse should expect to see impaired orientation ability and impaired visuospatial skills. Because of this, clients are unable to maintain orientation to their environment. Symptoms of anxiety, fear, and paranoia are not associated with this alteration.
   3. When there is an alteration in the hippocampus, the nurse should expect to see impaired memory. Because of this, clients initially experience short-term memory loss and later are unable to form new memories. Symptoms of anxiety, fear, and paranoia are not associated with this alteration.
   4. **When there is an alteration in the amygdala, the nurse should expect to see impaired emotions—depression, anxiety, fear, personality changes, apathy, and paranoia. The amygdala is a mass of gray matter in the anterior portion of the temporal lobe. It also is believed to play an important role in arousal.**

   TEST-TAKING HINT: To answer this question correctly, the test taker must be familiar with brain structure and function and the symptoms caused by alterations in these structures.

3. 1. Atrophy in the frontal and temporal lobe is associated with Pick's, not Parkinson's, disease.
   2. A transmissible agent known as a slow virus, or prion, is associated with Creutzfeldt-Jakob, not Parkinson's, disease.
   3. **In Parkinson's disease, there is a loss of nerve cells located in the substantia nigra. Diminished dopamine activity results in involuntary muscle movements, slowness, and rigidity. Tremor in the upper extremities is characteristic. Neurocognitive deficits, which closely resemble an NCD due to Alzheimer's disease, are observed in 60% of clients diagnosed with Parkinson's disease.**
   4. Damage in the basal ganglia and the cerebral cortex is associated with Huntington's, not Parkinson's, disease.

   TEST-TAKING HINT: The test taker must understand the pathophysiology of Parkinson's disease to answer this question correctly.

Nursing Process—Assessment

4. **The correct order is 7, 1, 2, 6, 5, 4, 3. The progressive nature of symptoms associated with NCD due to Alzheimer's disease is described in seven stages.**
   1. **Stage 1: No apparent symptoms—In this stage there is no apparent decline in memory.**

2. **Stage 2: Forgetfulness**—The individual begins to lose things or forget names of people. These symptoms are often not observed by others.

3. **Stage 3: Mild cognitive decline**—There is interference with work performance and the individual may get lost when driving.

4. **Stage 4: Mild to moderate cognitive decline**—The individual may forget major events in personal history, such as a child's birthday.

5. **Stage 5: Moderate cognitive decline**—Individuals need assistance to perform some activities of daily living (ADLs) independently, such as hygiene, dressing, and grooming.

6. **Stage 6: Moderate to severe cognitive decline**—Disorientation to surroundings is common, and the person may be unable to recall the day, season, or year.

7. **Stage 7: Severe cognitive decline**—The individual is most commonly bedfast and aphasic.

TEST-TAKING HINT: To answer this question correctly, the test taker must understand the progressive nature of symptoms associated with an NCD due to Alzheimer's disease and then recognize symptoms described in the seven stages.

5. 1. *Anhedonia*, not *aphasia*, is the term used when an individual is sad and has no ability to experience or even imagine any pleasant emotion.

2. *Cachexia*, not *aphasia*, is the term used when an individual is in ill health and experiencing malnutrition and wasting. This may occur in many chronic diseases, certain malignancies, and advanced pulmonary tuberculosis.

3. *Aphasia* is the term used when an individual is having difficulty communicating through speech, writing, or signs. This is often caused by dysfunction of brain centers. Aphasia is a cardinal symptom observed in an NCD due to Alzheimer's disease.

4. *Aphonia*, not *aphasia*, is the term used when an individual is no longer able to speak. This may result from chronic laryngitis, laryngeal nerve damage, brain lesions, or psychiatric causes, such as hysteria.

TEST-TAKING HINT: The test taker needs to understand the term *aphasia* and be able to recognize the client symptoms that reflect this problem.

6. The client in the question is using confabulation. Confabulation is the creation of imaginary events to fill in memory gaps.

1. Although the client is using confabulation, the underlying reason is to protect the ego by maintaining self-esteem, not to achieve secondary gains.

2. Clients diagnosed with an NCD due to Alzheimer's disease use confabulation to create imaginary events to fill in memory gaps. Referred to as *hiding*, this is actually a form of denial, which is a protective ego defense mechanism used to maintain self-esteem and avoid losing one's place in the world.

3. The client in the question is using confabulation, not perseveration. A client who exhibits perseveration persistently repeats the same word or idea in response to different questions.

4. Although maintaining self-esteem is important for individuals diagnosed with an NCD due to Alzheimer's disease, the use of perseveration does not increase self-esteem. The client in the question is using confabulation, not perseveration. A client who exhibits perseveration persistently repeats the same word or idea in response to different questions.

TEST-TAKING HINT: To answer this question correctly, the test taker first must understand the meaning of the terms *confabulation* and *perseveration*. Also, the test taker must note that when two concepts are presented in answer choices, both concepts must be correct. Knowing this, the test taker can eliminate answers 1 and 4 immediately.

7. A client's symptoms may mimic an NCD. This masquerade is sometimes referred to as pseudodementia (depression). A battery of psychological tests may be ordered to differentiate between the two diagnoses.

1. A slow progression of symptoms is associated with NCD. A rapid progression is associated with pseudodementia (depression).

2. Impaired attention and concentration are associated with NCD, whereas intact attention and concentration are characteristics of pseudodementia (depression).

3. Diminished appetite is a symptom of pseudodementia (depression). Appetite in clients diagnosed with NCD remains unchanged. Also, clients diagnosed with NCD appear unconcerned about their disorder, whereas a client diagnosed with pseudodementia (depression) communicates severe distress regarding this frightening development.

4. As the day progresses, a client diagnosed with pseudodementia (depression)

experiences a diminished severity of symptoms, whereas a client diagnosed with NCD experiences an increase in the severity of symptoms.

5. A client diagnosed with pseudodementia (depression) does not become lost in familiar surroundings and does not have to be oriented to time and place. A client diagnosed with NCD often seems lost in what should be familiar surroundings and is in need of continual orientation to time and place.

TEST-TAKING HINT: The test taker must understand that cognitive symptoms of depression may mimic NCD. To answer this question correctly, the test taker must differentiate between the symptoms of NCD and pseudodementia (depression).

8. 1. A nursing assessment of a client with an acute decrease in cognitive ability should include a family history, such as specific mental and physical changes, and the age at which the changes began. If the client is unable to relate this information, the data should be obtained from family or friends. A nurse may administer a mini-mental state examination (MMSE), which is a commonly used assessment tool to quantify an individual's cognitive ability. It assesses orientation, registration, attention and calculation, and language. Scoring is from 0 to 30, with 30 indicating intact cognition.

2. A nursing assessment should include vital signs and the results of diagnostic laboratory tests ordered by the physician. Blood and urine samples should be obtained to test for various infections, hepatic and renal function, diabetes or hyperglycemia, electrolyte imbalances, and the presence of toxic substances. Vital signs are measured to assess for physiological problems and to establish a baseline.

3. A nursing assessment should include the results of a toxicology report ordered by the physician. The nurse also should understand that even with a negative report, delirium might persist after substance intoxication or substance withdrawal.

4. To assess a client effectively, it is essential for a nurse to use good communication skills. To obtain important facts and specific details, close-ended, not open-ended, questions can be effective in focusing a client with an acute decrease in cognition.

5. Familiarizing the client with the milieu is important; however, this nursing action is an intervention, not an assessment.

TEST-TAKING HINT: It is important for the test taker to note keywords in the question, such as *assessment.* Answer 5 can be eliminated immediately because it is an intervention, not an assessment.

9. 1. Delirium is characterized by a disturbance of consciousness and a state of awareness that may range from hypervigilance to stupor or semi coma.

2. The onset of delirium usually is quite abrupt, not slow, and often results in confusion, disorientation, restlessness, hyperactivity, and agitation.

3. The onset of an NCD, not delirium, is insidious and relentless. The duration of delirium is usually brief.

4. The symptoms of NCD, not delirium, last for 1 month or longer, often continuing and progressing throughout the lifetime. The symptoms of delirium are usually short term, lasting 1 week and rarely more than 1 month. The age of the client and the duration of the delirium influence the rate of symptom resolution.

TEST-TAKING HINT: To answer this question correctly, the test taker must be able to differentiate between the assessment data associated with NCD and delirium.

10. 1. The enzyme acetyltransferase is needed to synthesize the neurotransmitter acetylcholine. Some theorists propose that the primary memory loss that occurs in an NCD due to Alzheimer's disease is the direct result of reduction in acetylcholine available to the brain.

2. Loss of purposeful movement despite intact motor function (ataxia) may be associated with a decrease in acetylcholine; however, the development of ataxia is not the primary result of this reduction. Dopamine, norepinephrine, serotonin, and other substances may play a role in this condition. Also, loss of purposeful movement is a psychomotor, not cognitive, deficit.

3. Loss of sensory ability to recognize familiar objects audibly, visually, or tactilely (agnosia) may be associated with a decrease in acetylcholine; however, the development of agnosia is not a primary result of this reduction. Dopamine, norepinephrine, serotonin, and other substances also may play a role in this condition.

4. Loss of language ability (aphasia) may be associated with a decrease in acetylcholine; however, the development of aphasia is not a primary result of this reduction. Dopamine, norepinephrine, serotonin, and other substances also may play a role in this condition.

TEST-TAKING HINT: When reading the question, the test taker needs to note the keyword *primarily*. Various cognitive deficits may be associated with reduced levels of acetylcholine in the brain, but only answer 1 is primarily associated with this reduction.

11. Major NCD runs a progressive, irreversible course. Mild NCD can be reversible. The reversibility of mild NCD is a function of the timeliness of interventions that address the underlying pathology.
    1. Concern of individual that there has been a significant decline in cognitive function is a criterion for the diagnosis of major, not mild, NCD.
    2. Cognitive deficits interfering with independence in everyday activities is a criterion for the diagnosis of major NCD.
    3. When cognitive deficits do not occur exclusively in the context of delirium, they can be classified as either mild or major NCD.
    4. When cognitive deficits cannot be better explained by another medical condition, they can be classified as either mild or major NCD.
    5. When neuropsychological testing shows substantial impairment in cognitive performance, the criteria for major, not mild, NCD has been met.

TEST-TAKING HINT: To answer this question correctly, the test taker needs to review the criteria for the diagnosis of both mild and major NCDs.

Nursing Process—Diagnosis

12. 1. The nursing diagnosis of disturbed thought processes is defined as the disruption of cognitive operations and activities. Although clients diagnosed with vascular NCD may experience disturbed thought processes, the symptoms of isolation, poor role performance, and loss of independent functioning are not reflective of this nursing diagnosis.
    2. The nursing diagnosis of risk for injury is defined as the result of interaction of (internal or external) environmental conditions with the client's adaptive and defense resources. Although clients diagnosed with vascular NCD are at risk for injury, the symptoms

noted in the question are not reflective of this nursing diagnosis. Also, a correctly written "risk for" nursing diagnosis does not contain an "as evidenced by" statement.
    3. The nursing diagnosis of disturbed body image is defined as confusion in mental picture of one's physical self. There is no information noted in the question that indicates this client is experiencing a disturbed body image.
    4. **The nursing diagnosis of low self-esteem is defined as a negative self-evaluation or feelings about self or self-capabilities. This client is experiencing social isolation, which is evidence of low self-esteem. Poor role performance and loss of independent functioning exacerbate this problem.**

TEST-TAKING HINT: To answer this question correctly, the test taker must pair the symptoms presented in the question with the nursing diagnosis that reflects the client's problem. Because the nursing diagnosis in answer 2 is incorrectly written, the test taker can eliminate this choice immediately.

13. Delirium is defined as a state of mental confusion or excitement characterized by disorientation for time and place, often with hallucinations, incoherent speech, and a continuous state of aimless physical activity.
    1. **The nursing diagnosis of disturbed sensory perception is defined as a change in the amount of patterning of incoming internal or external stimuli accompanied by a diminished, exaggerated, distorted, or impaired response to such stimuli. This client is experiencing symptoms of a urinary tract infection (UTI). The client's combativeness and visual hallucinations, caused by septicemia secondary to the UTI, are indicative of a disturbed sensory perception. In an elderly client, a UTI, if untreated, often leads to symptoms of delirium.**
    2. The nursing diagnosis of risk for violence: self-directed is defined as behaviors in which a client demonstrates that they can be physically, emotionally, or sexually harmful to self. No information is presented in the question that indicates this client is at risk for self-directed violence. Combativeness may place the client at risk for violence directed toward others.
    3. The nursing diagnosis of self-care deficit is defined as the impaired ability to perform or complete ADLs independently. No information is presented in the question

that indicates this client is experiencing a self-care deficit.

4. The nursing diagnosis of social isolation is defined as aloneness experienced by the individual and perceived as imposed by others and as a negative or threatened state. No information is presented in the question that indicates this client is experiencing social isolation.

TEST-TAKING HINT: To answer this question correctly, the test taker must pair the symptoms presented in the question with the nursing diagnosis that reflects the client's problem.

Nursing Process—Planning

14. **1. Remaining free from injury is an appropriate short-term outcome for the nursing diagnosis of risk for injury. This short-term outcome meets all the criteria for a correctly written outcome. It is specific (injury), positive (free from), measurable (during this shift), realistic, and client centered.**
    2. This outcome does not include a time frame, so it is not measurable.
    3. Verbalizing staff appreciation does not relate to the nursing diagnosis of risk for injury.
    4. Demonstrating ability to perform ADLs does not relate to the nursing diagnosis of risk for injury.

TEST-TAKING HINT: The test taker must be able to match the stated nursing diagnosis with the appropriate outcome. Outcomes need to be client specific, realistic, attainable, and measurable and contain a time frame.

15. All outcomes must be client-centered, realistic, specific, positive, and measurable and contain a time frame.
    1. **The client participating in ADLs is a short-term outcome related to the nursing diagnosis of self-care deficit. This outcome meets all the criteria listed in the rationale. It is specific (ADLs), positive (participate), measurable (by discharge), realistic, and client centered.**
    2. NCD due to Alzheimer's disease is irreversible. The client accomplishing ADLs without assistance after discharge is not a realistic outcome for this client.
    3. The client exhibiting feelings of self-worth does not relate to the nursing diagnosis of self-care deficit.
    4. Maintaining physical safety is an important outcome. However, this outcome is not

measurable and does not relate to the nursing diagnosis of self-care deficit.

TEST-TAKING HINT: To answer this question correctly, the test taker needs to pair outcomes with the stated nursing diagnosis. Outcomes need to be realistic, and because of the chronic and irreversible nature of the diagnosis of an NCD due to Alzheimer's disease, answer 2 can be eliminated immediately.

Nursing Process—Implementation

16. 1. Telling a client who is experiencing delirium to calm down and listen is unrealistic. The client's reasoning ability and goal-directed behavior are impaired, and the client is unable to calm down or listen.
    2. Acknowledging that the client is upset promotes understanding and trust, but the nurse in this situation can address the client's symptoms appropriately by frequent orientation to reality without calling the supervisor.
    3. **Empathetically expressing understanding of the client's situation promotes trust and may have a calming effect on the client. Delirious or confused clients may be at high risk for injury and should be monitored closely.**
    4. Requesting an explanation from a client regarding reasons for feelings, thoughts, or behaviors in any situation, especially a situation in which a client is experiencing delirium, is nontherapeutic.

TEST-TAKING HINT: The test taker must understand that in the situation presented the client is in need of empathy, support, and close observation. Only answer 3 provides these interventions. It is nontherapeutic to request an explanation by asking the client a "why" question, which eliminates answer 4 immediately. Also, if one part of the answer is incorrect, the whole answer is incorrect, as in answer 2.

17. 1. Questioning the client's perception shows contempt for the client's ideas or behaviors. Asking a client to provide reasons for thoughts can be intimidating and implies that the client must defend their behavior or feelings.
    2. Challenging the client belittles the client and discourages further interactions.
    3. **Orienting the client to person, place, and time, as necessary, refocuses the client to the here and now. Casually reminding the client of a noon meal**

redirects the client in a manner that is considerate and respectful. It is imperative to preserve the client's self-esteem.

4. At this time, prn medication would do nothing to reorient the client to the here and now; prn haloperidol would be appropriate if the client were exhibiting agitation or uncontrolled behavior, not confusion and disorientation.

TEST-TAKING HINT: When clients are diagnosed with NCD, it is important to preserve self-esteem. These clients do not have the capacity to correct impaired orientation. When the nurse challenges the client's thought processes, as in answers 1 and 2, the client's self-esteem is decreased. Medicating a client, as in answer 4, without pursuing other avenues of problem-solving is inappropriate.

18. Primary prevention is a true prevention and precedes disease or dysfunction. Secondary prevention focuses on individuals who are experiencing health problems or illnesses. Tertiary prevention attempts to reduce the residual effects when a defect or disability is permanent and irreversible.

1. **Because the client is experiencing alterations in cognition, reinforcing speech with nonverbal techniques, such as pointing to and touching items, is a secondary prevention intervention.**

2. Keeping surroundings simple by reducing clutter would prevent injury if a client's gait is impaired. Nothing in the question indicates that this client has an impaired gait.

3. Offering family ethics consultation or hospice assistance would be a tertiary, not secondary, prevention intervention.

4. **Placing a large, visible clock and calendar in the client's room addresses the client's current confusion. Because this addresses the client's actual problem of disorientation, this intervention would be considered secondary prevention.**

5. Talking to family members about their genetic predisposition to an NCD is a primary, not secondary, prevention intervention.

TEST-TAKING HINT: To answer this question correctly, the test taker needs to understand and differentiate the nursing actions that occur in primary, secondary, and tertiary prevention.

19. 1. **Nutritional deficits are common among clients diagnosed with a late-stage NCD due to Alzheimer's disease. These clients must be assisted in consuming fluids and food to prevent electrolyte imbalance.**

Meeting this physical need would be prioritized over meeting psychological needs.

2. Clients diagnosed with late-stage NCD due to Alzheimer's disease may have severely impaired speech and language, may no longer recognize family members, and may be socially withdrawn and unaware of environment and surroundings. Reorientation would not be an effective intervention at this time.

3. Clients diagnosed with late-stage NCD due to Alzheimer's disease are most commonly bedridden and aphasic. At this stage, caregivers need to complete the client's ADLs. Promoting dignity and comfort, not self-esteem, would be a priority intervention in this case.

4. It is common for clients diagnosed with late-stage NCD due to Alzheimer's disease to be confined to a wheelchair or bed; ambulation and the need for assistance would not be expected.

TEST-TAKING HINT: The test taker must recognize that nursing interventions need to be realistic. This eliminates answers 2 and 3 immediately. Because of the chronic nature and irreversibility of the client's disorder, the client cannot realistically achieve the goals of these interventions. Also, the term *late-stage* directs the test taker to appropriate interventions.

20. 1. Using tranquilizing medications and soft restraints might be a priority intervention if the client were a danger to self or others; however, there is no mention of violent behavior in the question. The least restrictive measures should be employed initially.

2. It is necessary first to assess the client's level of disorientation and confusion before initiating other interventions. Continually reorienting this client would not be an effective intervention because of the irreversible nature of the client's diagnosis.

3. **Assessing the client's level of disorientation and confusion should be the first nursing intervention. Assessment of a client diagnosed with an NCD is necessary to formulate a plan of care and to determine specific interventions and requirements for safety.**

4. Assessing the client's level of disorientation and confusion is necessary to determine specific requirements for safety. The nurse then may remove potentially harmful objects from the client's room, if needed.

TEST-TAKING HINT: The test taker needs to understand that assessment, the first step in

the nursing process, is the initial step in determining an appropriate plan of care for a client.

Nursing Process—Evaluation

21. 1. Delirium is characterized by symptoms developing rapidly over a short period of time.
    2. Delirium affects the ability to learn new information; however, this condition is temporary, not permanent. Because a client diagnosed with delirium is extremely distractible and must be reminded repeatedly to focus, the ability to learn is impaired.
    3. Aphasia, apraxia, and agnosia are cognitive deficits and symptoms of an NCD, not delirium.
    4. Delirium is characterized by a disturbance of consciousness and a change in cognition. Reasoning ability and goal-directed behaviors are temporarily impaired.
    5. Delirium is always secondary to another condition, such as a general medical condition, substance-induced delirium, substance-intoxication delirium, substance-withdrawal delirium, or simply a delirium due to multiple etiologies.

TEST-TAKING HINT: To answer this question correctly, the test taker must understand and recognize symptoms of delirium. Because of the temporary nature of delirium, noting the word *permanently* assists the test taker in eliminating answer 2 immediately.

22. An NCD is classified as either mild or major, with the distinction primarily being one of severity of symptoms.
    1. A modest decline in cognitive function indicates the presence of mild NCD. Early intervention can prevent or slow progression of mild NCD. A positive prognosis will depend on the underlying cause and the severity of the symptoms.
    2. This client's modest decline in cognitive function indicates the presence of mild, not major, NCD.
    3. Early intervention can prevent or slow progression of mild NCD. A positive prognosis will depend on the underlying cause and the severity of the symptoms.
    4. This client's modest decline in cognitive function indicates the presence of mild, not major, NCD. Major NCD is irreversible.

TEST-TAKING HINT: To answer this question correctly, the test taker must differentiate between mild and major NCD.

Psychopharmacology

23. 1. Although short-term treatment for insomnia may be prescribed for a client diagnosed with an NCD, donepezil hydrochloride is not a sedative/hypnotic and is not used for insomnia.
    2. Donepezil hydrochloride is a treatment for NCD due to Alzheimer's disease. A decrease in cholinergic function may be the cause of this disease, and donepezil is a cholinesterase inhibitor. This drug exerts its effect by enhancing cholinergic function by increasing the level of acetylcholine.
    3. Antipsychotics are sometimes used for the symptoms of NCD due to Alzheimer's disease, but donepezil hydrochloride is not an antipsychotic drug, and it is not used in this context.
    4. Although clients diagnosed with NCD due to Alzheimer's disease may need anxiolytic medications to decrease anxiety, donepezil hydrochloride is not an anxiolytic and would not be used in this context.

TEST-TAKING HINT: The test taker must know the classification and use of the drug donepezil hydrochloride to answer this question correctly.

24. Meclizine is a medication used for the management of motion sickness and vertigo.
    1. Meclizine is used to improve vertigo, not auditory hallucinations. An antipsychotic medication would be indicated for this symptom.
    2. Meclizine is used to improve vertigo, not sleep problems. A benzodiazepine would be an appropriate short-term intervention to improve sleep.
    3. Meclizine has central anticholinergic, central nervous system depressant, and antihistaminic properties and is used to improve vertigo. Maintaining balance is an indication that vertigo has improved.
    4. Meclizine is used to improve vertigo, not anorexia. An appetite stimulant would be indicated for this symptom.

TEST-TAKING HINT: To answer this question correctly, the test taker must recognize meclizine as a medication used for dizziness and vertigo.

25. The client will reach the target dose on day four. The client will receive 50 mg on day one, then 50 mg each additional day. Every 2 days, the medication will be increased by 100 mg, so it will take 4 days to reach 200 mg.

TEST-TAKING HINT: The test taker must factor in the increasing dosage of the medication to determine how many days are required to reach the target dosage.

Eating Disorders

KEYWORDS

The following words include English vocabulary, nursing/medical terminology, concepts, principles, or information relevant to content specifically addressed in this chapter or associated with topics presented in it. English dictionaries, your nursing textbooks, and medical dictionaries such as *Taber's Cyclopedic Medical Dictionary* are resources that can be used to expand your knowledge and understanding of these words and related information.

Amenorrhea

Anorexia nervosa

Binge-eating disorder

Binging

Body mass index (BMI)

Bulimia nervosa

Cachexia

Disturbed body image

Eating patterns

Emaciated

Hypothalamus

Nutritional deficits

Obesity

Purging

QUESTIONS

Theory

1. Which structure in the brain contains the appetite regulation center?
   1. Thalamus.
   2. Amygdala.
   3. Hypothalamus.
   4. Medulla.

2. The nurse is teaching about factors that influence eating patterns. Which of the following statements indicate that learning has occurred? **Select all that apply.**
   1. "Factors such as taste and texture can affect appetite."
   2. "The function of my digestive organs affects my eating behaviors."
   3. "High socioeconomic status determines nutritious eating patterns."
   4. "Social interaction contributes little to eating patterns."
   5. "Society and culture influence eating patterns."

3. Which anorexia nervosa etiology is from a neuroendocrine perspective?
   1. Anorexia nervosa is more common among sisters and mothers of clients with the disorder than among the general population.
   2. Altered structure and function of the thalamus is implicated in the diagnosis of anorexia nervosa.
   3. There is a higher-than-expected frequency of mood disorders among first-degree relatives of clients diagnosed with anorexia nervosa.
   4. Clients diagnosed with anorexia nervosa have elevated cerebrospinal fluid cortisol levels and possible alterations in the regulation of dopamine.

4. Which etiological implication for obesity is from a physiological perspective?
   1. Eighty percent of offspring of two obese parents become obese.
   2. Individuals who are diagnosed with obesity have unresolved dependency needs and are fixed in the oral stage of development.
   3. Hyperthyroidism interferes with metabolism and may lead to obesity.
   4. Lesions in the appetite and satiety centers in the hypothalamus lead to overeating and obesity.

Nursing Process—Assessment

5. A client is being admitted to the inpatient psychiatric unit with a diagnosis of bulimia nervosa. The nurse would expect this client to fall within which age range?
   1. 5 to 10 years old.
   2. 10 to 14 years old.
   3. 18 to 22 years old.
   4. 40 to 45 years old.

6. Which individual would be at highest risk for obesity?
   1. A black woman whose income is below the federal poverty level.
   2. A white woman who is wealthy.
   3. A white man who is wealthy.
   4. A black man who is well educated.

7. A client with a long history of bulimia nervosa is seen in the emergency department. The client is seeing things that others do not, is restless, and has dry mucous membranes. Which is most likely the cause of this client's symptoms?
   1. Mood disorders, which often accompany the diagnosis of bulimia nervosa.
   2. Nutritional deficits, which are characteristic of bulimia nervosa.
   3. Vomiting, which may lead to dehydration and electrolyte imbalance.
   4. Binging, which causes abdominal discomfort.

8. An 18-year-old female client weighs 95 pounds and is 70 inches tall. The client has not had a period in 4 months and states, "I am so fat!" Which statement is reflective of this client's symptoms?
   1. The client meets the criteria for a diagnosis of bulimia nervosa.
   2. The client meets the criteria for a diagnosis of anorexia nervosa.
   3. The client needs further assessment to be diagnosed.
   4. The client is exhibiting normal developmental tasks according to Erikson.

9. The nurse is assessing a client with a body mass index (BMI) of 35. The nurse would suspect this client to be at risk for which of the following conditions? **Select all that apply.**
   1. Hypoglycemia.
   2. Rheumatoid arthritis.
   3. Angina.
   4. Respiratory insufficiency.
   5. Hyperlipidemia.

10. The family of a client diagnosed with anorexia nervosa has cancelled the past two family counseling sessions. Which of the following could be reasons for this nonadherence? **Select all that apply.**
    1. The family is fearful of the social stigma of having a family member with emotional problems.
    2. The family is dealing with feelings of guilt because of the perception that they have contributed to the disorder.
    3. There may be a pattern of conflict avoidance, and the family fears conflict would surface in the sessions.
    4. The family may be attempting to maintain family equilibrium by keeping the client in the sick role.
    5. The client is now maintaining adequate nutrition, and the sessions are no longer necessary.

11. Which anorexia nervosa symptom is physical in nature?
    1. Dry, yellow skin.
    2. Perfectionism.
    3. Frequent weighing.
    4. Preoccupation with food.

12. Which of the following statements are true as they relate to obesity? **Select all that apply.**
    1. Obesity is a psychiatric disorder, and diagnostic criteria are similar to other eating disorders.
    2. Binge-eating disorder is described as an eating disorder in the *Diagnostic and Statistical Manual of Mental Disorders*, Fifth Edition, Text Revision (*DSM-5-TR*), and this disorder can lead to obesity.
    3. Obesity is currently evaluated for all clients as a psychological factor affecting medical conditions.
    4. Obesity is not classified as an eating disorder but can be considered as a psychological factor affecting other medical conditions.
    5. The World Health Organization (WHO) defines obesity as a BMI of 30.0 or greater.

13. After a routine dental examination on an adolescent, the dentist reports to the parents that bulimia nervosa is suspected. On which of the following assessment data would the dentist base this determination? **Select all that apply.**
    1. Extreme weight loss.
    2. Amenorrhea.
    3. Discoloration of dental enamel.
    4. Bruises of the palate and posterior pharynx.
    5. Dental enamel dysplasia.

Nursing Process—Diagnosis

14. A client diagnosed with anorexia nervosa has a short-term outcome that states, "The client will gain 2 pounds in 1 week." Which nursing diagnosis reflects the problem that this outcome addresses?
    1. Ineffective coping R/T lack of control.
    2. Altered nutrition: less than body requirements R/T decreased intake.
    3. Self-care deficit: feeding R/T fatigue.
    4. Anxiety R/T feelings of helplessness.

15. A client with cachexia states, "I don't care what you say; I am horribly fat and will continue to diet." The client is experiencing arrhythmias and bradycardia. Based on this client's symptoms, which nursing diagnosis takes priority?
    1. Ineffective denial.
    2. Imbalanced nutrition: less than body requirements.
    3. Disturbed body image.
    4. Ineffective coping.

Nursing Process—Planning

16. A client is leaving the inpatient psychiatric facility after 1 month of treatment for anorexia nervosa. Which outcome is appropriate during discharge planning for this client?
    1. Client will accept refeeding as part of a daily routine.
    2. Client will perform nasogastric tube feeding independently.
    3. Client will verbalize recognition of fat body misperception.
    4. Client will discuss importance of monitoring weight daily.

17. A client diagnosed with anorexia nervosa has a nursing diagnosis of imbalanced nutrition: less than body requirements. Which long-term, correctly written outcome addresses client problem improvement?
    1. The client's BMI will be 20 by the 6-month follow-up appointment.
    2. The client will be free of signs and symptoms of malnutrition and dehydration.
    3. The client will use one healthy coping mechanism during a time of stress by discharge.
    4. The client will understand a previous dependency role by the 3-month follow-up visit.

Nursing Process—Implementation

18. Which nursing intervention would directly assist a hospitalized client diagnosed with bulimia nervosa in avoiding the urge to purge after discharge?
    1. Locking the door to the client's bathroom.
    2. Holding a mandatory group after mealtime to assist in exploration of feelings.
    3. Discussing preplanned meals to decrease anxiety around eating.
    4. Educating the family to recognize purging side effects.

19. A client diagnosed with anorexia nervosa is newly admitted to an inpatient psychiatric unit. Which intervention takes priority?
    1. Assessment of family issues and health concerns.
    2. Assessment of early disturbances in mother–infant interactions.
    3. Assessment of the client's knowledge of selective serotonin reuptake inhibitors used in treatment.
    4. Assessment and monitoring of vital signs and laboratory values to recognize and anticipate medical problems.

20. When using a behavioral modification approach for the treatment of eating disorders, which nursing intervention would be most likely to produce positive results?
    1. Take a matter-of-fact, directive approach with the input of the entire treatment team.
    2. Clients should perceive that they are in control of clearly communicated treatment choices.
    3. Appropriate treatment choices are presented to the client's family for consideration.
    4. The treatment team develops a system of rewards and privileges that can be earned by the client.

21. A nurse sitting with a client diagnosed with anorexia nervosa notices that the client has eaten 80% of lunch. The client asks the nurse, "What do you like better, hamburgers or spaghetti?" Which is the best response by the nurse?
    1. "I'm Italian, so I really enjoy a large plate of spaghetti."
    2. "I'll weigh you after your meal."
    3. "Let's focus on your continued improvement. You ate 80% of your lunch."
    4. "Why do you always talk about food? Let's talk about swimming."

22. A client on an inpatient psychiatric unit has been diagnosed with bulimia nervosa. The client states, "I'm going to the bathroom and will be back in a few minutes." Which nursing response is most appropriate?
    1. "Thanks for checking in."
    2. "I will accompany you to the bathroom."
    3. "Let me know when you get back to the dayroom."
    4. "I'll stand outside your door to give you privacy."

23. A client diagnosed with binge-eating disorder has a nursing diagnosis of low self-esteem. Which nursing intervention would address this client's problem?
    1. Offer independent decision-making opportunities.
    2. Review previously successful coping strategies.
    3. Provide a quiet environment with decreased stimulation.
    4. Allow the client to remain in a dependent role throughout treatment.

24. A 5-foot 4-inch client, weighing 75 pounds, diagnosed with anorexia nervosa, has been assigned a nursing diagnosis of imbalanced nutrition: less than body requirements R/T altered body perception. Which nursing intervention would address this client's problem?
    1. Encourage the client to keep a diary of food intake.
    2. Plan exercise tailored to individual choice.
    3. Help the client to identify triggers to self-induced purging.
    4. Monitor physician-ordered nasogastric tube feedings.

Nursing Process—Evaluation

25. The instructor is teaching nursing students about the psychodynamic influences of eating disorders. Which statement indicates that more teaching is necessary?
    1. "Eating disorders result from very early and profound disturbances in father–infant interactions."
    2. "Disturbances in mother–infant interactions may result in retarded ego development."
    3. "When a mother meets the physical and emotional needs of a child by providing food, this behavior contributes to the child's ego development."
    4. "Poor self-image leads to a perceived lack of control. The client compensates for this perceived lack of control by controlling behaviors related to eating."

26. Which of the following nursing evaluations of a client diagnosed with anorexia nervosa would lead the treatment team to consider discharge? **Select all that apply.**
    1. The client participates in individual therapy.
    2. The client has a BMI of 16.
    3. The client consumes adequate calories as determined by the dietitian.
    4. The client is dependent on their mother for most basic needs.
    5. The client states, "I realize that I can't be perfect."

Psychopharmacology

27. A client diagnosed with bulimia nervosa has responded well to citalopram. Which is the possible cause for this response?
    1. There is an association between bulimia nervosa and dilated blood vessels and inactive alpha-adrenergic and serotoninergic receptors.
    2. There is an association between bulimia nervosa and the neurotransmitter dopamine.
    3. There is an association between bulimia nervosa and the neurotransmitters serotonin and norepinephrine.
    4. There is an association between bulimia nervosa and a malfunction of the thalamus.

28. Which medication is used most often in the treatment of clients diagnosed with anorexia nervosa?
    1. Fluphenazine.
    2. Clozapine.
    3. Fluoxetine.
    4. Methylphenidate.

29. Structures of the brain impact eating disorders. Identify the following structures of the brain on the provided diagram.
    1. _____ Thalamus.
    2. _____ Amygdala.
    3. _____ Hypothalamus.
    4. _____ Hippocampus.

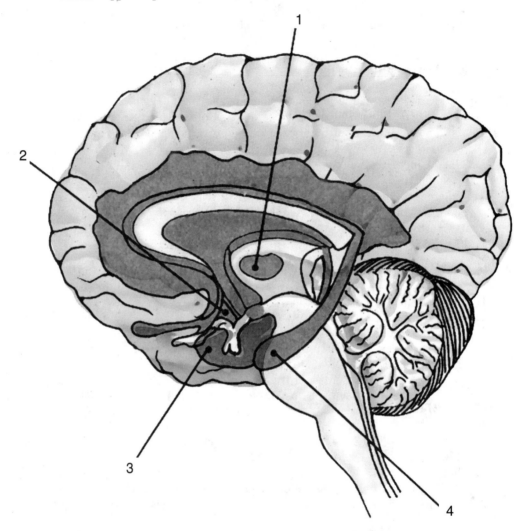

30. A client diagnosed with anorexia nervosa is admitted with dehydration. An IV of D_5W is ordered to run at 150 mL/hr. Using tubing that delivers 15 gtt/mL, the nurse should adjust the rate of flow to _____ gtt/min.

31. A client diagnosed with an eating disorder asks the nurse about medications to help with food cravings. The nurse should provide information on which of the following medications? **Select all that apply.**
    1. Bupropion-naltrexone.
    2. Lorcaserin.
    3. Orlistat.
    4. Phentermine-topiramate.
    5. Liraglutide.

The correct answer number and rationale for why it is the correct answer are given in **boldface blue type**. Rationales for why the other answer options are incorrect are given as well, but they are not in boldface type.

Theory

1. 1. The thalamus integrates all sensory input (except smell) on its way to the cortex and is involved with emotions and mood. It does not regulate appetite.
   2. The amygdala is located in the temporal lobe of the brain and may play a major role in memory processing and learned fear. It does not regulate appetite.
   3. **The hypothalamus exerts control over the actions of the autonomic nervous system and regulates appetite and temperature.**
   4. The medulla of the brain contains vital centers that regulate heart rate; blood pressure; respiration; and reflex centers for swallowing, sneezing, coughing, and vomiting. It does not regulate appetite.

TEST-TAKING HINT: The test taker must be familiar with the structure and function of the various areas of the brain to recognize the hypothalamus as the appetite regulation center.

2. Providing a social setting can improve eating patterns, whereas societal pressures may be detrimental.
   1. **Environmental factors, such as taste, texture, temperature, and stress, can affect eating behaviors.**
   2. **The function of the gastrointestinal tract affects eating behaviors and appetite. Physiological variables include the balance of neuropeptides and neurotransmitters, metabolic rate, the structure and function of the gastrointestinal tract, and the ability to taste and smell.**
   3. A high socioeconomic status does not determine healthy eating patterns. Many people in affluent cultures in the United States and all over the world have poor nutritional status because of poor eating choices.
   4. Social interactions *do* contribute to eating patterns. Eating is a social activity. Most special events revolve around the presence of food. Providing a social setting can improve appetite and eating behaviors.

5. Society and culture have a great deal of influence on eating behaviors and perceptions of ideal weight. Eating patterns are developed based on attempts to meet these societal norms.

TEST-TAKING HINT: The test taker must recognize the impact of the social activity of eating and the effect society has on eating patterns to answer this question correctly.

3. 1. Anorexia nervosa is more common among sisters and mothers of clients with the disorder than among the general population. However, this is an etiological implication from a genetic, not neuroendocrine, perspective.
   2. An altered structure and function of the hypothalamus, not thalamus, is implicated in the diagnosis of anorexia nervosa. This would support a physiological, not neuroendocrine, etiological perspective.
   3. There is a higher-than-expected frequency of mood disorders among first-degree relatives of clients diagnosed with anorexia nervosa. However, this is an etiological implication from a genetic, not neuroendocrine, perspective.
   4. **Research has shown that clients diagnosed with anorexia nervosa have elevated cerebrospinal fluid cortisol levels and possible alterations in the regulation of dopamine. This is an etiological implication from a neuroendocrine perspective.**

TEST-TAKING HINT: To answer this question correctly, the test taker should note the perspective required in the question. All answers except 2 are correct etiological implications for the diagnosis of anorexia nervosa; however, only answer 4 is from a neuroendocrine perspective.

4. 1. Eighty percent of offspring of two obese parents become obese. However, this etiological implication is from a genetic, not physiological, perspective.
   2. The psychoanalytic, not physiological, view of obesity proposes that obese individuals have unresolved dependency needs and are fixed in the oral stage of development.
   3. Hypothyroidism, not hyperthyroidism, decreases metabolism and is more likely to lead to obesity. Hyperthyroidism, because of increased metabolic rates, may lead to weight loss.

4. A theory of obesity from a physiological perspective is that lesions in the appetite and satiety centers in the hypothalamus lead to overeating and obesity.

TEST-TAKING HINT: To answer this question correctly, the test taker must look for a potential obesity cause from a physiological, or "physical," perspective. Answer 3 is physiologically based but contains inaccurate information and so can be eliminated.

Nursing Process—Assessment

5. The onset of bulimia nervosa commonly occurs in late adolescence or early adulthood. Bulimia nervosa is more prevalent than anorexia nervosa. Research suggests that bulimia occurs primarily in societies that place emphasis on thinness as the model of attractiveness for women and in which an abundance of food is available.
   1. These ages are not within the range of late adolescence to early adulthood.
   2. These ages are not within the range of late adolescence to early adulthood. Age 14 would be considered early, not late, adolescence.
   3. **These ages are within the range of late adolescence to early adulthood, in which the onset of bulimia nervosa commonly occurs.**
   4. These ages are not within the range of late adolescence to early adulthood. Age 40 falls in the category of late, not early, adulthood.

TEST-TAKING HINT: The test taker must recognize the age ranges for onset of bulimia nervosa to answer this question correctly.

6. 1. **Obesity is more common in black women than in white women, and the prevalence among lower socioeconomic classes is six times greater than among upper socioeconomic classes. Therefore, this individual is at highest risk for obesity compared with the others described.**
   2. Obesity is less common in white women than in black women, and the prevalence among lower socioeconomic classes is six times greater than among upper socioeconomic classes. Therefore, this client has a comparatively lower risk for obesity than the other clients presented.
   3. Obesity is more common in white men than in black men, but because the prevalence among lower socioeconomic classes is six times higher than among upper socioeconomic classes, this individual's risk is comparatively lower than the other clients presented.

4. Obesity is more common in white men than in black men, and there is an inverse relationship between obesity and education level. Therefore, this client has a comparatively lower risk for obesity than the other clients presented.

TEST-TAKING HINT: The test taker must be aware of the epidemiological factors that influence the prevalence rate of obesity to determine which of the individuals described is at highest risk for becoming obese.

7. 1. Mood disorders often accompany the diagnosis of bulimia nervosa, but the client symptoms described in the question do not reflect a mood disorder.
   2. Nutritional deficits are characteristic of bulimia nervosa, but the client symptoms described in the question do not reflect a nutritional deficit.
   3. **Purging behaviors, such as vomiting, may lead to dehydration and electrolyte imbalance. Hallucinations and restlessness can be signs of electrolyte imbalance. Dry mucous membranes indicate dehydration.**
   4. Binging large quantities of food can cause abdominal discomfort, but the client symptoms described in the question do not reflect abdominal discomfort.

TEST-TAKING HINT: To answer this question correctly, the test taker must recognize common signs and symptoms of electrolyte imbalance and dehydration.

8. 1. Included in the diagnostic criteria for bulimia nervosa are binge eating, self-induced vomiting, abuse of laxatives, and/or poor self-evaluation unduly influenced by body shape and weight. This client is not experiencing any binge eating, purging, or inappropriate use of laxatives. Although weight may fluctuate, clients diagnosed with bulimia nervosa can maintain weight within a normal range. This client does not meet the criteria for a diagnosis of bulimia nervosa.
   2. **Significantly low body weight in the context of age, sex, developmental trajectory, and physical health; disturbance in the way in which one's body weight is experienced; undue influence of body weight on self-evaluation; and lack of recognition of the seriousness of the current low body weight are all diagnostic criteria for anorexia nervosa. This client meets the criteria for this diagnosis.**
   3. Because the client meets the diagnostic criteria for anorexia nervosa, additional assessments are unnecessary.

4. Extreme weight loss, disturbed body image, and amenorrhea are not normal developmental tasks for an 18-year-old client, according to Erikson. Erikson identified the development of a secure sense of self as the task of the adolescent stage (12 to 20 years) of psychosocial development.

TEST-TAKING HINT: To answer this question correctly, the test taker must remember diagnostic criteria for anorexia nervosa and differentiate these from the criteria for bulimia nervosa.

9. Clients with a body mass index (BMI) of 30 or greater are classified as obese. It is important to learn the complications of obesity because, based on World Health Organization guidelines, half of all Americans are obese.
   1. Obese clients commonly have hyperglycemia, not hypoglycemia, and are at risk for developing diabetes mellitus.
   2. Osteoarthritis, not rheumatoid arthritis, results from trauma to weight-bearing joints and is commonly seen in obese clients.
   3. **Workload on the heart is increased in obese clients, often leading to symptoms of angina.**
   4. **Workload on the lungs is increased in obese clients, often leading to symptoms of respiratory insufficiency.**
   5. **Due to intake of increased amounts of fatty foods, obese clients often present with hyperlipidemia, particularly elevated triglyceride and cholesterol levels.**

TEST-TAKING HINT: To answer this question correctly, the test taker first must recognize that this client is obese as reflected by the BMI mentioned in the question.

10. Eating disorders are considered family disorders, and resolution of the disease cannot be achieved until dynamics within the family have improved.
    1. Support is given through family counseling as families deal with the existing social stigma of having a family member with emotional problems. This stigma also may discourage adherence with therapies, as the family copes with the stress by denying the illness.
    2. Families who are experiencing feelings of guilt associated with the perception that they have contributed to the onset of the disorder may avoid dealing with this guilt by being nonadherent with family therapy.
    3. Dysfunctional family dynamics may lead the family to avoid conflict by avoiding highly charged family sessions.
    4. Dysfunctional family systems often focus conflicts and stress on a scapegoat

family member. These families balance their family system by maintaining this member in a dependent, sick role. Because of disruption in the dysfunctional family system, there is little interest shown in changing the role of this member who is deemed to be sick.

5. Anorexia nervosa is a disease that requires long-term treatment for successful change to occur. It would be improbable that the client would begin eating spontaneously, maintain adequate nutrition, and no longer require treatment.

TEST-TAKING HINT: To select the correct answer, the test taker must recognize the deterrents to active participation in family therapy. It is vital to understand these deterrents to be able to encourage effective adherence with family therapy.

11. 1. **Dry, yellow skin is a physical symptom of anorexia nervosa. This is due to the release of carotenes as fat stores are burned for energy.**
    2. Perfectionism is often experienced by clients with a diagnosis of anorexia nervosa, but it is a behavioral, not physical, symptom.
    3. Frequent weighing is a behavioral, not physical, symptom of anorexia nervosa.
    4. Preoccupation with food is a cognitive, not physical, symptom of anorexia.

TEST-TAKING HINT: To select the correct answer, the test taker first must determine if the symptom presented is a symptom of anorexia nervosa, then be able to categorize this symptom accurately as physical.

12. 1. Obesity is not classified as a psychiatric disorder, but because of the strong emotional factors associated with the condition, it may be considered under "psychological factors affecting medical conditions."
    2. Binge-eating disorder is described as an eating disorder in the *Diagnostic and Statistical Manual of Mental Disorders*, Fifth Edition, Text Revision (*DSM-5-TR*). Obesity is a factor in binge-eating disorder because the individual binges on large amounts of food (as in bulimia nervosa) but does not engage in behaviors to rid the body of the excess calories.
    3. Because of the strong emotional factors associated with obesity, it may be considered under "psychological factors affecting medical conditions"; however, this evaluation does not apply to all clients.
    4. Obesity is not classified as an eating disorder. It is considered under

"psychological factors affecting medical conditions" in the *DSM-5-TR*.

5. Obesity is defined by the World Health Organization as a BMI of 30.0 or greater.

TEST-TAKING HINT: Note the words *all clients* in answer 3. Superlatives that are all inclusive or exclusive, such as *all*, *always*, and *never*, usually indicate that the answer choice is incorrect.

13. 1. Clients with bulimia nervosa can maintain a normal weight. Extreme weight loss would be a symptom of anorexia nervosa, not bulimia nervosa.
    2. Amenorrhea, due to estrogen deficiencies, is a symptom of anorexia nervosa, not bulimia nervosa. A dentist would not be in a position to evaluate this symptom during a routine dental examination.
    3. A client diagnosed with bulimia nervosa may show evidence of dental discoloration due to the presence of acidic gastric juices in the oral cavity during frequent vomiting.
    4. Bruises of the palate and posterior pharynx occur because of continual vomiting owing to purging behaviors by clients diagnosed with bulimia nervosa. This would be an indication to the dentist that bulimia nervosa should be suspected.
    5. Dental enamel dysplasia occurs because of the presence of gastric juices in the mouth from continual vomiting owing to purging behaviors by the client diagnosed with bulimia nervosa. This would be an indication to the dentist that bulimia nervosa should be suspected.

TEST-TAKING HINT: The test taker should consider the situation presented in the question to gain clues to the correct answer. What assessment data would a dentist gather? A dentist would not gather assessment information related to menstruation, so answer 2 can be eliminated quickly.

Nursing Process—Diagnosis

14. 1. The outcome of gaining 2 pounds in 1 week is not directly related to the nursing diagnosis of ineffective coping. Ineffective coping is defined as the inability to form a valid appraisal of the stressors, inadequate choices of practiced responses, or inability to use available resources. An appropriate outcome for ineffective coping for clients diagnosed with eating disorders would be to use healthy coping strategies effectively to deal with

anxiety or lack of control without resorting to self-starvation.

2. The outcome of gaining 2 pounds in 1 week is directly related to the nursing diagnosis of altered nutrition: less than body requirements. Altered nutrition: less than body requirements is defined as the state in which individuals experience an intake of nutrients insufficient to meet metabolic needs. Weight loss is characteristic of the diagnosis of anorexia nervosa, with weight gain being a critical outcome.

3. The outcome of gaining 2 pounds in 1 week is not directly related to the nursing diagnosis of self-care deficit: feeding R/T fatigue. Self-care deficit is related to the inability of the client to perform the acts of self-care, in this case feeding. Clients diagnosed with anorexia nervosa have the ability to feed themselves but choose not to because of impaired body image.

4. The outcome of gaining 2 pounds in 1 week is not directly related to the nursing diagnosis of anxiety R/T feelings of helplessness. Feelings of depression and anxiety often accompany the diagnosis of anorexia nervosa, but in the short term, weight gain would increase, not decrease, the anxiety experienced by the client.

TEST-TAKING HINT: To select the correct answer, the test taker must be able to pair the nursing outcome presented in the question with the correct nursing diagnosis. There always must be a correlation between the stated outcome and the problem statement.

15. Cachexia is a state of ill health, malnutrition, and wasting.

1. When clients diagnosed with eating disorders are unable to admit the effect of maladaptive eating behaviors on life patterns, they are experiencing ineffective denial. This is a valid nursing diagnosis for this client because there is an inability to admit emaciation. This diagnosis should be considered, however, only after resolution of life-threatening nutritional status.

2. The immediate and priority problem that this client faces is imbalanced nutrition: less than body requirements. Impaired nutrition causes complications of emaciation, dehydration, and electrolyte imbalance that can lead to death. When the physical condition is no longer life threatening, other problems may be addressed.

3. When emaciated clients diagnosed with eating disorders are negative about their

appearance and see themselves as overweight, they are experiencing disturbed body image. This is a valid nursing diagnosis for this client because the client views the body as "horribly fat" when in reality the client is critically thin. This diagnosis should be considered, however, only after resolution of life-threatening nutritional status.

4. Clients diagnosed with eating disorders cope ineffectively with stress and anxiety by maladaptive eating patterns. This is a valid nursing diagnosis because this client is choosing not to eat to deal with unconscious stressors. This diagnosis should be considered, however, only after resolution of life-threatening nutritional status.

TEST-TAKING HINT: To answer this question correctly, the test taker first must understand the terms used in the question, such as *cachexia*. Physiological needs must take priority over psychological needs. If physiological needs are not addressed, the client is at risk for life-threatening complications.

Nursing Process—Planning

16. 1. Accepting refeeding as part of a daily routine is an outcome that would be appropriate early in treatment and should have been accomplished before discharge planning consideration.
    2. Performing nasogastric tube feeding independently is an outcome that would be appropriate early in treatment and should have been accomplished before discharge planning consideration.
    3. **The outcome of verbalizing recognition of misperception involving fat body image is a long-term outcome, appropriate for discharge planning for a client diagnosed with anorexia nervosa.**
    4. Monitoring weight on a daily basis is an inappropriate outcome for a client diagnosed with anorexia nervosa. Obsession about food and weight gain is a characteristic symptom of the disease, and this outcome would reinforce this problem.

TEST-TAKING HINT: An outcome that is appropriate for discharge planning must be a long-term outcome. Answers 1 and 2 are short term in nature and should occur early in treatment. Answer 4 would be excessive and inappropriate. Answers 1, 2, and 4 can be eliminated immediately.

17. 1. A normal BMI range is 20 to 25. Achieving the outcome of a BMI of 20 would

indicate improvement for the stated nursing diagnosis of imbalanced nutrition: less than body requirements.
2. Experiencing no signs and symptoms of malnutrition and dehydration is an outcome related to the nursing diagnosis of imbalanced nutrition. However, this outcome is incorrectly written because it does not contain a time frame.
3. Improving the ability to demonstrate healthy coping mechanisms by discharge is a short-term outcome related to the nursing diagnosis of ineffective coping, not imbalanced nutrition.
4. Stating understanding of a previous dependency role by the 3-month follow-up appointment is a long-term outcome related to the nursing diagnosis of low self-esteem, not imbalanced nutrition.

TEST-TAKING HINT: To select the correct answer, the test taker must be able to pair the client problem presented in the question with the measurable outcome that is a realistic expectation of client improvement. Answers 3 and 4 may be appropriate outcomes for clients diagnosed with eating disorders, but only answer 1 indicates client improvement related to imbalanced nutrition: less than body requirements.

Nursing Process—Implementation

18. 1. Locking the client's door would be an appropriate behavioral approach to prevent purging in an inpatient setting but would not assist the client in avoiding the urge to purge when discharged.
    2. **Holding a mandatory group after meal-time to assist in exploration of feelings is an appropriate intervention to help the hospitalized client diagnosed with bulimia nervosa to avoid the urge to purge after discharge. If the client can become aware of feelings that may trigger purging, future purging may be avoided.**
    3. Discussing preplanned meals to decrease anxiety around eating is an intervention focused on binging, not purging.
    4. Educating the family to recognize purging side effects would not directly assist the client in avoiding purging after discharge. This intervention is focused on providing the family tools to use if purging behaviors continue, not on helping the client to avoid these behaviors.

TEST-TAKING HINT: To answer this question correctly, the test taker must note the time frame presented in the question. The client must be present on the unit for answer 1 to be a possible intervention. Although answer 2 occurs on the unit, the information presented in group therapy would help the client to avoid purging behaviors after discharge. Answer 4 can be eliminated because it focuses on the family instead of the client.

19. 1. It is important to assess family issues and health concerns, but because of the critical nature of physical problems experienced by clients diagnosed with anorexia nervosa, this intervention is not prioritized.
    2. It is important to assess early disturbances in mother–infant interactions, but because of the critical nature of physical problems experienced by clients diagnosed with anorexia nervosa, this intervention is not prioritized.
    3. It is important to assess the client's previous knowledge of selective serotonin reuptake inhibitors before any teaching, but because of the critical nature of physical problems experienced by clients diagnosed with anorexia nervosa, this intervention is not prioritized.
    4. **The immediate priority of nursing interventions in eating disorders is to restore the client's nutritional status. Complications of emaciation, dehydration, and electrolyte imbalance can lead to death. The assessment and monitoring of vital signs and laboratory values to recognize and anticipate these medical problems must take priority. When the physical condition is no longer life threatening, other treatment modalities may be initiated.**

TEST-TAKING HINT: To answer this question correctly, the test taker must note that the question requires a "priority" intervention. Physical needs that threaten life always take priority over psychological needs.

20. 1. A behavior modification program should be instituted with client input and involvement. A directive approach would not give the client the needed and sought-after control over behaviors. Typically, control issues are the underlying problem precipitating eating disorders.
    2. A behavior modification program for clients diagnosed with eating disorders should ensure that the client does not feel controlled by the program. Issues of control are central to the etiology of these disorders, and for a program to succeed, the client must perceive they

are in control of behavioral choices. This is accomplished by contracting with the client for privileges based on weight gain.
    3. A behavior modification program should be instituted with client input and involvement. Focusing on the family and excluding the client from treatment choices has been shown to be ineffective.
    4. It is important for staff members and clients to work jointly to develop a contract for rewards and privileges that can be earned by the client. It would be inappropriate for the treatment team to solely develop this contract. The client should have ultimate control over behavioral choices, including whether to abide by the contract.

TEST-TAKING HINT: To select the correct answer, the test taker must understand that issues of control are central to the etiology of eating disorders. Effective nursing interventions are client focused. Only answer 2 involves the client in developing the plan of care.

21. 1. Because clients diagnosed with anorexia nervosa are obsessed with food, the nurse should not discuss food or eating behaviors. Discussion of food or eating behaviors can provide unintended positive reinforcement for negative behaviors. This statement by the nurse also focuses on the nurse and not the client.
    2. The nurse should weigh the client daily, immediately on arising, following first voiding, and not after a meal.
    3. **It is important to offer support and positive reinforcement for improvements in eating behaviors. Because clients diagnosed with anorexia nervosa are obsessed with food, discussion of food can provide unintended positive reinforcement for negative behaviors. In this answer choice, the nurse is appropriately redirecting the client.**
    4. When the nurse requests an explanation that the client cannot give, the client may feel defensive. "Why" questions are blocks to therapeutic communication.

TEST-TAKING HINT: The test taker must understand the underlying obsession and preoccupation with food that clients diagnosed with eating disorders experience. When this is understood, it is easy to choose an answer that does not support this maladaptive behavior.

22. 1. The response "Thanks for checking in" does not address the nurse's responsibility to deter the client's self-induced vomiting

behavior. The nurse should accompany the client to the bathroom.

2. The response "I will accompany you to the bathroom" is appropriate. Any client suspected of self-induced vomiting should be accompanied to the bathroom for the nurse to be able to deter this behavior.

3. The response "Let me know when you get back to the dayroom" does not address the nurse's responsibility to deter the client's self-induced vomiting behavior. The nurse should accompany the client to the bathroom.

4. The response "I'll stand outside your door to give you privacy" does not address the nurse's responsibility to deter the client's self-induced vomiting behavior. The nurse should accompany the client to the bathroom. Providing privacy is secondary to preventing further nutritional deficits.

TEST-TAKING HINT: The test taker must understand that sometimes all client needs cannot be met. Although privacy is a client need, in this case the nurse must put aside the client's need for privacy to intervene to prevent further nutritional deficits resulting from self-induced vomiting.

23. 1. **Offering independent decision-making opportunities promotes feelings of control. Making decisions and dealing with the consequences of these decisions should increase independence and improve the client's self-esteem.**

2. Reviewing previously successful coping strategies is an effective nursing intervention for clients experiencing altered coping, not low self-esteem. Altered coping is a common problem for clients diagnosed with binge-eating disorder, but this nursing diagnosis is not stated in the question.

3. Providing a quiet environment with decreased stimulation is an effective nursing intervention for clients experiencing anxiety, not low self-esteem. Anxiety is a common problem for clients diagnosed with binge-eating disorder, but this nursing diagnosis is not stated in the question.

4. Allowing the client to remain in a dependent role throughout treatment would decrease, rather than increase, self-esteem. There is little opportunity for successful experiences and increased self-esteem when decisions and choices are made for the client.

TEST-TAKING HINT: To select the correct answer, the test taker must be able to pair the client problem presented in the question with the

nursing intervention that addresses this problem. Answers 2 and 3 may be appropriate interventions for clients diagnosed with binge-eating disorder, but only answer 1 correlates with the client problem of low self-esteem.

24. 1. Clients diagnosed with anorexia nervosa have a preoccupation with food. Focusing on food by encouraging the client to keep a food diary only reinforces maladaptive behaviors. Encouraging a food diary is an appropriate nursing intervention for clients designated as obese.

2. Clients diagnosed with anorexia nervosa are critically ill. They are not meeting their nutritional needs because of poor caloric intake. Exercise would increase the client's metabolic requirements further and exacerbate the client's problem.

3. Self-induced purging is typical of bulimia nervosa, not anorexia nervosa. Also, identifying triggers does not directly address the nursing diagnosis of imbalanced nutrition: less than body requirements.

4. **If clients are unable or unwilling to maintain adequate oral intake, the physician may order a liquid diet to be administered via nasogastric tube. This treatment is initiated because without adequate nutrition a life-threatening situation exists for these clients. Nursing care of a client receiving tube feedings should be based on established hospital procedures.**

TEST-TAKING HINT: To select the correct answer, the test taker must be able to pair the client problem presented in the question with the nursing intervention that addresses this problem. Only answer 4 correlates with the client problem of imbalanced nutrition: less than body requirements.

Nursing Process—Evaluation

25. 1. **Eating disorders result from very early and profound disturbances in mother–infant, not father–infant, interactions. This statement would indicate that more teaching is necessary.**

2. Disturbances in mother–infant interactions result in retarded ego development, which contributes to the development of an eating disorder. This is a correct statement and further teaching is not necessary.

3. Ego development can be attributed to a mother meeting the physical and emotional needs of a child by providing food. This is

a correct statement and further teaching is not necessary.

4. Poor self-image leads to a perceived lack of control. The client compensates for this perceived lack of control by controlling behaviors related to eating. This is a correct statement and further teaching is not necessary.

TEST-TAKING HINT: The question is asking for an incorrect statement about eating disorders, which would indicate that "more teaching is necessary."

26. 1. Willingness to participate in individual therapy is an indication that this client meets discharge criteria. Individual therapy encourages the client to explore unresolved conflicts and to recognize maladaptive eating behaviors as defense mechanisms used to ease emotional pain.
2. The BMI for normal weight is 20 to 25. Because this client's BMI is lower than the normal range, consideration for discharge may be inappropriate at this time.
3. **It is significant when a client diagnosed with anorexia nervosa consumes adequate calories to maintain metabolic needs. This assessment information would indicate that the client should be considered for discharge.**
4. Families of clients diagnosed with anorexia nervosa often consist of a passive father, a domineering mother, and an overly dependent child. This client's continued dependence on the mother may indicate that consideration for discharge is inappropriate at this time.
5. **A high value is placed on perfectionism in families of clients diagnosed with anorexia nervosa. These clients feel that they must satisfy these unrealistic standards, and when this is found to be impossible, helplessness results. Because this client shows insight into this problem by the recognition that perfection is impossible, consideration for discharge is appropriate.**

TEST-TAKING HINT: To answer this question correctly, the test taker must have an understanding of the basic problems underlying the diagnosis of anorexia nervosa. Remembering the BMI value for normal weight eliminates answer 2.

Psychopharmacology

27. Citalopram is a selective serotonin reuptake inhibitor (SSRI) and affects the neurotransmitter serotonin.

1. Vascular headaches, not bulimia nervosa, are caused by dilated blood vessels in the brain. Drugs such as ergotamine are used to treat vascular headaches by stimulating alpha-adrenergic and serotoninergic receptors.
2. There is an association between bulimia nervosa and the neurotransmitters serotonin and norepinephrine, not dopamine.
3. **There is an association between bulimia nervosa and the neurotransmitters serotonin and norepinephrine. Because citalopram is an SSRI, it would be useful in the treatment of bulimia nervosa and responsible for a positive client response.**
4. There is an association between bulimia nervosa and a malfunction of the hypothalamus, not thalamus.

TEST-TAKING HINT: To answer this question correctly, the test taker must recognize citalopram as an SSRI.

28. 1. Fluphenazine is an antipsychotic medication prescribed for thought disorders and is rarely used in the treatment of anorexia nervosa.
2. Clozapine is an antipsychotic medication prescribed for thought disorders and is rarely used in the treatment of anorexia nervosa.
3. **Fluoxetine is an antidepressant medication. Feelings of depression and anxiety often accompany anorexia nervosa, making antianxiety and antidepressant medications the treatments of choice for the disorder.**
4. Methylphenidate is a stimulant medication prescribed for attention deficit-hyperactivity disorder, not anorexia nervosa.

TEST-TAKING HINT: The test taker must note keywords in the question, such as *most often*, to answer this question correctly. Although antipsychotic medications can, on rare occasions, be used to treat selected clients diagnosed with anorexia nervosa, the most frequently used medications are antidepressants and antianxiety agents.

29. The labeling sequence is 1, 3, 2, 4.
1. **The thalamus is labeled "1" on the diagram of the brain. This structure of the brain integrates all sensory input except smell. The thalamus also is involved in emotions and mood.**
2. **The amygdala is labeled "3" on the diagram of the brain. This structure of the brain, located in the anterior portion of the temporal lobe, plays an important role in arousal.**

3. The hypothalamus is labeled "2" on the diagram of the brain. This structure of the brain regulates the anterior and posterior lobes of the pituitary gland, controls the auditory nervous system, and regulates appetite and temperature.
4. The hippocampus is labeled "4" on the diagram of the brain. This structure of the brain is part of the limbic system, which is associated with fear and anxiety, anger and aggression, love, joy, hope, sexuality, and social behavior.

TEST-TAKING HINT: To answer this question correctly, the test taker must be familiar with the location of various structures of the brain.

30. The nurse should adjust the rate of flow to **38 gtts/min.**
Use the following formula:

$$\frac{150 \text{ mL/hr}}{60 \text{ min}} \times 15 \text{ (gtt/mL)}$$

$$= 37.5 \text{ or } 38 \text{ gtt per min}$$

TEST-TAKING HINT: When calculating drip rates, the test taker must remember that there is no such thing as a half-drop, and drip rates must be rounded to the nearest whole number. Newer electronic pumps may accept less than whole-number calculations.

31. Clients diagnosed with eating disorders may be prescribed various medications to control symptoms. Nurses need to be aware of newly developed medications in order to provide clients with accurate information.
    1. Brupropion-naltrexone is believed to work in two areas of the brain, the hunger center and the reward system. This medication could be prescribed for this client, and the nurse should provide appropriate medication information.
    2. Lorcaserin works by controlling appetite, specifically by activating brain receptors for serotonin, a neurotransmitter that triggers feelings of fullness and satisfaction. This medication could be prescribed for this client, and the nurse should provide appropriate medication information.
    3. Orlistat is a gastrointestinal lipase inhibitor for obesity management that acts by inhibiting the absorption of dietary fats. This medication would not be prescribed for this client.
    4. Phentermine-topiramate affects the neurotransmitter gamma-aminobutyric acid (GABA), suppressing appetite and enhancing fullness. This medication could be prescribed for this client, and the nurse should provide appropriate medication information.
    5. Liraglutide is an injectable medication that mirrors a hormone the body produces naturally that regulates appetite, known as glucagon-like peptide-1 (GLP-1). By activating areas of the brain that regulate appetite, liraglutide reduces hunger. It is prescribed for clients with excess weight (BMI >27) who also have weight-related medical problems. This medication could be prescribed for this client, if they meet the other requirements listed above. If liraglutide is prescribed, the nurse should provide appropriate medication information.

TEST-TAKING HINT: In order to answer this question correctly, the test taker must first understand the mechanism of action for each medication listed. The nurse would only provide information regarding medications appropriate to address food cravings. Answer 3, orlistat, addresses weight loss by inhibiting the absorption of dietary fats, not decreasing cravings for food.

Children and Adolescents

16

KEYWORDS

The following words include English vocabulary, nursing/medical terminology, concepts, principles, or information relevant to content specifically addressed in this chapter or associated with topics presented in it. English dictionaries, your nursing textbooks, and medical dictionaries such as *Taber's Cyclopedic Medical Dictionary* are resources that can be used to expand your knowledge and understanding of these words and related information.

Attention deficit-hyperactivity disorder (ADHD)

Autism spectrum disorder

Conduct disorder

Intermittent explosive disorder

Mild intellectual developmental disorder (mild IDD)

Moderate intellectual developmental disorder (moderate IDD)

Oppositional defiant disorder (ODD)

Profound intellectual developmental disorder (profound IDD)

Separation anxiety disorder

Severe intellectual developmental disorder (severe IDD)

Tourette's disorder

QUESTIONS

Theory

1. Which is a description of the etiology of autism spectrum disorder from a genetic perspective?
   1. Parents who have one child diagnosed with autism spectrum disorder are at higher risk for having other children with the disorder.
   2. Amygdala abnormality in the anterior portion of the temporal lobe is associated with the diagnosis of autism spectrum disorder.
   3. Decreased levels of serotonin have been found in individuals diagnosed with autism spectrum disorder.
   4. Congenital rubella has been implicated in the predisposition leading to autism spectrum disorder.

2. Which is a predisposing factor in the diagnosis of autism spectrum disorder?
   1. Having a sibling diagnosed with intellectual developmental disorder (IDD).
   2. Congenital rubella.
   3. Dysfunctional family systems.
   4. Inadequate ego development.

3. Which factors does Mahler attribute to the etiology of attention deficit-hyperactivity disorder (ADHD)?
   1. Genetic factors.
   2. Psychodynamic factors.
   3. Neurochemical factors.
   4. Family dynamic factors.

4. The theory of family dynamics has been implicated as contributing to the etiology of conduct disorders. Which of the following are factors related to this theory? **Select all that apply.**
   1. Frequent shifting of parental figures.
   2. Birth temperament.
   3. Father absenteeism.
   4. Large family size.
   5. Fixation in the separation individuation phase of development.

5. Which is associated with the etiology of Tourette's disorder from a biochemical perspective?
   1. An inheritable component, as suggested by monozygotic and dizygotic twin studies.
   2. Abnormal levels of several neurotransmitters.
   3. Prenatal complications, including low birth weight.
   4. Enlargement of the caudate nucleus of the brain.

Nursing Process—Assessment

6. Which developmental characteristic would be expected of an individual with an IQ level of 40?
   1. Independent living with assistance during times of stress.
   2. Academic skill to the sixth-grade level.
   3. Little, if any, speech development.
   4. Academic skill to the second-grade level.

7. The nurse on an inpatient pediatric psychiatric unit is admitting a client diagnosed with autism spectrum disorder. Which would the nurse expect to assess?
   1. A strong connection with siblings.
   2. An active imagination.
   3. Abnormalities in physical appearance.
   4. Absence of language.

8. Which is a diagnostic criterion for the diagnosis of ADHD?
   1. Inattention.
   2. Recurrent and persistent thoughts.
   3. Physical aggression.
   4. Anxiety and panic attacks.

9. When admitting a child diagnosed with a conduct disorder, which symptom would the nurse expect to assess?
   1. Excessive distress about separation from home and family.
   2. Repeated complaints of physical symptoms such as headaches and stomachaches.
   3. History of cruelty toward people and animals.
   4. Confabulation when confronted with wrongdoing.

10. The nursing instructor is preparing to teach nursing students about oppositional defiant disorder (ODD). Which fact should be included in the lesson plan?
    1. Prevalence of ODD is higher in females than in males.
    2. The diagnosis of ODD occurs before the age of 3.
    3. The diagnosis of ODD occurs no later than early adolescence.
    4. The diagnosis of ODD is not a developmental antecedent to conduct disorder.

11. Which of the following signs and symptoms supports a diagnosis of depression in an adolescent? **Select all that apply.**
    1. Poor self-esteem.
    2. Insomnia and anorexia.
    3. Sexually acting out and inappropriate anger.
    4. Increased serotonin levels.
    5. Exaggerated psychosomatic complaints.

Nursing Process—Diagnosis

12. A child diagnosed with mild to moderate IDD is admitted to the hospital for an appendectomy. The nurse observes that the child is having difficulty making desires known. Which nursing diagnosis reflects this client's problem?
    1. Ineffective coping R/T developmental delay.
    2. Anxiety R/T hospitalization and absence of familiar surroundings.
    3. Impaired verbal communication R/T developmental alteration.
    4. Impaired adjustment R/T recent admission to hospital.

13. A child diagnosed with severe IDD displays failure to thrive related to neglect and abuse. Which nursing diagnosis would best reflect this situation?
    1. Altered role performance R/T failure to complete kindergarten.
    2. Risk for injury: self-directed R/T poor self-esteem.
    3. Altered growth and development R/T inadequate environmental stimulation.
    4. Anxiety R/T ineffective coping skills.

14. A child diagnosed with autism spectrum disorder makes no eye contact; is unresponsive to staff members; and continuously twists, spins, and head bangs. Which nursing diagnosis would take priority?
    1. Personal identity disorder R/T poor ego differentiation.
    2. Impaired verbal communication R/T withdrawal into self.
    3. Risk for injury R/T head banging.
    4. Impaired social interaction R/T delay in accomplishing developmental tasks.

15. A foster child diagnosed with ODD is spiteful, vindictive, and argumentative and has a history of aggression toward others. Which nursing diagnosis would take priority?
    1. Impaired social interaction R/T refusal to adhere to conventional social behavior.
    2. Defensive coping R/T unsatisfactory child-parent relationship.
    3. Risk for violence: directed at others R/T poor impulse control.
    4. Nonadherence R/T a negativistic attitude.

16. A child admitted to an inpatient psychiatric unit is diagnosed with separation anxiety disorder. This child is continually refusing to go to bed at the designated time. Which nursing diagnosis best documents this child's problem?
    1. Nonadherence with rules R/T low self-esteem.
    2. Ineffective coping R/T hospitalization and absence of major attachment figure.
    3. Powerlessness R/T confusion and disorientation.
    4. Risk for injury R/T sleep deprivation.

Nursing Process—Planning

17. Which short-term correctly written outcome would take priority for a client who is diagnosed with moderate IDD and who resorts to self-mutilation during times of peer and staff conflict?
    1. The client will form peer relationships by end of the shift.
    2. The client will demonstrate adaptive coping skills in response to conflicts.
    3. The client will take direction without becoming defensive by discharge.
    4. The client will experience no physical harm during this shift.

18. A client diagnosed with moderate IDD suddenly refuses to participate in supervised hygiene care. Which short-term outcome would be appropriate for this individual?
    1. The client will comply with supervised hygiene by day 3.
    2. The client will be able to complete hygiene without supervision by day 3.
    3. The client will be able to maintain anxiety at a manageable level by day 2.
    4. The client will accept assistance with hygiene by day 2.

19. Which short-term outcome would be considered a priority for a hospitalized child diagnosed with autism spectrum disorder who bites self when care is attempted?
    1. The child will initiate social interactions with one caregiver by discharge.
    2. The child will demonstrate trust in one caregiver by day 3.
    3. The child will not inflict harm on self during the next 24-hour period.
    4. The child will establish a means of communicating needs by discharge.

20. A child diagnosed with a conduct disorder is disruptive and nonadherent with rules in the milieu. Which correctly written outcome, related to this client's problem, should the nurse expect the client to achieve?
    1. The child will maintain anxiety at a reasonable level by day 2.
    2. The child will interact with others in a socially appropriate manner by day 2.
    3. The child will accept direction without becoming defensive by discharge.
    4. The child will contract not to harm self during this shift.

Nursing Process—Implementation

21. Which charting entry would document an appropriate nursing intervention for a client diagnosed with profound IDD?
    1. "Rewarded client with lollipop after independent completion of self-care."
    2. "Encouraged client to tie own shoelaces."
    3. "Kept client in line of sight continuously during shift."
    4. "Taught the client to sing the alphabet 'ABC' song."

22. A child diagnosed with autism spectrum disorder has a nursing diagnosis of impaired social interaction R/T withdrawal into self. Which of the following nursing interventions would be most appropriate to address this problem? **Select all that apply.**
    1. Prevent physical aggression by recognizing signs of agitation.
    2. Allow the client to behave spontaneously and shelter the client from peers.
    3. Remain with the client during initial interaction with others on the unit.
    4. Establish a procedure for behavior modification with rewards to the client for appropriate behaviors.
    5. Explain to other clients the meaning behind some of the client's nonverbal gestures and signals.

23. A child diagnosed with autism spectrum disorder withdraws into self and, when spoken to, makes inappropriate nonverbal expressions. The nursing diagnosis of impaired verbal communication is documented. Which intervention would address this problem?
    1. Assist the child in recognizing separateness during self-care activities.
    2. Use a face-to-face and eye-to-eye approach when communicating.
    3. Provide the child with a familiar toy or blanket to increase feelings of security.
    4. Offer self to the child during times of increasing anxiety.

24. A child diagnosed with ODD begins yelling at staff members when asked to leave group therapy because of inappropriate language. Which nursing intervention would be appropriate?
    1. Administer prn medication to decrease acting-out behaviors.
    2. Accompany the child to a quiet area to decrease external stimuli.
    3. Institute seclusion following agency protocol.
    4. Allow the child to stay in group therapy to monitor the situation further.

25. A child newly admitted to an inpatient psychiatric unit with a diagnosis of major depressive disorder has a nursing diagnosis of high risk for suicide R/T depressed mood. Which nursing intervention would be most appropriate at this time?
    1. Encourage the child to participate in group therapy activities daily.
    2. Engage in one-to-one interactions to assist in building a trusting relationship.
    3. Monitor the child continuously while no longer than an arm's length away.
    4. Maintain open lines of communication for expression of feelings.

Nursing Process—Evaluation

26. A client diagnosed with ODD has an outcome of learning new coping skills through behavior modification. Which client statement or question indicates that behavior modification has occurred?
    1. "I didn't hit Johnny. Can I have my Tootsie Roll?"
    2. "I want to wear a helmet like Jane wears."
    3. "Can I watch television after supper?"
    4. "I want a puppy right now."

27. A client diagnosed with Tourette's disorder has a nursing diagnosis of social isolation. Which charting entry documents a successful outcome related to this client's problem?
    1. "Compliant with instructions to use bathroom before bedtime."
    2. "Made potholder at activity therapy session."
    3. "Able to distinguish right hand from left hand."
    4. "Able to focus on TV cartoons for 30 minutes."

28. A child diagnosed with autism spectrum disorder has a nursing diagnosis of impaired social interaction. The child is currently making eye contact and allowing physical touch. Which statement addresses the evaluation of this child's behavior?
    1. The nurse is unable to evaluate this child's ability to interact socially based on the observed behaviors.
    2. The child is experiencing improved social interaction as evidenced by making eye contact and allowing physical touch.
    3. The nurse is unable to evaluate this child's ability to interact socially because the child has not experienced these behaviors for an extended period.
    4. The child making eye contact and allowing physical touch are indications of improved personal identity, not improved social interaction.

Psychopharmacology

29. A 10-year-old client prescribed dextroamphetamine has a nursing diagnosis of imbalanced nutrition: less than body requirements R/T a side effect of anorexia. Which of the following nursing interventions addresses this client's problem? **Select all that apply.**
    1. Monitor output and sleep patterns daily.
    2. Administer medications with food to prevent nausea.
    3. Schedule medication administration after meals.
    4. Increase fiber and fluid intake to prevent constipation.
    5. Encourage frequent high-calorie snacks.

30. A 7-year-old client has been prescribed atomoxetine. An appropriate nursing diagnosis is imbalanced nutrition: less than body requirements R/T a side effect of anorexia. Which short-term correctly written outcome is appropriate?
    1. The client will eat meals in the dining area while socializing.
    2. The client will maintain expected parameters of growth over the next 6 months.
    3. The client will verbalize the importance of eating 100% of all meals.
    4. The client will eat 80% of all three meals throughout the hospital stay.

31. A client diagnosed with ADHD and juvenile diabetes is prescribed methylphenidate. Which nursing intervention related to both diagnoses takes priority?
    1. Teach the client and family that methylphenidate should be taken in the morning because it can affect sleep.
    2. Teach the client and family to report restlessness, insomnia, and dry mouth.
    3. Teach the client and family to monitor fasting blood sugar levels daily at various times during treatment.
    4. Teach the client and family that methylphenidate should be taken exactly as prescribed.

32. Which of the following stimulant medications are prescribed in the treatment of ADHD? **Select all that apply.**
   1. Methylphenidate.
   2. Guanfacine.
   3. Lisdexamfetamine.
   4. Amphetamine/dextroamphetamine.
   5. Clonidine.

33. A 14-year-old client, diagnosed with ADHD, reports that by the end of the school day, the prescribed short-acting stimulant is less effective. Which of the following medications would the nurse expect the physician to order? **Select all that apply.**
   1. Evekeo (d- & l-amphetamine salt).
   2. Mydayis (mixed amphetamine based).
   3. Aptensio (methylphenidate).
   4. Zenzedi (d-amphetamine sulfate).
   5. ProCentra (d-amphetamine sulfate).

34. A client is diagnosed with intermittent explosive disorder. The clinic nurse should anticipate potentially teaching about which of the following medications? **Select all that apply.**
   1. Sertraline.
   2. Paliperidone.
   3. Buspirone.
   4. Phenelzine.
   5. Valproate sodium.

35. A client, diagnosed with attention deficit-hyperactivity disorder (ADHD), is complaining that the medication prescribed is not helping first thing in the morning. The practitioner prescribes methylphenidate HCL extended-release capsules (Jornay). Which client statement indicates that teaching is understood?
   1. "I have to take Jornay with my breakfast in order for the medication to be absorbed."
   2. "I must take Jornay at least 2 hours before I have to start to focus during school."
   3. "Jornay will work the best if I take it with my morning coffee."
   4. "I have to take Jornay at bedtime in order for it to be effective in the morning."

36. A client, diagnosed with attention-deficit hyperactivity disorder (ADHD), is told that they will be prescribed a nonstimulant medication to treat issues with focus. Which of the following medications could be prescribed? **Select all that apply.**
   1. Amphetamine (Dyanavel XR).
   2. Viloxazine hydrochloride.
   3. Dexmethylphenidate (Azstarys).
   4. Atomoxetine.
   5. Quanfacine XR.

The correct answer number and rationale for why it is the correct answer are given in **boldface blue type**. Rationales for why the other answer options are incorrect are given as well, but they are not in boldface type.

Theory

1. 1. **Research has revealed strong evidence that genetic factors may play a significant role in the etiology of autism spectrum disorder. Studies show that parents who have one child with this disorder are at an increased risk for having more than one child with the disorder. Also, monozygotic and dizygotic twin studies have provided evidence of genetic involvement.**
   2. Abnormalities associated with autism spectrum disorders have been found in the area of the amygdala; however, this finding supports a biological, not genetic, etiology.
   3. Elevated, not decreased, levels of serotonin have been found in individuals diagnosed with autism spectrum disorder. Alteration in serotonin levels would support a biological, not genetic, etiology.
   4. Congenital rubella may be implicated in the predisposition to autism spectrum disorder; however, this identification supports a biological, not genetic, etiology.

   TEST-TAKING HINT: To select the correct answer, the test taker must note the keywords *genetic perspective*. Answers 2 and 4 are correct about the etiology of autism spectrum disorder; however, only answer 1 is from a genetic perspective.

2. 1. Studies have shown that parents who have one child diagnosed with autism spectrum disorder, not intellectual developmental disorder (IDD), in general are at increased risk for having more than one child diagnosed with autism spectrum disorder.
   2. **Children diagnosed with congenital rubella, postnatal neurological infections, phenylketonuria, or fragile X syndrome are predisposed to being diagnosed with autism spectrum disorder.**
   3. Most clinicians now believe that ineffective parenting does not predispose a child to being diagnosed with autism spectrum disorder.

   4. No known psychological factors in the ego development of a child predispose the child to autism spectrum disorder.

   TEST-TAKING HINT: The test taker must understand that as a result of current research findings, some older psychosocial theories related to the development of autism spectrum disorder have lost credibility.

3. 1. Research shows that genetic factors are associated with the etiology of attention deficit-hyperactivity disorder (ADHD); however, these factors are not addressed in Mahler's theory.
   2. **Mahler's theory suggests that a child with ADHD has psychodynamic problems. Mahler describes these children as fixed in the symbiotic phase of development. They have not differentiated self from mother. Ego development is retarded, and impulsive behavior, dictated by the id, is manifested.**
   3. Research shows that neurochemical factors are associated with the etiology of ADHD. A deficit of the neurotransmitters dopamine and norepinephrine has been suggested as a causative factor. However, these factors are not addressed in Mahler's theory.
   4. Bowen, not Mahler, proposes that when a dysfunctional spousal relationship exists, the focus of the disturbance is displaced onto the child, whose behavior, in time, begins to reflect the pattern of the dysfunctional system. Family dynamics are a factor in the diagnosis of ADHD. However, these factors are not addressed in Mahler's theory.

   TEST-TAKING HINT: To select the correct answer, the test taker must be able to distinguish the concepts of Mahler's theory from the concepts of other theories that support the etiology of ADHD.

4. 1. **According to the theory of family dynamics, frequent shifting of parental figures has been implicated as a contributing factor in the predisposition to conduct disorder. An example of frequent shifting of parental figures may include, but is not limited to, divorce, death, and inconsistent foster care.**
   2. According to a physiological perspective, the term *temperament* refers to personality traits that become evident very early in life and may be present at birth. Evidence suggests

an association between difficult temperament in childhood and behavioral problems such as conduct disorder later in life. The concept of birth temperament is not a component of family dynamic theory.

3. **According to the theory of family dynamics, the absence of a father or the presence of a father diagnosed with alcohol use disorder has been implicated as a contributing factor to the diagnosis of conduct disorder.**

4. **According to the theory of family dynamics, large family size has been implicated as a contributing factor in the predisposition to conduct disorder. The quality of family relationships needs to be assessed for evidence of overcrowding, poverty, neglect, and abuse to determine this risk factor.**

5. Fixation in the separation individuation phase of development addresses conduct disorder from a psychodynamic, not family dynamic, perspective.

TEST-TAKING HINT: To select the correct answer, the test taker must be familiar with the theory of family dynamics and how this theory relates to the etiology of conduct disorder.

5. 1. Monozygotic and dizygotic twin studies suggest that there is an inheritable component to the diagnosis of Tourette's disorder; however, this is from a genetic, not biochemical, etiological perspective.

2. **Abnormalities in levels of dopamine, serotonin, dynorphin, gamma-aminobutyric acid, acetylcholine, and norepinephrine have been associated with Tourette's disorder. This etiology is from a biochemical perspective.**

3. Prenatal complications, which include low birth weight, have been noted to be an etiological implication in the diagnosis of Tourette's disorder; however, these are environmental, not biochemical, factors that contribute to the etiology of the disorder.

4. Enlargement of the caudate nucleus of the brain and decreased cerebral blood flow in the left lenticular nucleus have been found in individuals diagnosed with Tourette's disorder. However, these are structural, not biochemical, factors that contribute to the etiology of the disorder.

TEST-TAKING HINT: To select the correct answer, the test taker must note keywords in the question, such as *biochemical perspective*. All answers are correct related to the etiology of Tourette's disorder, but only answer 2 is from a biochemical perspective.

Nursing Process—Assessment

6. 1. Independent living with assistance during times of stress would be a developmental characteristic expected of an individual diagnosed with mild intellectual developmental disorder (IDD) (IQ level 50 to 70), not of an individual diagnosed with moderate IDD.

2. Academic skill to the sixth-grade level would be a developmental characteristic expected of an individual diagnosed with mild IDD (IQ level 50 to 70), not of an individual diagnosed with moderate IDD.

3. Little, if any, speech development would be a developmental characteristic expected of an individual diagnosed with profound IDD (IQ level <20), not of an individual diagnosed with moderate IDD.

4. **An IQ level of 40 is within the range of moderate IDD (IQ level 35 to 49). Academic skill to the second-grade level would be a developmental characteristic expected of an individual in this IQ range.**

TEST-TAKING HINT: To answer this question correctly, the test taker needs to know the developmental characteristics of the levels of IDD by degree of severity. These are categorized by IQ range.

7. 1. The nurse would expect to note a disconnection, not a connection, with siblings when assessing a child diagnosed with an autism spectrum disorder. Autism spectrum disorder usually is first noticed by the parent when the infant fails to be interested in, or socially responsive to, others.

2. The nurse would expect to note a lack of spontaneous make-believe and imaginative play with no active imagination ability when assessing a child diagnosed with an autism spectrum disorder. These children have a rigid adherence to routines and rituals, and minor changes can produce catastrophic reactions.

3. The nurse would assess a normal, not abnormal, physical appearance in a child diagnosed with autism spectrum disorder. These children have a normal appearance; however, on closer observation, no eye contact or facial expression is noted.

4. **One of the first characteristics that the nurse would note is the client's abnormal language patterning or total absence of language. Children diagnosed with autism spectrum disorder display an uneven development of intellectual skills.**

Impairments are noted in verbal and non-verbal communication. These children cannot use or understand abstract language, and they may make unintelligible sounds or say the same word repeatedly.

TEST-TAKING HINT: To select the correct answer choice, the test taker must recognize the characteristic impairments associated with the diagnosis of autism spectrum disorder.

8. The diagnostic criteria for ADHD are divided into three categories: inattention, hyperactivity, and impulsivity. The list of symptoms under each category is extensive. Six (or more) symptoms of inattention or hyperactivity-impulsivity, or both, must persist for at least 6 months to a degree that is maladaptive and inconsistent with developmental level.

   1. **Essential diagnostic criteria for ADHD includes inattention, along with hyperactivity and impulsivity. Children with this disorder are highly distractible and have extremely limited attention spans.**
   2. Recurrent and persistent thoughts are a diagnostic criterion for obsessive-compulsive disorder, not ADHD. A child diagnosed with ADHD would have difficulty focusing on a thought for any length of time.
   3. The classic characteristic of conduct disorder, not ADHD, is the use of physical aggression in the violation of the rights of others.
   4. Anxiety and panic attacks are not diagnostic criteria for a diagnosis of ADHD. Although children with this disorder are restless and fidgety and often act as if "driven by a motor," these behaviors are associated with their boundless energy, not anxiety or panic.

TEST-TAKING HINT: To select the correct answer, the test taker must understand the diagnostic criteria for ADHD.

9. 1. Children diagnosed with conduct disorder have poor peer and family relationships and little concern for others. They lack feelings of guilt and remorse and would not experience, or express distress related to separation from home and family.
   2. Children diagnosed with separation anxiety, not conduct disorder, have repeated complaints of physical symptoms, such as headaches and stomachaches, related to fear of separation. A child diagnosed with a conduct disorder is a bully, projects a tough image, and believes their aggressiveness is justified. Frequent somatic complaints would be uncharacteristic of a child diagnosed with conduct disorder.

3. A history of physical cruelty toward people and animals is commonly associated with conduct disorder. These children may bury animals alive and set fires intending to cause harm and damage.
4. Confabulation is defined as a creative way to fill in gaps in the memory with detailed accounts of fictitious events believed true by the narrator. A child diagnosed with conduct disorder has no memory problem and would most likely deny or lie, not confabulate, when confronted with wrongdoing.

TEST-TAKING HINT: To select the correct answer, the test taker must be familiar with the diagnostic criteria of conduct disorder.

10. 1. The prevalence of oppositional defiant disorder (ODD) is higher in males, not females.
    2. The symptoms of ODD typically are evident by 8, not 3, years of age.
    3. **The symptoms of ODD usually appear no later than early adolescence. A child diagnosed with ODD presents with a pattern of negativity, disobedience, and hostile behavior toward authority figures. This pattern of behavior occurs more frequently than is typically observed in individuals of comparable age and developmental level.**
    4. In a significant proportion of cases, ODD is a developmental antecedent to conduct disorder.

TEST-TAKING HINT: To select the correct answer, the test taker must be familiar with the various facts related to the diagnosis of ODD.

11. 1. A symptom of depression in adolescence is poor self-esteem. Puberty and maturity are gradual processes and vary among individuals. Adolescents may experience a lack of self-esteem when their expectations of maturity are not met or when they compare themselves unfavorably with peers.
    2. **Eating and sleeping disturbances are common signs and symptoms of depression in adolescents.**
    3. **Acting out sexually and expressing inappropriate anger are symptoms of depression in adolescence. The fluctuating hormone levels that accompany puberty contribute to these behaviors. A manifestation of behavioral change that lasts for several weeks is the best indicator of a mood disorder in an adolescent.**
    4. A decrease, not an increase, in serotonin levels occurs when an adolescent is experiencing depression.

5. Exaggerated psychosomatic complaints are symptoms of depression in adolescence. Between the ages of 11 and 16, normal rapid changes to the body occur, and psychosomatic complaints are common. These complaints must be differentiated from the exaggerated psychosomatic complaints that occur in adolescent depression.

TEST-TAKING HINT: To answer this question correctly, the test taker needs to differentiate between the symptoms of depression and the normal physical and psychological changes that occur during childhood and adolescence.

Nursing Process—Diagnosis

12. 1. Ineffective coping is described as the inability to form a valid appraisal of the stressors, inadequate choices of practiced responses, or inability to use available resources. This child's inability to communicate effectively is not related to ineffective coping.
2. A child diagnosed with mild to moderate IDD may experience anxiety because of hospitalization and the absence of familiar surroundings; however, the child in this question is not displaying symptoms of anxiety. This child's problem is an inability to communicate desires.
3. **Impaired verbal communication R/T developmental alteration is the appropriate nursing diagnosis for a child diagnosed with mild to moderate IDD who is having difficulties making needs and desires understood to staff members. Clients diagnosed with mild to moderate IDD often have deficits in communication.**
4. Impaired adjustment is defined as the inability to modify lifestyle or behavior in a manner consistent with a change in health status. Hospitalization of a child with mild to moderate IDD may precipitate impaired adjustment, but the client problem described in the question indicates impaired communication.

TEST-TAKING HINT: The test taker needs to understand that the selection of an appropriate nursing diagnosis for clients diagnosed with IDD depends largely on client behaviors, the extent of the client's capabilities, and the severity of the condition. The test taker must look at the client behaviors described in the

question to determine the appropriate nursing diagnosis. In this question, the keywords *difficulty making desires known* suggests a lack of verbal communication.

13. Altered growth and development is defined as the state in which an individual demonstrates deviations in norms from their age-group. This may result from IDD, neglect and abuse, or both.
1. A child with severe IDD (IQ level 20 to 34) cannot benefit from academic or vocational training, making this an inappropriate nursing diagnosis for this child.
2. Because of abuse and neglect, this child may aggressively act out to deal with frustration when needs are not met. However, there is nothing in the question that indicates this child is experiencing self-directed aggression.
3. **The nursing diagnosis of altered growth and development related to inadequate environmental stimulation would best address this child's problem of failure to thrive. Failure to thrive frequently results from neglect and abuse.**
4. A child diagnosed with severe IDD would not be expected to have any insight or coping skills. Lack of insight would prevent the child from experiencing anxiety and the need to cope.

TEST-TAKING HINT: To answer this question correctly, the test taker needs to match the problem presented in the question with the nursing diagnosis that reflects the client's problem. Other nursing diagnoses may apply to clients diagnosed with severe IDD, but only answer 3 addresses failure to thrive.

14. 1. Children diagnosed with autism spectrum disorder have difficulty distinguishing between self and others. Although the nursing diagnosis of personal identity disorder has merit for the future, potential injury from head banging would need to be addressed first.
2. Children diagnosed with autism spectrum disorder have a delayed or absent ability to receive, process, transmit, or use a system of symbols to communicate. Although the nursing diagnosis of impaired verbal communication has merit for the future, potential injury from head banging would need to be addressed first.
3. **Children diagnosed with autism spectrum disorder frequently head bang because of neurological alterations,**

increased anxiety, or catastrophic reactions to changes in the environment. Because the nurse is responsible for ensuring client safety, the nursing diagnosis of risk for injury takes priority.

4. Children diagnosed with autism spectrum disorder do not form interpersonal relationships with others and do not respond to or show interest in people. Although the nursing diagnosis of impaired social interaction has merit for the future, potential injury from head banging would need to be addressed first.

TEST-TAKING HINT: Although all nursing diagnoses presented may apply to clients diagnosed with autism spectrum disorder, the test taker needs to understand that client safety is always the nurse's primary responsibility. The keywords *head bangs* in the question should alert the test taker to choose the nursing diagnosis of risk for injury as the priority client problem.

15. 1. Impaired social interaction is defined as the state in which an individual participates in an insufficient or excessive quantity or ineffective quality of social exchange. A child diagnosed with oppositional defiant disorder (ODD) generally displays a negative temperament, including an underlying hostility. Impaired social interaction would be a valid nursing diagnosis for this client; however, because of this child's history of aggressive behavior, risk for violence: directed at others, not impaired social interaction, would be the priority nursing diagnosis.

2. Defensive coping is defined as the state in which an individual repeatedly projects a falsely positive self-evaluation based on a self-protective pattern that defends against underlying perceived threats to positive self-regard. Defensive coping would be a valid nursing diagnosis for this client; however, because of this child's history of aggressive behavior, risk for violence: directed at others, not defensive coping, would take priority.

3. Risk for violence: directed at others is defined as behaviors in which an individual demonstrates that they can be physically, emotionally, or sexually harmful to others. Children diagnosed with ODD have a pattern of negativistic, spiteful, and vindictive behaviors. The foster child described in the question also has a history of aggressive behaviors. Because maintaining safety

is a critical responsibility of the nurse, risk for violence: directed at others would be the priority nursing diagnosis.

4. Nonadherence is defined as the extent to which a person's behavior fails to coincide with a health-promoting or therapeutic plan agreed on by the person or family members (or both) and a health-care professional. A child diagnosed with ODD generally displays a negative temperament, denies problems, and exhibits underlying hostility. These characteristics may lead to nonadherence with treatment, but because maintaining safety is a critical responsibility of the nurse, risk for violence: directed at others would be the priority nursing diagnosis.

TEST-TAKING HINT: To answer this question correctly, the test taker needs to correlate the data collected during the nursing assessment with the appropriate nursing diagnosis in order of priority. Maintaining safety always is prioritized.

16. 1. Nonadherence is defined as the extent to which a person's behavior fails to coincide with a health-promoting or therapeutic plan agreed on by the person and family members (or both) and a health-care professional. A child diagnosed with separation anxiety may be reluctant or may refuse to obey rules regarding bedtime; however, this nonadherence would be associated with separation from a major attachment figure, not from low self-esteem.

2. **Ineffective coping is defined as the inability to form a valid appraisal of the stressors, ineffective choices of practiced responses, or inability to use available resources. A child diagnosed with separation anxiety often refuses to go to school or bed because of fears of separation from home or from individuals to whom the child is attached. The child in the question is refusing to go to bed as a way to cope with fear and anxiety. The nursing diagnosis of ineffective coping would be an appropriate documentation of this client's problem.**

3. Powerlessness is defined as the perception that one's own action would not significantly affect an outcome—a perceived lack of control over a current situation or immediate happening. The child in the question may be experiencing powerlessness and is thereby refusing to comply with bedtime rules in an effort to gain control.

However, this nursing diagnosis documents the cause of powerlessness as confusion and disorientation. No symptoms are presented in the question that indicate that the client is confused or disoriented.

4. Risk for injury is defined as the state in which the individual is at risk of injury as a result of environmental conditions interacting with the individual's adaptive and defensive resources. In the future, this could be a valid nursing diagnosis if refusal to sleep leads to sleep deprivation, thereby placing the client at risk for injury. However, this does not address the client's current problem. This client is coping ineffectively by refusing to adhere to bedtime rules because of separation anxiety.

TEST-TAKING HINT: The test taker must read this question carefully to recognize that the question is asking for documentation of the client problem presented in the question rather than asking which client problem takes priority.

Nursing Process—Planning

17. 1. Because this client is diagnosed with moderate intellectual developmental disorder (IDD), the client would have difficulty adhering to social conventions, which may interfere with the establishment of peer relationships. Expecting the client to form peer relationships by the end of the shift presents an unrealistic time frame. Also, this diagnosis does not address the self-mutilation behavior described in the question.

2. Even though self-mutilation is a maladaptive way to cope, clients diagnosed with moderate IDD (IQ level 35 to 49) would not be expected to make adaptive coping choices, so this outcome is unrealistic. Also, this short-term outcome does not have a time frame and is not measurable.

3. Because this client is diagnosed with moderate IDD, the client would have limited speech and communication capabilities, so taking directions would be an unrealistic short-term outcome.

4. **A child diagnosed with moderate IDD who resorts to self-mutilation during times of peer and staff conflict must be protected from self-harm. A realistic, measurable outcome would be that the client would experience no physical harm during this shift.**

TEST-TAKING HINT: To answer this question correctly, the test taker must be able to identify and select appropriate outcomes that are based on client behaviors described. Self-mutilation behaviors should lead the test taker to focus on safety-related outcomes.

18. 1. **With appropriately implemented interventions that direct the client back to previously supervised hygiene performance, the short-term outcome of client adherence and participation by day 2 can be a reasonable expectation. To achieve this outcome, interventions might include exploring reasons for nonadherence; maintaining consistency of staff members; or providing the client with familiar objects, such as an old versus a new toothbrush.**

2. This outcome is inappropriate because completing hygiene without supervision is an unrealistic expectation for a client diagnosed with moderate intellectual developmental disorder (IDD).

3. This outcome is inappropriate because nothing is presented in the question that indicates that the client is experiencing anxiety.

4. This outcome is inappropriate because clients diagnosed with moderate IDD can perform their own hygiene activities independently. Supervision, not assistance, would be required.

TEST-TAKING HINT: To answer this question correctly, the test taker needs to know the reasonable expectations of clients diagnosed with IDD. The level of severity of IDD should determine realistic outcomes for these clients.

19. 1. It would be unrealistic to expect a child diagnosed with autism spectrum disorder to initiate social interactions. This outcome also does not address the priority safety problem of self-mutilation.

2. Because of impaired social interaction, a child diagnosed with autism spectrum disorder would not trust another person easily. The child demonstrating trust in one caregiver would take considerable time, is unrealistic to expect by day 3, and does not address the priority safety problem of self-mutilation.

3. **A child diagnosed with autism spectrum disorder who bites self when care is attempted is at risk for injury R/T self-mutilation. Self-injurious behaviors, such as head banging and hand and arm biting, are used as a means to relieve tension. Considering that the nurse's**

primary responsibility is client safety, expecting the child to refrain from inflicting self-harm during a 24-hour period is the short-term outcome that should take priority.

4. A child diagnosed with autism spectrum disorder would experience difficulties in receiving, processing, transmitting, and using a system of symbols to communicate. Expecting a child to establish a means of communicating needs by discharge is a valid outcome; however, it does not address the priority problem of self-mutilation.

TEST-TAKING HINT: To select the correct answer, the test taker must remember that client safety is the nurse's primary responsibility. The client's self-mutilating behavior must be addressed as a priority.

20. All outcomes should be client centered, specific, realistic, positive, measurable, and contain a time frame.
   1. In the question, anxiety is not presented as the child's problem. Anxiety is not a characteristic of children diagnosed with conduct disorder because these children generally lack feelings of guilt or remorse that might, in other children, lead to anxiety. Also, a "reasonable" level of anxiety is neither specific nor measurable.
   2. It is unrealistic to expect this child to interact with others in a socially appropriate manner by day 2. This outcome would, it is hoped, be realized in a longer time frame.
   3. Accepting direction without becoming defensive by discharge is a specific, measurable, positive, realistic, client-centered outcome for this child. The disruption and nonadherence to rules on the milieu is this child's defensive coping mechanism. Helping the child to see the correlation between this defensiveness and the child's low self-esteem, anger, and frustration would assist in meeting this outcome.
   4. In the question, self-harm is not presented as the child's problem. Self-harm is not generally a characteristic of children diagnosed with conduct disorder. These children are far more likely to harm someone or something else and must be closely monitored.

TEST-TAKING HINT: To select the correct answer, the test taker must match the client behavior presented in the question with the appropriate outcome. In this question, recognizing that an outcome must be realistic should lead the test taker to eliminate answer 2.

Nursing Process—Implementation

21. Clients diagnosed with profound intellectual developmental disorder (IDD) have IQ levels that are <20 and have no capacity for independent functioning.
   1. A client diagnosed with profound IDD (IQ level <20) has no capacity for independent functioning and would require constant aid and supervision with hygiene care. Using a reward system as a nursing intervention would be appropriate for a child whose IQ level was 50 to 70, not for a child with an IQ level <20.
   2. A client diagnosed with profound IDD (IQ level <20) lacks fine and gross motor skills and would be unable to tie shoelaces. This nursing intervention would be appropriate for a child whose IQ level was 35 to 70, not for a child with an IQ level <20.
   3. A client diagnosed with profound IDD requires constant care and supervision. Keeping this client in line of sight continuously during the shift is an appropriate intervention for a child with an IQ level <20.
   4. A client diagnosed with profound IDD (IQ level <20) has little, if any, speech development and no capacity for singing. This nursing intervention would be appropriate for a child whose IQ level was 35 to 70, not for a child with an IQ level <20.

TEST-TAKING HINT: To select the correct answer choice, the test taker needs to understand the developmental characteristics of IDD by degree of severity and match client deficits with appropriate interventions.

22. 1. This intervention would be appropriate if the client were displaying physical aggression or agitation; however, this client is experiencing withdrawal into self.
   2. Allowing the client to behave spontaneously would hinder the ability of the client to interact with others in a socially appropriate manner and impair social interactions further.
   3. The nurse assumes the role of advocate and social mediator when the nurse remains with the client during initial interactions with others on the unit. The presence of a trusted individual provides a feeling of security and supports the client while appropriate socialization skills are learned.

4. Positive reinforcements can contribute to desired changes in socialization behaviors. These privileges are individually determined as staff members learn the client's likes and dislikes.
5. By explaining to peers the meaning behind some of the client's nonverbal gestures, signals, and communication attempts, the nurse facilitates social interactions. With this understanding, others in the client's social setting would be more receptive to social interactions.

TEST-TAKING HINT: To answer this question correctly, the test taker must look for interventions focused on correcting socialization problems. Other interventions may be appropriate for this client, but they do not address the client's shyness and withdrawal into self.

23. 1. Children diagnosed with autism spectrum disorder have difficulty distinguishing between self and others. Assisting the child in recognizing separateness is an intervention associated with the nursing diagnosis of disturbed personal identity. Although this nursing intervention is important for this child, it does not relate to the nursing diagnosis of impaired verbal communication.
2. A child diagnosed with autism spectrum disorder has impairment in communication affecting verbal and nonverbal skills. Nonverbal communication, such as facial expression, eye contact, or gestures, is often absent or socially inappropriate. Eye-to-eye and face-to-face contact expresses genuine interest in, and respect for, the individual and role-models correct nonverbal expressions.
3. When a child diagnosed with autism spectrum disorder becomes anxious and stressed, providing comfort and security is an appropriate and helpful nursing intervention. However, this intervention does not relate to the nursing diagnosis of impaired verbal communication.
4. When a child diagnosed with autism spectrum disorder demonstrates expressions of anxiety, such as head banging or hand biting, offering self to the child may decrease the need to self-mutilate and increase feelings of security. Although this nursing intervention is important for this individual, it does not relate to the nursing diagnosis of impaired verbal communication.

TEST-TAKING HINT: To select the correct answer, the test taker must be able to pair the nursing diagnosis presented in the question with the correct nursing intervention. There must always be a correlation between the stated problem and the nursing action that addresses the problem.

24. 1. Administering a prn medication, such as an anxiolytic, does not address this child's impaired social interaction, negative temperament, or underlying hostilities. Sedating medication is rarely, if ever, administered to a child for disturbances in behavior.
2. Accompanying the child to a quiet area to decrease external stimuli is the most beneficial action for this child. This action would aid in decreasing anger and hostility expressed by the child's outburst and inappropriate language. Later, the nurse may sit with the child and develop a system of rewards for adherence with therapy and consequences for nonadherence. This can be accomplished by starting with minimal expectations and increasing these expectations as the child begins to manifest evidence of control and adherence.
3. Instituting seclusion would be punitive and counterproductive. This action would serve only to increase this child's anger and hostility and may decrease adherence to further therapy. The nurse always should use interventions that are the least restrictive.
4. Allowing this child to remain in group therapy would not only disrupt the entire group but would also communicate that this behavior is acceptable.

TEST-TAKING HINT: To answer this question correctly, the test taker must understand that when managing a child diagnosed with oppositional defiant disorder, support, understanding, and firm guidelines are critical. These criteria are missing in answers 1, 3, and 4.

25. 1. This intervention would not be a priority at this time. A child diagnosed with major depressive disorder would be unable to concentrate on or participate in group therapy activities. Encouraging group therapy can be introduced when the child's mood is elevated and the risk for suicide has been addressed.
2. Although it is necessary to establish rapport and build a trusting relationship with this child, because a one-to-one interaction

does not address the safety of this client, it would be inappropriate at this time.

3. Keeping a child who is at high risk for suicide safe from self-harm would take immediate priority over any other intervention. Monitoring the child continuously while no longer than an arm's length away would be an appropriate nursing intervention. This observation would allow the nurse to note self-harm behaviors and intervene immediately if necessary.

4. Although it is necessary to maintain open lines of communication for expression of feelings with this child, because this intervention does not address the safety of this client, it would be inappropriate at this time.

TEST-TAKING HINT: To answer this question correctly, the test taker must remember that client safety is always the nurse's first priority, especially when clients are at high risk for suicide.

Nursing Process—Evaluation

26. Behavior modification is defined as a treatment modality aimed at changing undesirable behaviors by using a system of reinforcement to bring about the modifications desired.
   1. The question implies that the client defensively copes with frustration by lashing out and hitting people. New coping skills have been achieved through behavior modification when the client says, "I didn't hit Johnny. Can I have my Tootsie Roll?" The intervention used to achieve this outcome is a reward system that recognizes and appreciates appropriate behavior, modifying behavior that was previously unacceptable.
   2. The statement "I want to wear a helmet like Jane wears" indicates that the client recognizes and desires the belongings of another child. The statement does not reflect that behavior modification is being used or that new coping skills have been developed.
   3. "Can I watch television after supper?" is just a simple question asked by the client. The question does not reflect that behavior modification is being used or that new coping skills have been developed.

4. The client statement "I want a puppy right now" does not reflect that behavior modification is being used or that new coping skills have been developed.

TEST-TAKING HINT: To answer this question correctly, the test taker needs to recognize a statement or question that indicates that behavior modification is being used and that it has been used successfully. Only answer 1 meets both of these criteria.

27. 1. This charting entry documents that a client can cooperate by following instructions; however, the ability to cooperate does not address the client problem of social isolation.
   2. During activity therapy, clients interact with peers and staff. This participation in a social activity reflects a successful outcome for the nursing diagnosis of social isolation.
   3. The ability to distinguish right from left documents a client's cognitive ability; however, this cognitive ability does not address the client problem of social isolation.
   4. The ability to focus for 30 minutes documents a client's ability to concentrate; however, this ability does not address the client problem of social isolation.

TEST-TAKING HINT: To answer this question correctly, the test taker needs to correlate the nursing diagnosis presented in the question (social isolation) with the charting entry that documents a successful outcome. The only answer choice that addresses social isolation is answer 2.

28. 1. The nurse should have no difficulty in evaluating this child's social interaction based on the child's ability to make eye contact and allow physical touch. For a child diagnosed with autism spectrum disorder, this social interaction would represent a major accomplishment.
   2. By making eye contact and allowing physical touch, this child is experiencing improved social interaction, making this an accurate evaluative statement.
   3. Because the child has made significant progress in overcoming social impairment, as evidenced by making eye contact and allowing physical touch, the nurse should have no difficulty in evaluating this child's social interaction. A time frame should not be a factor in this evaluation.
   4. The nurse can accurately evaluate improved social interaction by observing

the client's ability to maintain eye contact and allow physical touch. These improved behaviors are associated with social interaction, not personal identity.

TEST-TAKING HINT: To select the correct answer, the test taker must understand that making eye contact and allowing physical touch are behaviors that evaluate improved social interaction in children diagnosed with autism spectrum disorder.

Psychopharmacology

29. Dextroamphetamine is a stimulant used in the treatment of ADHD. It is important for the nurse to monitor the client's development because stimulant medications can stunt growth.
    1. Monitoring output and sleep patterns would not assist in meeting this client's nutritional needs.
    2. In the stated situation, the imbalanced nutrition is due to the side effect of anorexia, not to nausea and vomiting. If the client were experiencing nausea and vomiting, taking the medication with food would be an appropriate intervention.
    3. **The nurse should administer stimulants after meals for clients to be able to consume a balanced diet before experiencing the potential side effect of anorexia.**
    4. The imbalanced nutrition in this situation is not being caused by constipation; it is being caused by the side effect of anorexia.
    5. **Encouraging frequent high caloric snacks would help the client achieve balanced nutrition if they were experiencing anorexia.**

TEST-TAKING HINT: To answer this question correctly, the test taker must pair the nursing intervention with the nursing diagnosis presented in the question.

30. Atomoxetine is a medication used in the treatment of ADHD.
    1. This outcome does not relate to the stated nursing diagnosis and does not contain a measurable time frame.
    2. This is a long-term, not short-term, outcome for the stated nursing diagnosis.
    3. This outcome does not have a time frame and is not measurable.
    4. **The outcome of the client eating 80% of meals is realistic, has a time frame, and is appropriate for the stated nursing diagnosis.**

TEST-TAKING HINT: To answer this question correctly, the test taker must pair the stated outcome with the nursing diagnosis presented in the question. Correctly stated outcomes are client centered, realistic, and measurable. Including a time frame in the outcome makes the outcome measurable.

31. 1. Methylphenidate can affect sleep; however, this answer does not relate to juvenile diabetes, and because the question clearly asks for interventions related to both diagnoses, the answer is incorrect.
    2. Reporting these potential side effects of methylphenidate is important, but it does not relate to juvenile diabetes. Because the question clearly asks for interventions related to both diagnoses, the answer is incorrect.
    3. **Methylphenidate lowers the client's activity level, which decreases the use of glucose and increases glucose levels. Because of this, it is necessary to monitor fasting blood sugar levels regularly.**
    4. It is important to take methylphenidate as prescribed, but this answer does not relate to juvenile diabetes; because the question clearly asks for interventions related to both diagnoses, the answer is incorrect.

TEST-TAKING HINT: The test taker must note keywords in the question, such as *both diagnoses*. If the answer choices address only one diagnosis, as in 1, 2, and 4, they can be eliminated.

32. 1. **Methylphenidate is a stimulant medication used in the treatment of ADHD.**
    2. Although guanfacine is used in the treatment of ADHD, it is an antihypertensive, not a stimulant, medication. Guanfacine can be used to treat ADHD as monotherapy or as adjunct therapy with stimulant medications.
    3. **Lisdexamfetamine is a stimulant medication used in the treatment of ADHD.**
    4. **Amphetamine/dextroamphetamine is a stimulant medication used in the treatment of ADHD.**
    5. Although clonidine is used in the treatment of ADHD, it is an antihypertensive, not a stimulant, medication. Clonidine can be used to treat ADHD as monotherapy or as adjunct therapy with stimulant medications.

TEST-TAKING HINT: To select the correct answer, the test taker must review different treatments of ADHD and then differentiate between stimulant and nonstimulant medications.

33. If a client's current ADHD medication is ineffective toward the end of the day, a longer acting stimulant may be the better drug of choice.
    1. Evekeo is a short-acting, not a long-acting, stimulant medication.
    2. **Mydayis is a long-acting stimulant medication.**
    3. **Aptensio is a long-acting stimulant medication.**
    4. Zenzedi is a short-acting, not a long-acting, stimulant medication.
    5. ProCentra is a short-acting, not a long-acting, stimulant medication.

TEST-TAKING HINT: To answer this question correctly, the test taker must note that the client's short-acting stimulant medication is not achieving the desired results. A long-acting stimulant may be required. The test taker must also be able to recognize the names of both short-acting and long-acting stimulant medications.

34. 1. An antidepressant medication such as sertraline is not the usual drug of choice for intermittent explosive disorder.
    2. **An antipsychotic medication such as paliperidone can be prescribed for intermittent explosive disorder.**
    3. An antianxiety medication such as buspirone is not the usual drug of choice for intermittent explosive disorder.
    4. A monoamine oxidase inhibitor such as phenelzine is not the usual drug of choice for intermittent explosive disorder.
    5. **A mood stabilizing medication such as valproate sodium can be prescribed for intermittent explosive disorder.**

TEST-TAKING HINT: To answer this question correctly, the test taker must have knowledge of various classifications of medications and which are commonly used to treat impulse control disorders such as intermittent explosive disorder.

35. Methylphenidate HCL extended-release capsules (Jornay) is a stimulant used to treat attention-deficit hyperactivity disorder (ADHD).
    1. Jornay does not have to be taken with food, and is taken in the evening, not morning.

2. Jornay does not have any immediate-release component in the formulation and will start being released in the colon approximately 10 hours after absorption. The client expecting the medication to be effective after two hours indicates that teaching has been misunderstood.
3. It is not recommended that any stimulants, including Jornay, be taken with caffeine, such as coffee, tea, or soda.
4. **Jornay needs to be taken approximately 10 hours before it is expected to start working. It is an extended-release medication and starts to release when it reaches the colon.**

TEST-TAKING HINT: To answer this question correctly the test-taker needs to review new medications prescribed for attention deficit-hyperactivity disorder (ADHD). Jornay is the only stimulant medication that is taken in the evening hours and has no immediate-release component in the formulation.

36. Attention deficit-hyperactivity disorder (ADHD) can be treated with behavioral interventions, nonstimulant medications, and two different classes of stimulant medications, methylphenidate-based and amphetamine-based stimulants.
    1. Amphetamine (Dyanavel XR) is a stimulant, not a nonstimulant, medication used to treat ADHD.
    2. **Viloxazine hydrochloride is a nonstimulant medication used to treat ADHD.**
    3. Dexmethylphenidate (Azstarys) is a stimulant, not a nonstimulant, medication used to treat ADHD.
    4. **Atomoxetine is a nonstimulant medication used to treat ADHD.**
    5. **Quanfacine XR is a nonstimulant medication used to treat ADHD.**

TEST-TAKING HINT: To answer the test question correctly the test taker must review the different medication classifications used to treat ADHD and then be able to recognize which are stimulant and which are nonstimulant medications.

Clinical Judgment Case Studies

17

This chapter presents various unfolding psychiatric case studies that test the six cognitive skills of the National Council of State Boards of Nursing's Clinical Judgment Measurement Model: recognizing cues, analyzing cues, prioritizing hypotheses, generating solutions, taking actions, and evaluating outcomes. It is important to practice and understand these steps in the unfolding case studies to develop strong clinical judgment skills and prepare for the Next Generation NCLEX® (NGN). The questions accompanying each case study follow these six steps (National Council of State Boards of Nursing [NCSBN], 2020):

1. Recognize cues: What matters most?
2. Analyze cues: What could it mean?
3. Prioritize hypotheses: Where do I start?
4. Generate solutions: What can I do?
5. Take action: What will I do?
6. Evaluate outcomes: Did it help?

For more information on the NGN, see https//www.ncsbn.org.

NCLEX questions assume the nurse has a provider's order for listed interventions unless noted otherwise.

ANXIETY: POSTTRAUMATIC STRESS DISORDER (PTSD) CASE STUDY

A nurse is caring for an ex-military client admitted from the emergency department (ED) to the psychiatric unit with orders for haloperidol IM prn, lorazepam, four-point restraints, and seclusion. This admission occurred after the client, with no provocation, assaulted someone in a parking lot. The client has a history of panic attacks and flashbacks, which led to violent behaviors. Currently, the client is physically threatening harm to staff personnel.

1. **Recognize cues: What matters most?** The client does not respond to verbal interventions or medications. Which nursing intervention should be prioritized?
   1. Offer the use of a urinal prior to administering restraints and seclusion.
   2. Apply four-point restraints and seclude the client.
   3. Offer staff safety information related to restraints and seclusion.
   4. Provide nourishment prior to applying restraints.

2. **Analyze cues: What could it mean?** The client is released from restraints and seclusion and is encouraged to participate in group activities. Which of the following client behaviors would indicate the need for further interventions to maintain safety? **Select all that apply.**
   1. The client is pacing the unit.
   2. The client is displaying pressured speech.
   3. The client is noted to have a flat affect.
   4. The client sits alone while eating.
   5. The client is muttering with unseen others.

3. **Prioritize hypotheses: Where do I start?** The client tells the nurse that the enemy is trying to storm the room. Which should be the nurse's initial intervention?
   1. Disagree with the client's observation.
   2. State, "You should know that no enemy is headed our way!"
   3. State, "You'll feel much better after you've had your dinner."
   4. Calmly present reality.

4. **Generate solutions: What can I do?** When caring for a client who is out of touch with reality, the nurse applies many interventions to reorient the client. For each potential nursing intervention, place a check mark in one appropriate box to indicate whether the intervention is *Indicated*, *Nonessential*, or *Contraindicated*.

Potential Intervention	Indicated	Nonessential	Contraindicated
1. Confront client with inappropriate ideations			
2. Apply restraints			
3. Orient to person, place, time, and situation			
4. Establish a trusting relationship			
5. Maintain suicide precautions			
6. Redirect inappropriate ideations			

5. **Take action: What will I do?** What is the nurse's immediate next step if the client's flashbacks lead to combative behavior?
   1. Objectively document behavior.
   2. Lead other clients on unit to safe area.
   3. Notify the client's physician for further orders.
   4. Bargain with client using off-unit privileges.

6. **Evaluate outcomes: Did it help?** Which of the following assessed client behaviors indicate that nursing interventions have led to the improvement of client symptoms? **Select all that apply.**
   1. Client looks forward to discussing details of flashbacks with counselor.
   2. Client has slept well without flashbacks for three nights.
   3. Client has participated in two off-unit activities without incident.
   4. Client has joined a veteran support group.
   5. Client focuses on other clients' problems during counseling.

ANXIETY: POSTTRAUMATIC STRESS DISORDER (PTSD) CASE STUDY ANSWERS AND RATIONALES

1.
   1. It is important to meet a client's physical needs while the client is being restrained, but when a client is exhibiting behaviors that are a danger to self or others, placing the client in the ordered physical restraint is the nurse's first priority.
   2. **Because the client is exhibiting aggressive behaviors that are a danger to others, the nurse's first priority is to provide a safe environment by restraining this client.**
   3. While it is important that all staff be familiar with restraint protocol, at this time, the safety of the environment must be prioritized.
   4. It is important to meet a client's physical needs while the client is being restrained, but when a client is exhibiting behaviors that are a danger to self or others, placing the client in the ordered physical restraint is the nurse's first priority.

2.

1. Pacing the unit is an indication that the client remains agitated and unsettled. Further assessment would determine whether additional interventions are indicated to maintain safety.
2. Pressured speech is an indication that the client remains agitated, and this behavior may cause unit disruption. Further assessment would determine whether additional interventions are indicated to maintain safety.
3. Flat affect is the virtual absence of an emotional response to a situation or condition. This is an important assessment; however, it would not indicate that additional interventions are needed to maintain safety.
4. Eating alone may be a preference, not an indication of aggressive or agitated behavior. No further interventions to maintain safety should be needed.
5. **The behavior of muttering with unseen others is an indication that the client is out of touch with reality. This behavior may indicate the need for further assessment to ensure unit safety.**

3.

1. Disagreeing with the client's ideation may increase agitation and aggression. Calmly presenting reality without confrontation is the more appropriate nursing intervention.
2. This statement indirectly confirms the client's delusions. Calmly presenting reality is the more appropriate nursing intervention.
3. This statement depreciates the client's feelings by not dealing directly with the client's concerns. This change of subject ignores the client's stated problem. Calmly presenting reality is the more appropriate nursing intervention.
4. **Reality is all that exists, as opposed to those ideas or mental images that are imagined. Calmly presenting reality can decrease this client's anxiety and should be the nurse's initial intervention.**

4. Answer:

Potential Intervention	Indicated	Nonessential	Contraindicated
1. Confront client with inappropriate ideations			X
2. Apply restraints			X
3. Orient to person, place, time, and situation	X		
4. Establish a trusting relationship	X		
5. Maintain suicide precautions		X	
6. Redirect inappropriate ideations	X		

1. Client confrontation is **contraindicated** because it puts the client on the defensive and impedes further nurse–client interactions.
2. Restraining the client is **contraindicated** because this client is not a danger to self or others.
3. When a client is out of touch with reality, orienting the client to person, place, time, and situation is **indicated.** This intervention will help the client understand the real world and their relationship to it.
4. The establishment of a trusting nurse–client relationship is **indicated** when a client is out of touch with reality. Trust is especially essential when the nurse is reorienting a client.

5. There is no indication that this client is considering self-harm, so this intervention would be **nonessential.**

6. The redirection of inappropriate ideations is **indicated** in order to present reality to a client who is experiencing thought disorders.

5.

1. It is very important to document this behavior objectively; however, the nurse's immediate next step needs to focus on maintaining a safe environment.

2. **The nurse's immediate next step must be to ensure the safety of the environment. Leading clients to a safe area should be the nurse's first priority.**

3. Notifying the physician of the client's behavior to attain further orders may be appropriate; however, the nurse's immediate next step is to ensure the safety of the unit.

4. Bargaining the use of off-unit privileges with a client is an inappropriate nursing intervention in any circumstance. The nurse's immediate next step is to ensure the safety of the unit.

6.

1. Counseling sessions should focus on reality, not details of flashbacks. Reality should be continually reinforced.

2. **A client sleeping well for three nights without flashbacks is an indication that nursing interventions have led to the improvement of client symptoms.**

3. **A client participating in off-unit activities without incident is an indication that nursing interventions have led to the improvement of client symptoms.**

4. **A client joining a veteran support group indicates that nursing interventions have led to the improvement of client symptoms.**

5. A client focusing on another client's issues during counseling indicates avoidance of personal issues and impedes the improvement of client symptoms.

BIPOLAR CASE STUDY

A client on an inpatient psychiatric unit is diagnosed with bipolar affective disorder type I (BPAD I). The treatment team is planning to start valproic acid treatment. Laboratory work results consist of white blood cell (WBC) count 6.5/L, red blood cell (RBC) count 5.1 mcL, platelets 250,000/mm^3, aspartate aminotransferase (AST) 45 U/L, and alanine transaminase (ALT) 56 U/L.

1. **Recognize cues: What matters most?** What laboratory result could impact initiation of valproic acid treatment?
   1. RBC count is too low to start valproic acid treatment.
   2. WBC count is too high to start valproic acid treatment.
   3. Platelets are too low to start valproic acid treatment.
   4. AST/ALT levels are too high to start valproic acid treatment.

2. **Analyze cues: What could it mean?** Based on these assessed laboratory values, what interventions would the nurse expect to implement? **Select all that apply.**
   1. The nurse will ask to add differential to the laboratory request.
   2. The nurse would notify the treatment team of the abnormal findings.
   3. The nurse will assess the client for bloating, nausea, and swelling.
   4. The nurse would compare current and past available laboratory work.
   5. The nurse will educate the client on the risks of a possible liver biopsy.

3. **Prioritize hypotheses: Where do I start?** The nurse assesses the client for further liver disease and notices bloating and swelling in the abdomen. The client's abdomen is soft upon palpation, and the client denies pain. During dinner, the client reports nausea. The client's skin is dry and flushed, and their eyes are white, with equal and reactive pupils. The nurse notes that current liver enzymes are slightly increased from past levels. The nurse anticipates which additional interventions would be indicated at this time? **Select all that apply.**
   1. After discussion, the treatment team decides a liver biopsy is necessary.
   2. The nurse will consult with a dietitian about a diet suitable for clients with liver disease.
   3. The nurse will turn and reposition the client every 2 hours to avoid skin breakdown.
   4. The nurse will initiate treatment for ascites.
   5. The nurse will assess the client for alcohol use and possible risks for hepatitis.

4. **Generate solutions: What can I do?** After further evaluation, it has been determined that valproic acid treatment will be started. When initiating and monitoring clients prescribed valproic acid, it is important to promote safety and monitor for complications. For each potential nursing intervention, place a checkmark in one appropriate box to indicate whether the intervention is *Indicated*, *Nonessential*, or *Contraindicated*.

Potential Intervention	Indicated	Nonessential	Contraindicated
1. Evaluate for excessive bleeding/bruising			
2. Monitor valproic acid levels			
3. Place on fall precautions			
4. Teach signs of valproic acid toxicity			
5. Remove suicide precautions			

5. **Take action: What will I do?** It is time for the next valproic acid dose. The nurse notices the client in the dining room struggling to eat. The client's tremor is impacting the ability to use utensils, resulting in spilled food. The nurse talks with the client and notices the client's slurred speech, confusion, and struggle to stay upright in the chair. What is the nurse's priority intervention?
   1. Hold the next dose of medication and assist the client with dinner.
   2. Administer the next dose of medication because of worsening symptoms.
   3. Hold the next dose of medication and contact the psychiatric medical provider.
   4. Administer the next dose of medication and initiate fall precautions.

6. **Evaluate outcomes: Did it help?** The nurse holds the following dose of valproic acid and calls the medical provider. The medical provider asks that the nursing staff hold the following two doses and orders a valproic acid level in 24 hours. The following day, the valproic acid level is 80 mcg/mL. The client is no longer tremulous, is calm, and is able to communicate without confusion. The client is getting ready for discharge. Which of the following client behaviors indicate that nursing interventions have been successful? **Select all that apply.**
   1. The client can give accurate feedback related to symptoms of valproic acid toxicity.
   2. The client is compliant and can recognize early signs of worsening symptoms.
   3. The client states, "I have to get my labs drawn 12 hours after I take my valproic acid."
   4. The client states, "I know I have to take the valproic acid on a full stomach."
   5. The client states, "After I'm discharged, I'll talk with my outpatient provider about a safety plan."

BIPOLAR CASE STUDY ANSWERS AND RATIONALES

1.

1. RBC count, whether high or low, will not impact initiating valproic acid treatment.
2. The WBC count is monitored before and during valproic acid treatment; however, the concern arises if the WBC is low. In the statement, the nurse must recognize the WBC is within normal limits (WNL), not high, and would not impact initiation of treatment.
3. Platelet count is monitored before and during valproic acid treatment. The concern arises if the platelets are too low. In the statement, the nurse must recognize that the platelet count is WNL, not low, and would not impact initiation of treatment.
4. **AST and ALT are monitored before and during valproic acid treatment to ensure that the medication is not impacting liver function. This client's AST and ALT values are elevated, which could impact the initiation of valproic acid treatment.**

2.

1. Concerns with the WBC count would precipitate the treatment team to order a differential added to the laboratory work. However, this WBC count is WNL, and therefore, a differential is not necessary.
2. **The nurse would want to notify the treatment team of the abnormal liver enzymes results.**
3. **The nurse will assess the client for bloating, nausea, and swelling because these are symptoms of liver disease. Other symptoms include fatigue, loss of appetite, electrolyte imbalances, yellow skin and eyes, mental confusion, bleeding, bruising, and itching.**
4. **The nurse would want to compare current and past laboratory work to determine if there is any change or worsening of liver enzyme levels.**
5. Although at some point the treatment team may want to obtain a liver biopsy, it is not indicated at this time.

3.

1. **If there are no other reasons for this client's enzymes to be elevated, a liver biopsy becomes necessary.**
2. **The nurse would consult with the dietitian about a diet specific for clients with liver disease.**
3. The nurse would not need to turn and reposition the client every 2 hours. The nurse assessed the client's skin to be dry and flushed. There is nothing to indicate the need for turning and repositioning the client.
4. The client does have bloating and swelling in the abdomen; however, when assessed, it is soft and without pain, and therefore shows no signs of ascites.
5. **The nurse should assess for all possible causes of liver disease, including alcohol and possible risks of hepatitis.**

4. Answer:

Potential Intervention	Indicated	Nonessential	Contraindicated
1. Evaluate for excessive bleeding/bruising	X		
2. Monitor valproic acid levels	X		
3. Place on fall precautions		X	
4. Teach signs of valproic acid toxicity	X		
5. Remove suicide precautions			X

1. Evaluating for excessive bleeding and bruising is **indicated** during valproic acid treatment. Laboratory work will include liver enzymes and a complete blood count to assess WBCs and platelets. When platelets are low, the client is at risk for excessive bleeding and bruising.
2. Monitoring valproic acid levels is **indicated** during treatment with valproic acid to ensure that levels remain within normal limits.
3. Placing a client on fall precautions is **nonessential** during valproic acid treatment unless otherwise clinically indicated. Valproic acid treatment in and of itself does not increase fall risk.
4. Teaching signs of valproic acid toxicity is **indicated** during valproic acid treatment. Signs of toxicity include tremor, excessive bleeding, bruising, confusion, dizziness, irritability, blurred or double vision, lethargy, nausea, vomiting, and myoclonus.
5. Removal of suicide precautions would be **contraindicated** until the client is assessed as physically and mentally stable.

5.

1. Holding the next dose of medication at this time would be appropriate; however, continuing with dinner would be unadvised. The client is experiencing signs of valproic acid toxicity and needs to be evaluated further.
2. The client is experiencing signs of valproic acid toxicity, not worsening symptoms. Therefore, administering more medication would worsen the situation.
3. **The nurse would want to hold the next dose of valproic acid and immediately call the psychiatric medical provider to report valproic acid toxicity.**
4. Due to worsening symptoms, initiating fall precautions would be necessary. However, the client's symptoms indicate valproic acid toxicity. Administering the next dose of valproic acid would exacerbate the situation.

6.

1. **An indication that nursing interventions have been successful is when the client can recognize the symptoms of valproic acid toxicity, hold the next medication dose, and notify the health-care provider.**
2. **An indication that nursing interventions have been successful is when the client is compliant and can recognize early signs of worsening symptoms.**
3. **An indication that nursing interventions have been successful is when the client recognizes that, to obtain an accurate level, blood for ordered laboratory tests must be drawn 12 hours after taking valproic acid.**
4. It is not necessary for the client to take valproic acid on a full stomach. This client statement indicates a need for further client teaching.
5. A safety plan should be formulated during in-patient therapy prior to discharge. This client statement indicates a need for further client teaching.

MEDICATIONS CASE STUDY

A hospitalized client, diagnosed with schizophrenia, is preparing to start clozapine treatment. The client's laboratory results show an absolute neutrophil count (ANC) of 1,900/mm^3.

1. **Recognize cues: What matters most?** What is the first action the nurse should perform?
    1. Double check the client's name band, ask for the date of birth, and administer the medication as prescribed.
    2. Review the client's entire complete blood count, because the white blood cell (WBC) count is equally important.
    3. Notify the prescriber, because the ANC is too low to administer clozapine as prescribed.
    4. Check past laboratory work and compare the ANC, because the client may be experiencing benign ethnic neutropenia (BEN).

2. **Analyze cues: What could it mean?** The medication has now been administered. Which of the following should the nurse implement at this time? **Select all that apply.**
   1. Implement fall precautions due to possible anorexia, bilirubinemia, jaundice, and coagulopathy.
   2. Implement seizure precautions.
   3. Monitor for unexplained fatigue, dyspnea, tachypnea, fever, and tachycardia.
   4. Assess fasting blood glucose and cholesterol levels initially and throughout therapy.
   5. Monitor for frequency and consistency of bowel movements and symptoms of hypomotility.

3. **Prioritize hypotheses: Where do I start?** The client is noted to be restless, tense, has trouble sitting still at breakfast, and has spilled orange juice all over the table. The nurse anticipates which additional intervention at this time? **Select all that apply.**
   1. Request someone to assist the client during meal time.
   2. Start utilizing the Abnormal Involuntary Movement Scale (AIMS).
   3. Initiate fasting blood sugar tests before every meal.
   4. Anticipate the addition of benztropine.
   5. Anticipate the addition of trihexyphenidyl.

4. **Generate solutions: What can I do?** When initiating and evaluating for treatment with clozapine, it is important to promote safety and monitor for complications. For each potential nursing intervention, place a checkmark in one appropriate box to indicate whether the intervention is *Indicated*, *Nonessential*, or *Contraindicated*.

Potential Intervention	Indicated	Nonessential	Contraindicated
1. Review the ANC weekly for first 6 months			
2. Restart the medication immediately if 3 days in a row are missed			
3. Explain the purpose of the risk evaluation and mitigation strategy (REMS)			
4. Inform the client that smoking can decrease clozapine levels			
5. Evaluate the positive and negative symptoms of schizophrenia			

5. **Take action: What will I do?** While the nurse is coming on shift, the nurse notices that the client is tired and experiencing diaphoresis. Vital signs consist of temperature of 101.3°F (38.5°C); respiratory rate of 20 breaths/min, short, labored; heart rate of 120 beats/min; and blood pressure 190/110 mm Hg. Based on this information, which nursing action takes priority?
   1. Administer the clozapine and notify the prescriber.
   2. Contact the prescriber to obtain an increased prescription of benztropine.
   3. Hold the clozapine dose and contact the prescriber.
   4. Hold the clozapine dose and monitor for worsening symptoms.

6. **Evaluate outcomes: Did it help?** After the nurse held the clozapine, the client was treated, and now the client's vitals are blood pressure, 128/78 mm Hg; pulse 68 beats/min; temperature 97.6°F (36.44°C); and respirations 16 breaths/min. The client expresses concern about rechallenging clozapine after experiencing neuroleptic malignant syndrome (NMS). Which nursing response is appropriate at this time? **Select all that apply.**
   1. Empathize with the client's concern and inform the prescriber the client has refused to restart clozapine.
   2. Acknowledge the client's concern, and remind them the rechallenge will be implemented slowly and monitored closely.
   3. Reassess vitals and monitor mental status, including both positive and negative symptoms.
   4. Remind the client to immediately share with the health-care team if symptoms return.
   5. Notify the prescriber that the client needs further education.

MEDICATION CASE STUDY ANSWERS AND RATIONALES

1.
   1. **The nurse should double check that they are administering the medication to the correct client and administer the medication. The ANC is above 1,500/mm3.**
   2. The WBC is no longer monitored before prescribing clozapine. The clozapine risk evaluation and mitigation strategy (REMS) is monitoring the ANC only.
   3. There is no need to notify the prescriber because the ANC is above 1,500/mm^3.
   4. BEN occurs when the ANC is lower than normal. Before a diagnosis of BEN can be made, there would need to be at least two baseline ANC levels greater than 1,000/mm^3.

2.
   1. Although the nurse should implement fall precautions, it is not related to anorexia, bilirubinemia, jaundice, or coagulopathy, which are signs of hepatotoxicity. The reason to implement fall precautions would be associated with side effects, including drowsiness, orthostatic hypotension, and possible motor and sensory instability.
   2. **The nurse will implement seizure precautions because clozapine does lower the seizure threshold, especially with clients who have a history of seizures.**
   3. **The nurse will monitor for unexplained fatigue, dyspnea, tachypnea, fever, and tachycardia, which are signs of myocarditis, a side effect of clozapine. Other signs of myocarditis include chest pain; palpitations; electrocardiogram (ECG) changes, such as ST-T wave abnormalities; arrhythmias; or tachycardia during the first month of therapy. If these occur, clozapine should be discontinued and not restarted.**
   4. **The nurse will monitor fasting blood glucose and cholesterol levels initially and throughout therapy because elevated blood glucose and cholesterol levels are side effects of clozapine.**
   5. **The nurse will monitor for frequency and consistency of bowel movements and symptoms of hypomotility because these are side effects of clozapine.**

3.
   1. Although the client is having difficulty with drinking, all the symptoms listed show the client is experiencing extrapyramidal side effects (EPS) and therefore will need interventions to address the concern.
   2. The client in the question is experiencing EPS, not tardive dyskinesia (TD). AIMS testing is done to monitor for TD. Symptoms of TD include uncontrolled rhythmic movement of the mouth, face, or extremities; lip smacking or puckering; puffing of cheeks; uncontrolled chewing; or rapid or wormlike movements of the tongue.

3. Although the client's blood sugar levels could be impacted by clozapine, that is not reflected in the client's symptoms and is therefore incorrect.

4. **The addition of benztropine would be expected because it is one of the medications that can treat EPS.**

5. **The addition of trihexyphenidyl would be expected because it is one of the medications that can treat EPS.**

4. Answer:

Potential Intervention	Indicated	Nonessential	Contraindicated
1. Review the absolute neutrophil count (ANC) weekly for the first 6 months	X		
2. Restart the medication immediately if medication is missed for 3 days			X
3. Explain the purpose of risk evaluation and mitigation strategy (REMS)		X	
4. Inform the client that smoking can decrease clozapine levels	X		
5. Evaluate the positive and negative symptoms of schizophrenia	X		

1. Reviewing the ANC weekly for the first 6 months is **indicated.** After the first 6 months, then biweekly ANC monitoring for 6 months; then, if maintained within acceptable parameters, monthly after 12 months.

2. Restarting the medication immediately if missing 3 days' worth of medication is **contraindicated.** The nurse should educate the client if they miss more than 2 days in a row, that the client must not restart the medication and must notify health-care professionals for new dosing instructions.

3. Explaining the purpose of REMS, including procedures, is **nonessential** at this time because it would have been completed before clozapine was started, not after the client has been prescribed medication for a period of time.

4. Informing the client that increased smoking can decrease clozapine levels is **indicated.** After the client leaves the facility, it will be important for the client to be aware of how a change in smoking can impact side effects as well as effectiveness of medications.

5. Evaluating both positive and negative symptoms of schizophrenia is **indicated** throughout clozapine treatment.

5.

1. Administering the clozapine is inappropriate and could worsen the symptoms; therefore, this nursing action is incorrect.

2. The client is experiencing NMS, not symptoms associated with EPS, and therefore benztropine would be inappropriate.

3. **The client is experiencing symptoms associated with NMS. Symptoms include fever, respiratory distress, tachycardia, possible seizures, diaphoresis, hyper- or hypotension, pallor, and tiredness. The nurse would want to hold the clozapine and contact the prescriber. Treatment of NMS includes withholding the agent, cooling the body, replacing lost fluids, possible mechanical ventilation, and giving medications to address other symptoms, such as arrhythmias or agitation.**

4. Although the nurse would want to hold the clozapine, it would be most important to notify the prescriber to initiate other treatment options. Monitoring for worsening symptoms could delay important interventions, harming the client.

6.

1. Although it is good for the nurse to empathize with the client's concern, the client is not refusing, they are voicing fear. At this time, it would be important for the nurse to educate the client, addressing concerns, then ask the client if they would like to refuse. Therefore, this is an incorrect response by the nurse.
2. **Acknowledging the client's concern and reminding them the rechallenge will be done slowly and monitored closely addresses the client's concern, and then the nurse should give the client information to help make the decision.**
3. If the client does take the medication, then at that time, it would be important to continue to reassess vitals, monitor mental status, and acknowledge positive and negative symptoms. But at this time, the client has voiced concern before the medication is administered, and therefore this answer is incorrect.
4. **Reminding the client that if the symptoms do return, they will need to immediately share with the health-care team is an appropriate intervention before administering the medication.**
5. The nurse is able to educate the client about the process and does not need to get the prescriber involved at this time. Therefore, this is an inappropriate response from the nurse.

PERSONALITY DISORDER CASE STUDY

A 14-year-old client, medically cleared in the emergency department, is admitted to the inpatient psychiatric unit following a suicide attempt by taking more than ten 200 mg tablets of ibuprofen. Upon assessment, the nurse notices scars on the client's lower arms and upper thighs.

1. **Recognize cues: What matters most?** The client currently denies suicidal ideations but expresses an urge for self-injurious behavior (SIB). Which nursing intervention should be prioritized?
   1. Place the client on elopement precautions.
   2. Administer prn medications to help with anxiety.
   3. Assess the client's plan to cut and monitor at irregular intervals.
   4. Teach the client first aid and signs of infection.

2. **Analyze cues: What could it mean?** The client expresses urges to use a found paperclip to cut both arms because of anger with their family. The nurse implements one-to-one observation and utilizes therapeutic communication. Which client behaviors indicate the beginning of a healthy nurse–client relationship? **Select all that apply.**
   1. Client returns the paperclip and stays with staff.
   2. Client attempts to split staff by criticizing the work ethic of the unit.
   3. Staff is attempting to engage the client and the client deliberately walks away.
   4. Client talks with nurse about relationships with others, including family.
   5. Client corners and attempts to hug the nurse.

3. **Prioritize hypotheses: Where do I start?** The client states, "I'm so mad at you. I'm going to tell all the other nurses how mean you are." The nurse anticipates which additional intervention at this time? **Select all that apply.**
   1. Set firm boundaries and refuse to work with the client.
   2. Directly discuss with the client their staff-splitting attempts.
   3. Redirect behaviors to help the client focus on own issues.
   4. Role model healthy communication skills to deal with conflict.
   5. Discuss the client's behavior with the treatment team to avoid splitting staff.

4. **Generate solutions: What can I do?** When caring for this client, the nurse applies many interventions to assist with the client's specific problems. For each potential nursing intervention, place a check mark in one appropriate box to indicate whether the intervention is *Indicated*, *Nonessential*, or *Contraindicated*.

Potential Intervention	Indicated	Nonessential	Contraindicated
1. Discuss the need for family therapy			
2. Monitor for self-injurious behavior (SIB)			
3. Scan the environment for objects that could be used for SIB			
4. Establish a trusting relationship			
5. Consult a nutritionist related to dietary needs			
6. Be compliant with the client's demands to promote self-esteem			

5. **Take action: What will I do?** The nurse is talking with the client about self-injurious behaviors. The client states, "The only way I can release my pain is to cut myself." What is the nurse's immediate next step?
   1. Ask the client, "Why do you have pain?"
   2. Suggest quiet time alone.
   3. State, "I am sure you don't really mean that."
   4. Explore alternative coping mechanisms.

6. **Evaluate outcomes: Did it help?** Which of the following assessed client behaviors indicate that nursing interventions have led to the improvement of client symptoms? **Select all that apply.**
   1. Client states, "I think I will try journaling as a way to express my emotions."
   2. Client starts avoiding socializing with others to prevent uncomfortable emotions.
   3. Client decides to talk with family about how family caused the client's issues.
   4. Client decides to attend intensive outpatient program upon discharge.
   5. Client expresses to staff their urges to cut and voluntarily stays in the milieu.

PERSONALITY DISORDER CASE STUDY ANSWERS AND RATIONALES

1.
   1. At some point, it may be necessary to place the client on elopement precautions, but there is nothing indicating necessity at this time. The nurse's first priority is to establish client safety and address urges to cut.
   2. It may be necessary for the nurse to administer prn medications to help with anxiety; however, at this time the nurse's first priority is to establish client safety and address urges to cut.
   3. **Assessing the client's plan to cut and monitoring the client at irregular intervals addresses the client's safety and is the nurse's first priority.**
   4. At some point, teaching first aid and signs of infection to a client who cuts is appropriate. However, at this time the nurse's first priority is to establish client safety and address urges to cut.

2.

1. The client's willingness to return the paperclip and stay with the nurse, indicates the beginning of a healthy nurse–client relationship.
2. A client criticizes the work ethic of the unit in order to redirect attention from their own behavior and disrupt the environment. This is called staff splitting and does not indicate the beginning of a healthy nurse–client relationship.
3. When staff is engaging a client and the client deliberately walks away, this behavior does not indicate the beginning of a healthy nurse–client relationship.
4. The client's willingness to converse with the nurse about family relationships displays trust in the nurse and indicates the beginning of a healthy nurse–client relationship.
5. When the client corners and attempts to hug the nurse, this demonstrates an unhealthy attachment and therefore does not indicate the beginning of a healthy nurse–client relationship.

3.

1. Setting firm boundaries with clients is always necessary and appropriate. However, refusing to work with a client does not address the client's behavior of staff splitting.
2. Directly discussing staff-splitting behaviors with the client would be an appropriate nursing intervention.
3. Redirecting behaviors to help the client focus on their own issues is a way to deter staff-splitting behavior and is an appropriate nursing intervention.
4. Role modeling health communication skills to deal with conflict is a way to address staff splitting and is an appropriate nursing intervention.
5. Discussing client behaviors with the treatment team is an appropriate nursing intervention to avoid further staff splitting by the client.

4. Answer:

Potential Intervention	Indicated	Nonessential	Contraindicated
1. Discuss the need for family therapy	X		
2. Monitor for self-injurious behavior (SIB)	X		
3. Scan the environment for objects that could be used for SIB	X		
4. Establish a trusting relationship	X		
5. Consult a nutritionist related to dietary needs		X	
6. Be compliant with the client's demands to promote self-esteem			X

1. The client has expressed family discord. The behavior of this teenage client impacts the entire family; therefore, family therapy is **indicated.**
2. A history of SIB and assessed arm and leg scarring would alert the nurse to continue to monitor for SIB. This intervention is **indicated.**
3. Scanning the environment for objects that could be used for SIB is **indicated** because removal of these objects will decrease the client's risk for self-harm.
4. The establishment of a trusting nurse–client relationship is **indicated** when working with clients experiencing traits associated with borderline personality disorder.

5. Consulting a nutritionist related to dietary needs is **nonessential** at this time. The client's symptoms and behaviors do not reflect a need for a dietary consultation.

6. Promoting self-esteem is essential. However, when clients exhibit traits associated with manipulation and staff splitting, it is important to maintain boundaries and avoid secondary gains. Being compliant with the client's demands is **contraindicated.**

5.

1. Asking the client, "Why do you have pain?" is a block to communication, places the client on the defense, and harms the nurse–client relationship.

2. Suggesting quiet time alone for a client who is experiencing SIBs to deal with pain would isolate the client and close further communication and is not appropriate.

3. The nurse stating, "I am sure you don't really mean that," is a block to communication, depreciates the client's feelings, and is not appropriate.

4. **Exploring alternative coping mechanisms would be the nurse's immediate next step. The client will need to learn new, healthier coping skills to replace cutting when feeling emotional pain.**

6.

1. **The client statement, "I think I will try journaling as a way to express my emotions," shows insight into reasons for SIBs and the need for healthy coping skills.**

2. The behaviors of avoiding socialization to prevent uncomfortable emotions are maladaptive and unrealistic. This behavior indicates that nursing interventions have not led to symptom improvement.

3. Nursing interventions have not led to symptom improvement when a client deflects and minimizes their behavior by blaming family for their mental health problems.

4. **Nursing interventions have led to improvement of client symptoms when a client exhibits an understanding of the need for continued outpatient treatment by attending an intensive outpatient program.**

5. **Although experiencing the urge to cut could be considered a setback, expressing the cutting urge to staff and voluntarily staying in the milieu show client behavior that indicates nursing interventions have led to improvement.**

SCHIZOPHRENIA CASE STUDY

The nurse is caring for a 45-year-old client diagnosed with schizophrenia. The client was admitted due to a suicide attempt related to command hallucinations. The client has been placed on suicide precautions and ordered ziprasidone IM and lorazepam IM. The client presents with a hostile affect and paranoid verbalizations and displays facial tics.

1. **Recognize cues: What matters most?** After administering prescribed medications, which nursing intervention should be prioritized?
   1. Maintain constant observation.
   2. Encourage hydration.
   3. Teach medication side effects.
   4. Encourage the client to recognize triggers for self-harm.

2. **Analyze cues: What could it mean?** After assessing that the client is experiencing facial and tongue movements, the nurse should anticipate the implementation of which additional interventions? **Select all that apply.**
   1. An order for valbenazine.
   2. Assessment using the Abnormal Involuntary Movement Scale (AIMS).
   3. An order for metoprolol.
   4. An order for a thyroid-stimulating hormone (TSH) level.
   5. Monitoring for uncontrollable, abnormal body movements.

3. **Prioritize hypotheses: Where do I start?** The client is uncooperative and refuses to take medications, insisting that "the voices tell me the pills will make me go blind." What should be the nurse's initial intervention?
   1. Implement forced medication protocols.
   2. State, "Why would you think this medication would affect your vision?"
   3. State, "This medication should help you by reducing the voices."
   4. Administer prn IM antianxiety medications.

4. **Generate solutions: What can I do?** When caring for a paranoid, hostile client, the nurse applies many interventions to promote safety. For each potential nursing intervention, place a check mark in one appropriate box to indicate whether the intervention is *Indicated*, *Nonessential*, or *Contraindicated*.

Potential Intervention	Indicated	Nonessential	Contraindicated
1. Promote self-esteem			
2. Increase the dosage of benztropine			
3. Apply restraints			
4. Closely monitor medication administration			
5. Establish a trusting relationship			

5. **Take action: What will I do?** What is the nurse's immediate next step if ideations of self-harm are assessed?
   1. Assess plan for self-harm.
   2. Note any involuntary movements.
   3. Administer any ordered medications.
   4. Meet with family to develop a discharge plan.

6. **Evaluate outcomes: Did it help?** Which assessed client behaviors indicate successful nursing interventions related to client improvement? **Select all that apply.**
   1. Client willingly takes ordered medications.
   2. Client verbalizes, "I can feel just as safe at home."
   3. Client implements a plan to deal with command hallucinations.
   4. Client participates in formulating a discharge plan.
   5. Client notifies staff that voices have returned.

SCHIZOPHRENIA CASE STUDY ANSWERS AND RATIONALES

1.
   1. Because this client is on suicide precautions due to a suicide attempt, the nurse should prioritize safety by maintaining constant client observation.
   2. Client hydration should always be encouraged; however, the nurse should prioritize safety by maintaining constant client observation.
   3. Teaching medication side effects is always an important nursing intervention; however, the nurse should prioritize safety by maintaining constant client observation.
   4. A client should always be encouraged to recognize triggers for self-harm including command hallucination; however, the nurse should prioritize safety by maintaining constant client observation.

2.

1. The nurse should recognize facial and tongue movements as signs of tardive dyskinesia (TD) and anticipate an order for valbenazine. Valbenazine is a specific treatment for TD, which is a side effect of antipsychotic medication.
2. The nurse should anticipate an order to administer the AIMS. AIMS is a rating scale that measures involuntary movements associated with tardive dyskinesia. Facial and tongue movements are symptoms of TD, which is a side effect of antipsychotic medications.
3. Metoprolol is an antihypertensive medication used to treat hypertension. Metoprolol would not be ordered to address facial and tongue movements.
4. A TSH level is used to measure thyroid activity and is not related to antipsychotic medications side effects.
5. The nurse should monitor for uncontrollable abnormal body movements, which are symptoms of TD, a side effect of antipsychotic medications.

3.

1. Forced medication protocols are never the nurse's initial intervention. All other interventions should be implemented prior to forced medication administration.
2. This nurse's statement challenges the client's thoughts and puts the client on the defensive by asking a "Why" question.
3. This nurse's statement presents a hopeful reality without challenging the client and should be the nurse's initial intervention.
4. It may be necessary to administer prn IM antianxiety medications; however, this intervention should be secondary to effective client communication.

4.

Potential Intervention	Indicated	Nonessential	Contraindicated
1. Promote self-esteem		X	
2. Increase the dosage of benztropine			X
3. Apply restraints			X
4. Closely monitor medication administration	X		
5. Establish a trusting relationship	X		

1. Although it is always important to encourage good self-esteem, this intervention is **nonessential** because it does not promote safety and may be misinterpreted by a paranoid and hostile client.
2. Benztropine is a medication used to decrease the extrapyramidal symptoms (EPS) that clients may experience as a side effect of antipsychotic medications. There is no indication that this client is experiencing EPS; therefore, increasing the dosage of benztropine would be **contraindicated.**
3. There is no indication that this client is experiencing behaviors that exhibit an immediate threat to self or others. Therefore, applying restraints would be **contraindicated.**
4. A client who is experiencing paranoid behavior is more likely to avoid swallowing their medications. By not taking medications, both hostility and paranoia may increase, leading to an unsafe environment. Closely monitoring medication administration may prevent "cheeking" (hiding medications between the gums and cheek); therefore, this intervention is **indicated.**
5. A paranoid and hostile client may misinterpret the nurse's attempts to communicate. It is **indicated** for the nurse to utilize therapeutic communication skills in building a trusting relationship.

5.

1. This client is already on suicide precautions. The nurse's immediate next step is to assess the client's plan for self-harm. Further interventions would depend on whether the client's plan is accessible and realistic.
2. Involuntary movements are indications of the side effects of psychotropic medications. Assessment of these side effects does not relate to client ideations of self-harm.
3. It is vital that any ordered medications are administered in a timely manner. However, the nurse's immediate next step would be to assess the client's plan for self-harm.
4. It is important to meet with the family to develop a discharge plan. However, the nurse's immediate next step would be to assess the client's plan for self-harm.

6.

1. A client who willingly takes ordered medications is participating in the plan of care, which indicates successful nursing interventions that have led to the client's improvement.
2. When the client verbalizes that safety can be obtained just as readily at home as in the hospital, the client is minimizing the need for treatment by using the defense mechanism of denial. This denial will hamper the client's overall recovery.
3. By implementing a plan to deal with command hallucinations, the client is participating in the plan of care, which indicates successful nursing interventions that have led to the client's improvement.
4. By participating in formulating a discharge plan, the client is cooperating in the plan of care, which indicates successful nursing interventions that have led to the client's improvement.
5. Even though having voices return may be considered a setback in treatment, the behavior of notifying staff shows recognition that the voices are part of the client's illness.

SUBSTANCE ABUSE CASE STUDY

A client has been using IV heroin daily for the last year. The police were called for a potential overdose. The client was brought to the emergency department via ambulance following administration of a dose of naloxone HCL. The client's vital signs consist of respiratory rate, 8 breaths/min; slow, shallow breaths; pulse, 42 beats/min; blood pressure, 60/48 mm Hg.

1. **Recognize cues: What matters most?** The client is difficult to arouse and is not oriented to person, place, time, or situation. Which nursing intervention should be prioritized?
   1. Place the client on suicide precautions.
   2. Reorient the client to situation.
   3. Assess the client for signs of infection.
   4. Administer a second dose of naloxone HCL.

2. **Analyze cues: What could it mean?**
   Which client behavior would indicate that the second dose of naloxone HCL has been effective? **Select all that apply.**
   1. The client's vital signs consist of respiratory rate, 14 breaths/min; pulse, 80 beats/min; blood pressure, 100/78 mm Hg.
   2. The client appears to be lethargic and starts vomiting.
   3. The client can follow simple commands and is oriented to situation.
   4. The client starts experiencing decreased level of consciousness, with limp arms and legs.
   5. The client talks about their experience leading to the intentional overdose.

3. **Prioritize hypotheses: Where do I start?** The client tells the nurse that they became addicted to pain pills following a motor vehicle crash and have been struggling with depression for years. During the last week, the client has been giving away belongings and saying goodbye to family. The nurse anticipates which additional intervention at this time? **Select all that apply.**
   1. Use open-ended questions and active listening to build rapport.
   2. Place the client on suicide precautions.
   3. Contact the family to gather further information.
   4. Tell the client how substance use is impacting their mental health.
   5. Administer prn medications to help with depression.

4. **Generate solutions: What can I do?** The client has been admitted to the inpatient psychiatric unit. When caring for this client, the nurse applies many interventions to assist in mental health and substance abuse treatment. For each potential nursing intervention, place a check mark in one appropriate box to indicate whether the intervention is *Indicated*, *Nonessential*, or *Contraindicated*.

Potential Intervention	Indicated	Nonessential	Contraindicated
1. Confront the client about behavior impacting family			
2. Monitor for worsening withdrawal symptoms			
3. Discuss the need for drug rehabilitation			
4. Establish a trusting relationship			
5. Maintain suicide precautions			
6. Encourage dual-diagnosis group attendance			

5. **Take action: What will I do?** Frustrated with the rules, on day 2, the client demands to leave. The client angrily states, "I already know all of this stuff." What is the nurse's immediate next step?
   1. Objectively document behavior.
   2. Place the client on elopement precautions.
   3. Discuss seclusion needs with treatment team.
   4. Offer extra snacks to stay in treatment.

6. **Evaluate outcomes: Did it help?** Which of the following assessed client behaviors indicate that nursing interventions have led to the improvement of client symptoms? **Select all that apply.**
   1. The client states, "When I wanted to leave, I was scared, and felt like using."
   2. The client calmly decides to go to the room and rest.
   3. The client decides to join a group in the milieu.
   4. The client watches the doors and paces the hall in front of the nursing station.
   5. The client focuses on other client's problems during group activities.

SUBSTANCE ABUSE CASE STUDY ANSWERS AND RATIONALES

1.

1. It may be necessary at some point to place the client on suicide precautions, but when a client is still exhibiting symptoms consistent with opiate overdose, administering a second dose of naloxone HCL is the nurse's first priority.
2. It is important to reorient a client to the situation, but when the client is still exhibiting symptoms consistent with opiate overdose, administering a second dose of naloxone HCL is the nurse's first priority.
3. It is important to monitor for signs of infections when clients are using IV heroin; however, when the client is exhibiting symptoms consistent with opiate overdose, administering a second dose of naloxone HCL is the nurse's first priority.
4. **The client is still exhibiting symptoms consistent with opiate overdose. Administering a second dose of naloxone HCL to reverse overdose symptoms is the nurse's first priority.**

2.

1. Vital signs consisting of a respiratory rate, 14 breaths/min; pulse, 80 beats/min; and blood pressure, 100/78 mm Hg indicate that the second dose of naloxone HCL has been effective.
2. When a client appears lethargic and vomits, they are exhibiting signs of continued opiate overdose. This would indicate that the second dose of naloxone HCL was not effective.
3. **A second dose of naloxone HCL has been effective when a client can follow simple commands and is oriented to situation. The nurse must recognize that even after naloxone HCL has been administered, the client could experience a return of overdose symptoms. The client would need to be continually monitored for at least 2 hours after the last administered dose.**
4. Decreased levels of consciousness and limp arms and legs are signs of continued opiate overdose, which indicate that the second dose of naloxone HCL was ineffective.
5. It is an indication that the second dose of naloxone HCL has been effective when the client is able to talk about their experience leading to the intentional overdose.

3.

1. **Using open-ended questions and active listening helps the client express their feelings. This builds rapport and establishes a nurse–client relationship. This nursing intervention can open lines of communication to help this client feel safe in expressing emotional pain.**
2. **This client is exhibiting behaviors that indicate thoughts of suicide. Placing the client on suicide precautions is a critical nursing intervention.**
3. Contacting the family to gather further information would be a breach of the Health Insurance Portability and Accountability Act of 1996 (HIPAA) and therefore would not be an appropriate intervention.
4. Substance use does impact mental health symptoms. However, by telling a client this information rather than exploring the subject with the client, the nurse blocks further therapeutic communication.
5. Prn medications may be necessary to help with withdrawal or anxiety symptoms. However, there are no prn medications prescribed to help with depression.

4. **Answer:**

Potential Intervention	Indicated	Nonessential	Contraindicated
1. Confront the client about behavior impacting family			X
2. Monitor for worsening with-drawal symptoms	X		
3. Discuss the need for drug rehabilitation		X	
4. Establish a trusting relationship	X		
5. Maintain suicide precautions	X		
6. Encourage dual-diagnosis group attendance	X		

1. Client confrontation is **contraindicated** because it puts the client on the defensive and impedes further nurse–client interactions.
2. Monitoring for worsening withdrawal symptoms is **indicated** because withdrawal symptoms from opiates can last for days and may require added continued nursing interventions.
3. During a crisis admission, discussing the need for drug rehabilitation is **nonessential.** It is too soon to expect the client to be able to focus on future plans.
4. The establishment of a trusting nurse–client relationship is **indicated** when working with all client populations. Trust is especially essential when discussing options for discharge.
5. Maintaining suicide precautions is **indicated** because the client stated that the overdose was intentional.
6. Encouraging the client to attend dual-diagnosis groups is **indicated.** This will assist the client to better understand the relationship between depression and substance use.

5.

1. It is very important to document this behavior objectively; however, the nurse's immediate next step is to ensure that the client remains on the unit.
2. **The nurse's immediate next step must be to ensure the client's safety by placing the client on elopement precautions.**
3. Discussing the situation with the treatment team is appropriate; however, there is no information that indicates that the client has escalated to the point where seclusion is needed. The nurse's immediate next step must be to ensure the client's safety by placing the client on elopement precautions.
4. Offering extra snacks to stay in treatment is an inappropriate nursing intervention in any circumstance. The nurse's immediate next step must be to ensure the client's safety by placing the client on elopement precautions.

6.

1. **There was an understanding of the underlying emotional cause of substance use when the client realized that the desire to leave the unit was based on fear. This behavior indicates that nursing interventions have led to improved client symptoms.**
2. **When the client shows the ability to calm down and redirect self to their room, this behavior is an indication that nursing interventions have led to the improvement of client symptoms.**

3. A client joining a group in the milieu without incident is an indication that nursing interventions have led to the improvement of client symptoms.

4. A client watching the doors and pacing the halls shows an escalation of tension and frustration. This behavior indicates that nursing interventions have not led to improved client symptoms.

5. A client focusing on another client's problems during group activities shows avoidance of personal issues. This behavior indicates that nursing interventions have not led to improved client symptoms.

Comprehensive Final Examination

18

1. Structure is a component of milieu therapy. Which description is reflective of this component?
   1. Affirmations of a client's individual self-worth promote self-esteem.
   2. Flexible patterns and varied schedules provide opportunities for growth.
   3. Level systems can provide clients with opportunities to earn privileges.
   4. Decreased demands on clients reduce stress.

2. A client diagnosed with panic disorder has a nursing diagnosis of social isolation R/T fear. Using a cognitive approach, which nursing intervention is appropriate?
   1. During a panic attack, remind the client to say, "I know this attack will last only a few minutes."
   2. Discuss what occurred prior to the panic attack in order to note cause and effect.
   3. Encourage the client to acknowledge two trusted individuals who can assist the client during a panic attack.
   4. Remind the client to use a journal to express feelings surrounding the panic attack.

3. A client diagnosed with neurocognitive disorder is becoming increasingly agitated and confused. Which intervention should the nurse implement first?
   1. Request a physician's order for laboratory tests to rule out infection.
   2. Assess the client's vital signs and any obvious physiological changes.
   3. Call the pharmacy to determine possible medication incompatibilities.
   4. Document the findings and notify the oncoming shift of the situation.

4. A nurse is discharging a client diagnosed with obsessive-compulsive personality disorder (OCD). Which employment opportunity is most likely to be recommended by the treatment team?
   1. Home construction.
   2. Air traffic controller.
   3. Night watchman at the zoo.
   4. Prison warden.

5. A client is discussing plans to have a serum lithium carbonate level taken on discharge. To obtain an accurate serum level, which discharge teaching information should be included?
   1. Remind the client to take lithium as prescribed just prior to having the serum level drawn.
   2. Remind the client to have the lithium carbonate serum level drawn after fasting at least 12 hours.
   3. Remind the client to notify the physician if they are exhibiting any signs and symptoms of toxicity.
   4. Remind the client to have a serum level drawn 12 hours after taking a dose of lithium carbonate.

6. A client diagnosed with an antisocial personality disorder is given a nursing diagnosis of defensive coping R/T a dysfunctional family system AEB denial of obvious problems and belligerence. Which client statement would confirm this nursing diagnosis?
   1. "I know what I did was wrong, and I understand the consequences."
   2. "I don't see how I can afford follow-up therapy."
   3. "I'm an angel compared with the rest of my family."
   4. "I go to church but only when it suits me."

7. Which client suicide plan would be considered most lethal?
   1. "While my spouse is sleeping, I will swallow 30 Zoloft pills."
   2. "Although I don't own a gun, I am going to shoot myself."
   3. "I plan to jump from a secluded bridge after midnight."
   4. "I will take 10 Tylenol with codeine right before my spouse comes home."

8. The nurse is teaching a 16-year-old female client, diagnosed with anorexia nervosa, about the potential risk for osteoporosis. Which statement by the client may indicate that further teaching about osteoporosis is necessary?
   1. "I have high estrogen levels, and that is why I am not having periods."
   2. "I have a high level of stress hormone, and this can affect my bones."
   3. "I am not taking in enough calcium, and my bones can be brittle."
   4. "I'm young, so my bone mass hasn't reached its peak. That puts me at risk."

9. A client on a psychiatric unit has continually told the treatment team, "I am not responsible for the breakup of my marriage." Which client statement would indicate that the client is ready to collaborate with the team?
   1. "Okay, I'll agree to talk about my spouse, but you have to know that this is their fault."
   2. "My mother supports me, and in my heart, I know you'll support me too."
   3. "You make me feel special. You kind of look like my spouse."
   4. "Okay, let's sit down and talk to my spouse and work out a counseling plan."

10. When assessing a client diagnosed with paranoid personality disorder, the nurse might identify which of the following characteristic behaviors? **Select all that apply.**
    1. A lack of empathy.
    2. Shyness and emotional coldness.
    3. Suspiciousness without justification.
    4. A lack of remorse for hurting others.
    5. Preoccupation with unjustifiable doubts.

11. Which statement is correct regarding clients with a dual diagnosis?
    1. The substance abuse issue must be addressed first.
    2. The mental health issue must be addressed first.
    3. Dual diagnosis is not possible. Only one diagnosis can be assigned.
    4. The primary focus must be on a holistic view of the client's problems.

12. Which etiological implication reflects social learning theory?
    1. Modeling and identification can be observed from early childhood in individuals exhibiting substance abuse behaviors.
    2. An individual is encouraged to continue using substances because of the pleasure experienced during intoxication.
    3. A child of a parent diagnosed with alcohol use disorder has a four times greater incidence of developing this disorder.
    4. Identical twins have twice the rate for concordance of alcohol use disorder compared with fraternal twins.

13. A nurse is completing a risk assessment on a newly admitted client with increased levels of anxiety. The nurse would document which of the following cognitive symptoms expressed by the client? **Select all that apply.**
    1. Gritting of the teeth.
    2. Changes in tone of voice.
    3. Increased energy.
    4. Misperceptions of stimuli.
    5. Difficulty concentrating.

14. The nurse would include which of the following biological interventions when caring for a client experiencing a panic attack? **Select all that apply.**
    1. Monitor blood pressure and pulse.
    2. Discuss situations surrounding past panic attacks.
    3. Stay with the client when signs and symptoms of a panic attack are present.
    4. Notify the client of the availability of alprazolam prn.
    5. Educate the client regarding how temperament affects anxiety disorders.

15. In which of the following situations would the nurse expect a client to exhibit symptoms of increased anxiety? **Select all that apply.**
    1. A client has a thyroid-stimulating hormone level of 0.03 mIU/L.
    2. A client has a fasting glucose level of 60 mg/dL.
    3. A client is experiencing caffeine intoxication.
    4. A client has a diagnosis of gastroesophageal reflux disease.
    5. A client is experiencing alcohol-induced withdrawal.

16. A client consistently chooses solitary activities, seems indifferent to praise and criticism, and has deficits in the ability to form meaningful personal relationships. Which diagnosis would the nurse expect to be documented?
    1. Schizotypal personality disorder.
    2. Paranoid personality disorder.
    3. Schizoid personality disorder.
    4. Histrionic personality disorder.

17. An adolescent diagnosed with major depression has a nursing diagnosis of social isolation. This client is currently attending groups and communicating with staff. Which statement evaluates this client's behavior accurately?
    1. The nurse is unable to evaluate this adolescent's ability to socialize, based on the observed behaviors.
    2. The client is experiencing a positive outcome exhibited by group attendance and communication with staff.
    3. The nurse is unable to evaluate this adolescent's ability to socialize because the client has not experienced these behaviors for an extended period.
    4. Attending group and communicating with staff are indications of improved self-esteem, not improved social isolation.

18. A client diagnosed with anorexia nervosa is forced into the emergency department (ED) by a family member. During the intake assessment, this family member answers all questions posed to the client. Which nursing intervention is appropriate at this time?
    1. Allow the family member to continue directing the conversation to gather critically needed information.
    2. Empathize with the family member and communicate the need to gain information directly from the client.
    3. Request that the physician ask the family member to wait outside during the assessment.
    4. Request an evaluation by a social worker to assist the client with interpersonal conflicts.

19. Using Kubler-Ross's model of the normal grief response, order the following stages of grief:
    1. _____ Depression.
    2. _____ Bargaining.
    3. _____ Acceptance.
    4. _____ Denial.
    5. _____ Anger.

20. While the nurse is completing an initial interview with a client in the emergency department, the client admits to recent drug use. Which area of assessment should take priority?
    1. The client's chief complaint.
    2. A complete history and physical examination.
    3. Type of drugs used.
    4. Family history.

21. Which of the following can be categorized as a benefit of alcohol use? **Select all that apply.**
    1. When alcohol enhances the flavor of food.
    2. When alcohol promotes celebration at special occasions.
    3. When alcohol is used in religious ceremonies.
    4. When alcohol helps mask stressful situations.
    5. When alcohol is used to cope with unacceptable feelings.

22. A client diagnosed with generalized anxiety disorder is getting ready for discharge. Which statement evaluates the client's cognitive response to nursing interventions?
    1. "The client appears calm; vital signs within normal limits; diaphoresis noted."
    2. "The client states that the breathing techniques used helped to decrease anxiety."
    3. "The client is able to recognize negative self-talk as a sign of increased anxiety."
    4. "The client uses journaling to express frustrations."

23. In which situation is a client at highest risk for lorazepam overdose?
    1. The client exhibits increased tolerance.
    2. The client experiences depression and anxiety.
    3. The client combines the drug with alcohol.
    4. The client takes the drug with antacids.

24. A hypomanic client diagnosed with bipolar II disorder chatters constantly and becomes disruptive in group. The client is forcibly placed in four-point restraints. Which of the following principles were violated in this scenario? **Select all that apply.**
    1. The principle of nonmaleficence.
    2. The principle of veracity.
    3. The principle of least restrictive treatment.
    4. The principle of beneficence.
    5. The principle of negligence.

25. A client diagnosed with bipolar disorder has been taking lithium carbonate for 3 months. Which assessment data would make the nurse request a lithium carbonate level?
    1. Blurred vision and vomiting.
    2. Increased thirst and urination.
    3. Drowsiness and dizziness.
    4. Headache and anorexia.

26. A client states, "I don't know why I'm depressed; my spouse takes care of all my needs. I don't even have to write a check or get a driver's license." Based on this statement, this client is most likely to be diagnosed with which personality disorder?
    1. Schizoid personality disorder.
    2. Histrionic personality disorder.
    3. Dependent personality disorder.
    4. Passive-aggressive personality disorder.

27. Which assessment data support the diagnosis of obsessive-compulsive disorder (OCD)?
    1. The client's thoughts, impulses, and/or images are expressed as worries concerning real-life problems and stressors.
    2. The client is aware at some point during the course of the disorder that the obsessions or compulsions are excessive, unreasonable, or both.
    3. The obsessions or compulsions experienced significantly interfere with only one area of functioning.
    4. The client represses thoughts, impulses, or images and then substitutes other thoughts or behaviors.

28. A client is experiencing hyperventilation, depersonalization, and palpitations. Which nursing diagnosis takes priority?
    1. Social isolation.
    2. Ineffective breathing pattern.
    3. Risk for suicide.
    4. Fatigue.

29. A child diagnosed with Tourette's disorder has a nursing diagnosis of impaired social interaction R/T aggressive behaviors. The child is currently threatening peers and manipulating staff. Which statement accurately evaluates this child's behavior?
    1. The nurse is unable to evaluate this child's ability to interact socially, based on the observed behaviors.
    2. The child is being assertive with peers and staff, which indicates improvement in social interaction.
    3. The nurse is unable to evaluate this child's ability to interact socially because the child has not experienced these behaviors for an extended period.
    4. Interacting with staff and peers by using threats and manipulation can be evaluated as an indication of continued social interaction impairment.

30. In which situation is a client at risk for delayed or inhibited grief?
    1. When a client's family expects the client to maintain normalcy.
    2. When a client experiences denial during the first week after the loss.
    3. When a client experiences anger toward the deceased within 1 month after the loss.
    4. When a client experiences preoccupation with the deceased for 1 year after the loss.

31. A client on an inpatient psychiatric unit is overheard stating, "I visited Miss Emma yesterday while I was out on a pass with my family." Which would the nurse expect to assess as a positive finding in this client's urine drug screen?
    1. Heroin.
    2. Oxycodone.
    3. Phencyclidine.
    4. Morphine.

32. The nurse is planning care for a recently admitted client with a long history of crack cocaine use. The nurse intentionally keeps the treatment plan simple. Which is the underlying rationale for this decision?
    1. The client would be unable to focus because of the use of denial.
    2. The client is at high risk for mild to moderate cognitive problems.
    3. Physical complications would impede learning.
    4. The client has arrested in developmental progression.

33. A client diagnosed with aquaphobia begins a therapeutic process in which they must stand in a pool for 1 hour. This is called _____ therapy.

34. A client diagnosed with schizophrenia is experiencing emotional ambivalence. When the nurse educates the client's family, which would best describe this symptom?
    1. An inward focus on a fantasy world.
    2. The simultaneous need for and fear of intimacy.
    3. Impairment in social functioning, including social isolation.
    4. The lack of emotional expression.

35. A client with extreme suicidal ideations needs to be admitted to the locked psychiatric unit. There are no beds available. Which client would the nurse anticipate that the treatment team would discharge?
    1. A client involuntarily committed 2 days ago with situational depression.
    2. A client voluntarily committed 2 days ago for alcohol detoxification.
    3. A client voluntarily committed 4 days ago with alterations in cognition related to a urinary tract infection.
    4. A client involuntarily committed 5 days ago due to experiencing command hallucinations.

36. A client admitted to an inpatient psychiatric unit has given written informed consent to participate in a medication research study. The client states, "I have changed my mind and don't want to take that medication." Which is the priority nursing intervention?
    1. Tell the client that once the forms are signed, the client must continue with the research.
    2. Tell the client that withdrawal from the research can be done at any time.
    3. Tell the client that they should have not been allowed to participate because of a thought disorder.
    4. Tell the client that they can withdraw only if the physician gives permission.

37. Which of the following rights are afforded to a client who is admitted to an inpatient psychiatric unit as a danger to self? **Select all that apply.**
    1. The right to refuse medications.
    2. The right to leave the locked facility at any time.
    3. The right to expect treatment that does no harm.
    4. The right to know the truth about their illness.
    5. The right to be treated equally.

38. Which situation reflects the defense mechanism of displacement?
    1. A disgruntled employee confronts and shouts at their boss.
    2. A disgruntled employee takes their boss and spouse out to dinner.
    3. A disgruntled employee inappropriately punishes their child.
    4. A disgruntled employee tells their child how much they like their job and boss.

39. A client diagnosed with alcohol use disorder has been recently diagnosed with peripheral neuropathy. Which nursing diagnosis addresses this client's problem?
    1. Altered coping R/T substance abuse AEB a long history of alcoholism.
    2. Pain R/T effects of alcohol AEB complaints of 6/10 pain.
    3. Powerlessness R/T substance abuse AEB no control over drinking.
    4. Altered sensory perception R/T effects of alcohol AEB visual hallucinations.

40. A physically abused child diagnosed with conduct disorder bullies and threatens peers on a psychiatric unit. Which nursing diagnosis would take priority?
    1. Risk for self-mutilation R/T low self-esteem.
    2. Ineffective individual coping R/T physical abuse.
    3. Impaired social interaction R/T neurological alterations.
    4. Risk for violence: directed at others R/T displaced anger.

41. A client is diagnosed with alcohol-induced neurocognitive disorder. Which intervention is appropriate for this client's nursing diagnosis of altered sensory perception?
    1. Assess vital signs.
    2. Decrease environmental stimuli.
    3. Maintain a nonjudgmental approach.
    4. Empathetically confront denial.

42. Of women who give birth, _____% to _____% experience postpartum blues.

43. The nurse is evaluating a client diagnosed with an antisocial personality disorder. Which client statement is reflective of this diagnosis?
    1. "I feel so guilty about hurting them, but I just lost control."
    2. "I'm very afraid when the voices tell me to kill myself."
    3. "I don't have a problem. It's your problem for misunderstanding."
    4. "I find it easier to be alone than with my family."

44. A client diagnosed with posttraumatic stress disorder after a rape states, "Even though I know it is important, I just can't go to my gynecologist." Which nursing diagnosis reflects this client's problem?
   1. Posttrauma syndrome R/T previous rape AEB unrealistic fear.
   2. Nonadherence R/T trauma AEB avoiding yearly examination.
   3. Knowledge deficit R/T importance of follow-up care AEB refusal to adhere to scheduled yearly appointment.
   4. Altered health maintenance R/T no yearly gynecological examination AEB canceled appointment.

45. The nurse focuses on exploration of alternatives rather than providing answers or advice. This is one of the many strategies of nonthreatening feedback. Which nursing statement is an example of this strategy?
   1. "You should sign up for the Alcoholics Anonymous (AA) meetings to help in your recovery."
   2. "Let's discuss past successful coping mechanisms that you can try after discharge."
   3. "I have found that others with problems like yours need an AA sponsor."
   4. "You need a hobby to get your mind off of alcohol."

46. Within the community, which nursing intervention is aimed at reducing the prevalence of psychiatric illness by shortening the duration of the illness?
   1. Teaching techniques of stress management.
   2. Providing classes on parenting skills.
   3. Providing education and support to the homeless.
   4. Staffing suicide hotlines.

47. A nurse is assessing a client being treated for a fractured leg. History reveals that the client's parent and grandparent died of complications of alcohol use disorder. The client admits using alcohol to reduce stress. Which statement is most likely true?
   1. The client is in the pre-alcoholic phase of drinking patterns and has a genetic predisposition to alcoholism.
   2. The client is in the early alcoholic phase of drinking patterns and has a biological tendency to drink.
   3. The client is in the crucial phase of drinking patterns and has learned from their family to reduce stress by drinking.
   4. The client is in the chronic phase of drinking patterns and needs medication to detox safely from alcohol.

48. A confused, tremulous, diaphoretic client with a short history of heavy drinking has a pulse rate of 120 beats/min, respirations of 24/min, and blood pressure of 180/90 mm Hg. Which would be the suspected cause of these symptoms?
   1. Wernicke-Korsakoff syndrome.
   2. Alcohol-induced neurocognitive disorder.
   3. Alcohol-induced withdrawal.
   4. Acute alcoholic myopathy.

49. Which of the following factors places a client at high risk for a suicide attempt? **Select all that apply.**
   1. A previous suicide attempt.
   2. Access to lethal methods.
   3. Isolation.
   4. Lack of a physical illness.
   5. Impulsive or aggressive tendencies.

50. Which disorder includes the diagnostic criteria of patterns of negativity, disobedience, and hostile behavior toward authority figures?
   1. Separation anxiety disorder.
   2. Oppositional defiant disorder (ODD).
   3. Narcissistic personality disorder.
   4. Autism spectrum disorder.

51. Which statement about attention deficit-hyperactivity disorder (ADHD) is true?
    1. ADHD is characterized by a persistent pattern of withdrawal into self.
    2. ADHD is frequently diagnosed before age 2.
    3. ADHD occurs equally among girls and boys.
    4. ADHD is characterized by a persistent pattern of inattention.

52. A client is diagnosed with somatic symptom disorder. When planning care, which nursing intervention should be included?
    1. Avoid discussing symptoms experienced.
    2. Encourage exploration of the source of anxiety.
    3. Remind the client about previous negative test results.
    4. Redirect the client to the physician when somatic complaints are expressed.

53. The nurse focuses on feedback that serves the needs of the client and not the needs of the nurse. This is one of the many strategies of nonthreatening feedback. Which nursing statement is an example of this strategy?
    1. "I had an eating disorder when I was 16. Let me tell you how I felt."
    2. "It upsets me to see your parent so worried about you."
    3. "Tell me about how you feel when you purge."
    4. "My friends teased me in high school, and I ignored them. Why not try that?"

54. A client monitored in an outpatient psychiatric clinic is taking clozapine 200 mg bid. The absolute neutrophil count (ANC) is 600 cells per microliter. Based on these values, which nursing intervention is appropriate?
    1. Stop the medication and call the physician because of the low ANC.
    2. Stop the medication and call the physician because of the high ANC.
    3. Give the medication because the ANC is within normal range.
    4. Give the medication but notify the physician about the abnormal ANC.

55. A client is diagnosed with obsessive-compulsive personality disorder. In which cluster would the *Diagnostic and Statistical Manual of Mental Disorders*, Fifth Edition, Text Revision *(DSM-5-TR)* categorize this personality?
    1. Cluster A.
    2. Cluster B.
    3. Cluster C.
    4. Cluster D.

56. During a nursing interaction, a client, although interacting appropriately, does not make eye contact. Which is a true statement about this nonverbal communication?
    1. Nonverbal communication is controlled by the conscious mind.
    2. Nonverbal communication carries less weight than what the client says.
    3. Nonverbal communication does not have the same meaning for everyone.
    4. Nonverbal communication generally is a poor reflection of what the client is feeling.

57. A nurse, administering a medication for ADHD, believes the client is cheeking the medication. Which of the following medications would limit cheeking? **Select all that apply.**
    1. Dyanavel XR (d- & l-amphetamine).
    2. Quillivant XR (methylphenidate).
    3. Contempla XR-ODT (methylphenidate extended base).
    4. Adzenys XR-ODT (d- & l-amphetamine).
    5. Kapvay (clonidine extended release).

58. The nurse is interacting with a client on the inpatient unit. The client states, "Most forward action grows life double plays circle uniform." Which charting entry should the nurse record about this client's statement?
    1. "Client is experiencing circumstantiality."
    2. "Client is communicating by the use of word salad."
    3. "Client is communicating tangentially."
    4. "Client is perseverating."

59. When a client experiences a manic episode, the nurse would expect to assess which of the following? **Select all that apply.**
    1. Grandiosity.
    2. Flight of ideas.
    3. Pressured speech.
    4. Frequent short naps for rest.
    5. Psychomotor agitation.

60. A client diagnosed with bipolar disorder states, "My mom has a history of depression." When the nurse uses a biological theory to teach about predisposing factors, which client statement indicates that teaching has been successful?
    1. "I am going to weigh the pros and cons before having children."
    2. "My negative thoughts about myself are making me worse."
    3. "It is entirely my mother's fault that I have this disorder."
    4. "I learned how to cope by watching my family interactions."

61. A client diagnosed with a schizophrenia spectrum disorder is having trouble expressing fears about impending discharge to the treatment team. Functioning in the role of an advocate, which is an appropriate nursing response?
    1. "Would you like me to explain how to increase your assertiveness skills?"
    2. "Let's see how you have effectively communicated to the team in the past."
    3. "I'll be with you when you talk to the team. I'll remind you of your concerns."
    4. "I can appreciate how stressful it is to talk to the team. Let's discuss it."

62. Which tool is used to assess for tardive dyskinesia?
    1. The CAGE assessment tool.
    2. Mini-Mental State Examination (MMSE).
    3. The Abnormal Involuntary Movement Scale (AIMS).
    4. Clock face assessment.

63. The student nurse is learning about dissociative identity disorder (DID). Which student statement indicates that learning has occurred?
    1. "Individuals with DID are unable to function in social or occupational situations."
    2. "The transition from one personality to another is usually sudden, often dramatic, and usually precipitated by stress."
    3. "DID is a personality disorder, commonly called multiple personality disorder."
    4. "All personalities are aware of one another, and events that take place are known by all the different personalities."

64. A client diagnosed with somatic symptom disorder who is experiencing pain is admitted to an inpatient psychiatric unit. Which client statement would the nurse assess as evidence of primary gain?
    1. "Experiencing severe back pain has taken my mind off my pending divorce."
    2. "My parent only listens to me when I am complaining about the pain."
    3. "Because of my pain disorder, I had to apply for disability."
    4. "When I tell people about my pain, they are very sympathetic to my situation."

65. A client is exhibiting sedation, auditory hallucinations, akathisia, and anhedonia. The client is prescribed haloperidol 5 mg tid and trihexyphenidyl 4 mg bid. Which statement about these medications is accurate?
    1. The trihexyphenidyl would address the client's auditory hallucinations.
    2. The trihexyphenidyl would counteract the akathisia.
    3. The haloperidol would address the anhedonia.
    4. The haloperidol would decrease the amount of sedation exhibited.

66. The nurse is interviewing a client who is experiencing a nihilistic delusion. Which client statement confirms the presence of this symptom?
    1. "The doctor says I'm not pregnant, but I know that I am."
    2. "Someone is trying to get a message to me through the articles in this magazine."
    3. "The world no longer exists."
    4. "The FBI has bugged my room, and they intend to kill me."

67. A client has an intelligence quotient (IQ) level of 30. Which client cognitive/educational capability would the nurse expect to observe?
    1. The client is capable of academic skills to a second-grade level.
    2. The client, with supervision, may respond to minimal training in self-help.
    3. The client would profit only from systematic habit training.
    4. The client is capable of academic skills to a sixth-grade level.

68. A client with anorexia who was recently deserted by a spouse is admitted to an inpatient psychiatric unit with a diagnosis of major depressive disorder. Which nursing diagnosis takes priority at this time?
    1. Social isolation R/T fear of failure.
    2. Imbalanced nutrition, less than body requirements R/T depressed mood.
    3. Powerlessness R/T a lifestyle of helplessness.
    4. Low self-esteem R/T fear of abandonment.

69. Which is the purpose of providing psychiatric/mental health nursing care?
    1. To recognize and address the client's patterns of response to actual or potential problems.
    2. To gather client data related to psychiatric illness, mental health problems, and potential comorbid physical illnesses.
    3. To focus nursing interventions on the diagnoses described in *DSM-5-TR*.
    4. To assist the physician in delivering comprehensive holistic client care.

70. Which is a behavioral influence on a client's sleep patterns?
    1. Sleep requirements increase during mental stress.
    2. During periods of intense learning, more sleep is required.
    3. Adolescents tend to sleep late, and older adults awaken early.
    4. Sleep can be used to avoid stressful situations.

71. The nurse is assessing a client diagnosed with an autism spectrum disorder. According to Mahler's theory of object relations, which describes the client's unmet developmental need?
    1. The need for survival and comfort.
    2. The need for awareness of an external source of fulfillment.
    3. The need for awareness of separateness of self.
    4. The need for internalization of a sustained image of a love object/person.

72. Thiamine deficiency is a major problem for clients diagnosed with alcohol use disorder. Of the presenting signs and symptoms caused by this deficiency, which is most life threatening?
    1. Paralysis of ocular muscles, diplopia, ataxia, somnolence, and stupor.
    2. Impaired mental functioning, apathy, euphoria or depression, sleep disturbance, and increasing confusion leading to coma.
    3. Nausea and vomiting, anorexia, weight loss, abdominal pain, jaundice, edema, anemia, and blood coagulation abnormalities.
    4. Impaired platelet production and risk for hemorrhage.

73. Which drug is commonly prescribed for clients diagnosed with narcolepsy?
    1. Barbiturates.
    2. Analgesics.
    3. Amphetamines.
    4. Benzodiazepines.

74. Difficulty initiating or maintaining sleep is to *insomnia* as parasomnia is to:
    1. Sleep disorders that are misaligned between sleep and waking behaviors.
    2. Excessive sleepiness or seeking excessive amounts of sleep.
    3. Unusual and undesirable behaviors that occur during sleep.
    4. Temporary cessation of breathing while sleeping.

75. Which factor is associated with the etiology of ADHD from a genetic perspective?
    1. Inborn error of metabolism.
    2. Having a sibling diagnosed with ADHD.
    3. A possible dopamine neurotransmitter deficit.
    4. Retarded id development.

76. A client diagnosed with an antisocial personality disorder has a nursing diagnosis of ineffective coping R/T parental neglect AEB "I broke the jerk's arm, but he deserved it." Which short-term correctly written outcome is appropriate for this client's problem?
    1. The client will be able to delay immediate gratification after discharge from the hospital.
    2. The client will verbalize understanding of unit rules and consequences for infractions by end of shift.
    3. The client will eventually have insight into negative behaviors and establish meaningful relationships.
    4. The client will verbalize personal responsibility for difficulties experienced in interpersonal relationships within the year.

77. A 60-year-old woman has been experiencing delusions of persecution, a depressed mood, and flat affect for 6 months. Which of the following factors would rule out a diagnosis of schizophrenia at this time? **Select all that apply.**
    1. A medical condition has not been assessed and ruled out.
    2. The client complains of depressed mood.
    3. The client's age is not typical.
    4. The client is experiencing the negative symptom of a flat affect.
    5. The client is a woman.

78. A client diagnosed with antisocial personality disorder is facing a 20-year prison term. The client has been prescribed sertraline for depressed mood. Which intervention would take priority?
    1. Monitor the client for suicidal ideations related to depressed mood.
    2. Discuss the need to take medications, even when symptoms improve.
    3. Instruct the client about the risks of stopping the medication abruptly.
    4. Remind the client that it takes 6 to 8 weeks for the medication's full effect to occur.

79. A client is newly admitted to an inpatient psychiatric unit. The following nursing diagnoses are formulated for this client. Which of these would the nurse prioritize?
    1. Defensive coping R/T dysfunctional family process.
    2. Risk for self-directed violence R/T depressed mood.
    3. Impaired social interactions R/T lack of social skills.
    4. Anxiety R/T fear of hospitalization.

80. Which describes the therapeutic communication technique referred to as *focusing?*
    1. Being fully present for a client as information is gathered.
    2. Verification of assumed meaning.
    3. Repetition of the main meaning.
    4. Concentration on one particular theme.

81. A 16-year-old client has a 6-month history of binge eating, abuse of laxatives, and feeling "down." Which statement most accurately describes this client's problem?
    1. The client meets the criteria for bulimia nervosa.
    2. The client meets the criteria for anorexia nervosa.
    3. The client meets the criteria for binge-eating disorder.
    4. The client is exhibiting normal developmental tasks according to Erikson.

82. What specific information is important to teach a client who has recently been prescribed ziprasidone?
    1. It may take 6 to 8 weeks to see the full effect on bothersome symptoms.
    2. Blood work needs to be drawn every 2 weeks to monitor for low neutrophil count.
    3. To ensure absorption, take this medication on a full stomach.
    4. Use diet and regular exercise to reduce the potential weight gain.

83. A nursing instructor is teaching the neurochemical effects of escitalopram. Which student statement indicates an understanding of the content presented?
    1. "Escitalopram increases the amount of norepinephrine available in the synapse."
    2. "Escitalopram encourages the reuptake of norepinephrine at the postsynaptic site."
    3. "Escitalopram encourages the reuptake of serotonin at the postsynaptic site."
    4. "Escitalopram increases the amount of serotonin available in the synapse."

84. Which client statement would best support the nursing diagnosis of ineffective coping R/T recent loss of spouse?
    1. "I use the gym to take my mind off of my loss."
    2. "A glass or two of wine before bedtime helps me sleep."
    3. "My doctor prescribed Ambien for 1 week to help me sleep at night."
    4. "I know I need help, and therapy can help me get through this rough time."

85. Which of the following situations would place a client at high risk for a life-threatening hypertensive crisis? **Select all that apply.**
    1. A client is prescribed phenelzine and fluoxetine.
    2. A client is prescribed phenelzine and warfarin sodium.
    3. A client is prescribed phenelzine and docusate sodium.
    4. A client is prescribed phenelzine and metformin.
    5. A client is prescribed phenelzine and diet pills.

86. A client states, "After retirement, my spouse divorced me, and my children left for college." The nurse responds, "It sounds to me like you are feeling pretty lonely." Which is a description of the therapeutic technique used by the nurse?
    1. Giving the client the opportunity to collect and organize thoughts.
    2. Helping the client to verbalize feelings that are being indirectly expressed.
    3. Striving to explain that which is vague or incomprehensible.
    4. Repeating the main idea of what the client has said.

87. A client diagnosed with major depression has a nursing diagnosis of low self-esteem. Which is an appropriate, correctly written short-term outcome related to this diagnosis?
    1. The client will verbalize two positive things about self by day 2.
    2. The client will exhibit increased feelings of self-worth by day 3.
    3. The client will set realistic outcomes and try to reach them.
    4. The client will demonstrate a decrease in fear of failure.

88. A client states, "I know that the night nurse has cast a spell on me." Which nursing diagnosis reflects this client's problem?
    1. Disturbed sensory perception.
    2. Disturbed thought process.
    3. Impaired verbal communication.
    4. Social isolation.

89. Which of the following situations would place a client at high risk for a life-threatening hypertensive crisis? **Select all that apply.**
    1. A client is prescribed isocarboxazid and drinks orange juice.
    2. A client is prescribed tranylcypromine and takes a diet pill.
    3. A client is prescribed isocarboxazid and has Cheerios for breakfast.
    4. A client is prescribed tranylcypromine and has a bowl of oatmeal.
    5. A client is prescribed tranylcypromine and eats miso soup.

90. A client diagnosed with body dysmorphic disorder has a nursing diagnosis of self-esteem disturbance. Which short-term outcome is appropriate for this nursing diagnosis?
    1. The client will participate in self-care by day 5.
    2. The client will express two positive attributes about self by day 3.
    3. The client will demonstrate one coping skill to decrease anxiety by day 4.
    4. The client will interact with peers in school during this fall semester.

91. A client diagnosed with AIDS becomes confused and has fluctuating memory loss, difficulty concentrating, and diminished motor speed. Which would be the probable cause of this client's symptoms?
    1. Impaired immune response.
    2. Persistent generalized lymphadenopathy.
    3. Kaposi's sarcoma (KS).
    4. Neurocognitive disorder due to HIV.

92. Believing in the dignity and worth of a client is to *respect* as acceptance and a nonjudgmental attitude is to:
    1. Trust.
    2. Rapport.
    3. Genuineness.
    4. Empathy.

93. A client diagnosed with major depressive disorder is prescribed bupropion and sertraline. The client states, "Why am I on two antidepressants?" Which is the best nursing response?
    1. "The bupropion assists with smoking cessation while the sertraline treats depressive symptoms."
    2. "Sertraline assists with the negative side effects of bupropion."
    3. "The medications treat the symptoms of depression through different mechanisms of action."
    4. "Both medications help with symptoms of anxiety along with depression."

94. Three weeks ago, a client suddenly developed a blunt affect and began exhibiting both eccentric behavior and impaired role functioning. These symptoms are reflective of which phase in the development of schizophrenia?
    1. Phase I—schizoid personality.
    2. Phase II—prodromal phase.
    3. Phase III—schizophrenia.
    4. Phase IV—residual phase.

95. Which intervention is a nurse's priority when working with a client suspected of having a conversion disorder?
    1. Avoid situations in which secondary gains may occur.
    2. Confront the client with the fact that anxiety is the cause of physical symptoms.
    3. Teach the client alternative coping skills to use during times of stress.
    4. Monitor assessments, laboratory reports, and vital signs to rule out organic pathology.

96. Which is an example of the therapeutic technique referred to as *exploring*?
    1. "Was this before or after . . . ?"
    2. "And after that, you . . . ?"
    3. "Give me an example of. . . ."
    4. "How does that compare with . . . ?"

97. A client becomes agitated in group therapy and yells, "You are all making me worse!" Which would be an appropriate response from the group leader?
    1. "You sound angry and frustrated. Can you tell us more about it?"
    2. "Maybe you would like to go to another group from now on."
    3. "We will talk more about this during our individual session."
    4. "What do the other group members think?"

98. A client admitted to an inpatient psychiatric unit following a manic episode is prescribed lithium carbonate 300 mg bid. Which serum lithium carbonate level would the nurse expect on discharge?
    1. 0.9 mEq/L.
    2. 1.4 mEq/L.
    3. 1.9 mEq/L.
    4. 2.4 mEq/L.

99. Which of the following are tasks of the orientation phase of the nurse–client relationship? **Select all that apply.**
    1. Establish a contract for intervention.
    2. Identify client's strengths and limitations.
    3. Problem-solve situational crises.
    4. Promote client's insight and perception of reality.
    5. Formulate nursing diagnostic statements.

100. A client has been admitted to an inpatient psychiatric unit expressing suicidal ideations, and complains of insomnia and feelings of hopelessness. During an admission assessment, which nursing intervention takes priority?
    1. Using humor in the interview to uplift the client's mood.
    2. Evaluating blood work, including thyroid panel and electrolytes.
    3. Teaching the client relaxation techniques.
    4. Evaluating any family history of mental illness.

The correct answer number and rationale for why it is the correct answer are given in **boldface blue type.** Rationales for why the other answer options are incorrect are given as well, but they are not in boldface type.

1. 1. Affirmation of a client's individual self-worth is a description of validation, another component of milieu therapy.
   2. Formal and informal structure is provided to assist the client in feeling secure. Flexible patterns and varied schedules may not provide this security.
   3. **Level systems can be used as a form of structure in milieu therapy.**
   4. The milieu provides an environment that decreases demands on the client and decreases stress. This is a description of support, another component of milieu therapy.

TEST-TAKING HINT: Reviewing the components of milieu therapy, which include meeting physiological needs, appropriate physical facilities, democratic self-government, assigned responsibilities, structure, and inclusion of family and community, assists the test taker in determining the correct answer to this question.

2. 1. **Reminding a client to challenge their thought process in ways such as "I know this attack will last only a few minutes" is an intervention that supports a cognitive approach.**
   2. Discussing what occurred prior to a panic attack in order to note cause and effect is a behavioral, not cognitive, approach.
   3. Encouraging the client to acknowledge two individuals the client trusts to assist them through a panic attack is an intervention that supports an interpersonal, not cognitive, approach.
   4. Reminding the client to use a journal to express feelings surrounding the panic attack is an intervention that supports an intrapersonal, not cognitive, approach.

TEST-TAKING HINT: When reviewing appropriate nursing interventions used during a panic attack, the test taker should pair the interventions being used with the theory that the intervention supports. This assists the test taker to be familiar with the theory that supports the intervention.

3. 1. Before requesting a physician's order for laboratory tests to rule out infection, it is important for the nurse to complete an initial physical assessment.
   2. **Assessing the client's vital signs and any obvious physiological changes alerts the nurse to immediate problems the client may be experiencing. The physician, when notified, would need access to the client's vital signs and presenting symptoms before formulating instructions and orders.**
   3. Calling the pharmacy to determine possible medication incompatibilities may be an important step in determining a client's problem, but this intervention would occur after an initial physical assessment.
   4. Accurate, comprehensive, and concise documentation is a vital aspect of nursing practice and should be completed in a timely manner. However, an initial physical assessment must be completed before documentation.

TEST-TAKING HINT: The test taker must recognize keywords in the question. In this case, the keyword is *first*. The first step of the nursing process is a complete client assessment; this information determines further appropriate interventions.

4. 1. The flexibility and mobility of construction work, which uses physical versus interpersonal skills, may be best suited for a client diagnosed with antisocial personality disorder. These clients tend to exploit and manipulate others, and construction work would provide less opportunity for the client to exhibit these behaviors. A client diagnosed with obsessive-compulsive personality disorder (OCD) would not be suited for this job.
   2. **Individuals diagnosed with OCD are inflexible and lack spontaneity. They are meticulous and work diligently and patiently at tasks that require accuracy and discipline. They are especially concerned with matters of organization and efficiency and tend to be rigid and unbending about rules and procedures, making them good candidates for the job of air traffic controller.**

3. Clients diagnosed with schizoid personality disorder experience an inability to form close, personal relationships. These clients are comfortable with animal companionship, making a night watchman job at the zoo an ideal occupation. This type of job would be unsuitable for a client diagnosed with OCD.

4. Individuals diagnosed with narcissistic personality disorder have an exaggerated sense of self-worth. They tend to exploit others to fulfill their own desires. Because they view themselves as superior beings, they believe they are entitled to special rights and privileges. Because the need to control others is inherent in the job of prison warden, this would be an appropriate job choice for a client diagnosed with narcissistic personality and inappropriate for a client diagnosed with OCD.

TEST-TAKING HINT: To answer this question correctly, the test taker must be familiar with the characteristics of the various personality disorders and how these traits would affect employment opportunities.

5. Lithium carbonate is a mood stabilizer that is used for individuals diagnosed with bipolar affective disorder. The margin between the therapeutic and toxic levels of lithium carbonate is very narrow.

1. If the client takes lithium carbonate just prior to having a serum level drawn, the results may be abnormally high, and the lithium dosage would be based on inaccurate data.

2. The client does not have to be fasting for the serum lithium level to be drawn.

3. It is important for the client to know the signs and symptoms of toxicity and to notify the physician if these occur; however, this statement does not answer the question. The question is asking for specific teaching regarding obtaining an accurate serum lithium carbonate level and not about general teaching needs regarding lithium carbonate treatment.

4. **The nurse needs to stress the importance of having the serum lithium carbonate level drawn 12 hours after the client's last dose for accurate monitoring. It is important that the client understand that the level can be altered if this instruction is not followed. If lithium carbonate dosage is based on inaccurate serum levels, clients can be in danger of relapse or toxicity.**

TEST-TAKING HINT: The test taker must understand the importance of timing in obtaining
accurate serum lithium carbonate levels to answer this question correctly.

6. The definition of *defensive coping* is the repeated projection of falsely positive self-evaluations, based on a self-protective pattern that defends against underlying perceived threats to positive self-regard.

1. Admitting guilt and accepting the consequences are not behaviors that would be expected from a client diagnosed with an antisocial personality disorder. Clients with antisocial personality disorders experience no guilt. No defensive coping is presented in this answer choice.

2. Realistically and honestly recognizing a problem is not a behavior that would be expected from a client diagnosed with an antisocial personality disorder. Clients with antisocial personality disorders are unrealistic with their expectations. No defensive coping is presented in this answer choice.

3. **Symptoms including denial of obvious problems, belligerence, and the projection of inappropriate behaviors onto others are indicative of defensive coping and would confirm this as an appropriate nursing diagnosis.**

4. A client diagnosed with antisocial personality disorder tends to be egocentric (focused on self); however, this statement does not reflect defensive coping behaviors.

TEST-TAKING HINT: To answer this question correctly, the test taker must recognize defensive coping as the client's need to protect their ego.

7. 1. Overdosing on a selective serotonin reuptake inhibitor (SSRI), such as sertraline (Zoloft), is less likely to be deadly. Also, if a spouse is sleeping in the same house, the client has an increased likelihood of being rescued.

2. Although a client's plan to shoot themselves is potentially lethal, this client does not own a gun. Clients without access to the means to commit suicide are less likely and able to carry out the plan.

3. **In this situation, the client has access to the bridge, the means to carry out the plan, and is less likely to be rescued. In relation to the other plans presented, this plan is the most lethal.**

4. Although overdosing on acetaminophen (Tylenol) and codeine is potentially lethal, the client's timing of taking the pills right before the spouse returns home increases the likelihood of the client being discovered and rescued.

TEST-TAKING HINT: To answer this question correctly, the test taker must recognize situations that increase the risk of a client completing a suicide attempt successfully.

8. 1. Female clients diagnosed with anorexia nervosa have low, not high, estrogen levels and experience amenorrhea. These low estrogen levels place clients at risk for osteoporosis. This client's statement does not indicate an understanding of this fact, and more teaching is necessary.

2. Increased levels of cortisol are present in clients diagnosed with anorexia nervosa. Based on the client's statement, the client understands that these increased levels put her at risk for osteoporosis.

3. Clients diagnosed with anorexia nervosa have inadequate vitamin and mineral intake, including calcium. Based on the client's statement, the client understands that calcium is essential for bone strength and prevention of osteoporosis.

4. In most women, anorexia nervosa is diagnosed before peak bone mass is achieved. Peak bone mass occurs at approximately age 24. Based on the client's statement, the client understands that reduced bone mass levels put her at risk for osteoporosis.

TEST-TAKING HINT: To answer this question correctly, the test taker must recognize incorrect information in the client's statement that would indicate the need for further instruction.

9. 1. This example of resistance is often caused by the client's unwillingness to change when the need for change is recognized. It also involves the client's reluctance to verbalize and/or accept troubling aspects of themselves.

2. This example of transference occurs when the client unconsciously displaces (or transfers) to the nurse feelings formed toward a person from their past. Transference also can take the form of overwhelming affection with unrealistic expectations of the nurse. When the nurse does not meet the expectations, the client may become angry and hostile. When a client is experiencing transference, it may hamper the client's openness to change.

3. In this example, transference refers to the client's behavioral and emotional response to the nurse. These feelings may be related to unresolved feelings toward the client's spouse. When a client is

experiencing transference, it may hamper the client's openness to change.

4. This example of collaboration reflects the treatment team and client working together and becoming involved in the client's goals and plan of care. Collaboration has great relevance in psychiatric nursing and encourages clients to recognize their own problems and needs.

TEST-TAKING HINT: To answer this question correctly, the test taker must be able to recognize a client statement that supports the readiness to collaborate with the treatment team.

10. 1. Clients diagnosed with narcissistic, not paranoid, personality disorder present with a pervasive pattern of grandiosity, a need for admiration, and a lack of empathy for others. Most individuals diagnosed with a cluster B personality disorder characteristically do not show empathy toward others.

2. Clients diagnosed with schizoid, not paranoid, personality disorder present with a pervasive pattern of detachment from social relationships and generally seem to be shy and emotionally cold.

3. **Clients diagnosed with paranoid personality disorder present with a pervasive distrust and suspiciousness of others and are preoccupied with unjustified doubts about the loyalty or trustworthiness of friends or associates.**

4. Clients diagnosed with antisocial, not paranoid, personality disorder present with a pervasive pattern of disregard for, and violation of, the rights of others. These individuals show a lack of remorse, as indicated by being indifferent to, or rationalizing, having hurt, mistreated, or stolen from others.

5. **Clients diagnosed with paranoid personality disorder experience a preoccupation with unjustified doubts about the loyalty or trustworthiness of friends or associates.**

TEST-TAKING HINT: To answer this question correctly, the test taker must pair characteristic behaviors with various personality disorders.

11. A dual diagnosis is defined as the presence of mental illness in a client with a history of concurrent substance use disorder.

1. In a dual-diagnosis situation, substance abuse and mental illness should be equally prioritized.

2. In a dual-diagnosis situation, mental illness and substance abuse should be equally prioritized.

3. Clients can be designated as having a variety of psychiatric diagnoses. Generalized anxiety disorder and major depressive disorder often occur together. Substance use and mood disorder could occur with any of these diagnoses, resulting in a dual diagnosis.

4. **Substance abuse and any other diagnosis of mental disorder must be treated concurrently to provide holistic client care. Both should be a priority consideration.**

TEST-TAKING HINT: To answer this question correctly, the test taker must recognize that the nursing focus is on holistic care of the client. The test taker should review terminology related to dual diagnosis.

12. 1. **This etiological implication is from a social learning perspective based on family influence.**
   2. This etiological implication is from a conditioning, not social learning, perspective based on the fact that many substances create a pleasurable experience that encourages the user to repeat the use of the substance.
   3. This etiological implication is from a genetic, not social learning, perspective based on the fact that hereditary factors are involved in the development of substance use disorders.
   4. This etiological implication is from a genetic, not social learning, perspective based on the fact that hereditary factors are involved in the development of substance use disorders.

TEST-TAKING HINT: Etiology is the cause or causative factors from which a disorder develops. All of the answer choices can be causes of substance use disorder development, but only answer 1 is from a social learning perspective.

13. 1. Gritting the teeth is a behavioral, not cognitive, sign that the nurse would want to document during a risk assessment.
   2. Changes in tone of voice are behavioral, not cognitive, signs that the nurse would want to document during a risk assessment.
   3. Increased energy is a behavioral, not cognitive, sign that the nurse would want to document during a risk assessment.
   4. **A misperception of stimuli, such as mistaking a handshake for an aggressive act, is a cognitive sign that the nurse would want to document during a risk assessment.**

5. Difficulty concentrating is a cognitive sign that the nurse would want to document during a risk assessment.

TEST-TAKING HINT: To answer this question correctly, the test taker must understand that cognitive symptoms consist of faulty, distorted, or counterproductive thinking patterns that accompany or precede maladaptive behaviors.

14. 1. **Blood pressure and pulse increase during panic attacks. Monitoring these vital signs is a biological intervention when caring for clients experiencing panic attacks.**
   2. Because of decreased levels of concentration and narrowed perceptions associated with panic attacks, this discussion is inappropriate at this time.
   3. Staying with the client when signs and symptoms of a panic attack are present is an interpersonal, not a biological, intervention.
   4. **Notifying the client of the availability of alprazolam prn is a biological intervention when caring for clients experiencing panic attacks.**
   5. Because of decreased levels of concentration and narrowed perceptions associated with panic attacks, teaching is an inappropriate intervention at this time.

TEST-TAKING HINT: The test taker must note the keyword *biological* in the question. Other interventions may be appropriate, but only a biological intervention will correctly answer this question.

15. 1. A thyroid-stimulating hormone level of 0.03 mIU/L is an indication of hyperthyroidism. A major symptom of hyperthyroidism is high levels of anxiety.
   2. A fasting blood glucose level of 60 mg/dL is an indication of hypoglycemia. One of the symptoms of hypoglycemia is a feeling of increased anxiety.
   3. A client diagnosed with caffeine toxicity would show signs of anxiety because of the stimulant effect of caffeine.
   4. Anxiety symptoms are not normally associated with a client diagnosed with gastroesophageal reflux disease. However, anxiety can be a cause or contribute to the exacerbation of this diagnosis.
   5. A client going through alcohol-induced withdrawal exhibits signs of increased anxiety due to rebound stimulation of the central nervous system.

TEST-TAKING HINT: To answer this question correctly, the test taker must be aware that clients with many physiological disease processes can present with signs and symptoms of anxiety. Before a diagnosis of anxiety can be determined, it is important to rule out a physiological cause.

16. 1. Individuals diagnosed with schizotypal personality disorder previously were described as *latent schizophrenics*. Their behavior is odd and eccentric but does not decompensate to the level of schizophrenia. More recent studies indicate that approximately 3% of the population has this disorder. The characteristics presented in the question do not reflect this disorder.
    2. Individuals diagnosed with paranoid personality disorder have a pervasive distrust and suspiciousness of others and interpret motives as malevolent. Prevalence is difficult to establish because individuals with this disorder seldom seek assistance for their problem or require hospitalization. This disorder is more commonly diagnosed in men than in women. The characteristics presented in the question do not reflect this disorder.
    3. **Individuals diagnosed with schizoid personality disorder display a lifelong pattern of social withdrawal, and their discomfort with human interaction is very apparent. Approximately 3% to 7.5% of the population has this disorder. The gender ratio of this disorder is unknown, although it is diagnosed more frequently in men.**
    4. Individuals diagnosed with histrionic personality disorder are excitable and emotional. They display colorful, dramatic, and extroverted behavior. Individuals with this disorder have difficulty maintaining long-lasting relationships because they require constant affirmation of approval and acceptance from others. The prevalence of this disorder is thought to be about 2% to 3% of the population, and it is more commonly diagnosed in women. The characteristics presented in the question do not reflect this disorder.

TEST-TAKING HINT: Nurses working in all types of clinical settings should be familiar with the characteristics associated with clients diagnosed with personality disorders. To answer this question correctly, the test taker must be able to differentiate among characteristics of various personality disorders.

17. 1. The nurse would have no difficulty evaluating this adolescent's socialization skills based on the adolescent's ability to attend group and communicate with staff.
    2. **When the adolescent attends group and communicates with staff members, the adolescent is experiencing improved socialization skills, making this an accurate and positive evaluative statement.**
    3. Because the adolescent has made significant progress in overcoming social isolation, as evidenced by the ability to attend groups and communicate with staff members, the nurse should have no difficulty in evaluating this client's socialization skills. A time frame should not be a factor in this evaluation.
    4. The nurse can accurately evaluate improved social isolation by observing the adolescent's ability to attend group and communicate with staff. These behaviors are associated with improved social isolation, not improved self-esteem.

TEST-TAKING HINT: To select the correct answer, the test taker must understand that attending group and communicating with staff members are behaviors that evaluate improved social isolation in clients diagnosed with major depression.

18. 1. It is important for the assessment data to be from the perspective of the client, not the family member. Privacy rights must be respected. If the client is uncooperative, with permission from the client, further data may be gained from family.
    2. **The family member is rightfully concerned about this client. The nurse should communicate understanding and empathy. It also is important to communicate the need to gain assessment information from the client's perspective, factoring in the client's right to privacy. Because clients diagnosed with anorexia nervosa have a distorted self-image, after obtaining client permission, it may be necessary to involve family to attain accurate information.**
    3. It would be the role of the nurse, not the physician, to intervene appropriately in this situation. The nurse must use knowledge of the disease process of anorexia nervosa and the client's rights to decide on an appropriate intervention.

4. It would be the role of the nurse, not the social worker, to intervene appropriately in this situation. The nurse must use knowledge of the disease process of anorexia nervosa and the client's rights to decide on an appropriate intervention. After further assessment data are collected, a consultation with a social worker may be obtained if necessary.

TEST-TAKING HINT: To answer this question correctly, the test taker must understand the role of the nurse in this setting. The scope of practice of the nurse includes the management of interpersonal conflicts. Knowing this assists the test taker to eliminate answers 3 and 4.

19. The stages of grief should be numbered as follows: 4, 3, 5, 1, 2. Kubler-Ross's five stages of grief consist of (1) denial, (2) anger, (3) bargaining, (4) depression, and (5) acceptance. Behaviors associated with each of these stages can be observed in individuals experiencing the loss of any concept of personal value. These stages typically occur in the order presented; however, there may be individualized variations in how grieving progresses.

TEST-TAKING HINT: To answer this question correctly, the test taker must be familiar with Elisabeth Kubler-Ross's model of the normal grief response.

20. 1. A client's chief complaint constitutes subjective data of the client's perception of symptoms or situations and is important to assess. The client's chief complaint does not take priority in this situation.
2. In an emergency situation, a focused assessment on critical and priority alterations in health status is more appropriate than a complete history and physical examination.
3. Symptoms of substance-induced overdose or withdrawal vary in intensity and can be life threatening. In this situation, it is critical to assess the specific substance used to provide individualized, safe, and effective care.
4. Gathering data on family history may assist the nurse in evaluating contributing factors related to client problems, but this does not take priority in this situation.

TEST-TAKING HINT: The keyword *priority* helps the test taker choose the correct answer for this question. Gathering data that may determine lifesaving interventions always should be an assessment priority.

21. Alcohol can be harmless and enjoyable, sometimes even beneficial, if it is used responsibly and in moderation.
1. Alcohol does enhance the flavor of foods and can be enjoyed with a good meal.
2. Alcohol is used at social gatherings to encourage relaxation and conviviality among guests. It can promote a feeling of celebration at special occasions, such as weddings, birthdays, and anniversaries.
3. An alcoholic beverage (wine) is used as part of the sacred ritual in some religious ceremonies.
4. When alcohol helps to mask stressful situations, it is being used as an indirect coping strategy to avoid situations that need to be dealt with directly with problem-solving techniques.
5. When alcohol is used to cope with unacceptable feelings, it is being used as an ineffective coping strategy by avoiding feelings that need to be directly addressed.

TEST-TAKING HINT: To eliminate incorrect answers in this question, it is important for the test taker to recognize altered coping (substance use). Using substances to deal with unacceptable feelings or stressful situations is a way to avoid handling these situations in a direct manner.

22. 1. A client's vital signs and the presence of diaphoresis are examples of a biological, not cognitive, response to nursing interventions.
2. A client successfully using a breathing technique to decrease anxiety is an example of a behavioral, not cognitive, response to nursing interventions.
3. A client recognizing negative self-talk as a sign of increased anxiety is an example of a cognitive response to nursing interventions.
4. A client using journaling to express frustrations is an example of an intrapersonal, not cognitive, response to nursing interventions.

TEST-TAKING HINT: To answer this question correctly, the test taker needs to review the potential biological, behavioral, cognitive, and intrapersonal client responses to nursing interventions related to generalized anxiety disorder.

23. Lorazepam, a benzodiazepine, is a central nervous system depressant used to assist clients with anxiety and during detoxification from alcohol.

1. Tolerance occurs when an individual's body needs an increased amount of medication to attain the same effect as the original dosage. Clients who increase their medication dosage because of tolerance are not at greater risk for overdose than the general population.

2. If a client is diagnosed with depression and anxiety, usually an SSRI is given for long-term use. Nurses need to assess clients with depression for suicidal ideations; however, the greatest potential for overdose is not in these specific clients.

3. **Alcohol has an additive central nervous system depressive effect with the benzodiazepine and can lead to overdose. Also, individuals who are under the influence of alcohol or any illicit drug tend to be more impulsive and make poor decisions, which places them at higher risk for overdose.**

4. Although using antacids may alter the absorption of the medication, it does not place the individual at higher risk for overdose.

TEST-TAKING HINT: To answer this question correctly, the test taker must note the words *highest risk* and must understand the concept of cumulative effect. Lorazepam and alcohol are both central nervous system depressants, and when combined, overdose is possible.

24. Health-care personnel must attempt to provide treatment in a manner that least restricts the freedom of the client. Restriction is based on the severity of symptoms and safety considerations. The behaviors noted in the question do not warrant four-point restraints. In this case, redirection, limit setting, and behavioral modifications should be implemented.
    1. **Nonmaleficence is the right to expect the health-care worker to do no harm. By unnecessarily placing the client in four-point restraints, psychological and potentially physical harm may occur.**
    2. Veracity is the right to expect the health-care worker to tell the client the truth. This is not represented in this situation.
    3. **The right to least restrictive treatment applies in this situation. If the client is not an imminent danger to self or others, four-point restraints are not warranted.**
    4. **Beneficence is the right to expect the health-care worker to promote the good of the client. When the client is not a danger to self or others, placing**

the client in four-point restraints does not promote the client's welfare.

5. **Negligence is the failure to do something that a reasonable individual, guided by considerations that ordinarily regulate human affairs, would do, or doing something that a prudent and reasonable individual would not do. By unnecessarily placing the client in four-point restraints, the nurse could be held responsible for committing a negligent act because four-point restraints are not indicated in this situation.**

TEST-TAKING HINT: The severity of the client's symptoms determines the correct answer to this question. Only the principle of veracity is not violated in this scenario.

25. 1. Blurred vision and vomiting are beginning signs of lithium carbonate toxicity. Other beginning signs include ataxia, tinnitus, persistent nausea, and severe diarrhea. These symptoms are seen at serum levels of 1.5 to 2 mEq/L.
    2. Increased thirst and urination are side effects of lithium carbonate, not signs of toxicity; a lithium carbonate level is unnecessary. The nurse may want to provide sugarless candy, ice, or frequent sips of water.
    3. Drowsiness and dizziness are side effects of lithium carbonate, not signs of toxicity; a lithium carbonate level is unnecessary. The nurse may want to ensure that the client does not participate in activities that require alertness.
    4. Headache and anorexia are side effects of lithium carbonate, not early signs and symptoms of toxicity, and therefore a lithium carbonate level is unnecessary.

TEST-TAKING HINT: To answer this question correctly, the test taker must distinguish between side effects of lithium carbonate and signs and symptoms of toxicity.

26. 1. Schizoid personality disorder (cluster A) is characterized by an inability to form close, personal relationships. The client has a spouse and thus is able to form close personal relationships.
    2. Histrionic personality disorder (cluster B) is characterized by a pervasive pattern of excessive emotionality and attention-seeking behavior. There are no histrionic symptoms in the statement by the client.
    3. Dependent personality disorder (cluster C) is characterized by allowing others to assume responsibility for major areas of life because of one's inability to function

independently. Although the client expresses satisfaction with their present situation, dependency lends itself to decreased self-esteem, self-worth, motivation, and, eventually, depression.

4. The *DSM-5-TR* describes passive-aggressive traits but does not include passive-aggressive personality disorder as a specific personality disorder. Passive-aggressive traits are characterized by a passive resistance to demands for adequate performance in occupational and social functioning. The client's statement does not indicate that they are using passive-aggressive behaviors.

TEST-TAKING HINT: To answer this question correctly, the test taker must recognize that the client's statement exhibits significant dependence on the client's spouse, which is a component of dependent personality disorder.

27. 1. The thoughts, impulses, and/or images experienced by a client diagnosed with OCD are not simply excessive worries concerning real-life problems and stressors. To warrant a diagnosis of OCD, worries must exceed the normal and be expressed in obsessions, compulsions, or both, that interfere with functioning in various areas of life.

 2. **At some point during the course of the disorder, a client diagnosed with OCD becomes aware that the obsessions or compulsions are excessive, unreasonable, or both.**

 3. The obsessions or compulsions experienced by a client diagnosed with OCD need to interfere significantly with more than one area of functioning.

 4. A client diagnosed with OCD consciously suppresses, not unconsciously represses, thoughts, impulses, or images by substituting other thoughts or behaviors, or both.

TEST-TAKING HINT: When answering this question, it is important to understand the difference between "unconscious repression" and "conscious suppression." Before diagnosis, a client may consciously suppress or deny the extent of the disorder; however, at some point during the course of the disorder, clients diagnosed with OCD become consciously aware that repetitive behaviors are unreasonable, excessive, or both. Recognizing this, the test taker can eliminate answer 4.

28. 1. Clients with anxiety disorders can experience social isolation. This problem is defined as aloneness experienced by the individual and perceived as imposed by others and as a negative or threatening state. No information is presented in the question that indicates symptoms of social isolation.

 2. **Ineffective breathing pattern is defined as inspiration or expiration that does not provide adequate ventilation. This is a life-threatening problem that must be prioritized immediately.**

 3. Risk for suicide is defined as a risk for self-inflicted, life-threatening injury. No information is presented in the question that indicates this client is exhibiting suicidal ideations.

 4. Fatigue is defined as an overwhelming sustained sense of exhaustion and decreased capacity for normal levels of physical and mental work. No information is presented in the question that indicates this client is exhibiting fatigue.

TEST-TAKING HINT: When prioritizing nursing diagnoses, the test taker needs to consider Maslow's hierarchy of needs. Physiological needs such as oxygen always take highest priority.

29. 1. The nurse would have no difficulty in evaluating this child's social interaction based on the child's interaction with staff members and peers.

 2. Assertive behaviors do not include threats and manipulation. When the child demonstrates inappropriate behaviors in interacting with staff members and peers, this child is experiencing continued impairment in social interaction. This is an inaccurate evaluation of this child's behavior.

 3. The nurse should have no difficulty in evaluating this child's current social interaction. A time frame should not be a factor in this evaluation.

 4. **The nurse can accurately evaluate social interaction by observing the child's ability to interact with staff members and peers. Threatening peers and manipulating staff is evidence of continued impairment in social interaction.**

TEST-TAKING HINT: To select the correct answer, the test taker must understand that inappropriate interactions with staff members and peers are behaviors that indicate continued impairment in social interaction in clients diagnosed with Tourette's disorder.

30. 1. Clients are at risk for delayed or inhibited grief when they do not have the

support of significant others to assist them through the mourning process. Instead of providing support to this client, this family, in an effort to meet their own needs, expects the client to maintain normalcy.

2. Clients experiencing denial during the first week after the loss is a normal part of the grieving process and is described in all theories of normal grief response. Denial occurs immediately on experiencing the loss and usually lasts 2 weeks.

3. Clients experiencing anger toward the deceased within the first month after the loss is a normal part of the grieving process and is described in all theories of normal grief response. Anger is directed toward self or others, and ambivalence or guilt, or both, may be felt toward the lost object.

4. Clients experiencing preoccupation with the deceased for 1 year after the loss is a normal part of the grieving process and is described in all theories of normal grief response. Preoccupation with the lost object and feelings of loneliness occur in response to realization of the loss.

TEST-TAKING HINT: To answer this question correctly, the test taker must recognize and understand the numerous factors influencing the normal grief response.

31. 1. Street names for heroin include horse, junk, brown sugar, smack, TNT, and Harry.
    2. Street names for oxycodone include perk, perkies, Oxy, and O.C.
    3. Street names for phencyclidine include angel dust, hog, peace pill, and rocket fuel.
    4. **Street names for morphine include Miss Emma, M., and white stuff.**

TEST-TAKING HINT: The test taker must be able to recognize common names for street drugs to answer this question correctly.

32. 1. Clients diagnosed with substance use disorders often use the defense mechanism of denial to avoid recognizing how substance use has changed their life in negative ways. The use of denial must be taken into consideration when planning client care but does not necessitate the use of a simple treatment plan by the nurse.
    2. **Approximately 40% to 50% of individuals diagnosed with substance use disorders have mild to moderate cognitive problems when actively using. These cognitive problems would**

necessitate the use of a simple treatment plan that would be more readily understood by the client.

3. Clients diagnosed with chronic substance use disorder most likely have poor general health. They may have nutritional deficits, be susceptible to infections, or be at risk for AIDS and hepatitis. In contrast to cognitive problems, these physical problems do not necessitate a simple treatment plan.

4. Clients diagnosed with chronic substance use disorder often arrest in developmental progression at the age when the abuse began. This alteration in developmental progression must be taken into consideration when planning client care but does not necessitate a simple treatment plan.

TEST-TAKING HINT: All of the answer choices are alterations in health experienced by clients diagnosed with substance use disorders. To answer this question correctly, the test taker must focus on which alteration directly affects the client's ability to learn, which necessitates the establishment of a simple treatment plan.

33. A client diagnosed with aquaphobia, the fear of water, begins the therapeutic process in which they must stand in a pool for 1 hour. This is called *implosion therapy*. Implosion therapy, also called *flooding*, is a therapeutic process in which the client must participate for a long time in real-life or imagined situations that they find extremely frightening. A session is terminated when the client responds with considerably less anxiety than at the beginning of the session.

TEST-TAKING HINT: To answer this question correctly, the test taker must review the many different phobias and the interventions that can be used to help treat specific phobias.

34. 1. When a client diagnosed with schizophrenia focuses inward on a fantasy world while distorting or excluding the external environment, they are experiencing autistic thinking, not ambivalence.
    2. **Emotional ambivalence experienced by the client diagnosed with schizophrenia refers to the coexistence of opposite emotions toward the same object, person, or situation. These opposing emotions may interfere with the client's ability to make a simple decision. The simultaneous need for and fear of intimacy interferes with the establishment of satisfying relationships.**

3. Impairment in social functioning including social isolation can be experienced by clients diagnosed with schizophrenia. These clients sometimes cling to others and intrude on the personal space of others, exhibiting behaviors that are not socially or culturally acceptable. These symptoms of schizophrenia are not reflective of emotional ambivalence.

4. Flat affect, not emotional ambivalence, is described as the lack of emotional expression. Emotional tone is weak, and the client seems to be void of emotional tone or expression.

TEST-TAKING HINT: The test taker must correctly identify the behaviors that indicate the symptom of schizophrenia presented in the question (emotional ambivalence) to answer this question.

35. Prioritization for discharge of any client is based on safety concerns.
   1. Clients who have been involuntarily committed need a court hearing to be discharged. This could take time and would affect a discharge decision.
   2. Alcohol-induced withdrawal can be a life-threatening situation for a client. Because this client was admitted only 2 days ago, the client is still at risk for detoxification complications and is an inappropriate candidate for discharge.
   3. **Delirium is a reversible condition. Because the urinary tract infection is the cause of the delirium, by day 4 antibiotics should have stabilized this client's condition, making this client a candidate for discharge.**
   4. Command hallucinations put a client at risk for harm to self or others. Also, a court hearing would be required for a client who was involuntarily committed to be discharged.

TEST-TAKING HINT: To determine the correct answer choice, the test taker needs to understand the importance of prioritizing safety issues when making decisions about client care.

36. A client has the option to participate or not to participate in medical research.
   1. The client can change their mind and drop out of a study at any time. Documentation of the client's consent does not make participation mandatory.
   2. **The client can change their mind and drop out of a study at any time.**

3. If a client can understand the risks and benefits of the research study, even if they are psychotic, the client can give informed consent and participate.
4. The client can change their mind and drop out of a study at any time. A physician's permission is not necessary.

TEST-TAKING HINT: To answer this question correctly, the test taker should understand that a nurse acts as an advocate to clarify information about research when a client is considering participating in a research study.

37. 1. It is the right of a competent individual, whether voluntarily or involuntarily committed, to refuse medications. Medications can be forced only when a client is assessed as an imminent danger to self or others or declared incompetent by the court.
   2. If a client is assessed as a danger to self or others, whether voluntarily or involuntarily committed, the client may be held for further evaluations for a time period determined by state law.
   3. **The ethical principle of nonmaleficence requires that health-care workers do no harm to their clients, either intentionally or unintentionally.**
   4. **The ethical principle of veracity requires that health-care providers tell the truth and not intentionally deceive or mislead clients.**
   5. **The ethical principle of justice requires that all clients be treated equally.**

TEST-TAKING HINT: The test taker must understand that a client who is voluntarily admitted has the right to leave an inpatient unit. If the client has been determined to be a danger to self or others, the client loses this right. When a client is an imminent danger to self or others, the right to refuse medications may also be lost.

38. 1. This is an example of direct confrontation and expression of anger, not the defense mechanism of displacement.
   2. By taking their boss out to dinner, the disgruntled employee suppresses the expression of their unacceptable anger toward their boss by expressing opposite behaviors. This would be considered the defense mechanism of reaction formation, not displacement.
   3. **The disgruntled employee considers their child less threatening than their boss and is transferring negative feelings**

from one target to another by using the defense mechanism of displacement.

4. The disgruntled employee is refusing to acknowledge the existence of the actual situation or the feelings associated with it. They are using the defense mechanism of denial, not displacement.

TEST-TAKING HINT: To answer this question correctly, the test taker needs to understand that displacement occurs when feelings are transferred from one target to another that is considered less threatening or neutral.

39. 1. Altered coping is an appropriate nursing diagnosis for clients diagnosed with substance use disorder, but this diagnosis does not address the peripheral neuropathy mentioned in the question.
    2. **Peripheral neuropathy is characterized by peripheral nerve damage resulting in pain, burning, tingling, or prickly sensations of the extremities. Pain R/T the effects of alcohol AEB rating pain as a 6 out of 10 on a pain scale is a nursing diagnosis that addresses this client's problem.**
    3. Powerlessness R/T substance abuse AEB no control over drinking is a common nursing diagnosis for clients diagnosed with alcohol use disorder, but it does not address the peripheral neuropathy mentioned in the question.
    4. Nothing is presented in the question that indicates a nursing diagnosis of altered sensory perception R/T effects of alcohol AEB visual hallucinations.

TEST-TAKING HINT: To be able to answer this question correctly, the test taker must know that pain is a symptom of peripheral neuropathy. Other nursing diagnoses may apply to this client, but they do not address the problem presented in the question.

40. 1. Children diagnosed with conduct disorder may project a tough image, but they have low self-esteem, low frustration tolerance, irritability, and temper outbursts. Because of their aggressive nature, these children direct their anger toward others and not toward themselves. They are not generally at risk for self-mutilation.
    2. Most children diagnosed with conduct disorder have a history of broken homes and parental rejection, experiencing inconsistent management with harsh discipline. Ineffective individual coping can be a valid nursing diagnosis for these

clients because they learn to cope through aggressive behavior and threats to others. However, compared with the other diagnoses presented, ineffective individual coping is not a priority at this time.
    3. Impaired social interactions for a client diagnosed with conduct disorder would involve bullying, intimidating, and fighting. Although impaired social interaction R/T neurological alteration is an appropriate nursing diagnosis for this child, it does not take priority at this time.
    4. **Studies reveal that children diagnosed with conduct disorder have a history of abuse, neglect, and the frequent shifting of parental figures, which then is displaced in aggression toward others. This aggression has been found to be the principal cause of peer rejection, contributing to a cycle of maladaptive behavior. Because the possibility of harm to others is so great, the nursing diagnosis of risk for violence: directed at others would take priority at this time.**

TEST-TAKING HINT: To select the correct answer, the test taker needs to know that when aggression is exhibited, safety is always the immediate nursing priority.

41. Altered sensory perception is the change in the amount or patterning of incoming stimuli (either internally or externally initiated) accompanied by a diminished, exaggerated, distorted, or impaired response to such stimuli.
    1. Cognitive problems due to alcohol-induced neurocognitive disorder are a result of the effects of alcohol on the brain. A client can maintain normal vital signs when experiencing altered sensory perception, making this assessment unnecessary.
    2. **Decreasing the amount of stimuli in the client's environment (e.g., by ensuring low noise level, few people, simple decor) lowers the possibility that a client diagnosed with alcohol-induced neurocognitive disorder will form inaccurate sensory perceptions.**
    3. It is always important to maintain a non-judgmental approach when dealing with any client under the nurse's care. However, this intervention does not address the client's problem of altered sensory perception.
    4. A client diagnosed with alcohol use disorder often uses the defense mechanism of denial. Because this client is diagnosed with alcohol-induced neurocognitive

disorder, they may have little insight related to the cause of symptoms. Confrontation would not be effective in this situation and might generate hostility and aggression. Also, this intervention does not address the client problem of altered sensory perception.

TEST-TAKING HINT: The correct answer choice must address the client's problem of altered sensory perception. The test taker must take the client's diagnosis into consideration when choosing the correct answer. Understanding that alcohol-induced neurocognitive disorder is a cognitive and not physical problem eliminates answer 1.

42. Of women who give birth, **50%** to **80%** experience postpartum blues. Moderate depression occurs in 10% to 16%, and severe or psychotic depression occurs in about 1% or 2% of every 1,000 postpartum women. Symptoms of the maternity or postpartum blues include tearfulness, despondency, anxiety, and subjectively impaired concentration occurring in the early puerperium. The symptoms usually begin 3 to 4 days after delivery, worsen at 5 to 7 days, and tend to resolve after 12 days. Symptoms of moderate postpartum depression have been described as depressed mood varying from day to day, with more bad days than good, tending to be worse toward evening and associated with fatigue, irritability, loss of appetite, sleep disturbances, and loss of libido.

TEST-TAKING HINT: To answer this question correctly, the test taker must understand the prevalence of postpartum depressive symptoms.

43. 1. Clients diagnosed with antisocial personality disorders are usually egocentric and find it difficult to empathize or experience guilt.
2. Hearing voices is a common problem with clients diagnosed with schizophrenia, not antisocial personality disorder.
3. **Clients diagnosed with antisocial personality disorders do not have insight into self-pathology and tend to blame other people and circumstances for their interpersonal problems.**
4. Clients diagnosed with schizoid personality disorders, not antisocial personality disorders, neither desire nor enjoy close relationships, including being part of a family.

TEST-TAKING HINT: To answer this question correctly, the test taker must recognize specific characteristics associated with antisocial personality disorder.

44. 1. **The client in the question is expressing unrealistic fears resulting from a previous trauma. The client's behaviors are being negatively influenced by these fears. This is evidence of the nursing diagnosis of posttrauma syndrome.**
2. The client understands the importance of the examination but is unable to follow through because of fear, not deliberate nonadherence.
3. The client verbalizes the importance of the gynecological examination, so they do not exhibit a knowledge deficit in this area.
4. Because the client has originally scheduled a gynecological appointment, there is evidence of a desire to maintain health. The cancellation of this appointment is the result of unrealistic fear.

TEST-TAKING HINT: To answer this question correctly, the test taker must understand the client's underlying problem. The client's statement reveals a desire to maintain health, so answers 2 and 4 can be eliminated.

45. 1. In this statement, the nurse is giving advice, which is a block to therapeutic communication. The nurse is providing a solution versus allowing the client to come to this conclusion on their own.
2. **This statement by the nurse helps the client focus on and explore alternatives rather than provide answers or solutions that may be unacceptable to the client.**
3. This statement by the nurse belittles the client's feelings by providing a solution that does not recognize the client's unique problems.
4. In this statement, the nurse is providing the solution without involving the client in the decision-making process.

TEST-TAKING HINT: The test taker must note that when the nurse is making the decision, as in answers 1 and 4, the answer is usually wrong.

46. 1. This nursing intervention, at the primary prevention level, is focused on targeting groups at risk and providing educational programs.
2. This nursing intervention, at the primary prevention level, is focused on targeting groups at risk and providing educational programs.
3. This nursing intervention, at the primary prevention level, is focused on targeting groups at risk and providing educational programs.

4. This nursing intervention, at the secondary prevention level, is focused on reducing the prevalence of psychiatric illness by shortening the duration of the illness. An individual calling a suicide hotline is experiencing suicidal ideations, and the staff member provides currently needed care to address the symptom.

TEST-TAKING HINT: Reviewing the functions of the nurse in all levels of community mental health prevention helps the test taker to distinguish interventions in each prevention category.

47. 1. In the pre-alcoholic phase, alcohol is used to relieve everyday stress and tension. This client, because of family history, has a genetic predisposition toward alcohol use disorder.
    2. In the early alcoholic phase, alcohol is no longer a source of pleasure or relief but a drug that is required by the individual. The information needed to determine this level of use has not been presented in the question. This client may have a biological tendency to drink, but drinking patterns have not progressed to the early alcoholic phase.
    3. Control is lost, and physiological dependence is evident in the crucial phase. The information needed to determine this level of use has not been presented in the question. The client may have learned drinking patterns from family members but drinking patterns have not progressed to the crucial alcoholic phase.
    4. The individual is usually intoxicated more often than sober, and emotional and physical disintegration occur in the chronic phase. This client's drinking patterns have not progressed to the chronic phase.

TEST-TAKING HINT: All parts of an answer must be correct for the answer to be the right choice. In this question, only answer 1 presents the correct phase of drinking pattern progression exemplified in the question.

48. 1. Wernicke-Korsakoff syndrome is a group of symptoms caused by chronic thiamine deficiency related to long-term, not short-term, alcohol use. Symptoms include paralysis of the ocular muscles, double vision, ataxia, somnolence, stupor, confusion, loss of recent memory, and confabulation. The situation presented in the question does not reflect these symptoms.

2. An alcohol-induced neurocognitive disorder is characterized by an inability to learn new information (short-term memory deficit) despite normal attention and an inability to recall previously learned information (long-term memory deficit). The situation presented in the question does not reflect these symptoms.
3. Alcohol-induced withdrawal is characterized by tremors, agitation, anxiety, diaphoresis, increased pulse and blood pressure, sleep disturbances, hallucinations, seizures, delusions, and delirium tremens. Delirium tremens is the most severe expression of alcohol-induced withdrawal. It is characterized by visual, auditory, or tactile hallucinations; extreme disorientation; restlessness; and hyperactivity of the autonomic nervous system. The client in the question is experiencing symptoms of alcohol-induced withdrawal.
4. Acute alcoholic myopathy is characterized by a sudden onset of muscle pain, swelling, and weakness. The situation presented in the question does not reflect these symptoms.

TEST-TAKING HINT: In this question, the test taker must match the symptoms presented with the possible diagnostic cause. Symptoms of various conditions sometimes overlap. The answer that best matches the symptoms presented should be chosen.

49. 1. A history of previous suicide attempts places a client at higher risk for future attempts.
    2. The ability to access a lethal means to commit suicide increases a client's risk for a suicide attempt.
    3. Withdrawal and isolative behaviors indicate the client is experiencing hopelessness and helplessness, which increases the client's risk for a suicide attempt.
    4. Physical illness, not a lack of physical illness, may lead to feelings of powerlessness and hopelessness, which increases a client's risk for a suicide attempt.
    5. A client is at an increased risk for suicide if the client's behaviors tend to be impulsive or aggressive. These personality characteristics may lead a client to hasty, reckless decisions, which may include suicide.

TEST-TAKING HINT: The test taker must recognize common suicide risk factors to answer this question correctly. It also is important to recognize that the list presented in this question is not comprehensive. Many factors place a client at risk for suicide.

50. 1. The essential feature of separation anxiety disorder is excessive anxiety concerning separation from the home or from those to whom the person is attached. A pattern of negativity, disobedience, and hostile behavior describes oppositional defiant disorder (ODD), not separation anxiety disorder.
    2. **A child diagnosed with ODD presents with a pattern of negativity, disobedience, and hostile behavior toward authority figures. This pattern of behavior occurs more frequently than is typically observed in individuals of comparable age and developmental level. ODD typically begins by 8 years of age and usually not later than adolescence. It is more prevalent in boys than in girls and is often a developmental antecedent to conduct disorder.**
    3. A narcissistic personality disorder is characterized by an exaggerated sense of self-worth. These individuals lack empathy and are hypersensitive to the evaluation of others. According to diagnostic criteria, the diagnosis of a personality disorder cannot be determined until an individual is 18 years old. A pattern of negativity, disobedience, and hostile behavior describes ODD, not narcissistic personality disorder.
    4. An autism spectrum disorder is characterized by withdrawal of the child into the self and into a fantasy world of their own creation. A pattern of negativity, disobedience, and hostile behavior describes ODD, not autism spectrum disorder.

TEST-TAKING HINT: To select the correct answer, the test taker must be familiar with the diagnostic criteria of ODD.

51. Children with ADHD show an inappropriate degree of inattention, impulsiveness, and hyperactivity, and the course of the disorder can be chronic, persisting into adulthood. ADHD may be diagnosed in 3% to 7% of school-age children.
    1. A persistent pattern of withdrawal into self is a characteristic of an autism spectrum disorder, not ADHD. Children diagnosed with ADHD are often disruptive and intrusive in group endeavors. Some ADHD children are very aggressive or oppositional and do not exhibit withdrawal behaviors.
    2. ADHD is difficult to diagnose in a child younger than 4-years-old because behavior in younger children is much more variable than that of older children. Frequently, the disorder is not recognized until the child enters school.
    3. ADHD is four to nine times more common in boys than in girls.
    4. **The essential feature of ADHD is a persistent pattern of inattention or hyperactivity-impulsivity, or both, that is more frequent and severe than is typically observed in individuals at a comparable level of development.**

TEST-TAKING HINT: To select the correct answer, the test taker must recognize that a persistent pattern of inattention or hyperactivity-impulsivity, or both, is characteristic of the diagnosis of ADHD.

52. 1. The nurse should not avoid discussing the client's symptoms. If the nurse avoids this discussion, an actual physiological problem may be overlooked.
    2. **The nurse must plan care that encourages exploration of the underlying anxiety experienced by the client. Because anxiety is unconsciously expressed through somatic symptoms, it is the nurse's responsibility to assist the client in beginning to understand the link between anxiety and somatic symptoms.**
    3. Reminding the client about previous negative test results would only increase the client's anxiety, which may lead to further somatic symptoms. The nurse needs to remember that somatic symptoms are real to the client. It is important for the nurse to respond to the client with respect to build a trusting relationship.
    4. The nurse avoids encouraging exploration of the client's anxiety when the client is redirected to the physician. This also may reinforce the validity of the somatic complaints.

TEST-TAKING HINT: To answer this question correctly, the test taker needs to recognize the nurse's role in client care when dealing with clients diagnosed with somatic symptom disorder.

53. 1. This statement focuses on the nurse's history and is not client centered.
2. This statement focuses on the nurse's feelings and is not client centered.
3. **This statement focuses on the needs of the client and not the needs of the nurse.**
4. This statement focuses on the nurse's history, the statement is not client centered, and giving advice is nontherapeutic.

TEST-TAKING HINT: To answer this question correctly, the test taker must be aware of the need to always focus on feedback that serves the needs of the client and not the needs of the nurse.

54. All clients taking clozapine need to have a complete blood count with differential ordered to monitor for neutropenia, a dangerous drop in the absolute neutrophil count (ANC). Treatment should be interrupted if neutropenia ANC less than 1,000 cells per microliter is suspected to be clozapine induced. For clients with benign ethnic neutropenia, treatment should be interrupted if neutropenia is suspected to be clozapine-induced for ANC less than 500 cells per microliter.
1. **An ANC of 600 cells per microliter is considered moderate neutropenia. Because of the low ANC, the medication must be held, and the laboratory value needs to be reported to the physician.**
2. The physician should be notified of the low, not high, ANC.
3. The ANC noted is not normal, so the medication should be held.
4. The nurse would need to recognize that the ANC was low, and that physician notification is indicated prior to giving clozapine.

TEST-TAKING HINT: To answer this question correctly, the test taker must be able to recognize that the ANC laboratory value in the question is less than normal and know that this would necessitate physician notification and the possible discontinuation of clozapine.

55. Personality disorders are grouped into three clusters as follows: cluster A—paranoid, schizoid, and schizotypal personality disorders; cluster B—antisocial, borderline, histrionic, and narcissistic personality disorders; and cluster C—avoidant, dependent, and obsessive-compulsive personality disorders. Personality disorders usually begin in childhood or adolescence and persist in a stable form into adulthood.
1. Paranoid, schizoid, and schizotypal, not obsessive-compulsive, personality disorders are grouped in cluster A.
2. Antisocial, borderline, histrionic, and narcissistic, not obsessive-compulsive, personality disorders are grouped in cluster B.
3. **Obsessive-compulsive personality disorder is grouped in cluster C.**
4. There is no cluster D grouping of personality disorders.

TEST-TAKING HINT: To answer this question correctly, the test taker must understand and review personality disorder clusters.

56. 1. Nonverbal behavior is controlled more by the unconscious than by the conscious mind.
2. Nonverbal behavior carries more, not less, weight than verbal interactions because nonverbal behavior is influenced by the unconscious.
3. **Interpreting nonverbal communication can be problematic. Sociocultural background is a major influence on the meaning of nonverbal behavior. Some cultures may consider eye contact intrusive, threatening, or harmful and minimize or avoid its use. Nonverbal communication includes all of the five senses and everything that does not involve the spoken word.**
4. Conversely, nonverbal behaviors often directly reflect feelings.

TEST-TAKING HINT: To answer this question correctly, the test taker must review concepts of nonverbal communication and sociocultural differences.

57. *Cheeking* means that a client hides a medication between the cheek and gums. Stimulant medications are controlled substances and can be misused or sold. When cheeking is suspected, the use of dissolvable or liquid medication may be indicated.
1. **Dyanavel XR (d- & l-amphetamine) is a long-acting liquid amphetamine-based stimulant. Liquid medications cannot be cheeked.**
2. **Quillivant XR (methylphenidate) is a long-acting liquid methylphenidate-based stimulant. Liquid medications cannot be cheeked. Quillichew ER is a chewable version of this medication that can also be prescribed.**

3. Contempla XR-ODT (d- & l-methyl-phenidate extended base) is a long-acting dissolvable methylphenidate-based stimulant. Dissolvable medications cannot be cheeked.

4. Adzenys XR-ODT (d- & l-amphet-amine) is a long acting dissolvable amphetamine-based stimulant. Dissolvable medications cannot be cheeked.

5. Kapvay (clonidine extended release) is an extended release blood pressure medication used to help treat ADHD. Because it is in tablet form, it can be cheeked.

TEST-TAKING HINT: To answer this question the test taker must understand the definition of cheeking medications. Knowing that liquid or dissolvable medications cannot be cheeked will assist the test taker in choosing the identified liquid or dissolvable medications.

58. 1. When experiencing circumstantiality, an individual delays in reaching the point of a communication because of the use of unnecessary and tedious details. The client statement presented is not reflective of circumstantiality.

2. Word salad is a group of words strung together in a random fashion, without any logical connection. The client's statement is an example of the use of word salad.

3. Tangentiality differs from circumstantiality in that the individual never gets to the point of the communication. Unrelated topics are introduced, and the original discussion is lost. The client's statement is not an example of the use of tangentiality.

4. Perseveration is the persistent repetition of the same word or idea in response to different questions. The client's statement is not an example of the use of perseveration.

TEST-TAKING HINT: The test taker can remember the meaning of word salad by visualizing a bowl of salad being tossed. The standalone ingredients of the salad are tossed together with little connection.

59. 1. Grandiosity is defined as irrational ideas regarding self-worth, talent, or power. Grandiosity is often assessed in clients experiencing manic states.

2. Flight of ideas is defined as a continuous but fragmentary stream of talk. The general train of thought can be followed, but the direction is frequently changed, often by chance stimuli from the environment. Flight of ideas is often assessed in clients experiencing acute manic states.

3. Pressured speech is defined as loud and emphatic speech that is increased in amount, accelerated, and usually difficult or impossible to interrupt. Pressured speech is often assessed in clients experiencing acute manic states.

4. Manic behaviors consist of psychomotor overactivity and increased levels of energy. This increased energy would prevent a client from taking short, frequent naps.

5. Psychomotor agitation is defined as excessive restlessness and increased physical activity. Psychomotor agitation is often assessed in clients experiencing acute manic states.

TEST-TAKING HINT: The test taker must recognize the signs and symptoms of mania to answer this question correctly.

60. 1. Genetic influences or predisposing factors are acquired through heredity. This client was at a higher risk because of family history. The client's statement indicates awareness of the biological theory of genetic predisposition.

2. Negative thoughts can contribute to learned responses, which influence normal adaptation responses. This would be related to the principles of cognitive, not biological, theory.

3. There are many influences on behavior and the development of mental disorders, heredity being one of them. Learned behaviors and cognitive perceptions are other influences. The client cannot blame the mother entirely for their diagnosis.

4. Past experiences influence learned patterns of behavior. This would be related to the principles of learning, not biological, theory.

TEST-TAKING HINT: To answer this question correctly, the test taker must understand that if an intervention or assessment is in the context of a theoretical construct, the answer must reflect the stated theory.

61. 1. When the nurse offers to present new information to the client, the nurse is functioning in the role of a teacher, not an advocate.

2. Assessing previously successful strategies is an effective intervention by the nurse but does not relate to the nurse functioning as an advocate.

3. Being present as a support person and offering to remind clients of their concerns is the functional role of the nurse advocate.

4. This is an empathizing statement but does not reflect the nurse's role as advocate.

TEST-TAKING HINT: To answer this question correctly, the test taker should understand the concept of advocacy and then determine which statement by the nurse reflects this role.

62. 1. The CAGE screening questionnaire is used to assess for alcohol use disorder, not tardive dyskinesia.

    CAGE: Have you ever
    C: felt the need to *Cut* down on your drinking/drugs?
    A: been *Annoyed* by the criticism of others about your drinking/drug use?
    G: felt *Guilty* about the amount of drinking/drugging you do?
    E: had an *Eye* opener drink first thing in the morning to steady your nerves?
    A positive response to two or more questions suggests an alcohol/substance use disorder.

    2. The Mini-Mental State Examination (MMSE) is a 30-point questionnaire used to measure cognitive impairment, not tardive dyskinesia.

    3. **The Abnormal Involuntary Movement Scale (AIMS) is a scale used to assess clients for tardive dyskinesia, a syndrome of symptoms characterized by bizarre facial and tongue movements, a stiff neck, and difficulty swallowing. AIMS is a comparative scale documenting changes over time.**

    4. The clock face assessment, or clock-drawing test, is sensitive to signs and symptoms of early neurocognitive disorder, not tardive dyskinesia. Clock face scoring is based on completion of the task of drawing the face of a clock. Much can be learned from this test about the client's ability to plan appropriately.

TEST-TAKING HINT: To answer this question correctly, the test taker must be aware of various assessment tools and how they can be used to identify specific client problems.

63. 1. Dissociative identity disorder (DID) is not always incapacitating. Some individuals with DID maintain responsible positions, complete graduate degrees, and are successful spouses and parents before diagnosis and during treatment.

    2. The transition from one personality to another is usually sudden, often dramatic, and usually precipitated by stress. The time during personality transition is usually a matter of seconds, and some behavioral symptoms, such as blinking of the eyes, facial changes, and changes in voice, may be present.

    3. DID is not a personality disorder. In the past, DID was referred to as multiple personality disorder. This terminology was changed to prevent confusion.

    4. The original personality usually has no knowledge of the other personalities; however, when two or more subpersonalities occur, they are usually aware of each other's existence. Only one personality is evident at any given moment, and generally there is amnesia regarding the events that occurred when another personality is in the dominant position. Often, however, one personality is not bound by such amnesia and retains complete awareness of the existence, qualities, and activities of the other personalities.

TEST-TAKING HINT: The test taker must be aware that *multiple personality disorder* is the older terminology for the diagnosis of DID. This should not be confused with an actual personality disorder. Understanding this, the test taker can immediately eliminate answer 3.

64. Primary gain enables the client to avoid unpleasant activities and feelings of anxiety associated with these activities. Secondary gains occur when clients obtain attention or support that they might not otherwise receive.

    1. This client is using pain as a method to avoid anxiety related to feelings of rejection associated with a pending divorce. This is an example of a primary gain.

    2. This client verbalizes that attention is received only when pain is expressed. This is an example of a secondary, not primary, gain.

    3. This client is receiving disability solely because of experiencing pain. Because this pain is related to a diagnosis of somatic symptom disorder, this would be an example of a secondary, not primary, gain.

    4. This client is receiving sympathy solely because of experiencing pain. Because this pain is related to a diagnosis of somatic symptom disorder, this is an example of a secondary, not primary, gain.

TEST-TAKING HINT: To answer this question correctly, the test taker must be able to differentiate between primary and secondary gains.

65. Trihexyphenidyl, an anticholinergic medication, is prescribed to counteract extrapyramidal symptoms, which are side effects of all antipsychotic medications. Haloperidol, an antipsychotic medication, is prescribed to assist individuals with psychotic symptoms, such as hallucinations.
    1. Antipsychotic medications such as haloperidol, and not trihexyphenidyl, are prescribed to address auditory hallucinations.
    2. **Akathisia, an extrapyramidal symptom, is restlessness, a side effect of the use of antipsychotic medications such as haloperidol. Trihexyphenidyl is prescribed to address uncomfortable restlessness.**
    3. Haloperidol is a typical antipsychotic medication that has minimal effects on the negative symptoms of schizophrenia, such as anhedonia.
    4. Haloperidol, a typical antipsychotic, does not decrease sedation. Sedation is a side effect of the use of haloperidol.

TEST-TAKING HINT: To answer this question correctly, the test taker must understand the terms *akathisia* and *anhedonia*.

66. 1. The client's statement, "The doctor says I'm not pregnant, but I know that I am," is an example of a somatic, not nihilistic, delusion.
    2. The client's statement, "Someone is trying to get a message to me through the articles in this magazine," is an example of a delusion of reference, not a nihilistic delusion.
    3. **The client's statement, "The world no longer exists," is an example of a nihilistic delusion. A nihilistic delusion is when an individual has a false idea that the self, a part of the self, others, or the world is nonexistent.**
    4. The client's statement, "The FBI has bugged my room, and they intend to kill me," is an example of a delusion of persecution, not a nihilistic delusion.

TEST-TAKING HINT: The root word of *nihilistic* is "annihilate," which means to reduce to nothing. An understanding of this word should lead the test taker to choose the correct answer.

67. 1. A client diagnosed with moderate intellectual developmental disorder (IDD) Intelligence Quotient (IQ level 35 to 49) would be capable of academic skills to a second-grade level. As an adult, this individual should be able to contribute to their own support in sheltered workshops.
    2. A client diagnosed with profound IDD (IQ level <20) would be unable to profit from academic or vocational training. This client may respond to minimal training in self-help if presented in the close context of a one-to-one relationship.
    3. **The client in the question has been diagnosed with severe IDD (IQ level 20 to 34). This client would be unable to profit from academic or vocational training but might benefit from systematic habit training.**
    4. A client diagnosed with mild IDD (IQ level 50 to 70) would be capable of academic skills to a sixth-grade level. As an adult, this client should be able to achieve vocational skills for minimum self-support.

TEST-TAKING HINT: To answer this question correctly, the test taker needs to understand the various behavioral manifestations and abilities associated with each level of intellectual developmental disorder.

68. 1. Social isolation is defined as aloneness experienced by the individual and perceived as imposed by others and as a negative or threatened state. Although withdrawal behaviors are typical of clients diagnosed with major depressive disorder, which can lead to social isolation, this diagnosis is not prioritized at this time.
    2. **Imbalanced nutrition, less than body requirements, is defined as the state in which an individual experiences an intake of nutrients insufficient to meet metabolic needs. Clients diagnosed with major depressive disorders experience poor self-esteem and fatigue, which can influence their ability to meet nutritional needs. Physiological needs must be addressed prior to meeting needs that are psychological in nature.**
    3. Powerlessness is defined as the perception that one's own action will not significantly affect an outcome—a perceived lack of control over a current situation or immediate happening. Although experiencing feelings of powerlessness is typical of clients diagnosed with major depressive disorder, this diagnosis is not prioritized at this time.
    4. Low self-esteem is defined as a long-standing negative self-evaluation or negative feelings about self or self-capabilities. Although feelings of low self-esteem are typical of clients diagnosed with major depressive disorder, this is not prioritized at this time.

TEST-TAKING HINT: To answer this question correctly, the test taker must understand that one way to prioritize client problems is to utilize Maslow's hierarchy of needs. Physiological needs must be prioritized prior to addressing psychological needs.

69. 1. The psychiatric/mental health nurse analyzes data to determine client problems. The problem statement, or nursing diagnosis, is the client's response to actual or potential problems, and assisting with resolution of these problems is the basis and underlying objective of nursing interventions. Just as the physician cannot treat a client without knowing the medical diagnosis, the nurse cannot provide care to a client without an understanding of the client's functional problems.
    2. The gathering of client data related to psychiatric illness, mental health problems, and potential comorbid physical illnesses is the nurse's assessment of the client's problems. This assessment is part of the process that leads to the formulation of client problem statements or nursing diagnoses.
    3. Nursing interventions are focused on recognition and identification of patterns of response to actual or potential client problems, not medical diagnoses described in the *DSM-5-TR*. The nurse must stay within the nursing scope of practice and focus on client functional problems with which the nurse can assist. A medical diagnosis is never a part of a nursing diagnosis, unless it is a collaborative problem.
    4. The scope of practice of the registered nurse is unique to nursing. It is important to give holistic care, but there should be recognition of the nurse's unique role, not merely as an assistant to the physician.

TEST-TAKING HINT: To answer this question correctly, the test taker must understand that client problems are described as functional patterns of response and stated as nursing diagnoses. These problem statements form the basis for providing psychiatric/mental health nursing care. A nursing diagnosis provides the basis for selection of nursing interventions to achieve outcomes for which the nurse is accountable.

70. 1. Mental stress is a situational, not behavioral, factor that influences sleep patterns.
    2. Intense learning is a cognitive, not behavioral, factor that influences sleep patterns.
    3. Developmental changes in sleep patterns occur across the life span. It is true that typically adolescents tend to sleep late, and older adults awaken early, but this is a developmental, not behavioral, factor that influences sleep patterns.
    4. The behavioral factor of using sleep to avoid stressful situations influences sleep patterns.

TEST-TAKING HINT: The test taker must look for keywords in the question to determine what is being asked. All answer choices influence sleep patterns, but only answer 4 is a behavioral factor.

71. According to Mahler's theory of object relations, the infant passes through six phases from birth to 36 months. If the infant is successful, a sense of separateness from the parenting figure is finally established. Freud, similar to Mahler, theorized the importance of meeting an infant's basic needs. Freud said that when the infant does not experience gratification of basic needs, a sense of mistrust and insecurity develops.
    1. Phase 1 (birth to 1 month) is the normal autism phase of Mahler's development theory. The main task of this phase is survival and comfort. Fixation in this phase may predispose a child to autism spectrum disorders.
    2. Phase 2 (1 to 5 months) is the symbiosis phase. The main task of this phase is the development of the awareness of an external source of need fulfillment. Fixation in this phase may predispose a child to adolescent or adult-onset psychotic disorders.
    3. Phase 3 (5 to 36 months) is the separation-individuation phase. The main task of this phase is the primary recognition of separateness from the mother figure. Fixation in this phase may predispose a child to borderline personality.
    4. Consolidation is the third subcategory of the separation-individuation phase. With the achievement of consolidation, a child is able to internalize a sustained image of the mothering figure as enduring and loving. The child also is able to maintain the perception of the mother as a separate person in the outside world.

TEST-TAKING HINT: The test taker first must understand Mahler's theory of object relations, and then recognize that clients diagnosed with autism spectrum disorders have deficits during the normal autism phase.

72. 1. Paralysis of ocular muscles, diplopia, ataxia, somnolence, and stupor all are symptoms of Wernicke's encephalopathy. This is the most serious form of thiamine deficiency in clients diagnosed with alcohol use disorder. If thiamine replacement therapy is not undertaken quickly, death results.

2. Impaired mental functioning, apathy, euphoria or depression, sleep disturbance, and increasing confusion leading to coma all are symptoms of hepatic encephalopathy. This is a complication of cirrhosis of the liver and not due directly to a thiamine deficiency.

3. Nausea and vomiting, anorexia, weight loss, abdominal pain, jaundice, edema, anemia, and blood coagulation abnormalities all are symptoms of cirrhosis of the liver and not due directly to a thiamine deficiency.

4. Impaired platelet production and risk for hemorrhage are complications of cirrhosis of the liver and not due directly to a thiamine deficiency.

TEST-TAKING HINT: The test taker must choose symptoms that are a direct result of thiamine deficiency to answer this question correctly. Other symptoms presented are indicative of cirrhosis of the liver resulting from alcohol use disorder, not specifically thiamine deficiency.

73. Narcolepsy is a syndrome characterized by sudden sleep attacks. There is no pain associated with narcolepsy.

1. Barbiturates are central nervous system (CNS) depressants. The depression of the CNS would exacerbate narcolepsy.

2. Analgesics are used for pain control. Common side effects of these medications are dizziness and drowsiness, making them inappropriate for the treatment of narcolepsy.

3. Amphetamines stimulate the CNS and are used in the management of narcolepsy, attention-deficit disorders, and weight control.

4. Benzodiazepines are classified as anxiolytic (antianxiety) drugs and depress the CNS. The depression of the CNS would exacerbate narcolepsy.

TEST-TAKING HINT: The test taker must understand the symptoms of narcolepsy and be able to distinguish among the effects of the drugs presented to choose the correct answer to this question. Any drug that would depress the CNS would be inappropriate for treatment of narcolepsy.

74. Insomnia is a disorder defined as the prolonged inability to sleep or abnormal wakefulness.

1. Sleep disorders that can be described as a misalignment between sleep and waking behaviors are referred to as circadian rhythm sleep disorders, not parasomnia. Examples include shift workers who experience rapid and repeated changes in their work schedules and the phenomenon of jet lag, in which individuals travel through a number of time zones in a short period of time.

2. Hypersomnia, or somnolence, not parasomnia, is defined as excessive sleepiness or seeking excessive amounts of sleep. One example of this disorder is narcolepsy, in which an individual experiences sleep attacks. These attacks may occur in the middle of a task or even in the middle of a sentence.

3. Parasomnias are unusual to undesirable behaviors that occur during sleep. Examples are nightmare disorder, in which an individual's frightening dream leads to an awakening from sleep, and sleepwalking, in which an individual may leave the bed and walk about, dress, go to the bathroom, talk, scream, or even drive. This motor activity is performed while the individual remains asleep.

4. Sleep apnea, not parasomnia, is defined as the temporary cessation of breathing while asleep. It is considered to be the most common sleep-related breathing disorder. To be so classified, the apnea must last for at least 10 seconds and must occur 30 or more times during a 7-hour period of sleep.

TEST-TAKING HINT: To answer this question correctly, the test taker must be familiar with the common types of sleep disorders, including insomnia, hypersomnia, parasomnia, circadian rhythm sleep disorders, and sleep apnea.

75. 1. Studies show that ADHD might be the result of a dopamine and norepinephrine deficit, not the result of inborn errors of metabolism. This etiology is from a biochemical, not genetic, perspective.

2. Children diagnosed with ADHD are more likely than children without this diagnosis to have siblings who also are diagnosed with the disorder. Studies also reveal that when one twin of an identical twin has ADHD, the other is likely to have it, too. Other studies have indicated that many parents of hyperactive children showed signs of hyperactivity during their own childhoods. These studies support a genetic etiology for the diagnosis of ADHD.

3. It is believed that certain neurotransmitters—particularly dopamine, norepinephrine, and possibly serotonin—are involved in producing the symptoms associated with ADHD; however, their involvement is still under investigation. Alterations in neurotransmitters support a biochemical, not genetic, etiology for the diagnosis of ADHD.

4. Mahler's theory suggests that ego, not id, development is retarded, and impulsive behavior dictated by the id is manifested in an individual with the diagnosis of ADHD. Mahler's theory suggests that a child with ADHD is fixed in the symbiotic phase of development and has not differentiated self from mother. This etiology is from a developmental, not genetic, perspective.

TEST-TAKING HINT: To select the correct answer, the test taker must recognize and understand various etiologies associated with the development of ADHD and determine which theory is from a genetic perspective.

76. All outcomes must be specific, realistic, measurable (including a time frame), positive, and client centered.
    1. Although this outcome is specific and measurable, it is a long-term, not a short-term, outcome.
    2. This short-term outcome is stated in observable and measurable terms. This outcome sets a specific time for achievement (by end of shift), it is specific (rules and consequences), and it is written in positive terms, all of which should guide nursing interventions to improve this client's ability to cope appropriately.
    3. Although gaining insight and establishing meaningful relationships are client-centered and specific, these outcomes are not stated in measurable terms (eventually).
    4. Although this outcome is specific and measurable, it is a long-term, not a short-term, outcome.

TEST-TAKING HINT: When choosing outcomes, the test taker must make sure the outcome relates to the stated problem or nursing diagnosis. The test taker must note keywords, such as *short-term outcome*. Noting this, the test taker can immediately eliminate answers 1 and 4.

77. 1. A possible medical condition has not been assessed, and this could potentially rule out the diagnosis of schizophrenia. To meet the diagnostic criteria for schizophrenia, thought disturbances cannot be due to the direct physiological effects of a substance or a general medical condition.
    2. Schizoaffective disorder and mood disorders with psychotic features must be ruled out for the client to meet the criteria for the diagnosis of schizophrenia. No major depressive, manic, or mixed episodes should have occurred concurrently with the active-phase symptoms. If mood episodes have occurred during the active-phase symptoms, their total duration should have been brief relative to the duration of the active and residual periods.
    3. Symptoms of schizophrenia generally appear in late adolescence or early adulthood. The client's age is outside this range and makes a diagnosis of schizophrenia unlikely.
    4. A client experiencing the negative symptom of a flat affect does not rule out the diagnosis of schizophrenia. Negative symptoms such as affective flattening, alogia, and avolition are included in the characteristic criteria for the diagnosis of schizophrenia.
    5. The gender of this client does not rule out the diagnosis of schizophrenia. Schizophrenia is diagnosed in men and women. The gender prevalence is about equal, but the symptoms occur earlier in men and are more severe in nature and expression.

TEST-TAKING HINT: To answer this question correctly, the test taker must recognize that positive and negative symptoms can be experienced by men and women diagnosed with schizophrenia. This knowledge would eliminate answers 4 and 5.

78. Sertraline, an antidepressant, is classified as an SSRI.
    1. Monitoring the client for suicidal ideations related to depressed mood would be the priority nursing intervention for a client experiencing depressed mood. Risk for client injury always should be prioritized. Assessing suicidal ideation is necessary for the nurse to intervene appropriately.
    2. Although discussing the need for medication adherence, even when symptoms improve, is an intervention that the nurse would need to implement with a client who is newly

prescribed sertraline, this intervention does not address safety and is not a priority.

3. Although instructing the client about the risk for discontinuation syndrome is an intervention the nurse needs to implement regarding newly prescribed sertraline, this intervention does not address safety and is not a priority.

4. Although reminding the client that sertraline's full effect does not occur for 6 to 8 weeks is an intervention the nurse needs to implement regarding newly prescribed sertraline, this intervention does not address safety and is not a priority.

TEST-TAKING HINT: To answer this question correctly, the test taker must recognize assessments as the initial intervention needed when planning care. All assessments are interventions; however, all interventions are not assessments.

79. 1. The client should try to be aware of and decrease defensive coping throughout hospitalization; however, this client problem is not a priority on admission.

2. **Safety is always a priority. Risk for self-directed violence, if not addressed, puts the client's safety at risk. This client problem is especially important to assess and provide appropriate interventions when an individual is newly admitted to an inpatient psychiatric unit.**

3. After the client is stabilized during hospitalization, the nurse and client would work on issues concerning social interactions. Socialization, although important, is not a priority when a client is at risk for self-harm.

4. Anxiety on admission is common and would need to be monitored throughout hospitalization; however, safety is the priority when a client is at risk for self-harm.

TEST-TAKING HINT: It is important for the test taker to note the keywords *newly admitted* in this question and consider timewise interventions. The interventions implemented for an individual newly admitted to an inpatient psychiatric unit may be quite different from what would be implemented for someone who is ready for discharge. Safety issues throughout hospitalization would need to be monitored and prioritized.

80. 1. Listening, not focusing, is a therapeutic communication technique that involves being fully present for the client as information is gathered. Listening is probably the most important therapeutic communication technique.

2. Restating, not focusing, is a therapeutic communication technique that allows the nurse the opportunity to verify the nurse's understanding of the client's message. Restating also lets the client know that the nurse is listening and wants to understand what the client is saying.

3. Reflection, not focusing, is a therapeutic communication technique that the nurse uses to repeat the nurse's understanding of the client's ideas, feelings, questions, and content. Reflection is used to put the client's feelings in the context of when or where they occur.

4. **Focusing is the therapeutic technique in which the nurse takes particular notice of a single idea, word, or theme. The nurse directs the communication exchange to draw the client's attention to the meaning and significance of a theme in the communication process.**

TEST-TAKING HINT: The test taker needs to review definitions and purposes of therapeutic communication techniques to answer this question correctly.

81. 1. **Included in the diagnostic criteria for bulimia nervosa is binge eating; inappropriate behavior to prevent weight gain, such as the abuse of laxatives; and altered body image. These symptoms must occur, on average, at least twice a week for 3 months. This client meets the diagnostic criteria for the diagnosis of bulimia nervosa.**

2. The symptoms of binge eating, and abuse of laxatives are not included in the criteria for the diagnosis of anorexia nervosa.

3. Although binge eating is a criterion for binge-eating disorder, it must not be associated with the recurrent use of inappropriate compensatory behavior, such as the abuse of laxatives, as in bulimia nervosa.

4. Binge eating, abuse of laxatives, and feeling "down" for the past 6 months are not normal developmental tasks for a 16-year-old client, according to Erikson. Erikson identified the development of a secure sense of self as the task of the adolescent (12 to 20 years) stage of psychosocial development.

TEST-TAKING HINT: To answer this question correctly, the test taker must remember the diagnostic criteria for the diagnosis of bulimia nervosa and differentiate this from the diagnostic criteria for anorexia nervosa and binge-eating disorder.

82. Ziprasidone is an atypical antipsychotic used in the treatment of schizophrenia spectrum disorders.
    1. Medications that take 6 to 8 weeks to see the full effect are antidepressants, not antipsychotics.
    2. Clozapine, not ziprasidone, is an atypical antipsychotic requiring the client to have laboratory tests drawn every 2 weeks to monitor for low neutrophil count (neutropenia).
    3. **Ziprasidone needs to be taken on a full stomach to ensure effective absorption.**
    4. Although some antipsychotic medications can cause weight gain and metabolic changes, in studies ziprasidone was shown to be *weight neutral*, meaning that individuals neither gain nor lose weight while taking this medication.

TEST-TAKING HINT: To answer this question correctly, the test taker must understand that ziprasidone is only 50% effective if taken on an empty stomach.

83. Escitalopram is an SSRI used to treat depressive disorders and for long-term treatment of anxiety.
    1. Escitalopram does not affect norepinephrine.
    2. Escitalopram does not affect norepinephrine.
    3. Escitalopram does not encourage the reuptake of serotonin at the postsynaptic site.
    4. **SSRIs inhibit the reuptake of serotonin and allow for more serotonin to be available in the synapse.**

TEST-TAKING HINT: The test taker must recognize that escitalopram is classified as an SSRI to understand the neurochemical effects of this classification of medications.

84. 1. Exercise increases beta-endorphins and is an effective, not ineffective, coping mechanism to elevate the mood.
    2. **This is an example of ineffective coping because alcohol is a central nervous system depressant that decreases mood and may lead to alcohol use disorder.**
    3. During crisis periods, prescribed short-term courses of hypnotics for sleep are indicated and beneficial because insomnia can exacerbate depression. Using prescribed medications supports effective, not ineffective, coping.
    4. The ability to appreciate the potential need for therapy supports effective, not ineffective, coping.

TEST-TAKING HINT: To answer this question correctly, the test taker must recognize the difference between effective and ineffective coping strategies. Only answer 2 is an example of ineffective coping.

85. Monoamine oxidase inhibitors (MAOIs), such as phenelzine, are used to treat depression. The nurse working with a client prescribed one of these medications needs to provide thorough instruction regarding interactions with other medications and foods. The nurse needs to remind all clients that they must talk with their physician before taking any medication, including over-the-counter medications, to avoid a life-threatening hypertensive crisis. Medications that need to be avoided when taking MAOIs include other antidepressants, sympathomimetics (e.g., epinephrine, dopamine, ephedrine, and over-the-counter cough and cold preparations), stimulants (e.g., amphetamines, cocaine, methyldopa, and diet drugs), antihypertensives (e.g., methyldopa, guanethidine, and reserpine), meperidine and possibly other opioid narcotics (e.g., morphine and codeine), and antiparkinsonian agents (e.g., levodopa).
    1. **Phenelzine is an MAOI and cannot be taken with other antidepressants, such as fluoxetine.**
    2. Warfarin sodium is safe to take with MAOIs such as phenelzine.
    3. Docusate sodium is safe to take with MAOIs such as phenelzine.
    4. Metformin is safe to take with MAOIs such as phenelzine.
    5. **Phenelzine is an MAOI and cannot be taken with diet pills.**

TEST-TAKING HINT: To answer this question correctly, the test taker must review important drug–drug and drug–food interactions related to MAOIs.

86. 1. This is a description of the therapeutic technique of *using silence*. In the communication exchange presented, the nurse has responded to the client rather than using silence.
    2. This is a description of the therapeutic technique of *verbalizing the implied*. When the nurse states, "You are feeling pretty lonely," the nurse is verbalizing the implied by presenting what the client has hinted at or suggested.
    3. This is a description of the therapeutic technique of *attempting to translate into feelings*. When a client presents

information symbolically, the nurse seeks to verbalize these indirect feelings. In the communication exchange presented, the client's feelings are not presented symbolically.

4. This is a description of the therapeutic technique of *restating*. In the communication exchange presented, the nurse is not repeating what the client has said.

TEST-TAKING HINT: To answer this question correctly, the test taker must be able to recognize the difference between "verbalizing the implied" and "attempting to translate into feelings." When the nurse verbalizes the implied, the nurse has made an implication related to the client's directly expressed content. When the nurse attempts to translate into feelings, the nurse attaches feelings to the client's directly expressed symbolism. Example: Client: "I'm lost in the woods." Nurse: "You must be feeling very lonely now."

87. 1. The verbalization of strengths is a short-term outcome related to a nursing diagnosis of low self-esteem. Clients first must be aware of what they like about themselves before other long-term outcomes are set.
2. To "exhibit increased feelings of self-worth" is a long-term outcome for low self-esteem and too general to be measured.
3. To "set realistic outcomes and attempt to reach them" is an outcome for low self-esteem but not specific enough to be measured. This outcome has no time frame.
4. To "demonstrate a decrease in fear of failure" is a long-term outcome for low self-esteem but not specific enough to be measured. This outcome has no time frame.

TEST-TAKING HINT: When choosing a short-term outcome, the test taker needs to look for something that is realistic to expect the client to accomplish during hospitalization. An outcome must be written so that it has a time frame and is measurable. How would the nurse know when a client demonstrates a decreased fear of failure? Instead, the nurse can formulate an outcome that states, "Client verbalizes a decreased fear of failure by day 3."

88. 1. Disturbed sensory perception is defined as a change in the amount or patterning of incoming stimuli (either internally or externally initiated) accompanied by a diminished, exaggerated, distorted, or

impaired response to such stimuli. An example of a disturbed sensory perception is an auditory hallucination. The statement by the client in the question is an example of an altered thought process, not a disturbed sensory perception.

2. **The nursing diagnosis of disturbed thought process is defined as the disruption in cognitive operations and activities. An example of a disturbed thought process is a delusion. The statement by the client in the question is an example of a persecutory delusion, which is one form of altered thought process.**

3. Impaired verbal communication is defined as the decreased, delayed, or absent ability to receive, process, transmit, and use a system of symbols. No impairment in verbal communication is being exhibited by the client in the question. The client can be understood and is able to use language effectively, but the client's beliefs are inconsistent with the reality of the situation.

4. Social isolation is defined as aloneness experienced by the individual and perceived as imposed by others and as a negative or threatened state. The statement in the question does not indicate that social isolation is the client's problem.

TEST-TAKING HINT: The test taker must differentiate disturbed thought processes from disturbed sensory perceptions to answer this question correctly. Altered thought processes refer predominantly to delusions, which are false beliefs. Altered sensory perceptions refer predominantly to hallucinations, which are false sensory perceptions not associated with real external stimuli.

89. MAOIs are used to treat depression. A nurse working with an individual prescribed one of these medications needs to provide thorough instruction regarding interactions with other medications and foods. While taking MAOIs, clients are unable to consume a long list of foods, which include, but are not limited to, the following: aged cheese, wine (especially Chianti), beer, chocolate, colas, coffee, tea, sour cream, beef/chicken livers, canned figs, soy sauce, overripe and fermented foods, pickled herring, preserved sausages, yogurt, yeast products, smoked and processed meats, cold remedies, or diet pills. Remind all clients that they must talk with their physician before taking any medication, including over-the-counter medications, to avoid a

life-threatening hypertensive crisis. If a client consumes these foods or other medications during or within 2 weeks after stopping treatment with MAOIs, a life-threatening hypertensive crisis could occur.

1. Drinking orange juice is safe when taking an MAOI such as isocarboxazid.
2. Tranylcypromine is an MAOI, and if taken with diet pills, a life-threatening hypertensive crisis could occur.
3. Eating Cheerios is safe when taking an MAOI such as isocarboxazid.
4. Eating oatmeal is safe when taking an MAOI such as tranylcypromine.
5. Tranylcypromine is an MAOI, and if taken with miso soup, which contains soy products, a life-threatening hypertensive crisis could occur.

TEST-TAKING HINT: To answer this question correctly, the test taker must review important drug–drug and drug–food interactions related to MAOIs.

90. 1. The client's ability to participate in self-care is an outcome that would relate to the nursing diagnosis of self-care deficit, not self-esteem disturbance.
    2. The client's ability to express two positive attributes about self by day 3 is a short-term, measurable outcome that is reflective of the nursing diagnosis of self-esteem disturbance.
    3. The client's ability to demonstrate one coping skill to decrease anxiety is an outcome that would relate to the nursing diagnosis of ineffective coping, not self-esteem disturbance.
    4. The client's ability to interact with peers in school during this fall semester is a long-term, not short-term, outcome for the nursing diagnosis of social isolation, not self-esteem disturbance.

TEST-TAKING HINT: The keyword in this question is *short-term*. The test taker can immediately eliminate answer 4 because it is a long-term, not short-term, outcome for the nursing diagnosis of social isolation, not self-esteem disturbance.

91. 1. Although clients diagnosed with AIDS have impaired immune responses, the symptoms described in the question are not associated with this impairment.
    2. Persistent generalized lymphadenopathy is diagnosed as a frequent manifestation of AIDS. This condition involves the enlargement of two or more extra-inguinal

lymph nodes lasting 3 or more months. Symptoms include tenderness in these areas. The symptoms described in the question are not associated with persistent generalized lymphadenopathy.

3. Kaposi's sarcoma (KS) is the most common cancer associated with AIDS. KS presents as vascular macules, papules, or violet lesions affecting the skin and viscera. In the early stages, KS is painless, but it may become painful as the disease progresses. The symptoms described in the question are not associated with KS.
4. Neurocognitive disorder due to HIV affects 40% to 60% of clients diagnosed with this disease and is a common cause of mental status change in clients diagnosed with HIV. Typical manifestations are confusion, fluctuating memory loss, decreased concentration, lethargy, and diminished motor speed.

TEST-TAKING HINT: To answer this question correctly, the test taker must understand the link between the symptoms described in the question and the possible cause for these symptoms.

92. Showing respect to clients helps them recognize that they are being unconditionally accepted as unique individuals. A show of respect can serve to elevate the client's feelings of self-worth and self-esteem while developing the nurse–client relationship.
    1. To trust another individual, one must feel confidence in that individual's presence, reliability, integrity, veracity, and sincere desire to provide assistance when required. Acceptance and a nonjudgmental attitude are not reflective of trust.
    2. Rapport is the development between two people in a relationship of special feelings based on mutual acceptance, warmth, a sense of harmony, and a nonjudgmental attitude. Establishing rapport creates a sense of harmony based on knowledge and appreciation of each individual's uniqueness. The ability to care for and about others is the core of rapport.
    3. Genuineness refers to the nurse's ability to be open, honest, and real in interactions with the client. When one is genuine, there is congruency between what is felt and what is being expressed. Acceptance and a nonjudgmental attitude are not reflective of genuineness.

4. When the nurse experiences empathy, the nurse accurately perceives or understands what the client is feeling and encourages the client to explore these feelings. Conversely, in sympathy, the nurse actually shares what the client is feeling and experiences a need to alleviate the client's distress. Acceptance and a nonjudgmental attitude are not reflective of empathy.

TEST-TAKING HINT: An analogy is a comparison. The test taker needs to look at what is being compared and choose an answer that provides information that reflects a similar comparison. The test taker should review the characteristics necessary to establish a nurse–client relationship.

93. Bupropion is an antidepressant medication that affects dopamine and norepinephrine and is prescribed to help treat depressive symptoms. Sertraline is an SSRI that increases the amount of serotonin in the synapse and is prescribed to treat depressive symptoms.

   1. Although bupropion, also marketed as Zyban, can be prescribed to assist with smoking cessation, there is nothing in the question commenting on the client's need to stop smoking.
   2. Sertraline is not used to assist with negative side effects of bupropion.
   3. **The practitioner prescribed one medication that affects only serotonin (sertraline) and a medication that affects norepinephrine and dopamine (bupropion). When the practitioner prescribes this combination of medications, all three neurotransmitters, believed to be altered in major depressive disorder, are affected.**
   4. Sertraline can assist with depression and anxiety, but there is no mention in the question of the diagnosis of anxiety. Also, bupropion is not approved by the Food and Drug Administration (FDA) to treat anxiety.

TEST-TAKING HINT: When choosing an answer, the test taker must be sure not to add information to the question. There is nothing in the question regarding smoking, so answer 1 can be eliminated.

94. The pattern of development of schizophrenia can be viewed in four phases: phase I, schizoid personality; phase II, prodromal phase; phase III, schizophrenia; and phase IV, residual phase.

   1. Individuals diagnosed with schizoid personality are typically loners who seem cold and aloof, and are indifferent to social relationships. The symptoms described in the question do not reflect symptoms of schizoid personality.
   2. **Characteristics of the prodromal phase include social withdrawal, impairment in role functioning, eccentric behaviors, neglect of personal hygiene and grooming, blunted or inappropriate affect, disturbances in communication, bizarre ideas, unusual perceptual experiences, and lack of initiative, interests, or energy. The length of this phase varies, and this phase may last for many years before progressing to schizophrenia. The symptoms described in the question are reflective of the prodromal phase of the development of schizophrenia.**
   3. In the active phase of schizophrenia, psychotic symptoms are prominent. Two or more of the following symptoms must be present for a significant portion of time during a 1-month period: delusions, hallucinations, disorganized speech, grossly disorganized or catatonic behavior, and negative symptoms (affective flattening, alogia, or avolition). The client in the question does not present with these symptoms and has experienced symptoms for only 3 weeks.
   4. Schizophrenia is characterized by periods of remission and exacerbation. A residual phase usually follows an active phase of the illness. Symptoms during the residual phase are similar to the symptoms of the prodromal phase, with flat affect and impairment in role function being prominent. There is no indication in the question that the client has recently experienced an active phase of schizophrenia.

TEST-TAKING HINT: The test taker should note the time frame of the duration of symptoms presented in this question. Because the client has experienced symptoms for less than 1 month, answer 3 is eliminated. Also, because the prodromal and residual phases share similar symptoms, it is important to note whether the client has recently experienced symptoms of active schizophrenia to differentiate these phases.

95. 1. Although it is important for the nurse to avoid situations in which secondary gains may occur, this is not the priority nursing intervention when working with a client suspected of a conversion disorder. The nurse's focus first must be on ruling out

any organic pathology, then helping the client to understand the link between anxiety and the expressed physical symptoms.

2. Typically, the physical condition that occurs during a conversion disorder is the client's unconscious expression of underlying anxiety. Forcing insight would increase anxiety and might generate more physical symptoms. Because this client has not been definitively diagnosed with a conversion disorder, discussing the link between anxiety and physical symptoms would be premature.

3. A conversion disorder occurs during times of extreme anxiety. This would be an inappropriate time to teach alternative coping skills because this anxiety would impede learning. Because this client has not been definitively diagnosed with a conversion disorder, teaching alternative coping skills would be premature.

4. **In this situation, it is a priority for the nurse to monitor assessments, laboratory tests, and vital signs to rule out organic pathology. It is important for the nurse not to presume that a psychological problem exists before a physical disorder is thoroughly evaluated.**

TEST-TAKING HINT: It is important to note the keywords *suspected of* and *priority* in the question. When suspecting a conversion disorder, the nurse's priority is to assist the medical team in ruling out organic causes. This needs to be done before the implementation of any other intervention.

96. 1. This is the therapeutic technique of *placing an event in time or in sequence*, not exploring. This communication technique clarifies the relationship of events in time.

2. This is the therapeutic technique of *offering general leads*, not exploring. This communication technique gives the client encouragement to continue.

3. **This is the therapeutic technique of *exploring*. Exploring delves further into a subject or an idea and allows the nurse to examine experiences or relationships more fully. Asking for an example can clarify a vague or generic statement.**

4. This is the therapeutic technique of *encouraging comparisons*, not exploring. This communication technique asks that similarities and differences be noted.

TEST-TAKING HINT: To answer this question correctly, the test taker must be able to recognize the use of the therapeutic communication technique of exploring.

97. 1. **The leader first wants to explore the client's feelings by using the therapeutic technique of *attempting to translate into feelings*. The group leader then asks a focusing question that assesses the situation further.**

2. The group members may look at this as punishment. Group is there for clients to voice their feelings, and the leader is there to assist them in understanding where their feelings originate.

3. This statement dismisses the client's feelings without gaining more information about the statement. If, after assessing the topic, the leader believes that it is an inappropriate matter to discuss in group, the leader would appreciate the client's feeling and ask that it be discussed in the next individual session.

4. The leader needs to assess further before deciding to ask the group. If the leader asks the group before assessing, the client may feel they are still not being heard.

TEST-TAKING HINT: To answer this question correctly, the test taker must understand the need first to empathize with the client's feelings and then to assess the situation further.

98. Lithium carbonate is a mood stabilizer that is used in clients diagnosed with bipolar affective disorder. The margin between the therapeutic and toxic levels of lithium carbonate is very narrow. Serum lithium carbonate levels should be monitored once or twice a week after initial treatment until dosage and serum levels are stable. Blood samples should be drawn 12 hours after the last dose of lithium carbonate.

1. The maintenance level for lithium carbonate is 0.6 to 1.2 mEq/L, and 0.9 mEq/L is within the normal maintenance range for this drug. However, the client in the question is experiencing an acute manic episode and should attain a higher lithium carbonate level.

2. **The lithium carbonate level necessary for managing acute mania is 1 to 1.5 mEq/L, and 1.4 mEq/L is within this range.**

3. When the serum lithium carbonate level is 1.5 to 2 mEq/L, the client could exhibit signs such as blurred vision, ataxia, tinnitus, persistent nausea, vomiting, and diarrhea. A lithium level of 1.9 mEq/L is

outside both the maintenance and acute mania treatment range.

4. When the serum lithium carbonate level is 2 to 3.5 mEq/L, the client could exhibit signs such as excessive output of diluted urine, increased tremors, muscular irritability, psychomotor retardation, mental confusion, and giddiness. A lithium carbonate level of 2.4 mEq/L is outside both the maintenance and acute mania treatment range.

TEST-TAKING HINT: To answer this question correctly, the test taker must recognize the laboratory value that reflects serum lithium carbonate levels needed to manage acute mania.

99. 1. A contract for intervention is a task of the orientation phase. The contract details the expectations and responsibilities of the nurse and the client.
2. The identification of the client's strengths and limitations occurs during the orientation phase. This assessment of the client's potential is necessary to intervene appropriately and in a timely manner.
3. Problem-solving in situational crises occurs, after client assessment, in the working phase of the nurse–client relationship. The nurse works with the client to discuss options for problem solutions.
4. Promoting the client's insight and perceptions of reality is a therapeutic task of the working phase.
5. The formulation of nursing diagnostic statements is one of the tasks that occurs in the orientation phase.

A nursing diagnosis is a statement of an assessed client problem.

TEST-TAKING HINT: To answer this question correctly, the test taker must recognize that the orientation phase is when the nurse and client become acquainted. Review of the tasks for this phase assists the test taker in choosing a correct answer.

100. 1. The use of humor belittles the feelings of the client. Humor always must be used with discretion. It is inappropriate to try to "cheer up" depressed client who is feeling hopeless.
2. Some comorbid disorders that contribute to depression, such as endocrine or electrolyte disturbances, need to be ruled out before a client can be diagnosed with a depressive disorder. If these imbalances are detected, solving these problems would take priority.
3. Although relaxation techniques can aid in alleviating mood and decreasing anxiety, it is inappropriate to attempt to teach this client at this time. Depression affects concentration and the client's ability to learn.
4. It is important to evaluate this client's family history of mental illness to understand the genetic and environmental factors that may affect the client's condition. However, assisting in ruling out physical causes is the nurse's priority.

TEST-TAKING HINT: To answer this question correctly, the test taker must be able to recognize priority interventions. Using Maslow's hierarchy of needs can assist the test taker with this determination.

Glossary of English Words Commonly Encountered on Nursing Examinations

Abnormality — defect, irregularity, anomaly, oddity

Absence — nonappearance, lack, nonattendance

Abundant — plentiful, rich, profuse

Accelerate — go faster, speed up, increase, hasten

Accumulate — build up, collect, gather

Accurate — precise, correct, exact

Achievement — accomplishment, success, reaching, attainment

Acknowledge — admit, recognize, accept, reply

Activate — start, turn on, stimulate

Adequate — sufficient, ample, plenty, enough

Angle — slant, approach, direction, point of view

Application — use, treatment, request, claim

Approximately — about, around, in the region of, more or less, roughly speaking

Arrange — position, place, organize, display

Associated — linked, related

Attention — notice, concentration, awareness, thought

Authority — power, right, influence, clout, expert

Avoid — keep away from, evade, let alone

Balanced — stable, neutral, steady, fair, impartial

Barrier — barricade, blockage, obstruction, obstacle

Best — most excellent, most important, greatest

Capable — able, competent, accomplished

Capacity — ability, capability, aptitude, role, power, size

Central — middle, mid, innermost, vital

Challenge — confront, dare, dispute, test, defy, face up to

Characteristic — trait, feature, attribute, quality, typical

Circular — round, spherical, globular

Collect — gather, assemble, amass, accumulate, bring together

Commitment — promise, vow, dedication, obligation, pledge, assurance

Commonly — usually, normally, frequently, generally, universally

Compare — contrast, evaluate, match up to, weigh or judge against

Compartment — section, part, cubicle, booth, stall

Complex — difficult, multifaceted, compound, multipart, intricate

Complexity — difficulty, intricacy, complication

Component — part, element, factor, section, constituent

Comprehensive — complete, inclusive, broad, thorough

Conceal — hide, cover up, obscure, mask, suppress, secrete

Conceptualize — to form an idea

Concern — worry, anxiety, fear, alarm, distress, unease, trepidation

Concisely — briefly, in a few words, succinctly

Conclude — make a judgment based on reason, finish

Confidence — self-assurance, certainty, poise, self-reliance

Congruent — matching, fitting, going together well

Consequence — result, effect, outcome, end result

Constituents — elements, component, parts that make up a whole

Contain — hold, enclose, surround, include, control, limit

Continual — repeated, constant, persistent, recurrent, frequent

Continuous — constant, incessant, nonstop, unremitting, permanent

Contribute — be a factor, add, give

Convene — assemble, call together, summon, organize, arrange

Convenience — expediency, handiness, ease

Coordinate — organize, direct, manage, bring together

Create — make, invent, establish, generate, produce, fashion, build, construct

Creative — imaginative, original, inspired, inventive, resourceful, productive, innovative

Critical — serious, grave, significant, dangerous, life threatening

Cue — signal, reminder, prompt, sign, indication

Curiosity — inquisitiveness, interest, nosiness, snooping

Damage — injure, harm, hurt, break, wound

Deduct — subtract, take away, remove, withhold

Deficient — lacking, wanting, underprovided, scarce, faulty

Defining — important, crucial, major, essential, significant, central

Defuse — resolve, calm, soothe, neutralize, rescue, mollify

Delay — hold up, wait, hinder, postpone, slow down, hesitate, linger

Demand — insist, claim, require, command, stipulate, ask

Describe — explain, tell, express, illustrate, depict, portray

Design — plan, invent, intend, aim, propose, devise

Desirable — wanted, pleasing, enviable, popular, sought after, attractive, advantageous

Detail — feature, aspect, element, factor, facet

Deteriorate — worsen, decline, weaken

Determine — decide, conclude, resolve, agree on

Dexterity — skillfulness, handiness, agility, deftness

Dignity — self-respect, self-esteem, decorum, formality, poise

Dimension — aspect, measurement

Diminish — reduce, lessen, weaken, detract, moderate

Discharge — release, dismiss, set free

Discontinue — stop, cease, halt, suspend, terminate, withdraw

Disorder — complaint, problem, confusion, chaos

Display — show, exhibit, demonstrate, present, put on view

Dispose — to get rid of, arrange, order, set out

Dissatisfaction — displeasure, discontent, unhappiness, disappointment

Distinguish — to separate and classify, recognize

Distract — divert, sidetrack, entertain

Distress — suffering, trouble, anguish, misery, agony, concern, sorrow

Distribute — deliver, spread out, hand out, issue, dispense

Disturbed — troubled, unstable, concerned, worried, distressed, anxious, uneasy

Diversional — serving to distract

Don — put on, dress oneself in

Dramatic — spectacular

Drape — cover, wrap, dress, swathe

Dysfunction — abnormal, impaired

Edge — perimeter, boundary, periphery, brink, border, rim

Effective — successful, useful, helpful, valuable

Efficient — not wasteful, effective, competent, resourceful, capable

Elasticity — stretch, spring, suppleness, flexibility

Eliminate — get rid of, eradicate, abolish, remove, purge

Embarrass — make uncomfortable, make self-conscious, humiliate, mortify

Emerge — appear, come, materialize, become known

Emphasize — call attention to, accentuate, stress, highlight

Ensure — make certain, guarantee

Environment — setting, surroundings, location, atmosphere, milieu, situation

Episode — event, incident, occurrence, experience

Essential — necessary, fundamental, vital, important, crucial, critical, indispensable

Etiology — assigned cause, origin

Exaggerate — overstate, inflate

Excel — to stand out, shine, surpass, outclass

Excessive — extreme, too much, unwarranted

Exertion — intense or prolonged physical effort

Exhibit — show signs of, reveal, display

Expand — get bigger, enlarge, spread out, increase, swell, inflate

Expect — wait for, anticipate, imagine

Expectation — hope, anticipation, belief, prospect, probability

Experience — knowledge, skill, occurrence, know-how

Expose — lay open, leave unprotected, allow to be seen, reveal, disclose, exhibit

External — outside, exterior, outer

Facilitate — make easy, make possible, help, assist

Factor — part, feature, reason, cause, think, issue

Focus — center, focal point, hub

Fragment — piece, portion, section, part, splinter, chip

Function — purpose, role, job, task

Furnish — supply, provide, give, deliver, equip

Further — additional, more, extra, added, supplementary

Generalize — to take a broad view, simplify, to make inferences from particulars

Generate — make, produce, create

Gentle — mild, calm, tender

Girth — circumference, bulk, weight

Highest — uppermost, maximum, peak, main

Hinder — hold back, delay, hamper, obstruct, impede

Humane — caring, kind, gentle, compassionate, benevolent, civilized

Ignore — pay no attention to, disregard, overlook, discount

Imbalance — unevenness, inequality, disparity

Immediate — insistent, urgent, direct

Impair — damage, harm, weaken

Implantation — to put in

Impotent — powerless, weak, incapable, ineffective, unable

Inadvertent — unintentional, chance, unplanned, accidental

Include — comprise, take in, contain

Indicate — point out, sign of, designate, specify, show

Ineffective — unproductive, unsuccessful, useless, vain, futile

Inevitable — predictable, to be expected, unavoidable, foreseeable

Influence — power, pressure, sway, manipulate, affect, effect

Initiate — start, begin, open, commence, instigate

Insert — put in, add, supplement, introduce

Inspect — look over, check, examine

Inspire — motivate, energize, encourage, enthuse

Institutionalize — to place in a facility for treatment

Integrate — put together, mix, add, combine, assimilate

Integrity — honesty

Interfere — get in the way, hinder, obstruct, impede, hamper

Interpret — explain the meaning of, to make understandable

Intervention — action, activity

Intolerance — bigotry, prejudice, narrow-mindedness

Involuntary — instinctive, reflex, unintentional, automatic, uncontrolled

Irreversible — permanent, irrevocable, irreparable, unalterable

Irritability — sensitivity to stimuli, fretful, quick excitability

Justify — explain in accordance with reason

Likely — probably, possible, expected

Liquefy — to change into or make more fluid

Logical — using reason

Longevity — long life

Lowest — inferior in rank

Maintain — continue, uphold, preserve, sustain, retain

Majority — the greater part of

Mention — talk about, refer to, state, cite, declare, point out

Minimal — least, smallest, nominal, negligible, token

Minimize — reduce, diminish, lessen, curtail, decrease to smallest possible

Mobilize — activate, organize, assemble, gather together, rally

Modify — change, adapt, adjust, revise, alter

Moist — slightly wet, damp

Multiple — many, numerous, several, various

Natural — normal, ordinary, unaffected

Negative — no, harmful, downbeat, pessimistic

Negotiate — bargain, talk, discuss, consult, cooperate, settle

Notice — become aware of, see, observe, discern, detect

Notify — inform, tell, alert, advise, warn, report

Nurture — care for, raise, rear, foster

Obsess — preoccupy, consume

Occupy — live in, inhabit, reside in, engage in

Occurrence — event, incident, happening

Odorous — scented, stinking, aromatic

Offensive — unpleasant, distasteful, nasty, disgusting

Opportunity — chance, prospect, break

Organize — put in order, arrange, sort out, categorize, classify

Origin — source, starting point, cause, beginning, derivation

Pace — speed

Parameter — limit, factor, limitation, issue

Participant — member, contributor, partaker, applicant

Perspective — viewpoint, view, perception

Position — place, location, point, spot, situation

Practice — do, carry out, perform, apply, follow

Precipitate — to cause to happen, to bring on, hasten, abrupt, sudden

Predetermine — fix or set beforehand

Predictable — expected, knowable

Preference — favorite, liking, first choice

Prepare — get ready, plan, make, train, arrange, organize

Prescribe — set down, stipulate, order, recommend, impose

Previous — earlier, prior, before, preceding

Primarily — first, above all, mainly, mostly, largely, principally, predominantly

Primary — first, main, basic, chief, most important, key, prime, major, crucial

Priority — main concern, giving first attention to, order of importance

Production — making, creation, construction, assembly

Profuse — a lot of, plentiful, copious, abundant, generous, prolific, bountiful

Prolong — extend, delay, put off, lengthen, draw out

Promote — encourage, support, endorse, sponsor

Proportion — ratio, amount, quantity, part of, percentage, section of

Provide — give, offer, supply, make available

Rationalize — explain, reason

Realistic — practical, sensible, reasonable

Receive — get, accept, take delivery of, obtain

Recognize — acknowledge, appreciate, identify, aware of

Recovery — healing, mending, improvement, recuperation, renewal

Reduce — decrease, lessen, ease, moderate, diminish

Reestablish — reinstate, restore, return, bring back

Regard — consider, look upon, relate to, respect

Regular — usual, normal, ordinary, standard, expected, conventional

Relative — comparative, family member

Relevance — importance of

Reluctant — unwilling, hesitant, disinclined, indisposed, adverse

Reminisce — to recall and review remembered experiences

Remove — take away, get rid of, eliminate, eradicate

Reposition — move, relocate, change position

Require — need, want, necessitate

Resist — oppose, defend against, keep from, refuse to go along with, defy

Resolution — decree, solution, decision, ruling, promise

Resolve — make up your mind, solve, determine, decide

Response — reply, answer, reaction, retort

Restore — reinstate, reestablish, bring back, return to, refurbish

Restrict — limit, confine, curb, control, contain, hold back, hamper

Retract — take back, draw in, withdraw, apologize

Reveal — make known, disclose, divulge, expose, tell, make public

Review — appraisal, reconsider, evaluation, assessment, examination, analysis

Ritual — custom, ceremony, formal procedure

Rotate — turn, go around, spin, swivel

Routine — usual, habit, custom, practice

Satisfaction — approval, fulfillment, pleasure, happiness

Satisfy — please, convince, fulfill, make happy, gratify

Secure — safe, protected, fixed firmly, sheltered, confident, obtain

Sequential — chronological, in order of occurrence

Significant — important, major, considerable, noteworthy, momentous

Slight — small, slim, minor, unimportant, insignificant, insult, snub

Source — basis, foundation, starting place, cause

Specific — exact, particular, detail, explicit, definite

Stable — steady, even, constant

Statistics — figures, data, information

Subtract — take away, deduct

Success — achievement, victory, accomplishment

Surround — enclose, encircle, contain

Suspect — think, believe, suppose, guess, deduce, infer, distrust, doubtful

Sustain — maintain, carry on, prolong, continue, nourish, suffer

Synonymous — same as, identical, equal, tantamount

Systemic — affecting the entire organism

Thorough — careful, detailed, methodical, systematic, meticulous, comprehensive, exhaustive

Tilt — tip, slant, slope, lean, angle, incline

Translucent — see-through, transparent, clear

Unique — one and only, sole, exclusive, distinctive

Universal — general, widespread, common, worldwide

Unoccupied — vacant, not busy, empty

Unrelated — unconnected, unlinked, distinct, dissimilar, irrelevant

Unresolved — unsettled, uncertain, unsolved, unclear, in doubt

Utilize — make use of, employ

Various — numerous, variety, range of, mixture of, assortment of

Verbalize — express, voice, speak, articulate

Verify — confirm, make sure, prove, attest to, validate, substantiate, corroborate, authenticate

Vigorous — forceful, strong, brisk, energetic

Volume — quantity, amount, size

Withdraw — remove, pull out, take out, extract

Index

A

B